IMMUNOLOGY OF THE EAR

Immunology of the Ear

Editors

Joel M. Bernstein, M.D., Ph.D.
Adjunct Professor
Department of Speech-Language Pathology and Audiology
State College of New York at Buffalo
and Clinical Assistant Professor of Otolaryngology and Pediatrics
State University of New York at Buffalo
Buffalo, New York

Pearay L. Ogra, M.D.
Professor of Pediatrics and Microbiology
State University of New York at Buffalo
School of Medicine
and Division of Infectious Diseases
Children's Hospital of Buffalo
Buffalo, New York

Raven Press New York

Raven Press, 1185 Avenue of the Americas, New York, New York 10036

Made in the United States of America

Library of Congress Cataloging-in-Publication Data

Immunology of the ear.

Includes bibliographies and index.
1. Ear—Diseases—Immunological aspects.
I. Bernstein, Joel M. II. Ogra, Pearay L.
[DNLM: 1. Ear Diseases—immunology. WV 200 I33]
RF121.I45 1987 617.8′079 85-42511
ISBN 0-88167-270-X

9 8 7 6 5 4 3 2 1

This book is dedicated to our wives
and to our children.

Preface

In the last decade, advances in the cellular and molecular analysis of immunological reactivity have been increasingly applied to diseases of the ear. Whereas in the early 1970s a few manuscripts addressed the role of "allergy" in otitis media, the otolaryngologic literature of this decade concerns itself with lymphocyte subpopulations, macrophage-lymphocyte interaction, chemical mediators of inflammation, and autoimmunity of both the middle ear and inner ear. The collaboration of otologists and infectious disease clinicians with scientists in the fields of immunobiology, biochemistry, and microbiology has revolutionized our thinking about disorders such as otitis media and sensorineural hearing loss. Furthermore, after three international symposia on otitis media with effusion and two international symposia on immunobiology in otolaryngology, the editors decided to collect the body of pertinent information available on these subjects and make it available in the form of a comprehensive textbook.

The first section of this book illuminates the basic principles of the anatomy and physiology of the eustachian tube, middle ear, and inner ear on the one hand and the fundamental concepts of the lymphoid system of the upper respiratory tract and local immunity on the other. This section emphasizes the role of the bronchopulmonary lymphoid tissue and the tonsils and adenoids as possible sites of origin of T and B cells for the middle ear and possibly inner ear. The concept of the middle ear as a part of the common mucosal immune system is also discussed.

The second section of the book is devoted to the immunobiology of otitis media following eustachian tube dysfunction. The bacteriological and virological aspects of otitis media precedes an in-depth discussion of immune mechanisms in this disorder. If appropriate drainage of the middle ear cleft is not obtained, complement components and other biochemical and inflammatory mediators persist and may result in permanent tissue injury. In editing this book, it has been our aim to present the opposing effects of the immune mechanisms in otitis media: The same mechanisms that serve a protective function may be amplified and result in immunopathology if they persist in a closed space for a long period of time.

The controversial roles of IgE-mediated hypersensitivity and immune deficiency are carefully discussed, and some new perspectives on the immunobiology of cholesteatoma conclude this portion of the book.

The final section of the text addresses some of the most exciting new advances in the entire field of otology and immunology, namely, autoimmunity and sensorineural deafness. Not only is the inner ear the possible site of autoimmune injury and the stria vascularis and the endolymphatic sac specific sites of immunological reactivity, but the inner ear may also develop immunological injury secondary to immunological disease.

The structure of this book reflects our desire to prepare a text that would be relevant to otolaryngologists, pediatricians, immunologists, and infectious disease clinicians.

JOEL M. BERNSTEIN
PEARAY L. OGRA

Acknowledgments

We wish to express our sincere gratitude to all the contributing authors for their expertise and cooperation in attempting to make this textbook a successful, state-of-the-art account on immunology of the ear. We are also grateful to Mrs. Irene Sullivan, our editorial assistant, for devoting her indefatigable energy to this project.

Contents

vii Preface

Part I. Basic Science and Structure of the Ear

1 Middle Ear and Inner Ear Structure and Function
David J. Lim

39 Eustachian Tube and Nasopharynx
Charles D. Bluestone

63 Immune Functions and Immunopathology of Palatine and Nasopharyngeal Tonsils
Per Brandtzaeg

107 Respiratory Tract Lymphoid Tissue and Other Effector Cells of Immunity
Raffaele Scicchitano, Peter Ernst, and *John Bienenstock*

135 Mucosal Immune System and Local Immunity
James C. Cumella and Pearay L. Ogra

153 Pharmacologic Mediators of Inflammation
Jeffrey P. Tillinghast and Dean D. Metcalfe

179 Immunobiology of Tympanoplasty
Jan E. Veldman and Wim Kuijpers

Part II. Immunobiology of the Tympanic Membrane and Middle Ear

205 The Effect of Eustachian Tube Obstruction on Middle Ear Mucosal Transformation
Wim Kuijpers and J.M.H. van der Beek

231 Bacteriology of Otitis Media
Tasnee Chonmaitree and Virgil M. Howie

249 Virologic Aspects of Middle Ear Disease
Peter F. Wright

259 Secretory Immunoglobulin in the Nasopharynx: Implications in Otitis Media
Chr. Hjort Sørensen

279 Immune Mechanisms in Otitis Media With Effusion
Goro Mogi and Joel M. Bernstein

301 Inflammatory Cell Subpopulations in Secretory Otitis Media
Tauno Palva, Eero Taskinen, Pekka Hayry, and Joel M. Bernstein

319 Biochemistry of Middle Ear Effusion
Steven K. Juhn, Yukiyoshi Hamaguchi, and Timothy T. K. Jung

331 Inflammatory Mediators in Middle Ear Disease
Paul B. van Cauwenberge and Joel M. Bernstein

345 Complement and Other Amplification Mechanisms
Karin Prellner

363 Immune Deficiency and Otitis Media
Britta Rynnel-Dagöö and Anders Freijd

381 Allergy and Middle Ear Effusions: Fact or Fiction?
Robert C. Welliver

391 Immunobiology of Acquired Aural Cholesteatoma
Bruce J. Gantz and Michael J. Hart

403 Animal Models of Otitis Media with Effusion
G. Scott Giebink

Part III. Immunobiology of the Inner Ear

419 The Immunobiology of Autoimmune Disease of the Inner Ear
Joel M. Bernstein

427 Autoimmune Inner Ear Disease
Brian F. McCabe

437 Immunopathology of the Inner Ear
Jeffrey P. Harris

453 Immunological Factors in Meniere's Disease
Allen F. Ryan

463 Animal Model of Autoimmune Ear Disease
T.J. Yoo, R.A. Floyd, and H. Kitano

481 Otologic Manifestations of Systemic Immunologic Diseases
Michael Schatz and Robert S. Zieger

489 Wegener's Granulomatosis and Other Granulomatous Diseases of the Ear
Howard S. Faden and Pedro Piedra

501 Subject Index

Contributors

Joel M. Bernstein, M.D., Ph.D., *Adjunct Professor, Department of Speech-Language Pathology and Audiology, State College of New York at Buffalo; and Clinical Assistant Professor of Otolaryngology and Pediatrics, State University of New York at Buffalo, Buffalo, New York 14214*

John Bienenstock, *Host Resistance Programme, Department of Pathology and Intestinal Disease Research Unit, McMaster University Health Sciences Centre, Hamilton, Ontario, Canada L8N 3Z5*

Charles D. Bluestone, M.D., *Professor of Otolaryngology, University of Pittsburgh School of Medicine; and Director, Department of Pediatric Otolaryngology, Children's Hospital of Pittsburgh, One Children's Place, 3705 Fifth Avenue at De Soto Street, Pittsburgh, Pennsylvania 15213*

Per Brandtzaeg, Ph.D., *Laboratory for Immunochemistry and Immunopathology, Institute of Pathology, University of Oslo, The National Hospital, Rikshospitalet 0027, Oslo 1, Norway*

Tasnee Chonmaitree, M.D., *Assistant Professor of Pediatrics, Division of Infectious Diseases, University of Texas Medical Branch, Galveston, Texas 77550*

James C. Cumella, M.D., *Research Assistant Professor of Pediatrics, State University of New York at Buffalo, Buffalo, New York 14214; and Division of Infectious Diseases and Allergy, Children's Hospital of Buffalo, Buffalo, New York 14222*

Peter Ernst, *Host Resistance Programme, Department of Pathology and Intestinal Disease Research Unit, McMaster University Health Sciences Centre, Hamilton, Ontario, Canada L8N 3Z5*

Howard S. Faden, M.D., *Department of Pediatrics, State University of New York at Buffalo, School of Medicine, Buffalo, New York 14214; and Children's Hospital of Buffalo, Buffalo, New York 14222*

R.A. Floyd, Ph.D., *Departments of Medicine, Microbiology and Immunology, and Pathology; and Neurosciences Program, University of Tennessee, 956 Court Avenue H300, Memphis, Tennessee 38163*

Anders Freijd, *Departments of Otorhinolaryngology and Clinical Immunology, Huddinge University Hospital, Karolinska Institute, Stockholm, Sweden*

Bruce J. Gantz, M.D., *Department of Otolaryngology—Head and Neck Surgery, University of Iowa, Iowa City, Iowa 52242*

G. Scott Giebink, M.D., *Department of Pediatrics, University of Minnesota Medical School, Box 483, Mayo Memorial Building, 420 Delaware Street S.E., Minneapolis, Minnesota 55455*

Yukiyoshi Hamaguchi, *Department of Otolaryngology, University of Minnesota Medical School, Minneapolis, Minnesota 55455*

Jeffrey P. Harris, M.D., Ph.D., *Associate Professor of Surgery, Division of Otolaryngology, University of California, San Diego, School of Medicine, La Jolla, California 92093; and Veteran's Administration Medical Center, San Diego, California 92161*

Michael J. Hart, M.D., *Department of Otolaryngology—Head and Neck Surgery, University of Iowa, Iowa City, Iowa 52242*

Pekka Hayray, M.D., *Professor of Transplantation Immunology, Transplantation Laboratory, University of Helsinki, Helsinki, Finland*

Virgil M. Howie, M.D., *Professor of Pediatrics, Division of Ambulatory Pediatrics, University of Texas Medical Branch, Galveston, Texas 77550*

Steven K. Juhn, M.D., *Department of Otolaryngology, University of Minnesota Medical School, Minneapolis, Minnesota 55455*

Timothy T. K. Jung, M.D., Ph.D., *Division of Otolaryngology, Loma Linda University School of Medicine, Loma Linda, California 92354*

H. Kitano, M.D., *Departments of Medicine, Microbiology and Immunology, and Pathology; and Neurosciences Program, University of Tennessee, 956 Court Avenue H300, Memphis, Tennessee 38163*

Wim Kuijpers, Ph.D., *Department of Otorhinolaryngology, University of Nijmegen, Philips van Leydenlaan 15, 6525 EX Nijmegen, The Netherlands*

David J. Lim, M.D., *Professor and Director, Otological Research Laboratories, Department of Otolaryngology, Ohio State University College of Medicine, 436 Clinic Drive, Columbus, Ohio 43210*

Brian F. McCabe, M.D., *Professor of Otolaryngology, Department of Otolaryngology—Head and Neck Surgery, University of Iowa, Iowa City, Iowa 52242*

Dean D. Metcalfe, M.D., *Mast Cell Physiology Section, Laboratory of Clinical Investigation, National Institute of Allergy and Infectious Diseases, National Institutes of Health, Bethesda, Maryland 20205*

Goro Mogi, M.D., *Department of Otolaryngology, Medical College of Oita, Oita 879-56 Japan*

Pearay L. Ogra, M.D., *Professor of Pediatrics and Microbiology, State University of New York at Buffalo, School of Medicine, Buffalo, New York 14214; and Division of Infectious Diseases, Children's Hospital of Buffalo, Buffalo, New York 14222*

Tauno Palva, M.D., *Professor of Otolaryngology, ENT Department, University of Helsinki, Helsinki, Finland*

Pedro Piedra, M.D., *Department of Pediatrics, State University of New York at Buffalo, School of Medicine, Buffalo, New York 14214; and Children's Hospital of Buffalo, Buffalo, New York 14222*

Karin Prellner, M.D., *Department of Otorhinolaryngology, University Hospital, 221 85 Lund, Sweden*

Allen F. Ryan, Ph.D., *Department of Surgery, Division of Otolaryngology, University of California, San Diego, Medical School; and Research Service, Veteran's Administration Medical Center, San Diego, California 92161*

Britta Rynnel-Dagöö, *Departments of Otorhinolaryngology and Clinical Immunology, Huddinge University Hospital, Karolinska Institute, Stockholm, Sweden*

Michael Schatz, M.D., *Department of Allergy-Immunology, Kaiser Permanente Group, 4647 Zion Avenue, San Diego, California 92120*

Raffaele Scicchitano, *Host Resistance Programme, Department of Pathology and Intestinal Disease Research Unit, McMaster University Health Sciences Centre, Hamilton, Ontario, Canada L8N 3Z5*

Chr. Hjort Sørensen, M.D., *E.N.T. Department, Gentofte University Hospital, DK-2900 Hellerup, Denmark*

Eero Taskinen, M.D., *Pathologist, Transplantation Laboratory, University of Helsinki, Helsinki, Finland*

Jeffrey P. Tillinghast, M.D., *Mast Cell Physiology Section, Laboratory of Clinical Investigation, National Institute of Allergy and Infectious Diseases, National Institutes of Health, Bethesda, Maryland 20205*

Paul B. van Cauwenberge, M.D., *Professor of Otolaryngology, State University Hospital, B-9000 Ghent, Belgium*

J.M.H. van der Beek, M.D., *Department of Otorhinolaryngology, University of Nijmegen, N1-6500 HB Nijmegen, The Netherlands*

Jan E. Veldman, M.D., Ph.D., *Department of Otorhinolaryngology, University of Utrecht, P.O. Box 16250, 3500 CG Utrecht, The Netherlands*

Robert C. Welliver, M.D., *Associate Professor of Pediatrics, Division of Infectious Diseases and Microbiology Laboratories, Children's Hospital of Buffalo, Buffalo, New York 14222*

Peter F. Wright, M.D., *Professor of Pediatrics, Assistant Professor of Microbiology, and Head, Department of Pediatric Infectious Diseases, Vanderbilt University, Nashville, Tennessee 37232*

T.J. Yoo, M.D., *Departments of Medicine, Microbiology and Immunology, and Pathology, and Neurosciences Program, University of Tennessee, 956 Court Avenue H300, Memphis, Tennessee 38163*

Robert S. Zieger, M.D., *Department of Allergy-Immunology, Kaiser Permanente Group, 4647 Zion Avenue, San Diego, California 92120*

IMMUNOLOGY OF THE EAR

Immunology of the Ear, edited by J. Bernstein and P. Ogra. Raven Press, New York © 1987.

Middle Ear and Inner Ear Structure and Biological Function

David J. Lim

Otological Research Laboratories, Department of Otolaryngology, Ohio State University College of Medicine, Columbus, Ohio 43210

TUBOTYMPANUM

Because of the importance of otitis media, the morphology and function of the eustachian tube and middle ear lining have been well investigated in recent years. Numerous laboratory and clinical data support the notion that local defense mechanisms, in addition to systemic immunity, protect the tubotympanum from the invading organisms. The purpose of this chapter is to review the available histological, histochemical, immunochemical, and ultrastructural data to provide a broad morphological and cellular basis for understanding the mechanisms involved in tubotympanal protection.

Eustachian Tube

In adult humans, a cartilaginous portion distinct from the bony portion can be seen (Fig. 1), but in young infants (and in some adults) the cartilage often extends to the bony portion, making it difficult to delineate the two. In laboratory animals, particularly rodents and felines, the tubal cartilage extends directly to the tympanum. In general, in humans and primates these two parts are joined by a narrowing known as the *tubal isthmus* (Fig. 1). The diameter of this isthmus is smaller in children (about 2.4 mm × 0.8 mm) than in adults (about 4.3 mm × 1.7 mm) and also varies from individual to individual.

The cartilaginous portion of the tube, when cross-sectioned, shows a slit-like lumen that is partially reinforced by cartilage that resembles a shepherd's crook (Fig. 1). The lower portion of the main body of the cartilage becomes thicker toward the pharyngeal orifice. The epithelial cells of this portion of the tube are formed mainly of pseudostratified tall columnar ciliated epithelium with secretory, nonsecretory, and basal cells (Fig. 2). Occasionally, simple squamous mucosal epithelium lines the lumen, particularly near the pharyngeal orifice and the upper part of the tubal lumen. The eustachian tubal epithelium is composed of pseudostrati-

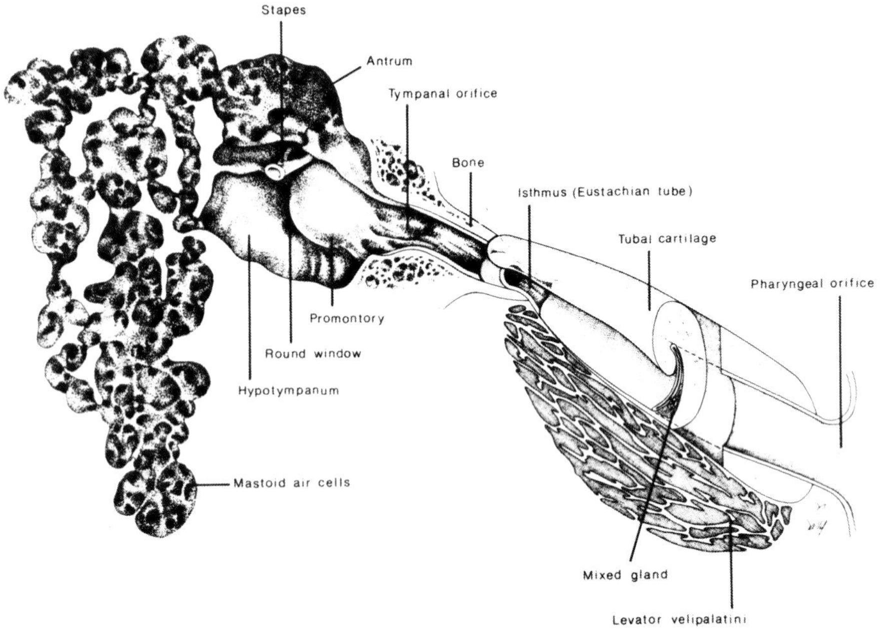

FIG. 1. Artist's view of the middle ear, mastoid, and eustachian tube, demonstrating anatomical landmarks. (From ref. 71.) (Drawing by Nancy Sally.)

fied columnar cells; interspersed among these cells are goblet cells and the underlying basal cells (Fig. 3).

The secretory cells are classified according to their morphological basis: light granulated cells, dark granulated cells, and mixed granulated cells. Further autoradiographic studies indicate that the light granulated cells are mucous, because radioisotope-labeled glucose is taken up largely by these cells, whereas the dark granulated cells are protein-secreting cells (serous), because they incorporate isotope-labeled amino acid leucine (70,87). The subepithelial connective tissue contains blood vessels, lymph capillaries, myelinated nerve fibers, fibrocytes, and occasional mast cells, macrophages, and plasma cells (Fig. 2).

The mucus-propelling cilia of the tube (columnar cells) are approximately 4 to 7 μm, whereas the cilia in the middle ear (often cuboidal or squamous type) are much shorter: 3 to 4 μm. Each ciliated cell in the tympanum possesses 40 to 60 cilia, whereas in the tubal lumen each can possess up to 250. The shape of the ciliated cells varies from tall columnar to cuboidal, or even squamous. The densities of the ciliated cell populations vary considerably. For example, in the human tubal lumen they compose over 80%; in the hypotympanum and near the tubal orifice of the tympanum they range between 51% and 80%; in the promontory and epitympanum, they are 11% to 60%; in the aditus, they are 1% to 19%; and in the

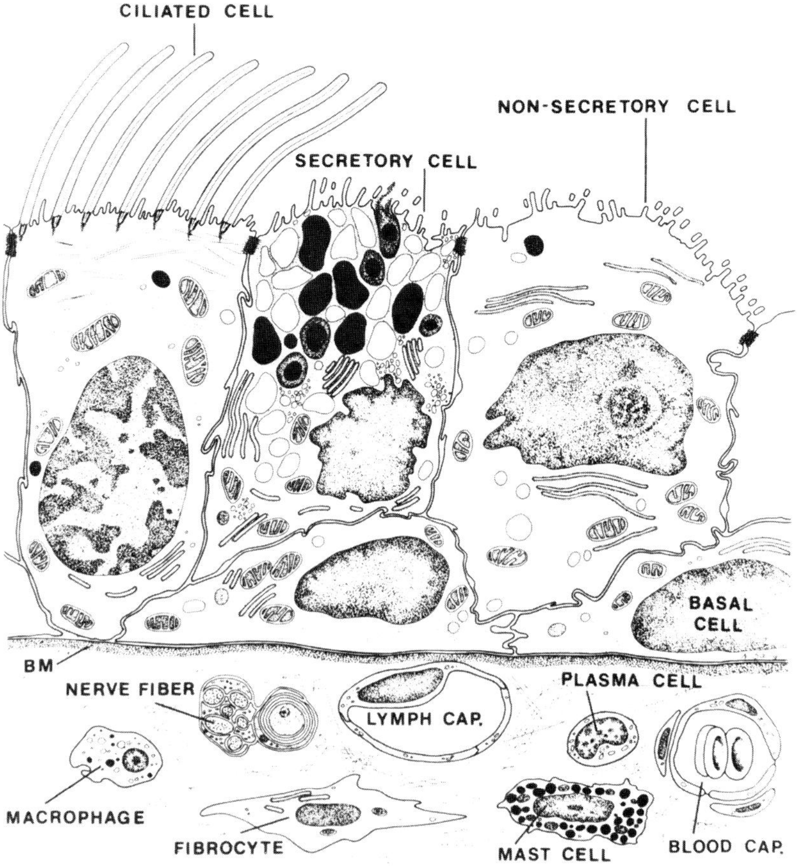

FIG. 2. Artist's view of the representative cells in the middle ear mucosa. (BM) Basement membrane. (From ref. 71.) (Drawing by Nancy Sally.)

mastoid, they are under 1% (Fig. 4) (141). In the hypotympanum, a major track formed of groups of ciliated cells is connected with the tubal lumen (141). A second track is formed of ciliated-cell clusters along the epitympanic recess and peripheral area of the tympanic membrane (pars tensa), which connects to the tubal opening area (74,75). It was later found that secretory cells always accompany the ciliated cells, even those that form an isolated island (86).

The cartilaginous part of the tube contains numerous seromucinous glands, and the serous acini are termed *demilunes* because of their half-moon shape due to compression by round mucous glands (Fig. 3). These mixed glands open to the tubal lumen through secretory ducts. Secreta pours out as viscous mucus droplets, or column, which then forms a thin mucous blanket.

There are two main tubal muscles: tensor veli palatini (TVP) muscle and levator

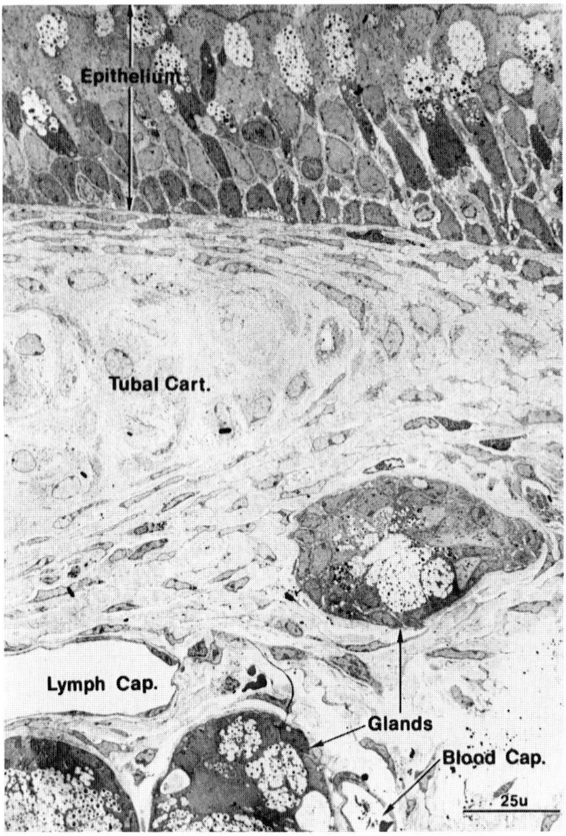

FIG. 3. Low-power transmission electron micrograph of a guinea pig eustachian tube at the cartilaginous portion showing stratified tall columnar epithelium, tubal cartilage, mixed glands, and capillaries. (From ref. 71.)

veli palatini (LVP) muscle (Fig. 1). The TVP muscle is attached to the hook end of the tubal cartilage; thus its contraction helps open the tubal lumen. The contraction of the LVP muscle is thought to elevate the lower luminar portion of the tube; thus the lower edge of the median side of the tubal cartilage is pushed upward, helping the opening of the tube in concert with the outward pulling motion of the TVP muscle action. These muscles are thought to be poorly developed in young children. The closing of the tubal lumen is provided by the relative stiffness of the tubal cartilage. In young children, this tubal cartilage is floppy because of its poor development, causing the collapse of the tube (18).

Although autonomic innervation (adrenergic and cholinergic) to the auditory tube is well established (57,155), the role it plays in tubal function is not clear. The stellate ganglion (superior cervical) block tends to reduce the patency of the

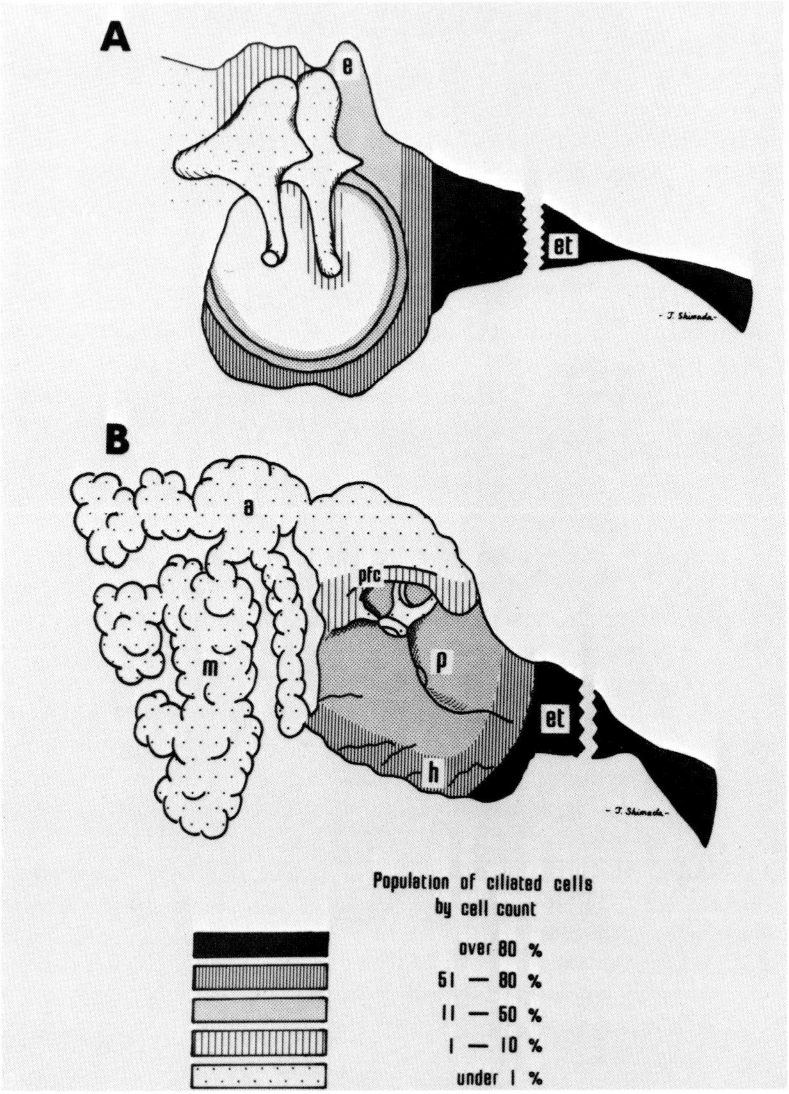

FIG. 4. Distribution of ciliated cells in the normal human ear, shown graphically. (et) Eustachian tube; (h) hypotympanum; (p) promontory; (e) epitympanic recess; (pfc) prominence of facial canal; (a) antrum; (m) mastoid air cells. (From ref. 141.) (Drawing by T. Shimada.)

tube, while the parasympathetic ganglion block tends to dilate the tube (65). A number of investigators (3,156) demonstrated that the tubal luminal tissue is richly endowed with adrenergic and cholinergic as well as peptidergic innervation, which may be involved in the regulation of local blood circulation, secretory activity, and even possibly the mucociliary activity.

Mucociliary Transporting System

There is unequivocal evidence that nonfunctioning or disrupted cilia of the tubotympanum lead to otitis media, because patients with immotile cilia syndrome, without exception, develop recurrent or chronic otitis media and maxillary sinusitis. Recent evidence suggests that influenza A virus causes destruction of the ciliated epithelium of the eustachian tube in the early stage of infection, leading to a secondary bacterial invasion (37; D. J. Lim et al., *unpublished data*). Within 48 hr after the introduction of the virus to the trachea, the cilia are virtually nonfunctioning, as judged by gross observation (L. O. Bakaletz et al., *unpublished data*). Functional investigation of the mucociliary apparatus in the tubotympanum has long been neglected, and only a few reports have been made in recent years. Therefore, the information obtained from other similar systems (e.g., trachea and maxillofacial sinus) provides a guide to understanding what may be occurring in the tubotympanal mucociliary system, and this information is largely relevant because there are clear similarities between the trachea and the maxillary sinuses. This will be reviewed here.

The *mucociliary system* is composed of motile epithelial cilia and the mucous blanket (Fig. 5A). The mucous blanket is suggested to be a nonhomogeneous mixture of different types of secretion (mucous and serous) forming a viscoelastic hydrophilic non-Newtonian gel (159). However, it has also been suggested that the mucous blanket (viscoelastic layer) is formed largely of secreted mucus, whereas the serous fluid (low viscosity layer) bathes the periciliary space (Fig. 5A), allowing free ciliary motion (90,132). Regulation of mucociliary transport depends on: (a) variations in the fluidic load produced by mucus on the cilia, (b) variations in the energy output of the ciliary engine, and (c) variations in the energy transfer from ciliary movement to mucus flow (159).

Because mucociliary coupling has a significant bearing on transport efficiency, the length of the cilium that penetrates the mucus and the thickness of the periciliary layer could have a ''clutching'' effect that regulates the degree of mechanical coupling between the mucus and the cilia during their active stroke (158). The tips of the cilia are known to penetrate about 0.5 μm into the mucous layer of the blanket during their effective stroke (144) so that the mucus is propelled forward. The recovery strokes, however, take place in the periciliary fluid. If the depth of the periciliary serous layer increases so that the tips of the cilia no longer hold (penetrate) the mucous layer, the mucus will not be propelled until excess fluid is removed. If the periciliary layer is made too shallow by loss of fluid or diminished secretion, the mucus propulsion will stop because the cilia are pressed down and can no longer complete their beat cycle properly (144) (Fig. 5B). This concept emphasizes the importance of the secretion of serous, as well as mucous, fluid. In this regard, it is important to note that even in the epithelial secretory cells of the tubotympanum there is a morphological as well as a biochemical heterogeneity (45,84), consistent with the concept mentioned above. To have a functioning mucociliary system, the serous fluid must be produced locally. A functioning mucocil-

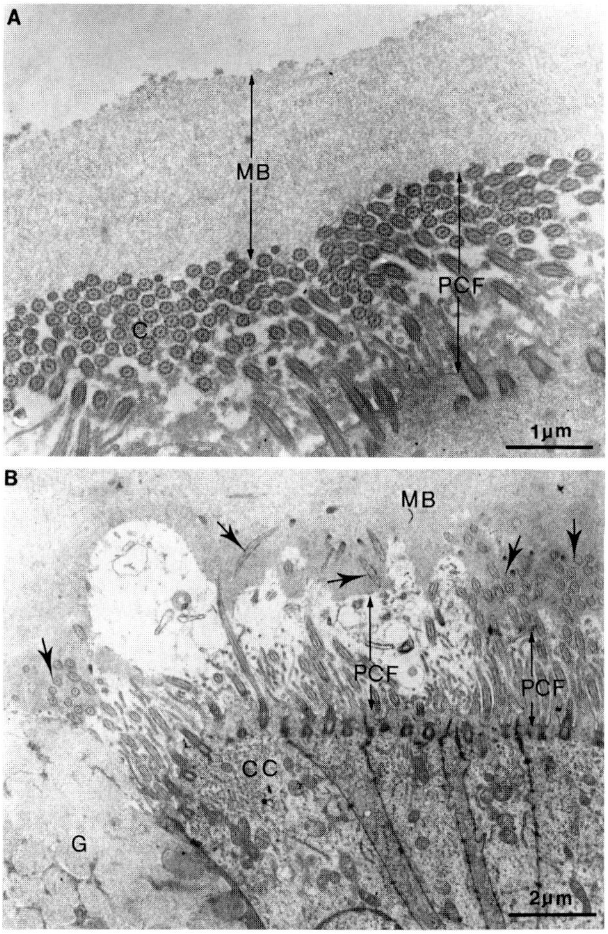

FIG. 5. A: Transmission electron micrograph showing the mucous blanket (MB) of a normal guinea pig eustachian tube, which is making contact with the cilia (C) of the ciliated cell. (PCF) Periciliary fluid space. **B:** Transmission electron micrograph of a chinchilla eustachian tube following viral (influenza A) infection, showing deep penetration (*arrows*) of the cilia into the mucous layer of the blanket (MB). This penetration occurred because of physicochemical changes of the mucus and/or reduction of the periciliary fluid due to the infection. Such penetration renders the mucociliary transportation ineffectual. (PCF) Periciliary fluid space; (G) goblet cell; (CC) ciliated cell. (From D.J. Lim et al., *unpublished data*.)

iary transporting system is known to exist in certain parts of the lining epithelium of the middle ear as well as in the bony tube, where no mixed glands are present.

Mucus is composed of (a) a solvent, water, containing various solutes of low molecular weight, and (b) a polymer network formed of glycoproteins of high molecular weight and consisting of a long protein core arranged as a random coil to which several oligosaccharide side chains are attached (19).

The viscoelastic properties of gels were thought to be dependent on the degree of disulfide cross-linkage between polymer chains in their molecular network (32) because disulfide bond-cleaving agents can disperse different kinds of mucus. However, a recent study using dynamic laser scattering ruled out the existence of a covalently cross-linked molecular network in mucus (159). Silberberg et al. (142) demonstrated that mucus can be spontaneously dispersed in water, supporting the above result. Therefore, solubilization of mucus by disulfide bond breakage must be due to ''crumbling'' of the fundamental fibrous backbone units rather than breakdown of a true interfibrillar covalently linked network (99). An alternative molecular model for the structure of the mucus is that of an entangled network of long, fibrillar, randomly coiled strands formed by aggregates of glycoprotein chains.

Recently, Tam and Verdugo (151) proposed that hydration of mucus resembles a Donnan equilibrium, in which the degree of swelling is dependent on the pH and ionic concentration of the swelling medium. This implies that the rheological properties of mucus might be controlled by exchange of water and ions across the ciliated epithelium. Transepithelial movement of water and ions is known to be hormonally regulated in the respiratory tract (108). The evidence of active osmotic exchange in the ciliated epithelium (108) and also the proposed dependence of the rheology of mucus upon the ionic composition of the periciliary fluid suggest that ciliated epithelium could autoregulate its mechanical load by controlling both the ionic composition and the volume of the fluid in the periciliary space (159).

Ciliary Motion

It is well known that ciliary motion is in metachrony, requiring a sequential coordination of the adjacent cilia. This coordination occurs because when a cilium begins to move among a group of stationary cilia, the clockwise swing of its recovery stroke brings it into contact with adjacent cilia, thereby stimulating the cilia on that side to commence their recovery strokes and causing them to excite their neighboring cilia. On living epithelia, such areas of metachronically coordinated activity can be seen to move for distances of a few tens of microns (not more than a few cell diameters) before disappearing, only to be followed by further waves propagated over the same group of cells. The whole epithelium is covered with many of these active areas, each acting independently of the others. Cilia of rabbit trachea epithelium commonly beat at 15 to 20 Hz (144).

In mammalian ciliated epithelial cells in culture, variations in the concentration of Ca^{2+} change the frequency of the ciliary beat; i.e., ethylene diaminetetraacetic acid-induced depletion of Ca^{2+} can arrest ciliary movement completely. This effect is reversible, and the maximum reactivation of ciliary beat is observed at 1 mM extracellular Ca^{2+}, whereas a concentration of only 1 μM of intracellular Ca^{2+} is needed to reactivate ciliary motion fully (159). In ciliated epithelia, calcium is important in the coupling of hormonal stimulation. The available evidence suggests that a pool of sequestered calcium is present in ciliated epithelial cells and that release of this calcium is responsible for the stimulus-response coupling of prostaglandin E_2 in ciliary activity (158).

The changes in ciliary beat, as well as the rheological properties of mucus, have significant consequences for the mucociliary transporting system. Changes in rheological properties of mucus as a mechanism of disturbed mucociliary clearance have been reported in secretory otitis media (133), whereas a significantly reduced rate of the ciliary beat has been reported in the case of chronic maxillary sinusitis (114), allergic rhinitis (113), and chronic otitis media with effusion (112).

Regulation of Ciliary Activity

Resting mucociliary activity continues for a long period in denervated *in vitro* preparations (42) and in *in vivo* experiments after vagotomy (91). Spontaneous activity is also present after blocking of (a) nicotinic receptors in autonomic ganglia, (b) postganglionic parasympathetic muscarinic receptors, and (c) postganglionic α- and β-adrenoreceptors (56). These findings can be interpreted to mean that the resting mucociliary activity is independent of sympathetic and parasympathetic innervation.

The parasympathomimetic drug methacholine caused acceleration of ciliary activity in the rabbit maxillary sinus (56), suggesting a parasympathetic nervous control of mucociliary activity. The effects of sympathomimetic agonists and antagonists on mucociliary activity in this model showed that the selective β_1-adrenoceptor agonist prenalterol did not influence the resting mucociliary activity. However, the β-adrenoceptor agonists salbutamol (β_2) and isoprenaline (β_1 and β_2) both gave a dose-dependent increase in the wave frequency, whereas the α-adrenoceptor agonists phenylepinephrine (α_1) and oxymetazoline (α_2) both provided a dose-dependent decrease in the mucociliary activity. According to this investigator, the nonselective β-adrenoceptor antagonist propranol did not, per se, influence the resting mucociliary activity, but it reduced the effects of both salbutamol and isoprenaline. It is concluded that the sympathomimetic agonists with selectivity to different groups of adrenoceptors have opposite effects on the mucociliary activity (e.g., acceleration by β_2-adrenoceptor agonists and reduction by α_1- and α_2-adrenoceptor agonists) (56). This finding is interpreted to mean that the resting mucociliary activity functions independently of sympathetic activity, at least in the anesthetized rabbit maxillary sinus, since β- and α-adrenoceptor antagonists on their own did not influence the resting mucociliary activity.

However, drugs acting on postganglionic muscarinic receptors (e.g., methacholine), on postganglionic β_2-adrenoceptors such as salbutamol and isoprenaline, and on ganglionic nicotinic receptors (e.g., nicotine) accelerate the mucociliary wave frequency in a dose-dependent manner (56). This accelerating effect is antagonized by receptor-blocking substances (e.g., atropine, propranol, and hexamethonium). These results can be interpreted to suggest that the autonomic innervation of the mucous membrane may have an influence in increasing the mucociliary activity (56), in addition to the known effects of the autonomic system on the mucus-secreting apparatus and blood vessels of the mucous membrane (5). *In vitro* studies using mucus-free monolayers of ciliated cells in culture have shown that β-adrenergic agonists stimulate ciliary activity in both respiratory and oviduct cilia (160).

Tubotympanal Secretions and Their Biological Functions

Secretion of the tubotympanum provides a multitude of biological substances essential for the function of the mucous membrane and its protection. Aside from the mucus it provides for the mucociliary blanket, the secretion also provides *tubal surface-active substances* to facilitate tubal opening (16,17,21,40,41,95,124).

Although there is good evidence suggesting that surface-active agents are present in the tubal lumen to facilitate tubal opening, as mentioned above, their biochemical characterization remains controversial. Many investigators likened the tubal surface-active agent to surfactant (41,166). Using rat eustachian tube *in vitro* preparations and radioisotope-labeled choline, Wheeler et al. (166) investigated the synthesis of phosphatidylcholine (PC). They found that the eustachian tube and lung synthesized PC significantly more than the control liver tissue of equal weight, suggesting that the tube may secrete a surfactant-like substance biochemically analogous to that of the lung. However, a study from the author's laboratory (95) demonstrated that the surface activity of the tubal washings resides primarily in the aqueous phase (glycoprotein or mucoprotein) rather than the lipid phase. Although an earlier cytochemical study (71) showed a secretory product and dark granules (of the serous cells) that reacted with tricomplex flocculation, suggesting the possible presence of phospholipids, secretory granules resembling the lamellar secretory granules of the alveolar type I secretory cells that produce surfactant (lecithin) have not been observed in the tubotympanum. Whether these different results are due to species differences or to methodological differences cannot be determined. Further study is needed to clarify this important question.

Immune System of the Tubotympanum

McMaster and Hudack (98) demonstrated, by injecting antigen into rat bullae, that the regional lymphatic tissue produces antibody. In these animals, antibody was recovered from the draining lymph nodes before it could be detected elsewhere. They injected two antigens into each ear, and the antibody to each of the antigens was detected first in the regional lymph nodes. There is also good clinical (13,15,20,60,68,101,105,145,146), immunohistochemical (12,13,14,72,75, 87,104), and experimental (36,131,163,169) evidence suggesting that the tubotympanum is protected by the local (humoral and cellular) (110) as well as the systemic immune system.

The human and animal studies are largely conducted in pathological or experimental conditions, where immune responses are enhanced. Only a few have been conducted in normal tubotympanums, namely, those of the developing guinea pig (103) and of the adult chinchilla (162,163). In the developing guinea pig tubotympanum, a few IgA- and IgM-forming cells were observed, but IgG-forming cells were rarely seen in the tubotympanums of 7th-postnatal-day animals. After antigenic stimulation, however, an increase in all classes of immunoglobulin-forming cells was seen in the tubotympanum (103). The tubal glands of developing guinea pigs (7 days old and older) produced secretory component and lactoferrin, suggesting that the immune system matures with advancing age. In the normal chinchilla tube, the glandular acini cells were positively stained with anti-IgA antibody, and a few IgA-forming immunocytes were observed in the tubal connective tissue, as well as in the bulla near the tube, but IgM- and IgG-forming immunocytes were rarely observed (162). However, after infection with *S. pneumoniae* (type 3 or 23), there was a dramatic increase in immunocytes in the submucosa in the bulla, the most being the IgG-forming cells, followed by IgM- and IgA-forming cells. The increase in immunocytes corresponded well with the increase in immunoglobulins in the middle ear effusions (163). These findings are consistent with results obtained in middle ear effusions. Liu et al. (89) demonstrated that IgG was the major immunoglobulin, followed by IgA and IgM, and they increased with advancing age.

The route of *antigenic absorption* has also been investigated, using a tracer. Lim and Hussl (81) demonstrated that horseradish peroxidase (HRP) instilled into the guinea pig bulla was transported actively via pinocytosis on the epithelial cell surface and into the intercellular space by reverse pinocytosis (Fig. 6). The intercellular HRP was then passively transported into the submucosal connective tissue and taken up by macrophages or by the lymphatics and venules. The tracer then found its way to the regional lymph nodes (deep cervical) within 15 min after tympanal instillation (81). These macromolecules were found in the macrophages in the lymph nodes. Thus, the regional lymph nodes seem to play an important role in the processing and presenting of the antigen to lymphocytes in the lymph nodes, thereby inducing the immune response to produce antibody and evoke cellular immunity to regional antigen.

The role of cellular immunity in protecting the tubotympanum against viral and bacterial agents has not been unequivocally established. However, natural killer cells (117) have been found in large numbers in mucous tissue together with mast cells (85). This finding suggests that local cellular immunity may be operative in the tubotympanum.

THE INNER EAR

The inner ear has a number of structural elements that are implicated in the local immune reaction (7,106,153) or autoimmunity (97,170). The nature of the normally functioning inner ear immune system has been established only recently, and the endolymphatic sac appears to be the immune organ required to protect the inner ear (153,154). The exact mechanisms involved in inner ear autoimmunity

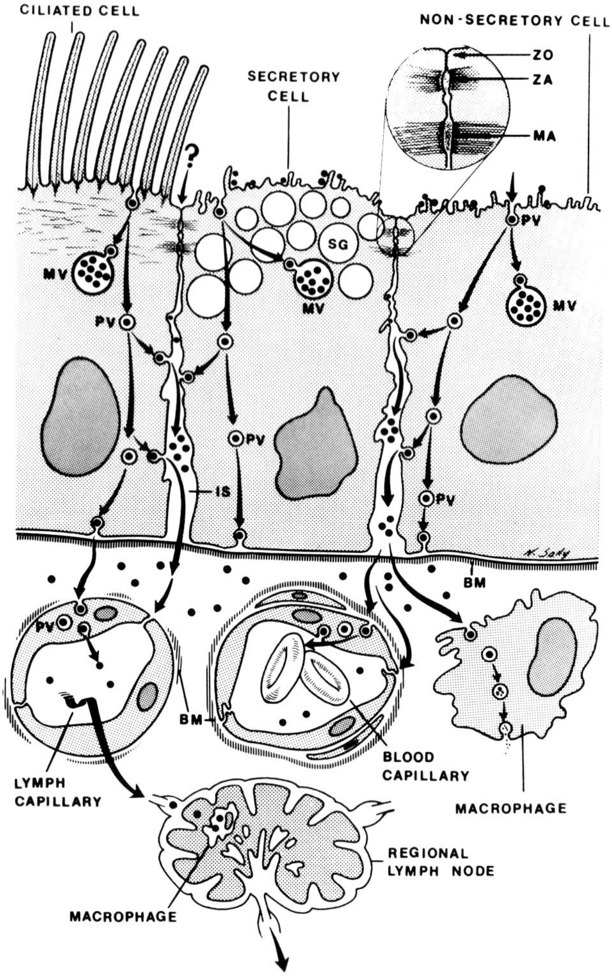

FIG. 6. Schematic diagram illustrating the mechanisms of cellular transport of macromolecules (HRP) by the middle ear mucosa. The major system for uptake of the macromolecules by the epithelium is accomplished by pinocytosis (PV) of the cellular membrane facing the middle ear cavity. They are then either stored in the multivesicular body (MV), or transported into the intercellular space (IS), or transported across the cell toward the basement membrane (BM). The HRP does not pass through the junctional complex, which includes zonula occludens (ZO), zonula adherens (ZA), or macula adherens (MA). However, it readily passes through the basement membrane of the epithelial cells. The tissue macrophages take up large quantities of HRP in the connective tissue layer. Some of the HRP enters into either the lymphatics or blood capillaries by pinocytosis and through the tight junctions. Once the particles enter the lymphatics, they are transported into the regional lymph nodes where the lymph macrophages take up most of the transported HRP. (From ref. 81.) (Drawing by Nancy Sally.)

have not been fully elucidated. However, abnormal cellular or humoral immune responsiveness has been reported in a number of inner ear disorders, such as idiopathic sensorineural hearing loss (96) and Meniere's disease (167). Yoo has reported the presence of autoantibodies against type II collagen in circulating blood significantly greater in Meniere's disease than in controls (171). The organs involved in such disorders are suggested to be the stria vascularis, ganglion cells, sensory cells, and endolymphatic duct and sac.

The inner ear is formed of two sensory organs: the auditory organs (or cochlea) and the balance organs (or vestibule). These sensory organs are made of mechanoreceptors specializing in transforming mechanical energy into electrical impulses.

Cochlea

The mammalian cochlea, including that of humans, is formed of a coiled membranous duct, containing a sensory organ known as the *organ of Corti,* which is located on the basilar membrane. This membrane is tapered along its length: in the apex it is wider and thinner, and in the base it is thicker and narrower. This anatomic gradation is thought to be responsible for the frequency resolution of the cochlea (11). The organ of Corti consists of one row of inner hair cells and three rows of outer hair cells, which are separated by the inner and outer pillar cells (Fig. 7). Surrounding the inner hair cells on the lateral side and sandwiched between the inner hair cells and the inner pillar cells are the inner phalangeal cells; medial to the inner hair cells are the border cells, which are next to the inner sulcus cells. The outer hair cells are supported by three rows of Deiters' cells (external phalangeal cells), and the last rows of Deiters' cells are bordered by Hensen's cells and Claudius' cells. The pillar cells and Deiters' cells contain bundles of tonofilaments; thus these cells are thought to provide mechanical support of the organ, which has to be moving constantly as a result of sound wave propagation along the basilar membrane.

At the top of the sensory cells are stereociliary (hair) bundles arranged in a "W" formation (Fig. 8), which is critical for the directional sensitivity of the hair cells (31). For example, the bending of the ciliary bundles toward the tip of the "W" is excitatory, and the reverse bending is inhibitory. This bending of the stereociliary bundles is caused by the shearing motion of the tectorial membrane and the reticular lamina of the organ of Corti as a result of basilar membrane motion. It is generally agreed that the tallest row of the stereociliary bundles of the outer hair cells is firmly attached (or coupled) to the overlying tectorial membrane, whereas the inner-hair-cell stereocilia are thought to be freestanding or at least not as firmly attached as those of the outer hair cells (76,77). Dallos (24) suggested that the outer hair cells are stimulated by the displacement of the tectorial membrane by virtue of their close coupling, whereas the inner-hair-cell stereociliary bundles are stimulated by the endolymph drag caused by the displacement of the tectorial membrane. However, this coupling of the inner-hair-cell stereocilia with the tectorial membrane remains controversial.

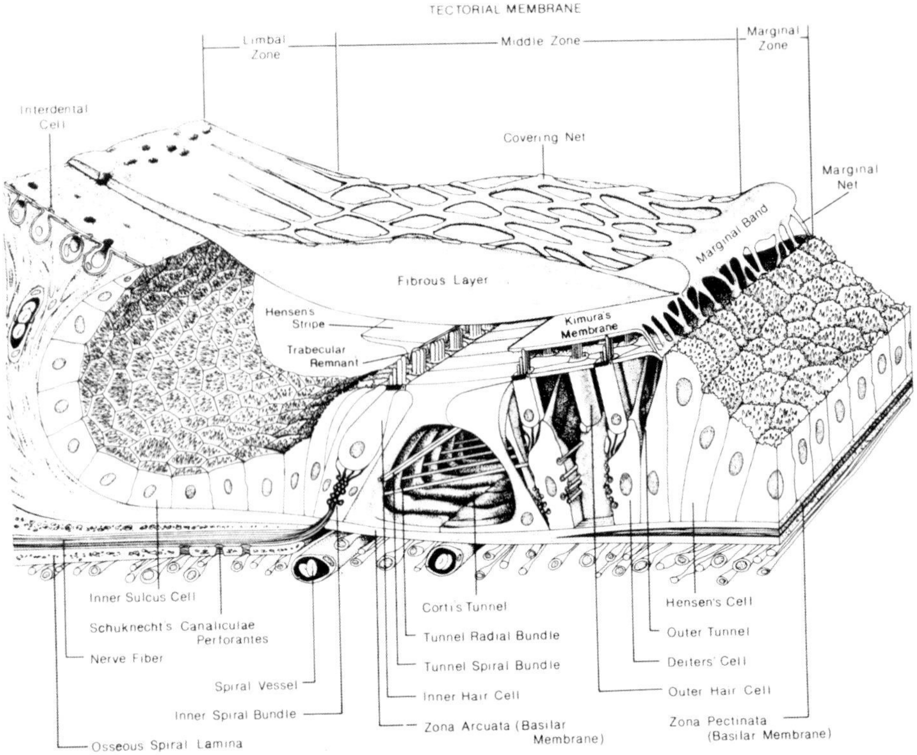

FIG. 7. Artist's conception of the organ of Corti. (From ref. 76.) (Drawing by Nancy Sally.)

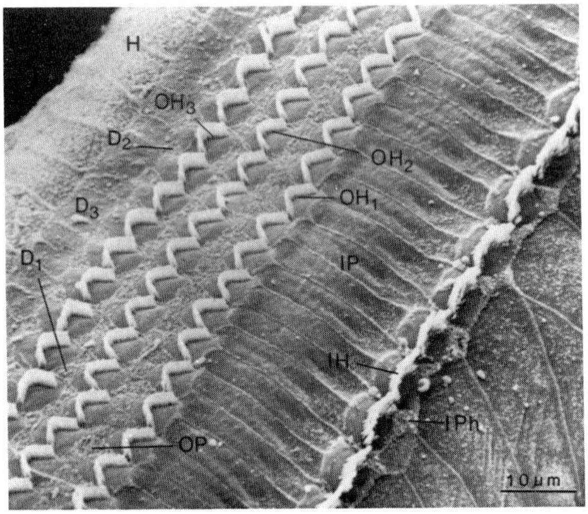

FIG. 8. Surface view of the organ of Corti showing inner hair cells (IH), head plates of the inner pillar cells (IP), inner phalangeal cell (IPh), three rows of the outer hair cells (OH_1, OH_2, OH_3), phalanges of the outer pillar cells (OP), phalanges of the three rows of Deiters' cells (D_1, D_2, D_3), and Hensen's cells (H). (From ref. 77.)

The inner and outer hair cells differ in a number of other aspects. For example, the outer hair cells are cylindrical and formed of an intricate organization of lamellar endoplasmic reticulum (subsurface cistern) on the entire circumference of the inner surface of the cell membrane, which is connected to the subsynaptic cistern—a membranous structure apposed to the efferent nerve endings. Numerous mitochondria are closely associated with the subsurface cisternae (Fig. 9A). This cisternal organization has been likened to the sarcoplasmic reticular system of muscles (83). In contrast, the inner hair cells are goblet shaped with narrow necks and wide bodies and are filled with tubulovesicular endoplasmic reticulum and mitochondria. The subsurface cistern is poorly developed or inconspicuous (Fig. 9B).

Another important difference between the inner and outer hair cells is their pattern of innervation. Most (95%) of the afferent nerves innervate the inner hair cells; only 5% of the afferent nerves innervate the outer hair cells, even though their number is three times greater than that of the inner hair cells. The efferent nerves, on the other hand, largely innervate the outer hair cells, and the inner hair cells receive a small portion. The afferent nerves make synapses directly on the sensory cells, whereas the efferent nerves to the inner hair cells have largely indirect axodendritic synapses on the afferent nerves innervating the inner hair cells (150). Furthermore, the efferent fibers innervating the inner and outer hair cells are distinct in their origins. Small lateral olivocochlear neurons innervate the inner hair cells, and large medial olivocochlear neurons innervate the outer hair cells. The medial efferent nerves commonly innervate on the afferent nerves whereas the lateral efferent nerves innervate directly on the outer hair cells (161). The afferent nerves innervating the inner hair cells are thought to be relayed via the type I ganglion cells, whereas those of the outer hair cells are thought to be relayed through the type II ganglion cells (149).

Despite these differences, the inner and outer hair cells have important features in common in their sensory ciliary organization. Both ciliary bundles are tonotopically organized, meaning that their stereociliary heights are graded along the length of the cochlea (76,135,152,168). The important role the sensory cilia may play in the sensory transduction process has been recently recognized (30,53,69). Recent evidence indicates that the stereocilia from different hair cells in the auditory organ of the alligator lizard are mechanically tuned to the frequencies to which those cells respond (34,50). Therefore, both inner and outer hair cells are considered mechanoreceptors capable of transducing mechanical energy into neural impulses.

It is well known that the endolymph contains a high concentration of K^+ and a high (+80 mV) electrical potential, in contrast to the high negative (−60 mV) intracellular potential of the hair cells. Recent evidence suggests that *calcium-sensitive potassium channels* exist on the apical portion of the stereociliary bundles in the frog saccule (52). This finding implies that mechanical bending of the stereocilia would open or close the potassium channels present on the apical surface of the stereocilia. In fact, a linkage system connecting the tips of the stereocilia to the sides of the tall neighboring stereocilia has been discovered, and it has been

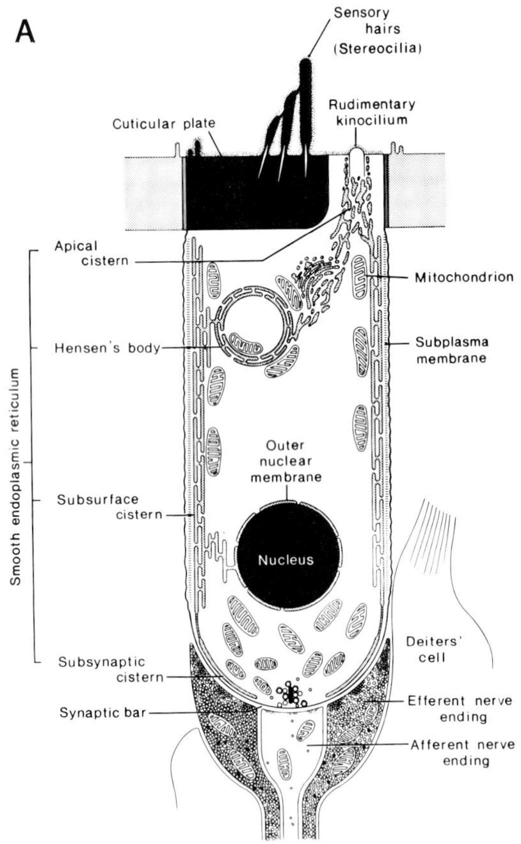

FIG. 9. A: Schematic representation of the cellular organization of the outer hair cells, indicating the intricate network of the endoplasmic reticulum, the end of which (subsynaptic cistern) is located directly apposed to the afferent nerve ending. (From ref. 79.) (Drawing by Nancy Sally.)

suggested that these structures may be associated with the aforementioned ion channels (115,119). Modulated K^+ ion passage through the stereociliary bundles would increase the intracellular K^+ ions, requiring their elimination through the basolateral side of the hair cells (52). Crawford and Fettiplace (23) reported that in the turtle auditory organ the sensory cells themselves have a *resonant membrane potential* to the injecting current, and that each cell has a best resonant frequency. This membrane resonance is most likely mediated by the efflux of K^+ ions through the cell membrane.

A number of clinical (54,97) and experimental (48,172) studies indicate that inner ear autoimmunity may result in sensorineural hearing loss. How this hearing loss comes about is not yet understood, and the exact target structures of the inner ear have not been established. However, sensory cell degeneration, ganglion cell

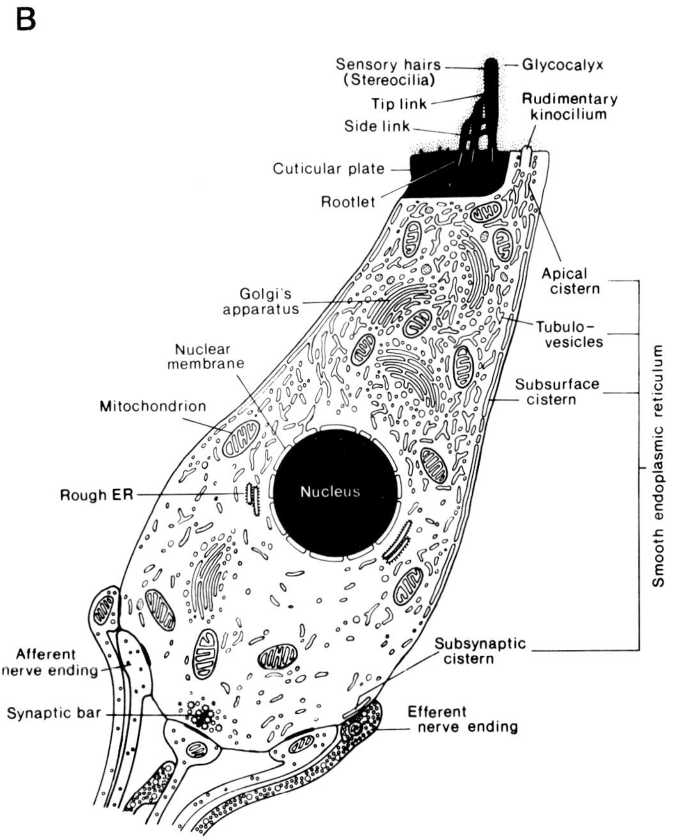

FIG. 9. B: Schematic diagram of the inner-hair-cell cellular organization, showing the complex network of tubulovesicular endoplasmic network filling the entire cell. The subsurface cistern is poorly developed, and when present it is usually a single layer and often interrupted. (From ref. 79.) (Drawing by Nancy Sally.)

degeneration, and arteritis have been observed in an animal model using type II collagen sensitization and challenge. Whether such pathologies also occur in human conditions is not known. One can postulate that the autoimmunity affects the strial cells or strial vasculature, which may adversely affect the electrolyte balance in the endolymph, thus affecting the transduction process. This concept is entirely speculative at present, in the absence of any supporting evidence.

Stria Vascularis

The lateral wall of the cochlear duct is formed of the stria vascularis and spiral ligament. The former is composed of three cell layers: marginal cells facing the endolymph, intermediate cells, and basal cells bordering the spiral ligament (Fig. 10). The stria vascularis is so named because of the abundant capillary network penetrating this epithelial structure so that the marginal cell and intermediate cell make direct contact with the capillaries. The capillaries are not the fenestrated type; but macromolecular tracers (HRP) can pass through the capillary wall by pinocytosis, whereas HRP does not pass from the capillaries of the spiral ligament and spiral prominence when injected intravenously.

The marginal cell is an epithelial cell characterized by well-developed basolateral infoldings. This polarized organization of the marginal cell conforms with the ion/water transporting epithelium. Recent immunocytochemical studies demonstrated the localization of Na^+,K^+-ATPase (61), adenyl cyclase (136), and carbonic anhydrase (51,82). A number of diuretics that are known to cause hearing loss also affect the strial marginal cells, such as causing swelling and increased extracellular-space fluid accumulation. Thus, the marginal cell is considered the most likely fluid/ion transporting epithelial cell, similar to the kidney tubule cell. The function of the intermediate cell is not known; however, it is suggested to be involved in phagocytosis (26). This cell also often degenerates following acoustic trauma and ototoxic insult with aminoglycosides and loop diuretics (79). However, the role played by the basal cells in ion/fluid regulation is not known.

Because of the morphological similarities, the often concurrent ototoxicity and nephrotoxicity of aminoglycosides, and the coexisting congenital anomalies in the kidney and inner ear (Alport's syndrome), Quick et al. (123) have suggested that a common structural basis or shared antigenic determinants of these two organs may be a cause of these disorders. When guinea pigs and rats were sensitized with

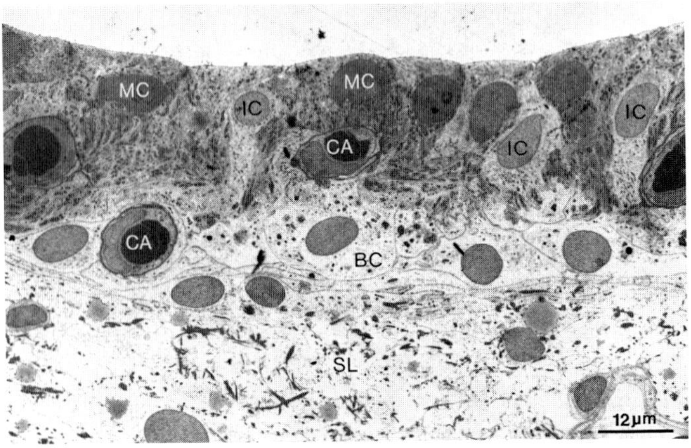

FIG. 10. Transmission electron microscope micrograph of a chinchilla stria vascularis, composed of marginal cells (MC), intermediate cells (IC), and basal cells (BC). (CA) Capillary; (SL) spiral ligament.

crude emulsified tissue of cochlear lateral walls or glomerular basement-membrane protein and then challenged, these authors found that anticochlear serum reacted specifically with connective tissue and vascular and epithelial elements of the kidney. In contrast, antiglomerular antibody reacted with vascular elements of both the stria and spiral ligament but was nonreactive to epithelial elements of the lateral cochlear wall. These authors inferred that these paradoxical results were probably due to the differences in antigens used, because the cochlear antigen was prepared from the entire lateral wall, including epithelial cells, whereas the kidney preparation was limited to the basement membrane. Thus, no firm conclusion can be drawn from their study.

Harada et al. (46) demonstrated IgG Fc receptor on the basolateral surface of the strial marginal cell and were able to induce hydrops in four of 11 guinea pigs following sensitization via the footpad using sonicated rabbit stria vascularis tissue. The hydrops did not occur in four complement-deficient guinea pigs following sensitization with rabbit strial tissue. They suggested that immune complex formation due to antigen-antibody reaction is the basis for the hydrops observed, based on their observation of a small amount of IgG and complement (C3 and C4) in the endolymph. In a follow-up study, Matsunaga et al. (94) demonstrated that this sensitization procedure and anaphylatoxin infusion induced strial vascular permeability. Of interest is the strial atrophy caused by the anaphylatoxin infusion. Strial atrophy has been reported in a number of other conditions, such as labyrinthitis due to measles, aging, and congenital syphilis (137).

Vestibular Labyrinth

The vestibular organs are composed of the gravity receptors (utricle and saccule) and cristae ampullaris, with their semicircular canals.

Macula

The saccule is located on the bony wall (elliptical recess) and connected to the cochlear duct through the ductus reuniens and to the endolymphatic duct through the saccular duct. The utricle is located on the spherical recess and connected to the cristae ampullaris. The sensory organs are composed of sensory epithelium and the otoconial membrane, which comprises the otoconial layer and the gelatinous layer, with which the stereocilia of the sensory cells are in contact. The otoconia in mammals are made of calcium carbonate in calcite form (Fig. 11).

There are two types of sensory cells: the type I cell has a flask-shaped body that is surrounded by the nerve chalice (afferent ending); the type II cell has a cylindrical-shaped body and is innervated by button-type nerve endings of both afferent and efferent nerves (Fig. 12) (55,164). The efferent nerves make synapses with the afferent fibers (147).

The sensory cells are packed with supporting cells that contain specific granules.

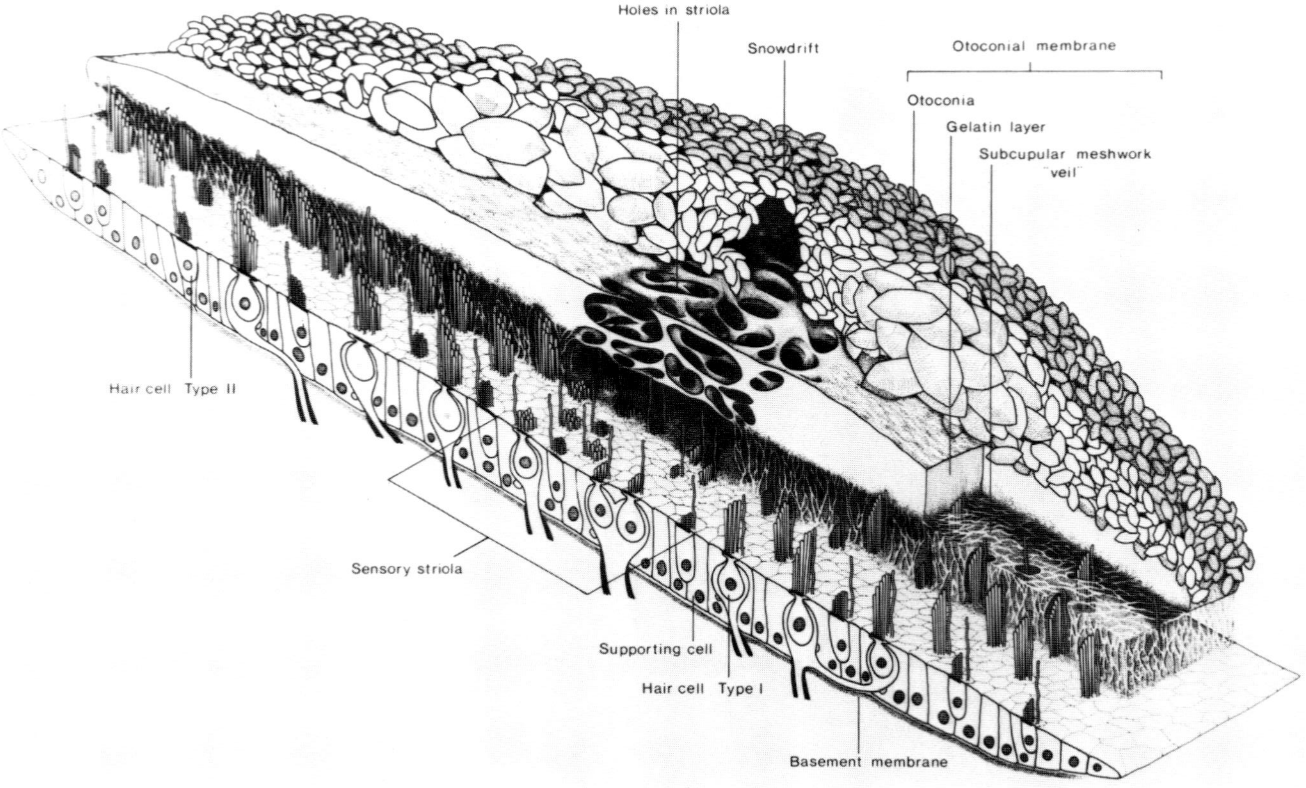

FIG. 11. Artist's conception of the saccule, illustrating the relationship between the otoconial membrane and the sensory epithelium. (From ref. 77.) (Drawing by Nancy Sally.)

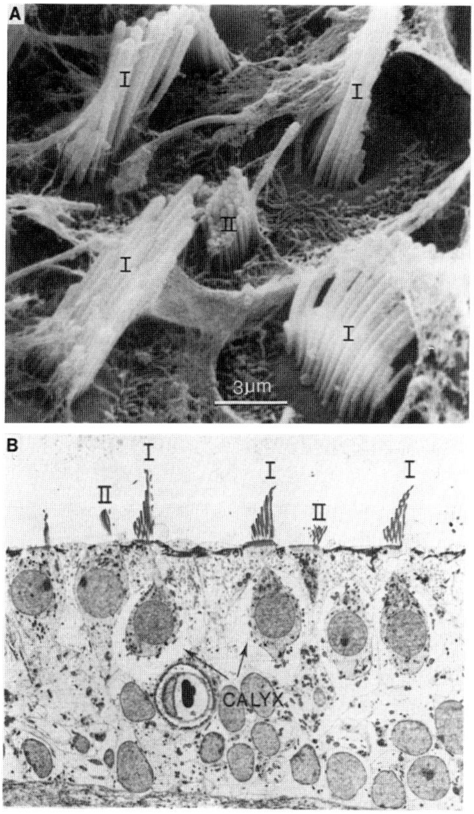

FIG. 12. A: Scanning electron microscope view of type I and type II cell stereocilia in a guinea pig utricle. Note the dramatic size and height differences between the two types. **B:** Transmission electron microscope micrograph of a cat utricle, showing: type I cells, which have tall, thick stereocilia; and type II cells, which have short, slender stereocilia.

Although the specific functions of the supporting cells have not been established, it has been suggested that they may be involved in the production and maintenance of the gelatinous materials needed to form the otoconial membrane or cupula in the crista.

The sensory epithelium of the saccule is hook-shaped and the central portion appears slightly indented due to its shorter stereociliary bundles. This central area is known as the *striola*. The utricular sensory epithelium is shaped like a shell or fan, and the striola is U-shaped.

The sensory epithelium of the saccule is hook-shaped, and the central portion appears slightly indented due to its shorter stereociliary bundles. This central area is known as the *striola*. The utricular sensory epithelium is shaped like a shell or fan, and the striola is U-shaped.

The sensory bundles of the vestibule are formed of 20 to 90 stereocilia in an organ-pipe-like arrangement of graded heights in steps and rows. The single kinocilium is found near the longest stereocilia, which are reported to be about 20 to discharge with stereociliary bending. The bending of the ciliary bundles in the opposite direction is inhibitory (165). The polarization of the sensory-cell stereociliary arrangement is demarcated along the striola, and in the saccule they are opposed to each other. In the utricle, however, the directional arrangement of the stereociliary bundles is toward the striola. This arrangement ensures spatial information even when only one ear is functioning.

Crista Ampullaris

The crista ampullaris contains a sensory crista that is saddle-shaped, with each end slightly fanned out. The central zone is analogous to the striola in the macula. The sensory ciliary height is considerably shorter in the central zone than in the peripheral zone, which was about 35 to 45 μm in guinea pigs (148). As in the macula, there are two types of sensory cells. Type II cells, in general, have longer, slender stereocilia; those of the type I cells are, in general, shorter and stubbier.

The *cupula* is made up of filamentous gelatin and contains numerous tubules into which some stereociliary bundles may penetrate. The stereociliary bundles in the peripheral zone, particularly the tall ones, may penetrate, whereas in the central zone, where the stereociliary bundles are short, they may be freestanding, because the cupular canals in this area are larger than the cupulary tubules (73,80).

The supporting cells of the cristae are morphologically identical, and they are thought to be involved, together with the cells of the planum semilunatum, in the secretion and maintenance of the cupula.

Dark Cells

Some portions of the walls of the utricle and crista ampullaris contain dark cells, so called because of their osmiophilic nature. This cell also has a well-developed basolateral infolding and is considered analogous to the strial marginal cells involved in the production and maintenance of the endolymph in the pars superior (utricle and semicircular canals). This cell is often associated with melanocytes.

Inner Ear Fluids and Their Regulating Organs

The inner ear membranous structures are subdivided into two fluid compartments: the endolymphatic and perilymphatic spaces. The endolymphatic space is self-contained and connected to the intradural blind sac, known as the *endolymphatic sac,* via the vestibular aqueduct, whereas the perilymphatic space communicates with the cerebrospinal fluid (CSF) through the cochlear aqueduct (Fig. 13). The endolymph is divided into two separate compartments: one occupying the pars superior and the other filling the pars inferior (cochlea and saccule).

Although the exact site of endolymph production remains unsettled, two opposing hypotheses have been proposed. The longitudinal flow theory, advocated by Guild (39), maintains that the stria is the primary source of endolymph that is absorbed by the endolymphatic sac. Results of experiments using trace particles

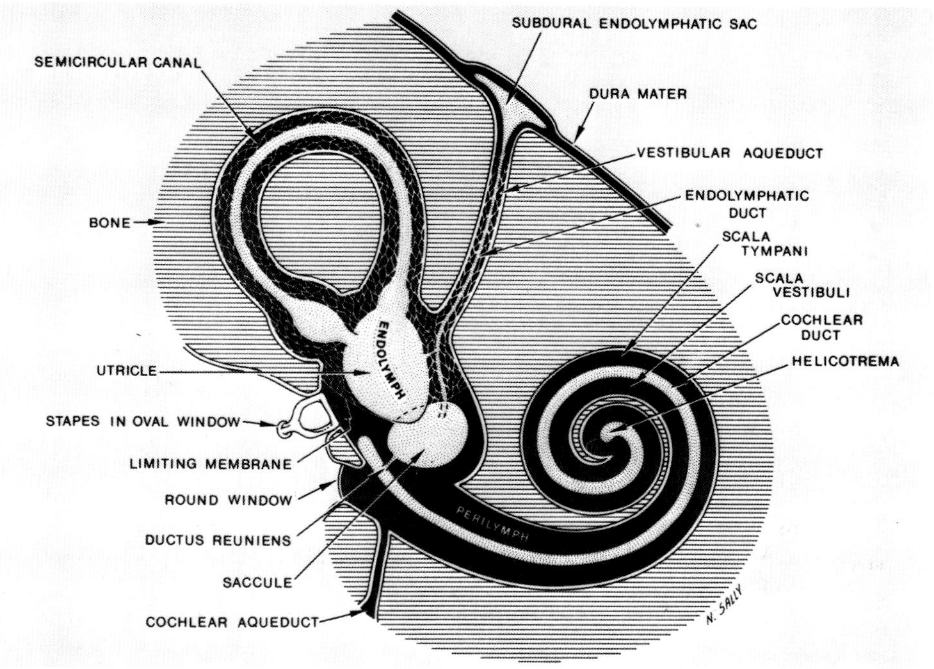

FIG. 13. Schematic diagram of the inner ear fluid system. (From ref. 77.) (Drawing by Nancy Sally.)

(2,4,39,58,92) and obstruction of the endolymphatic duct (64) strongly suggest that the endolymph flows in a longitudinal direction. The radial flow theory advocated by Naftalin and Harrison (109) is, however, supported by a trace-particle study (49) and an experiment creating small surgical holes in Reissner's membrane (67). In view of the evidence supporting both theories, it has been suggested that the flow of endolymph is longitudinal but that the exchange or balance of chemicals is radial across Reissner's membrane and other walls of the endolymphatic system (29,66); however, the endolymph from both areas is absorbed at the common endolymphatic sac, as demonstrated by experimentally injecting particles into the cochlear duct (2,38,93). When dyes were injected by an intravenous, intraperitonal, or subcutaneous route, they were subsequently found in the endolymphatic sac and perisaccular tissue. But the interpretation of this result has differed among investigators. Andersen (4) and Engström and Hjorth (28) interpreted it as evidence of endolymph resorption by the sac, whereas Seymour (140) and Van Egmond and Brinkman (157) considered it evidence of the secretion of endolymph by the sac.

The perilymph is biochemically similar to CSF in that it contains high sodium (150 meq/liter) and low potassium (6.0 meq/liter) content, whereas the endolymph contains low sodium (30 meq/liter) and high potassium (120 meq/liter) content.

The ionic concentration of endolymphatic sac fluid is reported to be similar to that of the endolymph of the cochlear duct (128,143); however, recent studies indicate that the endolymph of the sac is similar to the perilymph (107), presumably due to a leaky epithelium of the endolymphatic duct (125). In addition to its unusually high potassium concentration, the endolymph in the cochlear duct possesses a unique, high positive electric potential (+80 mV), and this endocochlear potential is believed to be generated by the stria vascularis.

The protein concentration of endolymph in the cochlear duct is reported to be 126 mg%, whereas that in the endolymphatic sac is 5,200 mg%. The protein concentration of the perilymph is 200 to 400 mg%, and that of the CSF is only 20 to 50 mg% (137,139,143). The exact nature of the proteins in these fluids is not fully known. A number of studies have attempted to measure the immunoglobulins in the inner ear fluids (largely perilymph) (22,35,46,47,102,116). The predominant immunoglobulin appears to be IgG in both perilymph (47,102) and endolymph (46), but IgA and IgM were also found in human perilymph (116). However, in guinea pigs and chinchillas, IgM was not found in the perilymph or CSF, although IgA and IgG were found (102).

The source of immunoglobulins in perilymph was examined by studying the transfer of serum antibodies to perilymph in chinchillas and guinea pigs (102). These authors found that the mean values of IgG and albumin in the perilymph were two to four times greater than those in CSF and suggested that the greater portion of the immunoglobulins in perilymph is probably derived from perilymphatic blood vessels as a filtrate and that the perilymphatic immune system is independent of the CSF. However, recent studies (106,153) showed that the endolymphatic sac contributes to the perilymphatic immunoglobulins, which are produced locally (see below).

Endolymphatic Duct and Sac

The *endolymphatic duct* system generally encompasses the saccular and utricular ducts and the endolymphatic sac. The ductus reuniens is included as part of this system because it links the cochlear and endolymphatic ducts through the saccule (Fig. 14).

The rate of fluid transport between the endolymphatic sac and pars superior or pars inferior is not yet established. A review of the interconnecting ductal system is relevant for gaining insight into this question. The ductus reuniens is a straight tube measuring about 2.5 mm long and 0.5 mm wide in the chinchilla. At the cochlear end it is continuous with Reissner's membrane, which becomes funnel-shaped. At the saccular end the ductus widens, resembling a trumpet, and is continuous with the saccular wall on one side and the saccular duct on the other. The saccular duct is short, resembling the ductus reuniens, and measures about 0.5 mm long and 0.4 mm wide in the chinchilla.

The diameter of the *ductus reuniens* and saccular duct is about six times greater than that of the utricular duct. Therefore, more endolymph circulation is expected

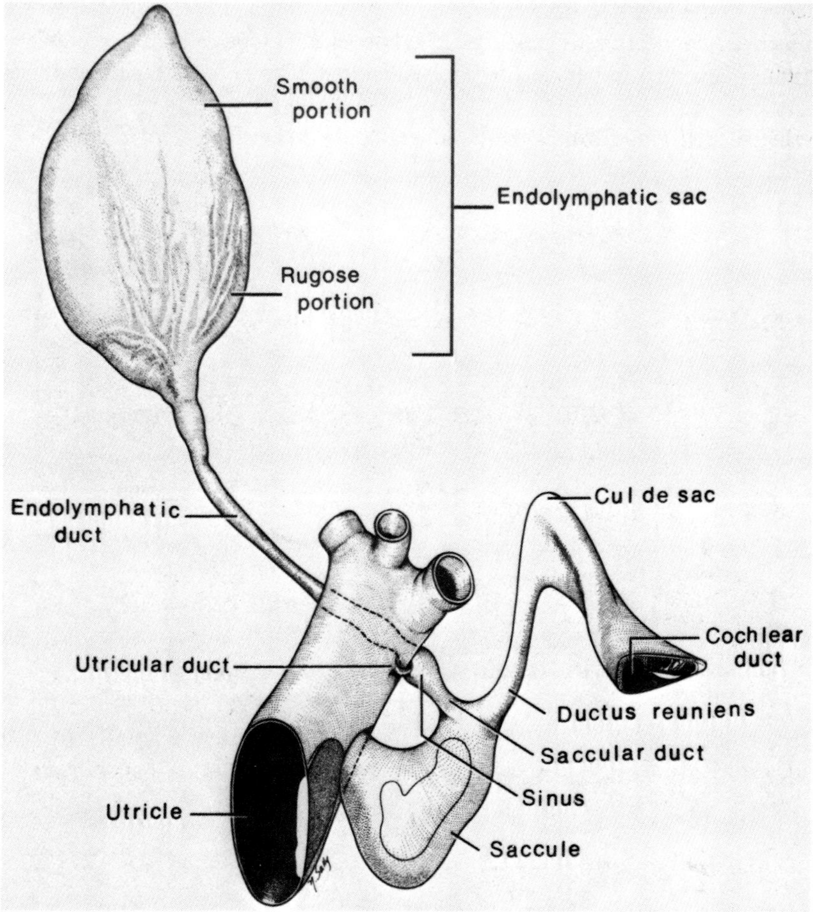

FIG. 14. Artist's conception of the endolymphatic duct system. (From ref. 86.) (Drawing by Nancy Sally.)

between the pars inferior and endolymphatic sac than between the pars superior and sac. In addition to the size differences mentioned above, the utricular duct at its utricular opening is slit-like and is formed partly by the utriculoendolymphatic valve (9), which may also impede the free flow of endolymph between the pars superior and endolymphatic duct. The *sinus* portion of the endolymphatic duct is slightly dilated and measures about 0.9 mm long and 0.7 mm wide in the chinchilla. The *utricular duct* is an ovoid or collapsed-hose-like structure slightly curved along the utricular wall, measuring about 0.2 mm long and 0.06 mm wide in the chinchilla.

The endolymphatic duct is housed in the vestibular aqueduct and measures about 5.1 mm long and 0.2 mm wide in the chinchilla (Fig. 15). The vestibular aqueduct contains loose connective tissue possessing square fibrils characteristic of inner-ear connective tissue (Fig. 15). Numerous blood vessels accompany the vestibular aqueduct in paravestibular canaliculi similar to those Ogura and Clemis (111) described.

Whether perilymph bathes the periductal and perisaccular areolar spaces is still

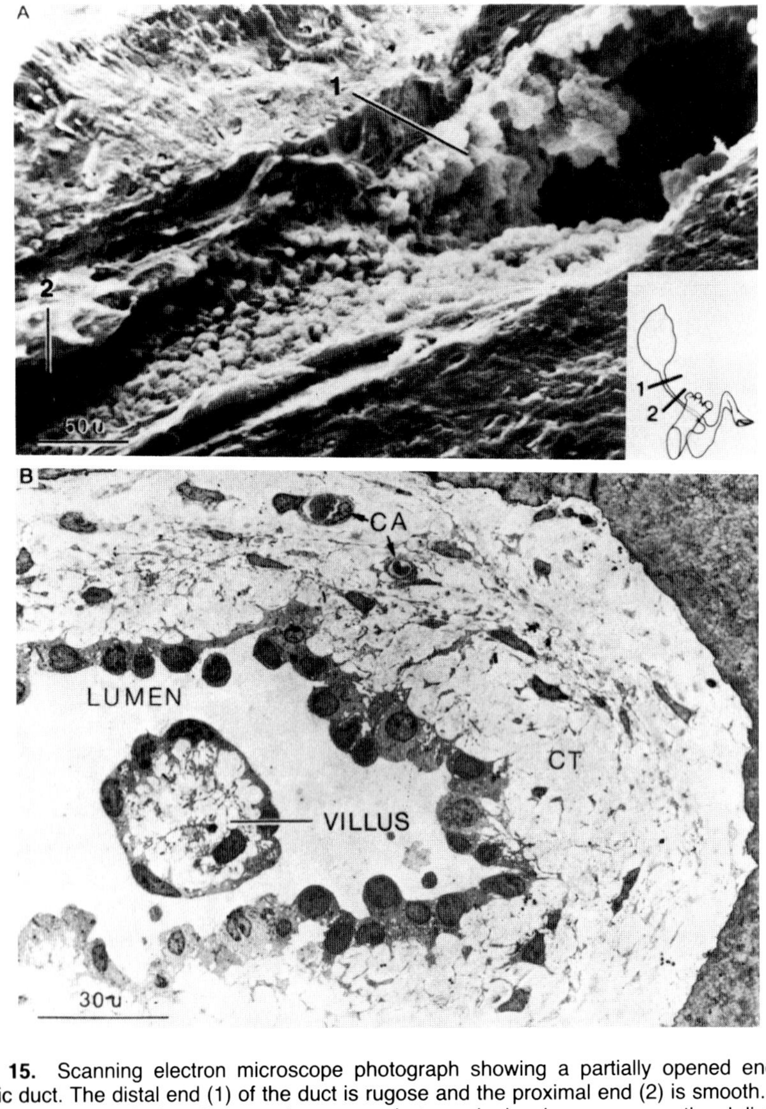

FIG. 15. Scanning electron microscope photograph showing a partially opened endolymphatic duct. The distal end (1) of the duct is rugose and the proximal end (2) is smooth. (From ref. 86.) **B:** Transmission electron microscope photograph showing a cross-sectional distal end of the tube. Loose connective tissue (CT) fills the vestibular aqueduct. (CA) Capillaries. (From ref. 86.) (Drawing by Nancy Sally.)

unsettled. Portmann (120) was of the opinion that this space is filled with perilymph in the guinea pig. Ogura and Clemis (111), on the basis of osmic acid staining, suggested that the perilymphatic space extends partly down the vestibular aqueduct, only reaching the proximal sac. Guild (39) observed the perisaccular areolar space but reserved any conclusion as to whether it communicates with the perilymphatic space.

In mammals the *endolymphatic sac* remains as an intradural sac formed of two morphologically distinct portions: smooth and rugose (10) (Fig. 13). It has been generally accepted that it is involved in equilibration of hydrostatic pressure in the labyrinth (1,10) and that it is engaged in resorption of endolymph and phagocytosis (28,39,59,64,92). The resorptive function of the sac has drawn considerable interest among investigators due to its implication in Meniere's disease (6,27,43,62,63,121,122,138). Although it has been suspected that the endolymphatic sac is a possible immune organ because of the presence of macrophages and immune cells (plasma cells and lymphocytes) (7,8,85,127), recent experimental evidence strongly supports its being a major immune organ for the inner ear (106,153,154).

The endolymphatic sac varies slightly in size and shape. In general, the sac is an ovoid intradural structure that measures about 3 mm long and 1 mm wide in the chinchilla (Figs. 13 and 15). The rugose portion is a widened chamber surrounded by bone and exhibits a rugose surface with numerous villi. Because of the rugosity, this portion is referred to as the *pars rugosa* by Zechner and Altmann (173).

The epithelial cells are often anchored to the basement membrane by a small stem, whereas the main body protrudes into the lumen due to exaggerated intercellular spaces, as observed earlier by Guild (39), providing a large surface that makes contact with the endolymph. Such exaggerated intercellular spaces in the sac epithelium are considered an expression of active fluid transportation across the epithelial cells, as suggested by Lim and Silver (86).

The epithelial cells are of two basic types in chinchillas: They are light and dark cells (Fig. 16), which are similar to those described in guinea pigs by Lundquist (92). These cells are either cuboidal or columnar. The light cell is generally larger than the dark cell. It is characterized by numerous mitochondria and long microvilli. The nucleus is round with little infolding. The cytoplasm occasionally contains vacuoles and lysosomal bodies. The basal portion of the cell is smooth, with few exceptions. The dark cell is generally smaller than the light cell. It is characterized by osmiophilic cytoplasm and an infolded nucleus. The base of the cell is also infolded and the basement membrane follows the irregular cell membrane. The microvilli are unusually short and sparsely distributed.

As noted above, the surface of the light cells appears to be provided with numerous long microvilli; this is in contrast to the dark cells, which are covered with short, sparse microvilli (92,100). The meaning of these findings is not known; however, it is speculated that the cells that possess numerous microvilli may be more actively involved in fluid transport. It is interesting to note that in the turtle

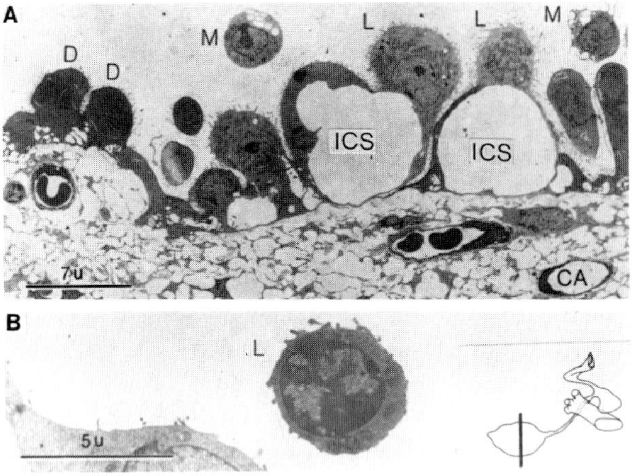

FIG. 16. **A:** Transmission electron microscope view of the rugose portion of a chinchilla endolymphatic sac, showing exaggerated intercellular space (ICS) of the epithelial cells, which are composed of dark cells (D) and light cells (L). Free macrophages (M) are also seen in the lumen. Observe spongy connective tissue. (CA) Capillary. **B:** A free lymphocyte (L) can be seen in the lumen of the rugose portion of a chinchilla. (From ref. 86.)

bladder the epithelial cells that are covered with numerous microvilli contain a high level of the enzyme carbonic anhydrase, which is involved in hydrogen ion and electrolyte transport, whereas the bare epithelial cells lack this enzyme (130). Introducing silver particles and bacteria into the cochlear duct, Lundquist (92) examined the endolymphatic sac and concluded that it has resorptive, as well as phagocytic, function. He further suggested that the light epithelial cells are mainly involved in fluid transport, whereas the dark epithelial cells are primarily phagocytic.

This subepithelial connective tissue, in the pars rugosa, is formed of three substrata in chinchillas; spongeous, elastic, and collagenous layers (Fig. 16) (85). The spongeous layer is so named because of its complex spongeous arrangement of cytoplasmic processes of fibrocytes. This layer is continuous with the areolar subepithelial connective tissue layer of the vestibular aqueduct. It is not possible to conclude whether this periductal and perisaccular areolar space is bathed with perilymph on the basis of morphologic study alone. However, it can be suggested that the connective tissue in the spongeous layer in the duct and sac has a common origin with the perilymphatic tissue. It has been speculated that this space is connected with the perilymphatic space (33,85,111). This suggestion is compatible with the observation that macromolecular tracers introduced into the middle ear cavity were found in the endolymphatic sac (78,134) and, furthermore, that when the duct was obliterated such transport failed to occur (134).

The *smooth portion* of the sac is a continuum of the rugose portion, and its surface gradually becomes smooth. As in the guinea pig (39), the lateral sinus is located near the sac in chinchillas. The epithelial cells are cuboidal or squamous and resemble the dark cells. The nuclei are generally infolded and their cytoplasm is osmiophilic due to the presence of abundant ribosomes and tonofilaments. They also contain lysosomal granules. The intercellular spaces contain numerous slender cytoplasmic processes and infoldings, indicating active fluid transport. The microvilli are short and scanty in number. Free-floating cells are not as numerous as in the rugose portion. The subepithelial connective tissue lacks the spongeous layer. It is composed of elastic and collagenous layers that are continuous with dura. The square fibers are not seen in this area. Since the distal portion is completely surrounded by dura, this portion is also called the *pars intraduralis* by Zechner and Altmann (173).

Free Cells in the Sac

Later investigations (85,127) confirmed earlier reports (39,92) that there are numerous free-floating cells in the endolymphatic sac. The majority of free-floating cells are macrophages. On rare occasions a free-floating lymphocyte was also seen (Fig. 16B) (85). The origin of macrophages in the endolymphatic sac is not yet settled. It is known that blood monocytes, bone-marrow stem cells, and histiocytes can transform into macrophages under certain conditions (118). It has been proposed that the dark cells are fixed epithelial phagocytes and can become free macrophages (92). Drastic morphologic changes can occur in macrophages following stimulation, and macrophages can fuse to form an epithelioid giant cell. There is a striking resemblance between the epithelioid cell and the dark cell with double nuclei (85).

Subepithelial Connective Tissue

The subepithelial connective tissue can be subdivided into three layers: spongeous, elastic, and collagenous. The spongeous layer contains a capillary network and is composed primarily of a loose cytoplasmic meshwork and scanty fibers that are square in cross-sectional view. The meshwork spaces are empty; therefore, it is assumed that they are filled with fluid. These meshwork cells are slender with scanty cell organelles and are often closely associated with the basement membrane of the epithelial cells. This phenomenon is more pronounced in the villi. Unmyelinated nerve fibers near capillaries and epithelial cells of the sac have been observed (85). The elastic layer is an extension of the spongeous layer but contains large numbers of elastic fibers. The collagenous layer is formed of well-arranged collagen fibers packed in stacks.

It is known that the fibrils found in the perilymphatic connective tissue are unique in that they are square when cross-sectioned (44). The same square fibers are also found in the periductal and perisaccular subepithelial connective tissue of the pars rugosa, suggesting that it is related to the perilymphatic connective tissue. Such square fibers do not appear to be found in the cochlear aqueduct (25). It is also interesting to note that this perilymphatic connective tissue thins out toward the distal portion of the sac. The subepithelial connective tissue in this portion is composed primarily of elastic fibers and collagen fibers. This arrangement supports the earlier notion that the distal portion of the sac is distensible and participates in hydrostatic pressure regulation of the endolymph, whereas the rugose portion is involved primarily in fluid resorption and phagocytosis (1,10).

There are a number of *migrating cells* in the perisaccular connective tissue. The most common ones found are macrophages, lymphocytes, occasional plasma cells, and even PMNs (126,127). A few plasma-cell-like cells have also been observed in human perisaccular connective tissue (8). Although rather abundant migratory cells have been found in the guinea pig (126,127), these cells were rare in chinchilla perisaccular tissue (85). A dramatic increase in macrophages, lymphocytes, and plasma cells into the endolymphatic sac has been demonstrated following perilymphatic challenge via the round window of guinea pigs that has been systematically sensitized by the potent immunogen keyhole limpet hemocyanin (153). An important result is that no cellular infiltration or fibrosis in the cochlea were observed in ears in which the endolymphatic sac had been obliterated, but they were seen in those on which the sham operation was performed. On this basis, the investigators concluded that the endolymphatic sac is required for the inner ear to mount an immune response. Morgenstern (106) earlier reported that the increase of immunoglobulins in the inner ear requires the endolymphatic sac. A significant increase in round cells has also been observed in chinchilla endolymphatic sac tissue following experimental otitis media (Lim, unpublished data).

In summary, the endolymphatic sac possesses all the cellular machinery needed to process antigens (macrophages) and produce antibodies (plasma cells), as suggested earlier (85,126). The fact that lymphocytes are also found in the sac lumen (85) and in the perisaccular tissue (127) may suggest that this organ also can mount a local humoral and cellular immune response.

ACKNOWLEDGMENT

This work was supported in part by grants from the NINCDS/NIH (NS08854) and Deafness Research Foundation. The invaluable assistance of Nancy Sally, Barbara Vogel, Shakuntala Lamgaday, Smokey Lynn Bare, and Katherine Adamson is gratefully acknowledged. Drs. Thomas F. DeMaria and Lauren O. Bakaletz critically reviewed the manuscript.

REFERENCES

1. Allen, G.W. (1964): Endolymphatic sac and cochlear aqueduct. *Arch. Otolaryngol.*, 79:322–327.
2. Altmann, F., and Waltner, J.G. (1950): Further investigations on the physiology of the labyrinthine fluids. *Ann. Otol. Rhinol. Laryngol.*, 59:657–686.
3. Amano, H., Yamashita, T., Kitajiri, M., Kumazawa, T., Tanaka, C., and Ibata, Y. (1984): Adrenergic innervation in the eustachian tube of the guinea pig: histochemical and electron mi-

croscopic observations. In: *Recent Advances in Otitis Media with Effusion,* edited by D.J. Lim, C.D. Bluestone, J.O. Klein, and J.D. Nelson, pp. 74–76. B.C. Decker, Philadelphia and Toronto.
4. Andersen, H.C. (1948): Passage of trypan blue into the endolymphatic system of the labyrinth. *Acta Otolaryngol.,* 36:273–283.
5. Änggard Å. (1974): Autonomic nervous control of blood circulation and secretion in the nasal mucosa. An experimental study in the cat. Thesis, Karolinska Institutet, Stockholm.
6. Arenberg, I.K., Marovitz, W.F., and Shambaugh, G.E., Jr. (1970): The role of the endolymphatic sac in the pathogenesis of endolymphatic hydrops in man. *Acta Otolaryngol.* (Suppl.), 275:1–49.
7. Arnold, W.W., and Altermatt, H.J. (1985): Presence of immunoglobulins (IgA, IgG) and secretory component in the human endolymphatic sac. In: *New Dimensions in Otorhinolaryngology—Head and Neck Surgery, Vol. 2,* edited by E. Myers, pp. 128–129. Elsevier Science Publishers, Amsterdam.
8. Arnold, W., Morgenstern, C., and Miyamoto, H. (1981): Morphology and function of the endolymphatic sac. In: *Ménière's Disease: Pathogenesis, Diagnosis, and Treatment,* edited by K.-H. Vosteen, H. Schuknecht, C.R. Pfaltz, J. Wersäll, R.S. Kimura, C. Morgenstern, and S.K. Juhn, pp. 110–114. Georg Thieme, Stuttgart.
9. Bast, T.H. (1928): The utriculo-endolymphatic valve. *Anat. Rec.,* 40:61.
10. Bast, T.H., and Anson, B.J. (1960): The ear and the temporal bone: development and adult structure. In: *Otolaryngology,* edited by G.M. Coates and H.P. Schenk. W.F. Prior, Hagerstown, Md.
11. von Békésy, G. (1960): *Experiments in Hearing,* translated and edited by E.G. Wever, pp. 703–710. McGraw-Hill, New York.
12. Bernstein, J.M., Hayes, E.R., Ishikawa, T., Tomasi, T.B. Jr., and Herd, J.K. (1972): Secretory otitis media: a histopathological and immunochemical report. *Trans. Am. Acad. Ophthalmol. Otolaryngol.,* 76:1305–1318.
13. Bernstein, J.M., and Ogra, P.L. (1980): Mucosal immune system: implications in otitis media with effusion. *Ann. Otol. Rhinol. Laryngol.,* 89 (Suppl. 68):326–332.
14. Bernstein, J.M., Tomasi, T.B. Jr., and Ogra, P. (1974): The immunochemistry of middle ear effusions. *Arch. Otolaryngol.,* 99:320–326.
15. Bernstein, J.M., Yamanaka, T., Cumella, J., Ogra, P.L., and Park, B. (1985): Some observations on lymphocyte and macrophage function in middle ear effusions. In: *Immunobiology, Autoimmunity and Transplantation in Otorhinolaryngology,* edited by J.E. Veldman, B.F. McCabe, E.H. Huizing, and N. Mygind, pp. 51–61. Kugler, Amsterdam.
16. Birken, E.A., and Brookler, R.H. (1973): Surface-tension lowering substance of the eustachian tube in non-suppurative otitis media: an experiment with dogs. *Laryngoscope* 83:255–258.
17. Birken, E.A., and Brookler, R.H. (1977): Surface-tension lowering substance of the canine eustachian tube. *Ann. Otol. Rhinol., Laryngol.,* 81:268–271.
18. Bluestone, C.D., Paradise, J.L., and Beery, Q.C. (1972): Symposium on prophylaxis and treatment of middle ear effusions. IV. Physiology of the eustachian tube in the pathogenesis and management of middle ear effusions. *Laryngoscope,* 82:1654–1670.
19. Boat, T.F., Cheng, P.W., Iver, R.N., Carlson, D.M., and Polony, I. (1976): Human respiratory tract secretions. *Arch. Biochem. Biophys.,* 177:95–104.
20. Branefors-Helander, P., Nylén, O., and Jeppsson, J.-H. (1973): Acute otitis media: Assay of complement-fixing antibody against *Haemophilus influenzae* as a diagnostic tool in acute otitis media. *Acta Pathol. Microbiol. B,* 81:508–518.
21. Brookler, R.H., and Birken, E.A. (1971): Surface-tension lowering substance of the canine eustachian tube. *Laryngoscope,* 81:1673–1781.
22. Chevance, L.G., Galli, A., and Jeanmaire, M.J. (1960): Immuno-electrophoretic study of the human perilymph. *Acta Otolaryngol.,* 52:41–46.
23. Crawford, A.C., and Fettiplace, R. (1981): An electrical tuning mechanism in turtle cochlear hair cells. *J. Physiol.,* 312:377–412.
24. Dallos, P. (1973): *The Auditory Periphery: Biophysics and Physiology.* Academic, New York and London.
25. Duckert, L. (1974): The morphology of the cochlear aqueduct and periotic duct of the guinea pig—a light and electron microscopic study. *Trans. Am. Acad. Ophthalmol. Otolaryngol.,* 78:ORL21–48.
26. Duvall, A.J. III, Quick, C.A., and Sutherland, C.R. (1971): Horseradish peroxidase in the lat-

eral cochlear wall: an electron microscopic study of transport. *Arch. Otolaryngol.*, 93:304–316.
27. Egami, T., Sando, I., and Black, F.O. (1978): Hypoplasia of the vestibular aqueduct and endolymphatic sac in endolymphatic hydrops. *J. Otorhinolaryngol. Relat. Spec.*, 86:327–339.
28. Engström, H., and Hjorth, S. (1951): On the distribution and localization of injected dyes in the labyrinth of the guinea pig. *Acta Otolaryngol.* (Suppl.), 95:149–158.
29. Fernández, C. (1967): Biochemistry of labyrinthine fluids: inorganic substances. *Arch. Otolaryngol.*, 86:222–233.
30. Flock, Å., Ulfendahl, M., and Flock, B. (1985): Motility in outer hair cells and its structural substrate. *Abstracts of the Eighth Midwinter Research Meeting,* Association for Research in Otolaryngology, pp. 175–176.
31. Flock, Å., and Wersäll, J. (1963): Morphological polarization and orientation of the hair cells, in the labyrinth and the lateral organ. *J. Ultrastruct. Res.*, 8:193–194.
32. Flory, P.J. (1969): Rubber elasticity. In: *Principles of Polymer Chemistry,* edited by P.J. Flory, pp. 432–492. Cornell University Press, Ithaca and London.
33. Friberg, U., Rask-Andersen, H., and Bagger-Sjöbäck, D. (1984): Human endolymphatic duct: an ultrastructural study. *Arch. Otolaryngol.*, 110:421–428.
34. Frishkopf, L.S., and DeRosier, D.J. (1983): Mechanical tuning of freestanding stereociliary bundles and frequency analysis in the alligator lizard cochlea. *Hear. Res.*, 12:393–404.
35. Fritsch, J.H., and Jolliff, C.R. (1966): Protein components of human perilymph. I. Preliminary study. *Ann. Otol. Rhinol. Laryngol.*, 75:1070–1076.
36. Giebink, G.S., and Quie, P.G. (1977): Comparison of otitis media due to types 3 and 23 *Streptococcus pneumoniae* in the chinchilla model. *J. Infect. Dis.* (Suppl.), 136:S191–S195.
37. Giebink, G.S., Ripley, M.L., and Wright, P.F. (1987): Eustachian tube histopathology during experimental influenza A virus infection in the chinchilla. *Ann. Otol. Rhinol. Laryngol.*
38. Guild, S.R. (1927): Circulation of the endolymph. *Laryngoscope,* 37:649.
39. Guild, S.R. (1927): Observations upon the structure and normal contents of the ductus and saccus endolymphaticus in the guinea-pig *(Cavia cobaya)*. *Am. J. Anat.*, 39:1–56.
40. Hagan, W.E. (1977): The mucous blanket of the eustachian tube: a morphologic and surface property demonstration. *Trans. Am. Acad. Ophthalmol. Otolaryngol.*, 84:242–268.
41. Hagan, W.E. (1977): Surface-tension lowering substance in eustachian tube function. *Laryngoscope,* 87:1033–1045.
42. Håkanson, C.H., and Toremalm, N.G. (1965): Studies on the physiology of the trachea. I. Ciliary activity indirectly recorded by a new "light beam reflex" method. *Ann. Otol. Rhinol. Laryngol.*, 74:954–969.
43. Hallpike, C.S., and Cairns, H. (1938): Observations on the pathology of Meniere's syndrome. *J. Laryngol. Otol.*, 53:625–654.
44. Hamilton, D.W. (1967): Perilymphatic fibrocytes in the vestibule of the inner ear. *Anat. Rec.*, 157:627–639.
45. Hanamure, Y., and Lim, D.J. (1986): Normal distribution of lysozyme and lactoferrin secreting cells in the chinchilla tubotympanum. *Am. J. Otolaryngol.*, 7:410–425.
46. Harada, T., Matsunaga, T., Hong, K., and Inoue, K. (1984): Endolymphatic hydrops and III type allergic reaction. *Acta Otolaryngol.*, 97:450–459.
47. Harris, J.P. (1983): Immunology of the inner ear: response of the inner ear to antigen challenge. *Otolaryngol. Head Neck Surg.*, 91:18–23.
48. Harris, J.P., Low, N.C., and House, W.F. (1985): Contralateral hearing loss following inner ear injury: sympathetic cochleolabyrinthitis? *Am. J. Otol.*, 6:371–377.
49. Hinojosa, R. (1971): Transport of ferritin across Reissner's membrane. *Acta Otolaryngol.* (Suppl.), 292:1–27.
50. Holton, T., and Hudspeth, A.J. (1983): A micromechanical contribution to cochlear tuning and tonotopic organization. *Science,* 222:508–510.
51. Hsu, D.-J., and Nomura, Y. (1984): Carbonic anhydrase activity in the inner ear. *Ear Res. Jpn,* 15:213–215.
52. Hudspeth, A.J. (1985): The cellular basis of hearing: the biophysics of hair cells. *Science,* 230:745–752.
53. Hudspeth, A.J., and Corey, D.P. (1977): Sensitivity, polarity, and conductance changes in the response of vertebrate hair cells to controlled mechanical stimuli. *Proc. Natl. Acad. Sci. USA,* 74:2407–2411.
54. Hughes, G.B., Kinney, S.E., Barna, B.P., and Calabrese, L.B. (1985): Autoimmune Meniere's

syndrome. In: *Immunobiology, Autoimmunity and Transplantation in Otorhinolaryngology,* edited by J.E. Veldman, B.F. McCabe, E.H. Huizing, and N. Mygind, pp. 119–129. Kugler, Amsterdam.
55. Hunter-Duvar, I.M., and Hinojosa, R. (1984): Vestibule: sensory epithelia. In: *Ultrastructural Atlas of the Inner Ear,* edited by I. Friedmann and J. Ballantyne, pp. 211–244. Butterworths, London.
56. Hybbinette, J.-C. (1981): On the pharmacological control of mucociliary activity in the rabbit maxillary sinus *in vivo.* Doctoral dissertation, Dept. of Otorhinolaryngology, University of Lund.
57. Ishii, T., and Kaga, K. (1976): Autonomic nervous system of the cat middle ear mucosa. *Ann. Otol. Rhinol. Laryngol.,* 85 (Suppl. 25):51–57.
58. Ishii, T., Silverstein, H., and Balogh, K. Jr. (1966): Metabolic activities of the endolymphatic sac: an enzyme histochemical and autoradiographic study. *Acta Otolaryngol.,* 62:61–73.
59. Iwata, N. (1924): Über das Labyrinth der Fledermaus mit besonder Berucksichtigung des statischen Apparates. *Aichi J. Exp. Med.,* 1:41.
60. Juhn, S.K., Giebink, G.S., Huff, J.S., and Mills, E.L. (1980): Biochemical and immunochemical characteristics of middle ear effusions in relation to bacteriological findings. *Ann. Otol. Rhinol. Laryngol.,* 89 (Suppl. 68):161–167.
61. Kerr, T.P., Ross, M.D., and Ernst, S.A. (1982): Cellular localization of Na^+,K^+-ATPase in mammalian cochlear duct: significance for cochlear fluid balance. *Am. J. Otolaryngol.,* 3:332–338.
62. Kimura, R.S. (1967): Experimental blockage of the endolymphatic duct and sac and its effect on the inner ear of the guinea pig: a study on endolymphatic hydrops. *Ann. Otol. Rhinol. Laryngol.,* 76:664–687.
63. Kimura, R.S. (1981): Recent observations on experimental endolymphatic hydrops. In: *Ménière's Disease: Pathogenesis, Diagnosis and Treatment,* edited by K.-H. Vosteen, H. Schuknecht, C.R. Pfaltz, J. Wersäll, R.S. Kimura, C. Morgenstern, and S.K. Juhn, pp. 15–23. Georg Thieme, Stuttgart.
64. Kimura, R.S., and Schuknecht, H.F. (1965): Membranous hydrops in the inner ear of the guinea pig after obliteration of the endolymphatic sac. *Pract. Otorhinolaryng.,* 27:343–354.
65. Kumazawa, T. (1985): Autonomic nerve regulation in the eustachian tube function. *Auris-Nasus-Larynx (Tokyo),* 12 (Suppl. I): S5–S7.
66. Lawrence, M. (1973): Inner ear physiology. In: *Otolaryngology, Vol. 1,* edited by M.M. Paparella and D.A. Shumrick, pp. 275–298, W.B. Saunders, Philadelphia.
67. Lawrence, M., Wolsk, D., and Litton, W.B. (1961): Circulation of the inner ear fluids. *Ann. Otol. Rhinol. Laryngol.,* 70:753–776.
68. Lewis, D.M., Schram, J.L., Birck, H.G., and Lim, D.J. (1979): Antibody activity in otitis media with effusion. *Ann. Otol. Rhinol. Laryngol.,* 88:392–396.
69. Liberman, M.C., and Dodds, L.W. (1984): Single neuron labeling and chronic cochlear pathology. III. Stereocilia damage and alterations of threshold tuning curves. *Hear. Res.,* 16:55–74.
70. Lim, D.J. (1970): Protein secreting cells in the normal middle ear mucosa of the guinea pig: an autoradiographic investigation. *Ann. Otol. Rhinol. Laryngol.,* 79:82–94.
71. Lim, D.J. (1974): Functional morphology of the lining membrane of the middle ear and eustachian tube: an overview. *Ann. Otol. Rhinol. Laryngol.,* 83 (Suppl. 11):5–18.
72. Lim, D.J. (1976): Functional morphology of the mucosa of the middle ear and eustachian tube. *Ann. Otol. Rhinol. Laryngol.,* 85 (Suppl. 25):36–43.
73. Lim, D.J. (1977): Ultra anatomy of sensory end-organs in the labyrinth and their functional implications. In: *Proceedings of the Shambaugh Fifth International Workshop on Middle Ear Microscopy and Fluctuant Hearing Loss,* edited by G.E. Shambaugh, Jr., and J.J. Shea, pp. 16–27. The Strode Publishers, Huntsville, Ala.
74. Lim, D.J. (1979): Anatomy and functional morphology of the middle ear and eustachian tube—a review. In: *Proceedings of the Second National Conference on Otitis Media,* edited by R.J. Wiet and S.W. Coulthard, pp. 35–39. Ross Laboratories, Columbus, Ohio.
75. Lim, D.J. (1979): Normal and pathological mucosa of the middle ear and eustachian tube. *Clin. Otolaryngol.,* 4:213–234.
76. Lim, D.J. (1980): Cochlear anatomy related to cochlear micromechanics. A review. *J. Acoust. Soc. Am.,* 67:1686–1695.
77. Lim, D.J. (1980): Scanning electron microscopic morphology of the ear. In: *Textbook of Otolar-*

yngology, Vol. 1, Basic Sciences and Related Disciplines, edited by M.M. Paparella and C.A. Shumrick, pp. 439–469. W.B. Saunders, Philadelphia.
78. Lim, D.J. (1985): Functional morphology of the tympanic membrane and tubotympanum: with the emphasis on immunobiology. In: *Immunobiology, Autoimmunity and Transplantation in Otorhinolaryngology,* edited by J.E. Veldman, B.F. McCabe, E.H. Huizing, and N. Mygind, pp. 11–25. Kugler, Amsterdam.
79. Lim, D.J. (1986): Effects of noise and ototoxic drugs at the cellular level in the cochlea: a review. *Am. J. Otolaryngol.,* 7:73–99.
80. Lim, D.J., and Anniko, M. (1985): Development morphology of the mouse inner ear: a scanning electron microscopic observation. *Acta Otolaryngol.* (Suppl.), 442:1–69.
81. Lim, D.J., and Hussl, B. (1975): Macromolecular transport by the middle ear and its lymphatic system. *Acta Otolaryngol.,* 80:19–31.
82. Lim, D.J., Karabinas, C., and Trune, D.R. (1983): Histochemical localization of carbonic anhydrase in the inner ear. *Am. J. Otolaryngol.,* 4:33–42.
83. Lim, D.J., and Melnick, W. (1971): Acoustic damage of the cochlea: a scanning and transmission electron microscopic observation. *Arch. Otolaryngol.,* 94:294–305.
84. Lim, D.J., and Shimada, T. (1971): Secretory activity of normal middle ear epithelium: scanning and transmission electron microscopic observations. *Ann. Otol. Rhinol. Laryngol.,* 80:319–329.
85. Lim, D.J., Shimada, T., and Yoder, M. (1973): Distribution of mucus-secreting cells in normal middle ear mucosa. *Arch. Otolaryngol.,* 98:2–9.
86. Lim, D.J., and Silver, P.: The endolymphatic duct system: a light and electron microscopic observation. In: *Proceedings of Bárány Society Meeting, Anaheim, 1974,* edited by J. Pulec *(in press).*
87. Lim, D.J., Viall, J., Birck, H., and St. Pierre, R. (1972): The morphological basis for understanding middle ear effusions. An electron microscopic, cytochemical, and autoradiographic investigation. *Laryngoscope,* 82:1625–1642.
88. Lindeman, H.H. (1969): Studies on the morphology of the sensory regions of the vestibular apparatus. *Adv. Anat. Embryol. Cell Biol.,* 42:1:1–113.
89. Liu, Y.S., Lim, D.J., Lang, R.W., and Birck, H.G. (1975): Chronic middle ear effusions: Immunochemical and bacteriological investigation. *Arch. Otolaryngol.,* 101:278–286.
90. Lucas, A.M., and Douglas, L.C. (1932): Principles underlying ciliary activity in the respiratory tract. *Arch. Otolaryngol.,* 20:518–541.
91. Lucas, A.M., and Douglas, L.C. (1935): Principles underlying ciliary activity in the respiratory tract. III. Independence of tracheal cilia in vivo of drug and neurogenous stimuli. *Arch. Otolaryngol.,* 21:285–296.
92. Lundquist, P.-G. (1965): The endolymphatic duct and sac in the guinea pig: an electron microscope and experimental investigation. *Acta Otolaryngol.* (Suppl.), 201:1–108.
93. Lundquist, P.-G., Kimura, R., and Wersäll, J. (1964): Experiments in endolymph circulation. *Acta Otolaryngol.* (Suppl.), 188:194–201.
94. Matsunaga, T., Harada, T., Inoue, K., and Hong, K. (1985): The role of stria vascularis in the development of allergenic endolymphatic hydrops of guinea pigs. In: *New Dimensions in Otorhinolaryngology—Head and Neck Surgery, Vol. 1,* edited by E. Myers, pp. 318–321. Elsevier Science Publishers, Amsterdam.
95. Maves, M.D., Patil, G.S., and Lim, D.J. (1981): Surface-active substances of the guinea pig tubotympanum: a chemical and physical analysis. *Otolaryngol. Head and Neck Surg.,* 89:307–316.
96. McCabe, B.F. (1985): Autoimmune inner ear disease. In: *Immunobiology, Autoimmunity and Transplantation in Otorhinolarygology,* edited by J.E. Veldman, B.F. McCabe, E.H. Huizing, and N. Mygind, pp. 107–110. Kugler, Amsterdam.
97. McCabe, B.F. (1979): Autoimmune sensorineural hearing loss. *Ann. Otol. Rhinol., Laryngol.,* 88:585–589.
98. McMasters, P.D., and Hudack, S. (1935): The formation of agglutinins within lymph nodes. *J. Exp. Med.,* 61:783.
99. Meyer, F.A., and Silberberg, A. (1978): Structure and function of mucus. In: *Ciba Foundation Symposium,* pp. 203–211. Elsevier North-Holland, Amsterdam and New York.
100. Mitani, Y., Kosaka, N., Konishi, S., and Ogura, Y. (1973): Observation of luminal surface of the endolymphatic sac in guinea pig. *Acta Otolaryngol.,* 76:149–156.

101. Mogi, G. (1976): Secretory IgA and antibody activities in middle ear effusions. *Ann. Otol. Rhinol. Laryngol.*, 85 (Suppl. 25):97–102.
102. Mogi, G., Lim, D.J., and Watanabe, N. (1982): Immunologic study on the inner ear: immunoglobulins in perilymph. *Arch. Otolaryngol.*, 108:270–275.
103. Mogi, G., Maeda, S., and Watanabe, N. (1980): The development of mucosal immunity in guinea pig middle ears. *Int. J. Pediatr. Otorhinolaryngol.*, 1:331–349.
104. Mogi, G., Maeda, S., Yoshida, T., and Watanabe, N. (1976): Immunochemistry of otitis media with effusion. *J. Infect. Dis.*, 133:125–136.
105. Mogi, G., Yoshida, T., Honjo, S., and Maeda, S. (1973): Middle ear effusions—quantitative analysis of immunoglobulins. *Ann. Otol. Rhinol. Laryngol.*, 82:196–202.
106. Morgenstern, C. (1984): Antibody production in experimental endolymphatic hydrops. Results presented on invitation of the International Collegium Oto-Rhino-Laryngologicum Amicitiae Sacrum, Corfu, Sept. 9–12.
107. Morgenstern, C., Amano, H., and Orsulakova, A. (1982): Ion transport in the endolymphatic space. *Am. J. Otolaryngol.*, 3:323–327.
108. Nadel, J.A., Davis, B., and Phipps, R.J. (1979): Control of mucus secretion and ion transport in airways. *Ann. Rev. Physiol.*, 41:369–381.
109. Naftalin, L., and Harrison, M.S. (1958): Circulation of labyrinthine fluids. *J. Laryng.*, 72:118–136.
110. Ogra, P.L., Bernstein, J.M., Yurchak, A.M., Coppola, P.R., and Tomasi, T.J. Jr. (1974): Characteristics of secretory immune system in human middle ear: implications in otitis media. *J. Immunol.*, 112:488–495.
111. Ogura, Y., and Clemis, J.D. (1971): A study of the gross anatomy of the human vestibular aqueduct. *Ann. Otol. Rhinol. Laryngol.*, 80:813–825.
112. Ohashi, Y., Nakai, Y., Kihara, S., and Ikeoka, H. (1987): Effects of *Staphylococcus aureus* on the ciliary activity of the middle ear lining. *Ann. Otol. Rhinol. Laryngol.*
113. Ohashi, Y., Nakai, Y., Kihara, S., Ikeoka, H., Takano, H., Imoto, T. (1985): Ciliary activity in patients with nasal allergies. *Arch. Otorhinolaryngol.*, 242:141–147.
114. Ohashi, Y., Nakai, Y., Zushi, K., Muraoka, M., Minowa, Y., Harada, H., and Masutani, H. (1983): Functional and morphological studies on chronic sinusitis mucous membrane. *Acta Otolaryngol.* (Suppl.), 397:1–59.
115. Osborne, M.P., Comis, S.D., Pickles, J.O. (1984): Morphology and cross-linkage of stereocilia in the guinea-pig labyrinth examined without the use of osmium as a fixative. *Cell Tissue Res.*, 237:43–48.
116. Palva, T., and Raunio, V. (1967): Disc electrophoretic studies of human perilymph and endolymph. *Acta Otolaryngol.*, 63:128–137.
117. Palva, T., Taskinen, E., and Häyry, P. (1985): T lymphocytes in secretory otitis media. In: *Immunobiology, Autoimmunity and Transplantation in Otorhinolaryngology,* edited by J.E. Veldman, B.F. McCabe, E.H. Huizing, and N. Mygind, pp. 45–50. Kugler, Amsterdam.
118. Pearsall, N.N., and Weiser, R.S. (1970): *The Macrophage,* pp. 21–30. Lea & Febiger, Philadelphia.
119. Pickles, J.O., Comis, S.D., and Osborne, M.P. (1984): Cross-links between stereocilia in the guinea-pig organ of Corti, and their possible relation to sensory transduction. *Hear. Res.*, 15:103–112.
120. Portmann, G. (1919): Recherches sur le sac et le canal endolymphatiques: sac et canal endolymphatiques du cobaye. *C. Soc. Biol. (Paris),* 82:1384.
121. Portmann, G. (1927): Recherches sur le sac endolymphatique: retultats et applications chirurgicale. *Acta Otolaryngol.*, 11:110.
122. Portmann, M. (1964): Decompressive opening of endolymphatic sac. *Arch. Otolaryngol.*, 79:328–337.
123. Quick, C.A., Fish, A., and Brown, C. (1973): The relationship between cochlea and kidney. *Laryngoscope,* 83:1469–1482.
124. Rapport, P.N., Lim, D.J., and Weiss, H.S. (1975): Surface-active agent in eustachian tube function. *Arch. Otolaryngol.*, 101:305–311.
125. Rask-Andersen, H., Bredberg, G., and Stahle, J. (1981): Structure and function of the endolymphatic duct. In: *Ménière's Disease: Pathogenesis, Diagnosis and Treatment,* edited by K.-H. Vosteen, H. Schuknecht, C.R. Pfaltz, J. Wersäll, R.S. Kimura, C. Morgenstern, and S.K. Juhn, pp. 99–109. Georg Thieme, Stuttgart.

126. Rask-Andersen, H., and Stahle, J. (1979): Lymphocyte-macrophage activity in the endolymphatic sac: an ultrastructural study of the rugose endolymphatic sac in the guinea pig. *J. Otorhinolaryngol. Relat. Spec.*, 41:177–192.
127. Rask-Andersen, H., and Stahle, J. (1980): Immunodefence of the inner ear? Lymphocyte-macrophage interaction in the endolymphatic sac. *Acta Otolaryngol.*, 89:283–294.
128. Rauch, S. (1964): *Biochemie des Hörorgans: Einführung in Methoden und Ergenbnisse*, pp. 286–308. Georg Thieme, Stuttgart.
129. Retzius, G. (1884): *Das Gehörorgan der Wirbelthiere. II. Das Gehörorgan der Reptilien, der Vögel und der Säugetiere*, p. 356. Der Centraldruckerei, Stockholm.
130. Rosen, S. (1970): Localization of carbonic anhydrase in transporting urinary epithelia. *J. Histochem. Cytochem.*, 18:668.
131. Ryan, A.F., and Vogel, C.-W. (1984): Complement depletion by cobra venom factor: effect on immune mediated middle ear effusion and inflammation. In: *Recent Advances in Otitis Media with Effusion*, edited by D.J. Lim, C.D. Bluestone, J.O. Klein, and J.D. Nelson, pp. 166–168. B.C. Decker, Philadelphia and Toronto.
132. Sadé, J. (1970): The muco-ciliary system in relation to middle ear pathology and sensorineural hearing loss. In *Sensorineural Hearing Loss*, edited by G.E.W. Wolstenholme and J. Knight, pp. 79–99. Churchill, London.
133. Sadé, J., Meyer, F.A., King, M., and Silberberg, A. (1975): Clearance of middle ear effusions by the mucociliary system. *Acta Otolaryngol.*, 79:277–282.
134. Saijo, S., and Kimura, R.S. (1984): Distribution of HRP in the inner ear after injection into the middle ear cavity. *Acta Otolaryngol.*, 97:593–610.
135. Saunders, J.C., Schneider, M.E., and Dear, S.P. (1985): The structure and function of actin in hair cells. *J. Acoust. Soc. Am.*, 78:299–311.
136. Schacht, J. (1982): Adenylate cyclase and cochlear fluid balance. *Am. J. Otolaryngol.*, 3:328–331.
137. Schuknecht, H.F. (1974): *Pathology of the Ear*. Harvard University Press, Cambridge, Mass.
138. Schuknecht, H.F. (1981): The pathophysiology of Ménière's disease. In: *Ménière's Disease: Pathogenesis, Diagnosis and Treatment*, edited by K.-H. Vosteen, H. Schuknecht, C.R. Pfaltz, J. Wersäll, R.S. Kimura, C. Morgenstern, and S.K. Juhn, pp. 10–15. Georg Thieme, Stuttgart.
139. Schuknecht, H.F., Griffin, W.L. Jr., Davies, G., and Silverstein, H. (1968): Chemical evaluation of inner ear fluid as a diagnostic aid. *Acta Otolaryngol.*, 65:169–173.
140. Seymour, J.C. (1954): Observations on the circulation in the cochlea. *J. Laryng.*, 68:689–711.
141. Shimada, T., and Lim, D.J. (1972): Distribution of ciliated cells in the human middle ear: electron and light microscopic observations. *Ann. Otol. Rhinol. Laryngol.*, 81:203–211.
142. Silberberg, A., Meyer, F.A., Gibbon, A., and Golman, R.A. (1977): Function and properties of epithelial mucus. *Adv. Exp. Med. Biol.*, 89:171–180.
143. Silverstein, H., and Schuknecht, H.F. (1966): Biochemical studies of inner ear fluid in man. *Arch. Otolaryngol.*, 84:395–402.
144. Sleigh, M.A. (1982): Movement and coordination of tracheal cilia and the relation of these to mucus transport. In: *Mechanism and Control of Ciliary Movement*, edited by C.J. Brokaw and P. Verdugo, pp. 19–24. Alan R. Liss, New York.
145. Sloyer, J.L. Jr., Cate, C.C., Howie, V.M., Ploussard, J.H., and Johnston, R.B. Jr. (1975): The immune response to acute otitis media in children. II. Serum and middle ear fluid antibody in otitis media due to *Haemophilus influenzae*. *J. Infect. Dis.*, 132:685–688.
146. Sloyer, J.L. Jr., Ploussard, H.J., and Howie, V.M. (1976): Immunology and microbiology in acute otitis media. *Ann. Otol. Rhinol. Laryngol.*, 85 (Suppl. 25):130–134.
147. Smith, C.A. (1967): Utricle and saccule. In: *Submicroscopic Structure of the Inner Ear*, edited by S. Iurato, pp. 175–195. Pergamon Press, Oxford and London.
148. Smith, C.A., and Tanaka, K. (1975): Some aspects of the structure of the vestibular apparatus. In: *The Vestibular System*, edited by R.W. Naunton, pp. 3–20. Academic Press, New York.
149. Spoendlin, H. (1978): The afferent innervation of the cochlea. In: *Evoked Electrical Activity in the Auditory Nervous System*, edited by R.W. Naunton and C. Fernandez, pp. 21–41. Academic, New York.
150. Spoendlin, H. (1984): Primary neurons and synapses. In: *Ultrastructural Atlas of the Inner Ear*, edited by I. Friedmann and J. Ballantyne, pp. 165–183. Butterworths, London.
151. Tam, P.Y., and Verdugo, P. (1981): Control of mucus hydration as a Donnan equilibrium process. *Nature*, 292:340–342.

152. Tilney, L.G., and Saunders, J.C. (1983): Actin filaments, stereocilia, and hair cells of the bird cochlea. I. Length, number, width, and distribution of stereocilia of each hair cell are related to the position of the hair cell on the cochlea. *J. Cell Biol.*, 96:807–821.
153. Tomiyama, S., and Harris, J.P. (1986): The endolymphatic sac: its importance in inner ear immune responses. *Laryngoscope*, 96:685–691.
154. Tomiyama, S., and Harris, J. P. (1986): The role of the endolymphatic sac in the generation of inner ear immune response. *Abstracts of the Ninth Midwinter Research Meeting*, Association for Research in Otolaryngology, p. 140.
155. Uddman, R., Aluments, J., Densert, O., Ekelund, M., Håkanson, R., Lorén, I., and Sundler, F. (1979): Innervation of the feline eustachian tube. *Ann. Otol. Rhinol. Laryngol.*, 88:557–561.
156. Uddman, R., Kitajiri, M., and Sundler, F. (1984): Autonomic innervation of the tubotympanum. In: *Recent Advances in Otitis Media with Effusion*, edited by D.J. Lim, C.D. Bluestone, J.O. Klein, and J.D. Nelson, pp. 76–78. B.C. Decker, Philadelphia and Toronto.
157. Van Egmond, A.J., and Brinkman, W.B. (1956): On the function of the saccus endolymphaticus. *Acta Otolaryngol.*, 46:285–289.
158. Verdugo, P. (1980): Ca^{2+}-dependent hormonal stimulation of ciliary activity. *Nature (London)*, 283:764–765.
159. Verdugo, P. (1982): Introduction: Mucociliary function in mammalian epithelia. In: *Mechanism and Control of Ciliary Movement*, edited by C.J. Brokaw and P. Verdugo, pp. 1–5. Alan R. Liss, New York.
160. Verdugo, P., Johnson, N.T., and Tam, P.Y. (1980): Beta-adrenergic stimulation of respiratory ciliary activity. *J. Appl. Physiol.*, 33:193–196.
161. Warr, W.B. (1978): The olivocochlear bundle: its origins and terminations in the cat. In: *Evoked Electrical Activity in the Auditory Nervous System*, edited by R.F. Naunton and C. Fernandez, pp. 43–65. Academic Press, New York.
162. Watanabe, N., Briggs, B.R., and Lim, D.J. (1982): Experimental otitis media in chinchillas. I. Baseline immunological investigation. *Ann. Otol. Rhinol. Laryngol.*, 91 (Suppl. 93):3–8.
163. Watanabe, N., DeMaria, T.F., Lewis, D.M., Mogi, G., and Lim, D.J. (1982): Experimental otitis media in chinchillas. II. Comparison of the middle ear immune responses to *S. pneumoniae* types 3 and 23. *Ann. Otol. Rhinol. Laryngol.*, 91 (Suppl. 93):9–16.
164. Wersäll, J., Engström, H., and Hjorth, S. (1954): Fine structure of the guinea pig macula utriculi. A preliminary report. *Acta Otolaryngol.*, 116:298–303.
165. Wersäll, J., Gleisner, L., Lundquist, P.-G. (1967): Ultrastructure of the vestibular end organs. In: *Myotatic, Kinesthetic and Vestibular Mechanisms*, edited by A. DeReuck and J. Knight, pp. 105–120. Little, Brown, Boston.
166. Wheeler, S.L., Pool, G.L., and Lumb, R.H. (1984): Rat eustachian tube synthesizes disaturated phosphatidylcholine. *Biochim. Biophys. Acta*, 794:348–349.
167. Williams, L.L., Lowery, H.W., and Glaser, R. (1985): Sudden hearing loss following infectious mononucleosis: possible effect of altered immunoregulation. *Pediatrics*, 75:1020–1027.
168. Wright, A. (1984): Dimensions of the cochlear stereocilia in man and the guinea pig. *Hear. Res.*, 13:89–98.
169. Yamaguchi, T., DeMaria, T.F., and Lim, D.J. (1987): Cross-reactive antibodies in type b and nontypable *H. influenzae*-induced experimental otitis media. *Ann. Otol. Rhinol. Laryngol.*
170. Yoo, T.J., Floyd, R.A., and Tomoda, K. (1985): Immunologically induced temporal bone lesions. An animal model. In: *Immunobiology, Autoimmunity and Transplantation in Otorhinolaryngology*, edited by J.E. Veldman, B.F. McCabe, E.H. Huizing, and N. Mygind, pp. 147–158. Kugler, Amsterdam.
171. Yoo, T.J., Stuart, J.M., Kang, A.H., Townes, A.S., Tomoda, K., and Dixit, S. (1982): Type II collagen autoimmunity in otosclerosis and Meniere's disease. *Science*, 217:1153–1155.
172. Yoo, T.J., Tomoda, K., Stuart, J.M., Cremer, M.A., Townes, A.S., and Kang, A.H. (1983): Type II collagen-induced autoimmune sensorineural hearing loss and vestibular dysfunction in rats. *Ann. Otol. Rhinol., Laryngol.*, 92:267–271.
173. Zechner, G., and Altmann, F. (1969): Histological studies on the human endolymphatic duct and sac. *Pract. Otorhinolaryngol.*, 31:65–83.

Immunology of the Ear, edited by J. Bernstein
and P. Ogra. Raven Press, New York © 1987.

Eustachian Tube and Nasopharynx

Charles D. Bluestone

*Department of Otolaryngology, University of Pittsburgh School of Medicine, and
Department of Pediatric Otolaryngology, Children's Hospital of Pittsburgh,
Pittsburgh, Pennsylvania 15213*

The eustachian tube should be considered as part of a system, which consists of the palate, nasopharynx, eustachian tube, middle ear, and mastoid air cells (Fig. 1). The structure and function of the tube will be reviewed first, followed by a discussion of current concepts of the various pathophysiologic conditions that can result in the disease state.

ANATOMY OF THE SYSTEM

In adults the eustachian tube lies at an angle of 45° in relation to the horizontal plane, whereas in infants this inclination is only 10° (36). The length of the tube in the adult varies with race; it has been reported to be as short as 30 mm (47) and as long as 40 mm (4), but the usual range of length reported in the literature is 31 to 38 mm (1,2,20,25,31,36). It is generally accepted that the posterior third (11–14 mm) of the adult tube is osseous and the anterior two-thirds (20–25 mm) is composed of membrane and cartilage (26,36).

The morphology of the eustachian tube and relation to other structures are presented in Fig. 2. As can be seen, the protympanum (osseous eustachian tube) lies completely within the petrous portion of the temporal bone and is directly continuous with the anterior wall of the superior portion of the middle ear. Graves and Edwards (26) report the juncture of the protympanum and epitympanum to lie 4 mm above the floor of the tympanic cavity. This relationship, although valid, is misrepresented in the more popular descriptions and depictions of the tubal-middle ear juncture and is of some importance to the functional clearance of middle ear fluids. The course of the osseous tube is linear anteromedially, following the petrous apex and deviating little from the horizontal plane. The lumen is roughly triangular, measuring 2 to 3 mm vertically and 3 to 4 mm along the horizontal base. The continued patency of the osseous lumen represents a functional distinction not characteristic of the fibrocartilaginous portion (26,46). The osseous and cartilaginous portions of the eustachian tube meet at an irregular bony surface and form an angle of about 160° with each other.

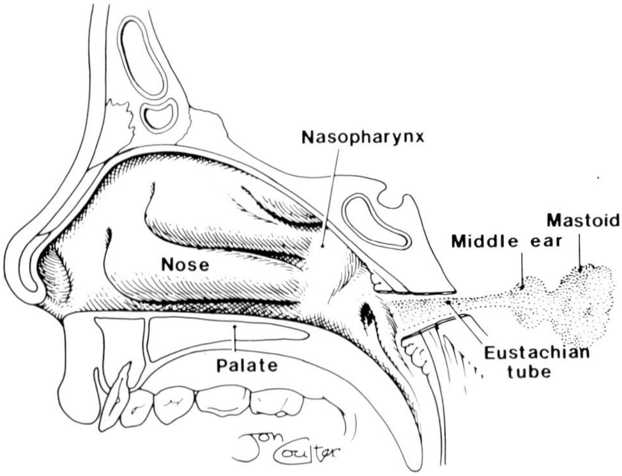

FIG. 1. Eustachian tube, which connects the middle ear and mastoid air cells to the nasopharynx.

The cartilaginous tube then courses anteromedially and inferiorly, angled in most cases 30° to 40° to the transverse plane and 45° to the sagittal plane (26), although these angles do exhibit some variability (20). The tube is closely applied to the basal aspect of the skull and is fitted to a sulcus (sulcus tubarius) between the greater wing of the sphenoid bone and the petrous portion of the temporal bone. The cartilaginous tube is firmly attached at its posterior end to the osseous orifice by fibrous bands and usually extends some distance (3 mm) into the osseous portion of the tube. At its inferomedial end it is attached to a tubercle on the posterior edge of the medial pterygoid lamina (2,15,20,26,36,43).

The cartilaginous tube has a crook-shaped mediolateral superior wall (see Fig. 2). It is completed laterally and inferiorly by a veiled membrane (1,36). Terracol (49) described the crook-like portion of cartilage as consisting of two cartilaginous laminae hinged by fibrous and elastic connective tissue. However, Rood and Doyle (43) described a single cartilaginous lamina with superior and medial aspects to be the more usual condition. Graves and Edwards (26), Rood (41), and Simkins (46) have described accessory cartilages, which are relatively common and probably representative of an incomplete chondrogenesis of the laminar segments (43). The veiled membrane is divisible into at least two layers: an inner membranous layer and an outer fibrous layer. The latter serves as the site for the attachment of the fibers of the dilator tubae, or tensor veli palatini muscle (15,42). Citelli (18) describes three layers of elastic fibers which invade the membranous portion of the tube and are more abundant in the tubal floor than in its lateral wall. The deepest layer follows all the folds and diverticuli of the lumen and supports the tubal epithelium. The middle layer is a collection of loosely bound elastic tissues, and the most superficial layer forms the fibrous floor of the eustachian tube. The tubal lumen is shaped like two cones joined at their apexes. The juncture of

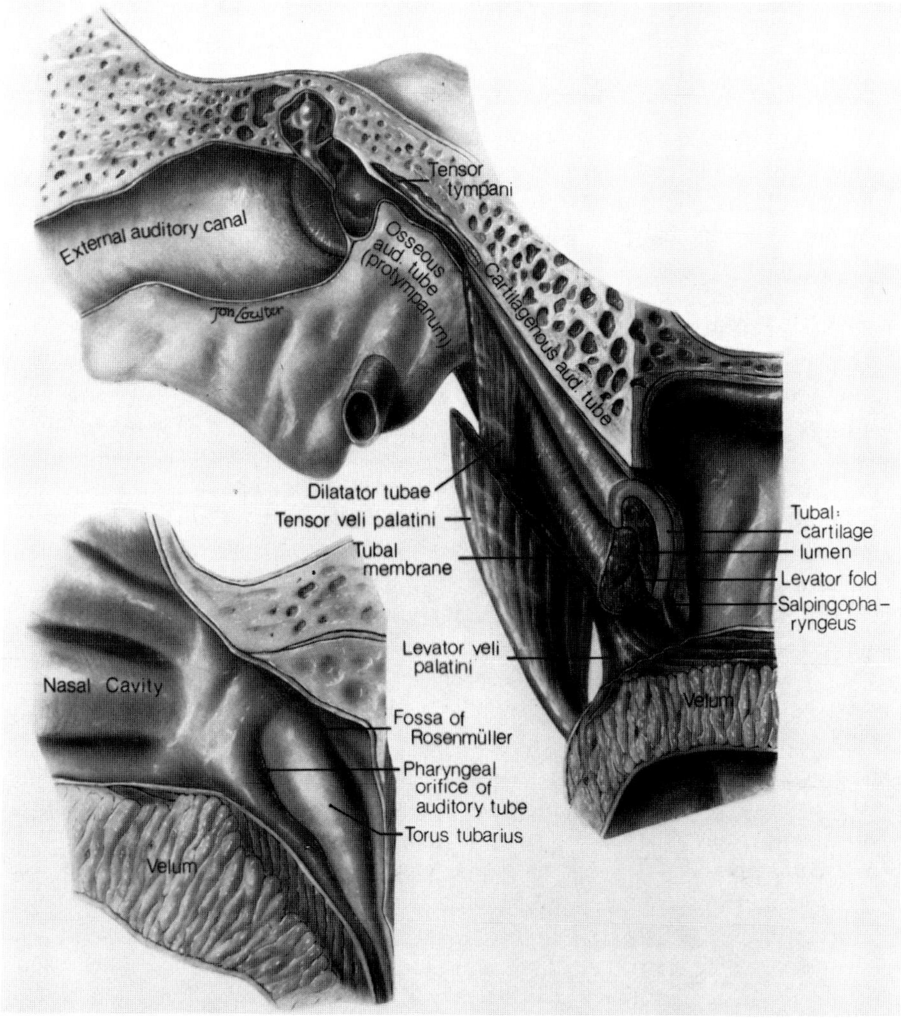

FIG. 2. **Right:** Illustration of a complete dissection of the eustachian tube and middle ear. Especially evident are the relations of the eustachian tube, paratubal muscles, and cranial base, as well as the positioning of the juncture between the protympanum and middle ear. **Left:** Appearance of the nasopharyngeal orifice of the eustachian tube. Note the large torus tubarius and its inferior continuation at the salpingopharyngeal fold. (From ref. 12.)

the cones is the narrowest point of the lumen and has been called the *isthmus,* the position of which is usually described as at or near the juncture of the osseous and cartilaginous portions of the tube. The lumen at this point is approximately 2 mm high and 1 mm wide (36). From the isthmus, the lumen expands to approximately 8 to 10 mm in height and 1 to 2 mm in diameter at the pharyngeal orifice (38).

The cartilaginous eustachian tube does not follow a straight course in the adult, but rather extends along a curve from the juncture of the osseous and cartilaginous portions to the medial pterygoid plate, approximating the cranial base for the greater part of its course. The eustachian tube crosses the superior border of the superior constrictor muscle immediately posterior to its terminus within the nasopharynx. The thickened anterior fibrous investment of the medial cartilage of the tube presses against the pharyngeal wall to form a prominent fold known as the *torus tubarius,* which measures 10 to 15 mm in thickness (36). Simkins (46) described the torus to be the site of origin of the salpingopalatine muscle, whereas Rosen (44) noted the torus as the point of origin of the salpingopharyngeus muscle, which lies within the inferoposteriorly directed salpingopharyngeal fold.

The mucosal lining of the eustachian tube is continuous with that of the nasopharynx and middle ear and may be characterized as respiratory epithelium. Structural differentiation of this mucosal lining is evident, with mucous glands predominating at the nasopharyngeal orifice grading to a mixture of goblet, columnar, and ciliated cells near the tympanum.

The fossa of Rosenmüller is a deep pocket within the nasopharynx extending under the eustachian tube posterolaterally and emerging behind the posterior edge of the levator veli palatini muscle. The fossa varies in height from 8 to 10 mm and in depth from 3 to 10 mm. Adenoid tissue usually extends into this pocket and adds to the soft tissue support of the eustachian tube (36). This network drains into either the retropharyngeal nodes medially or the deep cervical nodes laterally (26). Early investigators (Gerlach, 1874, cited in ref. 36) described a lymphoid mass within the tube of a 6-month-old infant. However, Wolf (52), in an examination of 250 subjects, and Aschan (3), in a histologic study of 39 eustachian tubes, failed to find such a structure. Further, in a more recent unpublished study (cited in ref. 43) of the developmental anatomy of the tubal system, Rood and Doyle failed to find this lymphoid mass and concluded with Wolf (52) and Aschan (3) that this tubal tonsil was a rare pathologic abnormality.

Innervation of the Eustachian Tube

The pharyngeal orifice is innervated by a branch from the otic ganglion, the sphenopalatine nerve, and the pharyngeal plexus. The remainder of the tube receives its sensory innervation from the tympanic plexus and the pharyngeal plexus. The glossopharyngeal nerve probably plays the predominant role in tubal innervation. Sympathetic innervation of the eustachian tube is dependent on the sphenopalatine ganglion, the otic ganglion, paired glossopharyngeal nerves, the petrosal nerves, and the caroticotympanic nerve (36). Mitchell (33) suggests that the parasympathetic nerve supply is derived from the tympanic branch of the glossopharyngeal nerve. More recently, Nathanson and Jackson (35) provided experimental evidence for a secondary parasympathetic innervation via the vidian nerve from the sphenopalatine ganglion.

Muscles Associated with Tubal Function

Traditionally there are four muscles that are commonly cited as being associated with the eustachian tube: the tensor veli palatini, the levator veli palatini, the salpingopharyngeus, and the tensor tympani. Each has at one time or another been directly or indirectly implicated in tubal function (1,14,15,25,41,50,51).

Usually the eustachian tube is closed, opening during such actions as swallowing, yawning, or sneezing and thereby permitting the equalization of middle ear and atmospheric pressures. Although controversy still exists as to the mechanism of tubal dilation, most anatomic and physiologic evidence supports active dilation induced solely by the tensor veli palatini muscle as the mechanism involved (17,39). Closure of the tube has been attributed to passive reapproximation of tubal walls by extrinsic forces exerted by the surrounding, deformed tissues and/or by the recoil of elastic fibers within the tubal wall. More recent experimental and clinical data suggest that, at least for certain abnormal populations, the closely applied internal pterygoid muscle may assist tubal closure by an increase in its mass within the pterygoid fossa, which applies medial pressure to the tensor veli palatini muscle and consequently to the lateral membranous wall of the eustachian tube (17,21).

The tensor veli palatini is composed of two fairly distinct bundles of muscle fibers divided by a layer of fibroelastic tissue. The bundles lie mediolateral to the tube. The more lateral bundle (the tensor veli palatini proper) is of an inverted triangular design, taking its origin from the scaphoid fossa and entire lateral osseous ridge of the sulcus tubarius for the course of the eustachian tube. The bundles descend anteriorly, laterally, and inferiorly to converge in a tendon that rounds the hamular process of the medial pterygoid lamina about an interposed bursa. This fiber group then inserts into the posterior border of the horizontal process of the palatine bone and into the palatine aponeurosis of the anterior portion of the velum. The more posteroinferior muscle fibers lack an osseous origin, extending instead into the semicanal of the tensor tympani muscle. Here, the latter group of muscle fibers receive a second muscle slip, which originates from the tubal cartilages and sphenoid bone. These muscle masses converge to a tendon that rounds the cochleariform process and inserts into the malleolar manubrium. This arrangement imposes a bipennate form to the tensor tympani muscle (30,42).

The medial bundle of the tensor veli palatini muscle lies immediately adjacent to the lateral membranous wall of the eustachian tube and is termed the *dilator tubae muscle* (25,42). It takes its superior origin from the posterior third of the lateral membranous wall of the eustachian tube. The fibers descend sharply to enter and blend with the fibers of the lateral bundle of the tensor veli palatini muscle. It is this inner bundle that is responsible for active dilation of the tube by inferolateral displacement of the membranous wall (41,42,45). This tripartite muscle is innervated by the mandibular division of the trigeminal nerve (17,40).

The levator veli palatini muscle arises from the inferior aspect of the petrous apex and from the lower border of the medial lamina of the tubal cartilage. The fibers pass inferomedially, paralleling the tubal cartilage and lying within the vault of the tubal floor. They fan out and blend with the dorsal surface of the soft palate (15,26,41). Most investigators deny a tubal origin for this muscle and believe that in fact it is related to the tube only by loose connective tissue (32,46). The muscle is innervated by the looped pharyngeal branch of the vagus nerve (cranial nerve X) (26,40).

The salpingopharyngeus muscle arises from the medial and inferior borders of the tubal cartilage via slips of muscular and tendinous fibers. The muscle then courses inferoposteriorly to blend with the mass of the palatopharyngeus muscle (26,32). Rosen (44) examined 10 hemisected human heads and identified the muscle in nine specimens. However, in all cases the muscle fibers were few in number and appeared to lack any ability to perform physiologically. This muscle is also innervated by a branch of the pharyngeal trunk of the vagus nerve (26,37).

Developmental Anatomy

The eustachian tube in the infant is about half as long as that in the adult, averaging about 18 mm. The cartilaginous tube represents somewhat less than two-thirds of this distance, whereas the osseous portion is relatively longer and wider in diameter than it is in the adult. The height of the pharyngeal orifice of the infant eustachian tube is about one-half that of the adult, whereas the width is similar. The ostium of the tube is more exposed in the infant than it is in the adult because in the infant it lies lower in the shallower nasopharyngeal vault. The direction of the tube varies, ranging from horizontal to an angle of about 10° to the horizontal, and the tube is not angulated at the isthmus but merely narrows (26). Holborow (27) demonstrated that in infants the medial cartilaginous lamina is relatively shorter and that there is a relatively greater amount of glandular tissue than in adults. He suggested that these differences may be related to a less efficient mechanism of active tubal dilation in this age group.

PHYSIOLOGY OF THE SYSTEM

The eustachian tube has at least three physiologic functions with respect to the middle ear: (a) equilibration of air pressure *(ventilation)* in the middle ear with atmospheric pressure; (b) *protection* from nasopharyngeal sound pressure and secretions; and (c) *drainage* (and clearance) into the nasopharynx of unwanted secretions and secretions produced within the middle ear (7) (Fig. 3). The normal eustachian tube is functionally obstructed or collapsed at rest, with probably a slight negative pressure existing in the middle ear. In ideal tubal function, intermittent *active* opening of the eustachian tube is due only to contraction of the tensor veli palatini muscle during swallowing (17,29,39).

It has been the belief in the past that ambient pressure is maintained in the middle ear by frequent opening of the tube, but, under normal conditions, there probably is infrequent exchange of gas from the nasopharynx to the middle ear, since the middle ear gas composition, even though still not defined, is most likely not the same as air (53). However, when there is a large pressure difference between the nasopharynx and the middle ear, the tube can either open actively to equalize the middle ear pressure or, if the gradient is large enough, the normal tube can passively open (e.g., ascent in an airplane, Valsalva maneuver).

The protective function of the eustachian tube presents unwanted nasopharyngeal foreign material from entering the middle ear and mastoid air cells. The protective function is dependent on: (a) length of the tube; (b) radius of its lumen; (c) compliance of its walls; (d) pressure differential across the tube; and (e) viscosity of the fluid.

The drainage function is enhanced by the pump-like action of the tube during acute opening and closing (28). Even though limited information is available con-

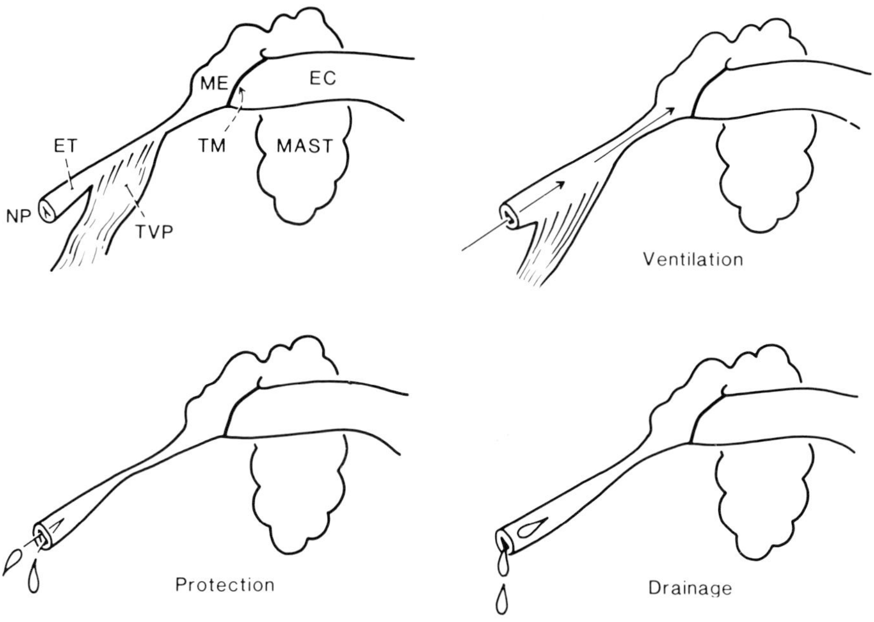

FIG. 3. Physiologic functions of the eustachian tube as related to the middle ear. (NP) Nasopharynx; (ET) eustachian tube; (TVP) tensor veli palatini; (ME) middle ear; (TM) tympanic membrane; (EC) ear canal; (MAST) mastoid air cells.

cerning the clearance function of the mucociliary transport system of the lining of the eustachian tube (and a small portion of the middle ear mucosa), clearance of secretions by this mechanism probably also aids in preventing middle ear disease.

Pathophysiology

There appear to be two types of eustachian tube *dysfunction* which could result in otitis media: *obstruction* and *abnormal patency*. Obstruction may be either *functional* or *mechanical* (Fig. 4). Functional obstruction could result from persistent collapse of the eustachian tube due to increased tubal compliance or an inadequate active opening mechanism, or both. Mechanical obstruction of the eustachian tube may be intrinsic or extrinsic, or both. *Intrinsic* obstruction can be the result of abnormal geometry or intraluminal or mural factors that compromise the lumen of the tube. *Extrinsic* obstruction can be the result of increased extramural pressure, such as when we are lying down, which is physiologic; but when there is extramural compression, the tube may be obstructed, irrespective of our body position. The other major type of dysfunction of the eustachian tube is *abnormal patency*. In its extreme form, the tube is open even at rest, i.e., patulous. Lesser degrees of abnormal patency would result in a semipatulous eustachian tube, which would be closed at rest but would have low resistance in comparison to the normal tube.

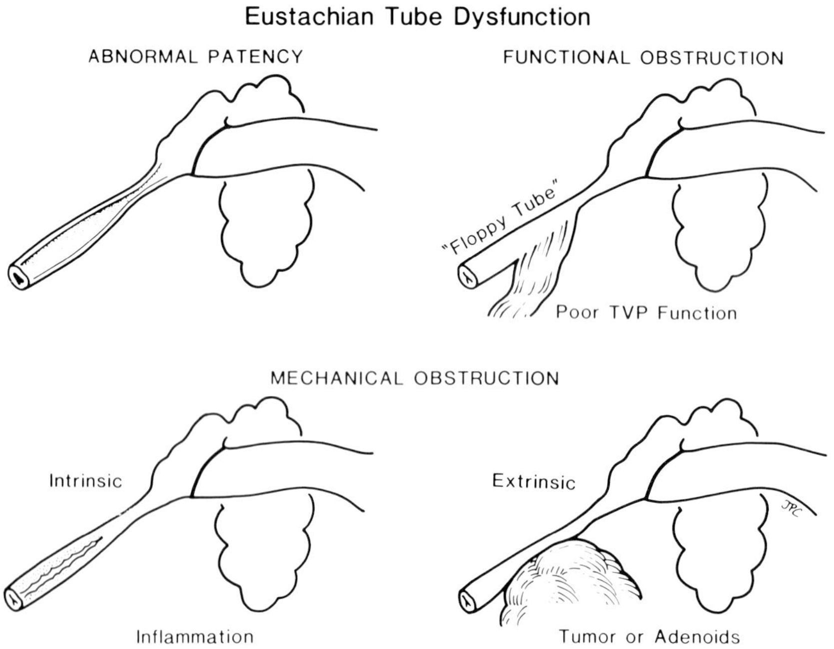

FIG. 4. Pathophysiology of the eustachian tube showing that the tube may be abnormally patent or obstructed.

Increased patency of the tube may be due to abnormal tube geometry or to a decrease in the extramural pressure (such as occurs with weight loss).

Tubal Function Related to Pathogenesis of Otitis Media

Functional obstruction may result in persistent high negative middle ear pressure. If middle ear pressure equilibration does not occur, persistent functional eustachian tube obstruction could result in *atelectasis* of the tympanic membrane or a sterile otitis media with effusion, or both (Fig. 5). If a large bolus of air enters the middle ear from the nasopharynx when there is high negative middle ear pressure, nasopharyngeal secretions could be *aspirated* into the middle ear and result in an acute otitis media with effusion. Functional eustachian tube obstruction is common in infants and younger children, since the amount and stiffness of the cartilage support of the eustachian tube is less than in older children and adults and since there appear to be marked age differences in the craniofacial base which render the tensor veli palatini muscle less efficient prior to puberty. In addition, the eustachian tube in the infant and young child is *shorter* than in the adult, which would make their tube less protective when secretions enter the nasopharyngeal end. This developmental difference would also explain why the tympanic membrane in the crying infant can be seen to bulge with positive middle ear pressure;

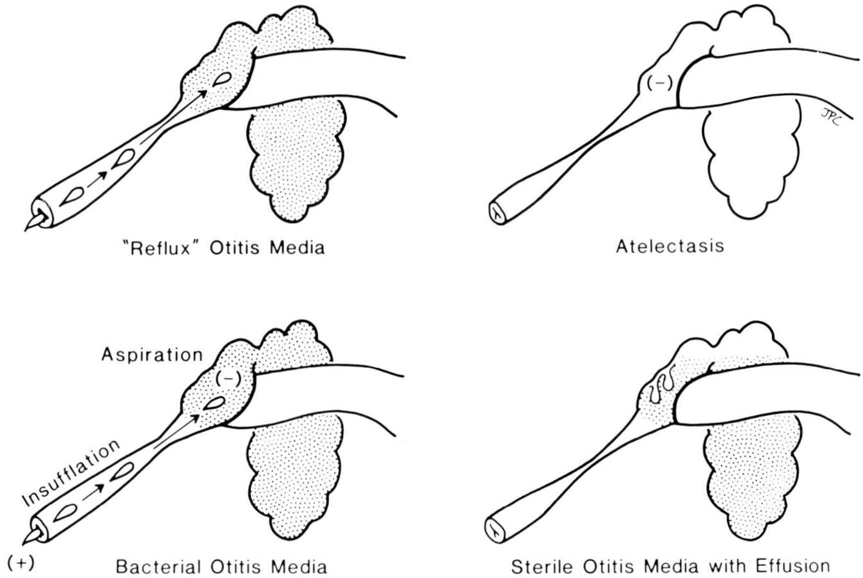

FIG. 5. Pathogenesis of otitis media and atelectasis. Reflux occurs when the tube is abnormally patent, whereas atelectasis and sterile middle ear effusions can occur from functional/mechanical obstruction. When the tube is patent, nasopharyngeal secretions can be aspirated/insufflated into the middle ear.

infants have the highest incidence of otitis media of any age group. All infants with unrepaired palatal clefts and many children with repaired palates have otitis media with effusion as a result of functional obstruction of the eustachian tube (6). Children with cleft palate are at high risk of developing cholesteatoma. Functional obstruction can be the result of denervation or direct interference with the action of the tensor veli palatini muscle, such as can occur with neurologic disease, trauma, surgery (34) or tumor (48).

Intrinsic mechanical obstruction of the eustachian tube may be due to inflammation. Most ears at risk for developing otitis media with effusion when inflammation is present probably have a significant degree of functional obstruction. An upper respiratory tract infection in such children has been shown to significantly decrease eustachian tube function (11). Periods of upper respiratory tract infection may then result in either (a) atelectasis of the tympanic membrane-middle ear or (b) bacterial or sterile otitis media with effusion due to swelling of the eustachian tube lumen. The mechanisms are similar to those described for functional eustachian tube obstruction. Tumor can also invade the lumen of the eustachian tube and result in otitis media (54).

Extrinsic mechanical obstruction of the eustachian tube may be the result of extrinsic compression by nasopharyngeal tumors (19) or adenoids (7–9). Partial eustachian tube obstruction may only result in atelectasis of the middle ear or a bacterial otitis media, but more severe obstruction could result in a sterile otitis media with effusion.

Abnormally patent eustachian tubes usually permit air to flow readily from the nasopharynx into the middle ear, which thus remains well ventilated; also, however, unwanted nasopharyngeal secretions can traverse the tube and result in "*reflux otitis media*." A semipatulous eustachian tube may be obstructed functionally, and the middle ear may even have negative pressure, an effusion, or both. Since the tubal walls are *distensible* (compliant), nasopharyngeal secretions may readily be *insufflated* into the middle ear even with modest positive nasopharyngeal pressures, e.g., as a result of noseblowing, sneezing, crying, or closed-nose swallowing. Some American Indians have been shown to have tubal resistances that are lower than those of the average Caucasian (5). They seem to have an increased incidence of reflux of nasopharyngeal secretion into the middle ear and frequently suffer from recurrent otitis media, which is often associated with perforation and discharge. However, American Indians have a low incidence of cholesteatoma. This type of eustachian tube function and middle ear disease is different from those in individuals who have a cleft palate.

Nasal obstruction may also be involved in the pathogenesis of otitis media with effusion. Swallowing when the nose is obstructed (due to inflammation or obstructed adenoids) results in an initial positive nasopharyngeal air pressure, followed by a negative pressure phase. When the tube is pliant, positive nasopharyngeal pressure might insufflate infected secretions into the middle ear, especially when the middle ear has a negative middle ear pressure; alternatively, with negative nasopharyngeal pressure, such a tube could be prevented from opening and could become further obstructed functionally (the "Toynbee phenomenon") (9).

ALLERGY AND EUSTACHIAN TUBE FUNCTION

The role of allergy in the etiology and pathogenesis of acute otitis media and otitis media with effusion may be related to one or more of the following mechanisms: (a) middle ear functioning as a targt organ; (b) inflammatory swelling of the eustachian tube; (c) inflammatory obstruction of the nose; or (d) reflux, insufflation, or aspiration of bacteria-laden nasopharyngeal secretions into the middle ear cavity (Fig. 6). The latter three mechanisms would be associated with abnormal function of the eustachian tube.

Even though there is a lack of convincing evidence that allergy plays a significant role in the etiology of otitis media, there may be a relation between upper respiratory tract allergy and eustachian tube dysfunction (22). A prospective study of children who had recurrent or chronic middle ear disease, and who had evidence of functional obstruction of the eustachian tube, had more severe obstruction (mechanical) of the tube when an upper respiratory tract infection developed (11). A similar relationship has been reported between upper respiratory tract allergy and eustachian tube function. In a study of adult volunteers who had normal tympanic membranes and a negative otologic history and had normal eustachian tube function prior to an intranasal challenge with an antigen to which they were sensitive, all developed partial eustachian tube obstruction following the challenge (24). However, otitis media did not develop in these subjects. Recently, animals that had been passively sensitized had eustachian tube dysfunction following intranasal challenge (22,23).

From these studies, the following sequence of events is postulated in patients who have allergy and otitis media. Most likely, a basic eustachian tube dysfunction is present which becomes clinically evident in the presence of upper respiratory tract allergy in a manner similar to eustachian tube obstruction caused by an

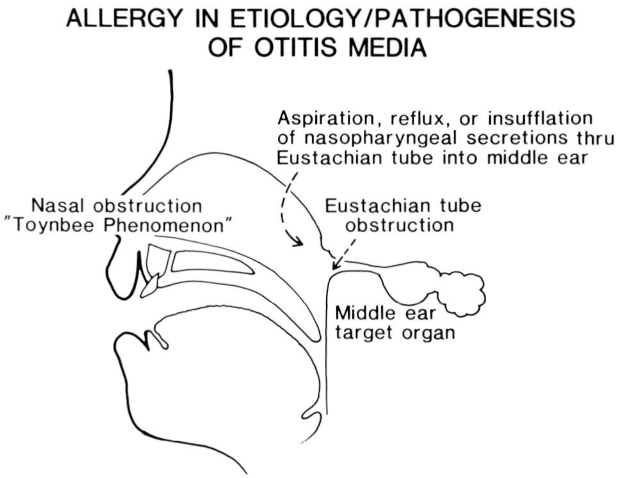

FIG. 6. The possible role that allergy plays in eustachian tube dysfunction and allergy.

upper respiratory tract infection. Upper respiratory tract allergy may cause some intrinsic mechanical obstruction in patients who have normal eustachian tube function, but their normal active opening mechanism, i.e., tensor veli palatini muscle pull, is able to overcome the obstruction (Fig. 7). Therefore, patients who have functional obstruction due to poor muscular opening would be at highest risk for developing sufficient mechanical obstruction to develop middle ear disease. Since many children have difficulty actively opening their eustachian tubes, they are a population who are at high risk. If the eustachian tube obstruction is minimal, then the patient will have only signs and symptoms of *eustachian tube dysfunction* such as otalgia (''popping'' and ''snapping'' sounds in the ear), mild hearing loss, tinnitus, or even vertigo. Often these symptoms will be fluctuating and only present during the worst periods of the patient's allergic rhinitis.

Even though there is no evidence that allergic nasopharyngeal secretions can be *aspirated* into the middle ear, this concept seems reasonable. Acute otitis media resulting from the aspiration of bacteria from the nasopharynx has been documented in animal models, which would lend credence to this pathogenic mechanism. Likewise, it is possible that nasopharyngeal secretions containing bacteria

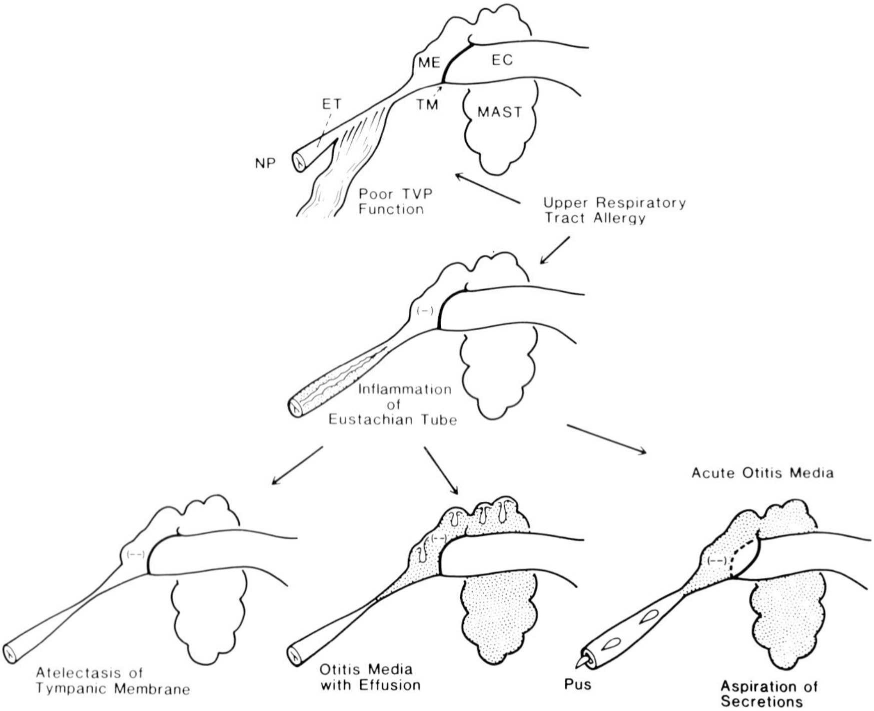

FIG. 7. Schema showing how allergy may be a possible cause of mechanical obstruction of eustachian tube and the proposed sequence of events leading to atelectasis or otitis media, or both. (NP) Nasopharynx; (ET) eustachian tube; (TVP) tensor veli palatini muscle; (ME) middle ear; (TM) tympanic membrane; (EC) external canal; (MAST) mastoid air cells (see text).

could be *refluxed* into the middle ear if the eustachian tube is abnormally patent, which could result in "reflux otitis media" (Fig. 8). *Insufflation* of bacteria-laden nasopharyngeal secretions secondary to allergy into the middle ear is also possible (a) during noseblowing, (b) while jumping or diving into water when swimming, (c) in the infant who is crying, or (d) during closed-nose swallowing, i.e., the "Toynbee phenomenon."

Allergic rhinitis, which is severe enough to cause nasal obstruction, might cause middle ear disease due to the "Toynbee phenomenon." If nasal obstruction exists, the nasopharyngeal pressure during closed-nose swallowing is first positive, due to the elevation of the soft palate and closing off of the velopharyngeal space, followed by negative pressure when the soft palate is in a lower position. These pressures are similar to pressure changes that occur in the lower pharynx during physiologic swallowing. If the eustachian tube opens during the positive phase of closed-nose swallowing, allergic nasopharyngeal secretions could be insufflated into the middle ear, resulting in otitis media. More likely, however, the eustachian tube is prevented from opening due to the high negative pressure developed in the nasopharynx during the second phase of closed-nose swallowing. This could cause eustachian tube obstruction and negative middle ear pressure, which would be

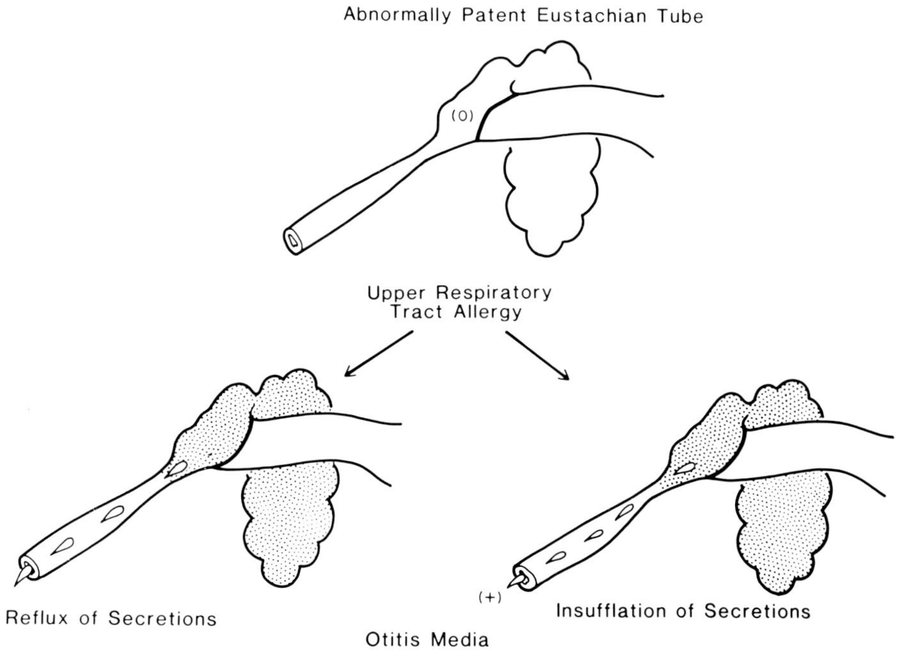

FIG. 8. Schema showing how allergic (and possibly bacterial) secretions may be refluxed or insufflated into the middle ear, causing otitis media if the eustachian tube is abnormally patent. See Fig. 7 and its legend for identification and definitions of the various elements in the upper diagram.

manifested by signs and symptoms of eustachian tube dysfunction (fluctuating or sustained otalgia, hearing loss, tinnitus, or vertigo), atelectasis of the tympanic membrane-middle ear, or possible development of otitis media. ''Locking'' of the eustachian tube, where it would be difficult for the patient to open the tube even after swallowing, could also be possible. Aspiration of allergic nasopharyngeal secretions in which bacteria were present could also be possible with this type of mechanism.

However, at present, there is no scientific proof in animals or humans that the ''Toynbee phenomenon'' is involved in the pathogenesis of otitis media, but the mechanism seems reasonable (10). Likewise, there is no conclusive evidence that upper respiratory tract allergy can cause otitis media when there is an associated eustachian tube dysfunction, but the study of adult volunteers which showed partial eustachian tube obstruction when they were challenged with antigen indicated that the eustachian tube certainly may be involved with allergy. Even though conclusive proof of this relationship is lacking, it would appear that in the individual with upper respiratory allergy and eustachian tube dysfunction, otitis media could be a result of this combination. Future studies are needed to define the role of allergy in the pathophysiology of the eustachian tube and the pathogenesis of otitis media. Randomized clinical trials will be required to determine the efficacy of the currently popular forms of immunotherapy and allergy control in the prevention of otitis media.

CLINICAL EUSTACHIAN TUBE FUNCTION TESTING

The following methods to test the function of the eustachian tube are available in the clinical setting (13).

Tympanometry

The use of an electroacoustic impedance instrument to obtain a tympanogram is an excellent way of determining the status of the tympanic membrane-middle ear system and can be helpful in the assessment of eustachian tube function. The presence of a middle ear effusion or high negative middle ear pressure as determined by this method usually indicates impaired eustachian tube function; however, unlike the otoscopic evaluation, the tympanogram is an objective way of determining the degree of negative pressure present in the middle ear. Unfortunately, assessing the abnormality of values of negative pressure is not so simple: High negative pressure may be present in some patients, especially children, who are asymptomatic and who have relatively good hearing, whereas in others, symptoms such as hearing loss, otalgia, vertigo, and tinnitus may be associated with modest degrees of negative pressure or even with normal middle ear pressures. Normal middle ear pressure for adults is between +50 and −50 mm H_2O and in children may be as low as −175 to −200 mm H_2O. However, these values depend on the time of day, season of the year, or the condition of the other parts of the system, such as the presence of an upper respiratory tract infection. For instance, a young child with a common cold may have transitory high negative pressure within the middle ear while he has the cold, but may be otherwise otologically normal. The decision as to whether or not high negative pressure is abnormal or is only a physiologic variation should be made taking into consideration the presence or absence of signs and symptoms of middle ear disease. If severe atelectasis or adhesive otitis of the tympanic membrane-middle ear system is present, the tympanogram may not be a reliable indicator of the actual pressure within the middle ear. Therefore, a resting pressure that is high negative is associated with some degree of eustachian tube obstruction, but the presence of normal middle ear pressure does not necessarily indicate normal eustachian tube function.

Manometry

The pump-manometer system of the electroacoustic impedance bridge is usually adequate to assess eustachian tube function clinically when the tympanic membrane is not intact. However, because of the limitations of the manometric systems of all of the commercially available instruments, a controlled syringe and manometer (a water manometer will suffice) should be available when these limitations are exceeded, e.g., when eustachian tube opening pressure is in excess of +400 to +600 mm H_2O.

Classic Tests of Tubal Patency

Valsalva and Politzer have developed methods to assess patency of the eustachian tube; eustachian tube catheterization achieves the same results (12). When the tympanic membrane is intact and the middle ear inflates following one of these tests, then the tube is not totally mechanically obstructed. Likewise, if the tympanic membrane is not intact, passage of air into the middle ear would indicate patency of the tube. The success of these tests can be determined subjectively by the use of the otoscope, a Toynbee tube, or a stethoscope at the middle ear end of the system. The assessment is more objective when a tympanogram is obtained when the tympanic membrane is intact, or when the manometer on the impedance instrument is observed when the tympanic membrane is not intact. However, inflation of the eustachian tube-middle ear from the nasopharynx end of the system by one of these classic methods only is an assessment of tubal patency and not function, and failure to inflate the middle ear does not necessarily indicate a lack of patency of the eustachian tube.

The Valsalva and Politzer maneuvers are more beneficial as management options in selected patients than they are as methods to assess tubal function.

Toynbee Test

One of the oldest and still one of the best tests of eustachian tube function is the Toynbee test. The test is usually considered positive when an alteration in middle ear pressure results. More specifically, if negative pressure (even transitory in the absence of a patulous tube) develops in the middle ear during closed-nose swallowing, the eustachian tube function can be considered most likely to be normal. When the tympanic membrane is intact, the presence of negative middle ear pressure must be determined by pneumatic otoscopy or, more accurately, by obtaining a tympanogram before and immediately following the test. When the tympanic membrane is not intact, the manometer of the impedance bridge can be observed to determine middle ear pressure.

The test is more valuable in determining normal versus abnormal eustachian tube function in adults than in children. The test is still of considerable value since, regardless of age, if negative pressure develops in the middle ear during or following the test, the eustachian tube function is most likely normal, since the eustachian tube actively opens and is sufficiently stiff to withstand nasopharyngeal negative pressure, i.e., it does not "lock." If positive pressure is noted or no change in pressure occurs, the function of the eustachian tube still may be normal and other tests of eustachian tube function should be performed.

Patulous Eustachian Tube Test

If a patulous eustachian tube is suspected, the diagnosis can be confirmed by otoscopy or objectively by tympanometry when the tympanic membrane is intact. One tympanogram is obtained while the patient is breathing normally, and a second is obtained while the patient holds his breath. Fluctuation of the tympanometric trace that coincides with breathing confirms the diagnosis of a patulous tube. Fluctuation can be exaggerated by asking the patient to occlude one nostril with the mouth closed during forced inspiration and expiration or by performing the Toynbee maneuver. When the tympanic membrane is not intact, a patulous eustachian tube can be identified by the free flow of air into and out of the eustachian tube using the pump-manometer portion of the electroacoustic impedance bridge. These tests should not be performed while the patient is in a reclining position since the patulous eustachian tube will close.

Nine-Step Inflation-Deflation Tympanometric Test

Another method of assessing the function of the eustachian tube when the tympanic membrane is intact is called the *nine-step inflation-deflation tympanometric test,* although the applied middle ear pressures are very limited in magnitude (Fig. 9). The middle ear must be free of effusion. The nine-step tympanometry procedure may be summarized as follows:

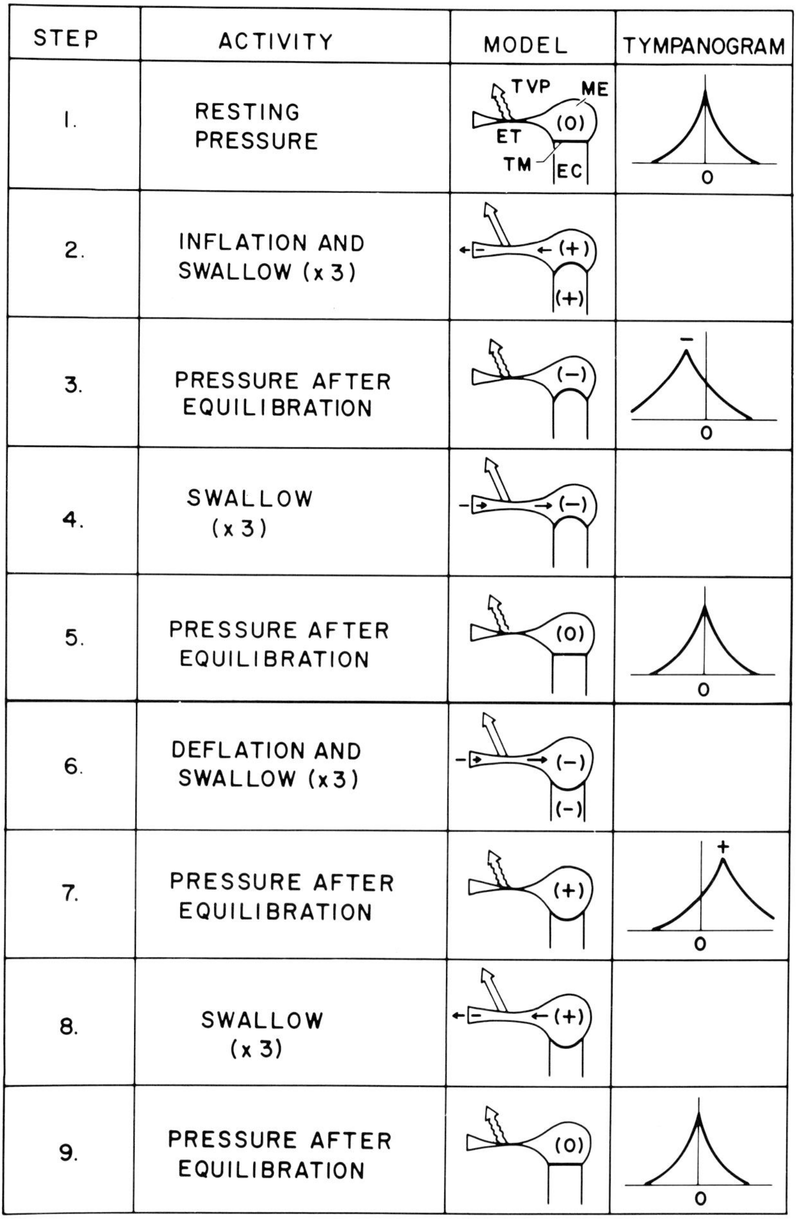

STEP
ACTIVITY
MODEL
TYMPANOGRAM
1.
RESTING PRESSURE
TVP
ME
(0)
ET
TM
EC
0
2.
INFLATION AND SWALLOW (x 3)
(+)
(+)
3.
PRESSURE AFTER EQUILIBRATION
(−)
−
0
4.
SWALLOW (x 3)
(−)
5.
PRESSURE AFTER EQUILIBRATION
(0)
0
6.
DEFLATION AND SWALLOW (x 3)
(−)
(−)
7.
PRESSURE AFTER EQUILIBRATION
(+)
+
0
8.
SWALLOW (x 3)
(+)
9.
PRESSURE AFTER EQUILIBRATION
(0)
0

FIG. 9. Nine-step tympanometry test of eustachian tube function (see text).

1. The tympanogram records resting middle ear pressure.
2. Ear canal pressure is increased to +200 mm H_2O, with medial deflection of the tympanic membrane and a corresponding increase in middle ear pressure. The subject swallows to equilibrate middle ear overpressure.
3. While the subject refrains from swallowing, ear canal pressure is returned to normal, thus establishing a slight negative middle ear pressure (as the tympanic membrane moves outward). The tympanogram documents the established middle ear underpressure.
4. The subject swallows in an attempt to equilibrate negative middle ear pressure. If equilibration is successful, airflow is from nasopharynx to middle ear.
5. The tympanogram records the extent of equilibration.
6. Ear canal pressure is decreased to −200 mm H_2O, causing a lateral deflection of the tympanic membrane and a corresponding decrease in middle ear pressure. The subject swallows to equilibrate negative middle ear pressure; airflow is from the nasopharynx to the middle ear.
7. The subject refrains from swallowing while external ear canal pressure is returned to normal, thus establishing a slight positive pressure in the middle ear as the tympanic membrane moves medially. The tympanogram records the overpressure established.
8. The subject swallows to reduce overpressure. If equilibration is successful, airflow is from the middle ear to the nasopharynx.
9. The final tympanogram documents the extent of equilibration.

The test is simple to perform and can give useful information regarding eustachian tube function and should be part of the clinical evaluation of patients with suspected eustachian tube dysfunction. In general, most normal adults can perform all or some parts of this test, but even normal children have difficulty in performing this test.

Modified Inflation-Deflation Test (Nonintact Tympanic Membrane)

When the tympanic membrane is not intact, the pump-manometer system of the electroacoustic impedance bridge can be used to perform the modified inflation-deflation eustachian tube function test, which assesses passive as well as active functioning of the eustachian tube. The middle ear should be free of any drainage for an accurate assessment of eustachian tube function using this test. The middle ear is inflated, i.e., positive pressure is applied, until the eustachian tube spontaneously opens. At this time, the pump is manually stopped and air is discharged through the eustachian tube until the tube closes passively. The pressure at which the eustachian tube is passively forced open is called the *opening pressure,* and the pressure at which it closes passively is called the *closing pressure*. The patient is then instructed to equilibrate the middle ear pressure actively by swallowing. The residual pressure remaining in the middle ear after swallowing is recorded.

The active function is also recorded by applying over- and underpressure to the middle ear, which the patient then attempts to equilibrate by swallowing. The residual pressure in the middle ear following equilibration of +200 mm H_2O (i.e., half of the passive opening pressure) is recorded. The residual negative pressure that remains in the middle ear after the attempt to equilibrate applied negative pressure of −200 mm H_2O is also noted. This procedure is not performed in patients who cannot equilibrate applied overpressure. If the eustachian tube does not open following application of positive pressure using the electroacoustic impedance bridge, and no reduction in positive pressure occurs during swallowing, then the eustachian tube must be assessed using a manometric system other than the electroacoustic impedance bridge manometric system. The opening pressure may be higher than 400 to 600 mm H_2O pressure, or not present at all (severe mechanical obstruction).

Failure to equilibrate the applied negative pressure may indicate locking of the eustachian tube during the test. This type of tube is considered to have increased compliance or to be "floppy" in comparison to a tube with perfect function. The tensor veli palatini muscle is unable to open (dilate) the tube. The speed of application of the positive and negative pressures is an important variable in testing eustachian tube function with the inflation-deflation test. The faster the positive pressure is applied, the higher the opening pressure. During the deflation phase of the study, the faster the negative pressure is applied, the more likely it is that the locking phenomenon will occur.

Even though the inflation-deflation test of eustachian tube function does not strictly duplicate physiologic functions of the tube, the results are helpful in differentiating normal from abnormal function. The mean opening pressure for apparently normal subjects with a traumatic perforation and negative otologic history reported by Cantekin and co-workers (16) is 330 mm H_2O (±70 mm H_2O). If (a) the test results reveal passive opening and closing within the normal range, (b) residual positive pressure can be equilibrated by swallowing, and (c) applied negative pressure can also be equilibrated completely, then the eustachian tube can be considered to have normal function. However, if the tube does not open to a pressure of 1,000 mm H_2O, one can assume that total mechanical obstruction is present. This pressure is not hazardous to the middle ear or inner ear windows if the pressure is applied slowly. An extremely high opening pressure (e.g., greater than 500–600 mm H_2O) would indicate a semipatulous eustachian tube. Inability to maintain even a modest positive pressure within the middle ear would be consistent with a patulous tube, i.e., one that is open at rest. Complete equilibration by swallowing of applied negative pressure is usually associated with normal function, but partial equilibration, or even failure to reduce any applied negative pressure, may or may not be considered abnormal since even a normal eustachian tube will lock when negative pressure is rapidly applied. Therefore, inability to equilibrate applied negative pressure may not indicate poor eustachian tube function, especially when it is the only abnormal parameter.

Clinical Indications for Testing Eustachian Tube Function

One of the most important reasons for assessing eustachian tube function is the need to make a differential diagnosis in a patient who has an intact tympanic membrane without evidence of otitis media but has symptoms that might be related to eustachian tube dysfunction (such as otalgia, snapping or popping in the ear, fluctuating hearing loss, tinnitus, or vertigo). An example of such a case would be a patient who has a complaint of fullness in the ear without hearing loss at the time of the examination, a symptom which could be related to abnornal functioning of the eustachian tube or could be due to inner ear pathology. A tympanogram that reveals a high negative pressure (-50 mm H_2O or less) is presumptive evidence of tubal obstruction, whereas normal resting middle ear pressure is not diagnostically significant. However, when the resting intratympanic pressure is within normal limits and the patient can develop negative middle ear pressure following Toynbee's test or can perform all or some of the functions in the nine-step inflation-deflation tympanometric test, the eustachian tube is probably functioning normally. Unfortunately, failure to develop negative middle ear pressure during the Toynbee test or inability to pass the nine-step test does not necessarily indicate poor eustachian tube function. Tympanometry is not only of value in determining if eustachian tube obstruction is present: It can also identify abnormality at the other end of the spectrum of eustachian tube dysfunction; the presence of an abnormally patent eustachian tube can be confirmed by the results of the tympanometric patulous tube test.

Tympanometry appears to be a reliable method for detecting the presence of high negative pressure as well as the presence of otitis media with effusion in children. The identification of high negative pressure without effusion in children is indicative of some degree of eustachian tube obstruction. These children as well as those with middle ear effusion should have follow-up serial tympanograms since they may be at risk of developing otitis media with effusion.

However, the most direct method available to the clinician today for testing eustachian tube function is the inflation-deflation test. A perforation of the tympanic membrane or a tympanostomy tube must be present in order to perform this test. The test uses the simple apparatus described earlier, with or without the electroacoustic impedance bridge pump-manometer system. This test will aid in determining (a) the presence or absence of a dysfunction and (b) the type and severity of dysfunction (obstruction versus abnormal patency) when one is present. No other test procedures may be needed if the patient has either functional obstruction of the eustachian tube or an abnormally patent tube. However, if there is a mechanical obstruction, especially if the tube appears to be totally blocked anatomically, then further testing may be indicated. In such instances, computed tomography of the tubal area should be obtained to determine the site and cause of the blockage. In most cases in which mechanical obstruction of the tube is found, inflammation is present at the middle ear end of the eustachian tube (protympanic or bony portion), which usually resolves with medical management or middle ear surgery. Serial inflation-deflation studies show resolution of the mechanical obstruction. However, if no middle ear cause is obvious, other studies should be performed to rule out the possibility of neoplasm in the nasopharynx.

Even though the testing of eustachian tube function is not an exact science and more research on such testing is needed, the methods presently available to the clinician provide useful information related to the diagnosis and management of middle ear disease (12).

ACKNOWLEDGMENTS

William J. Doyle, Ph.D., assisted in the preparation of the section on anatomy. Thomas Masley and Sandra K. Arjona, M.L.S., provided invaluable aid in the preparation of this manuscript.

REFERENCES

1. Anson, B. (1967): *Morris' Human Anatomy*. Blakiston Division, McGraw-Hill, New York.
2. Anson, B., and Donaldson, J. (1967): *The Surgical Anatomy of the Temporal Bone and Ear*. W. B. Saunders, Philadelphia.
3. Aschan, G. (1954): The eustachian tube. *Acta Otolaryngol. (Stockh.)*, 44:295–311.
4. Bacher, J.A. (1912): The applied anatomy of the eustachian tube. *Laryngoscope*, 22:21–37.
5. Beery, Q.C., Doyle, W.J., Cantekin, E.I., Bluestone, C.D., and Weit, R.J. (1980): Eustachian tube function in an American Indian population. *Ann. Otol. Rhinol. Laryngol.*, 89:28–33.
6. Bluestone, C.D. (1971): Eustachian tube obstruction in the infant with cleft palate. *Ann. Otol. Rhinol. Laryngol.*, 80:1–30.
7. Bluestone, C.D., Paradise, J.L., and Beery, Q.C (1972): Physiology of the eustachian tube in the pathogenesis and management of middle ear effusions. *Laryngoscope*, 82:1654–1670.
8. Bluestone, C.D., Witter, R.A., Paradise, J.L., and Felder, H. (1972): Eustachian tube function as related to adenoidectomy for otitis media. *Trans. Am. Acad. Ophthalmol. Otolaryngol.*, 76:1325–1339.
9. Bluestone, C.D., Cantekin, E.I., and Beery, Q.C. (1975): Certain effects of adenoidectomy on eustachian tube ventilatory function. *Laryngoscope*, 85:113–127.
10. Bluestone, C.D., and Beery, Q.C. (1976): Concepts on the pathogenesis of middle ear effusions. *Ann. Otol. Rhinol. Laryngol.*, 85:182–186.
11. Bluestone, C.D., Cantekin, E.I., and Beery, Q.C. (1977): Effect of inflammation on the ventilatory function of the eustachian tube. *Laryngoscope*, 87:493–507.
12. Bluestone, C.D., and Klein, J.O. (1983): Otitis media with effusion, atelectasis, and eustachian tube dysfunction. In: *Pediatric Otolaryngology*, edited by C.D. Bluestone and S.E. Stool, pp. 356–512. W. B. Saunders, Philadelphia.
13. Bluestone, C.D., and Klein, J.O. (1983): Otitis media with effusion, atelectasis, and eustachian tube dysfunction. In: *Pediatric Otolaryngology*, edited by C.D. Bluestone and S.E. Stool, pp. 366–402. W. B. Saunders, Philadelphia.
14. Brash, J., editor (1951): *Cunningham's Textbook of Anatomy*. Oxford University Press, London.
15. Bryant, W.S. (1907): The eustachian tube: its anatomy and its movement: with a description of the cartilages, muscles, fasciae, and the fossa of Rosenmuller. *Med. Rec.*, 71:931–934.
16. Cantekin, E.I., Bluestone, C.D., Saez, C., Doyle, W.J., and Philips, D. (1977): Normal and abnormal middle ear ventilation. *Ann. Otol. Rhinol. Laryngol.*, 86(Suppl. 41):1–15.
17. Cantekin, E.I., Doyle, W.J., Reichert, T.J., Phillips, D.C., and Bluestone, C.D. (1979): Dilation of the eustachian tube by electrical stimulation of the trigeminal nerve. *Ann. Otol. Rhinol. Laryngol.*, 88:40–51.
18. Citelli, S. (1905): Sulla struttura della trumba d'eustachio nell-uoma. *Arch. Ital. Otol.*, 16:404–418, 441–452.

19. Cundy, R.L., Sando, I., and Hemenway, W.G. (1973): Middle ear extension of nasopharyngeal carcinoma via eustachian tube. *Arch. Otolaryngol.*, 98:131–133.
20. Doyle, W.J., editor (1977): *A functiono-anatomic description of eustachian tube vector relations in four ethnic populations—an osteologic study*. Ph.D. Dissertation, University of Pittsburgh.
21. Doyle, W.J., Cantekin, E.I., Bluestone, C.D., Phillips, D.C., Kimes, K.K., and Siegel, M.I. (1980): A nonhuman primate model of cleft palate and its implications for middle ear pathology. *Ann. Otol. Rhinol. Laryngol.*, 89(68):41–46.
22. Doyle, W.J., Friedman, R., Fireman, P., and Bluestone, C.D. (1984): Eustachian tube obstruction after provocative nasal antigen challenge. *Arch. Otolaryngol.*, 110:508–511.
23. Doyle, W.J., Takahara, T., and Fireman, P. (1985): The role of allergy in the pathogenesis of otitis media with effusion. *Arch. Otolaryngol.*, 111:502–506.
24. Friedman, R.A., Doyle, W.J., Casselbrant, M.L., Bluestone, C.D., and Fireman, P. (1983): Immunologic-mediated eustachian tube obstruction: a double-blind crossover study. *J. Allergy Clin. Immunol.*, 71:442–447.
25. Goss, C., editor (1967): *Gray's Anatomy of the Human Body*. Lea & Febiger, Philadelphia.
26. Graves, G.O., and Edwards, L.F. (1944): The eustachian tube: review of its descriptive, microscopic, topographic, and clinical anatomy. *Arch. Otolaryngol.*, 39:359–397.
27. Holborow, C. (1975): Eustachian tube function: changes throughout childhood and neuro-muscular control. *J. Laryngol. Otol.*, 89:47–55.
28. Honjo, I. (1981): Experimental study of the pumping function of the eustachian tube. *Acta Otolaryngol.*, 91:85.
29. Honjo, I., Okazaki, N., and Kumazawa, T. (1979): Experimental study of the eustachian tube function with regard to its related muscles. *Acta Otolaryngol. (Stockh.)*, 87:84–89.
30. Lupin, A.J. (1969): The relationship of the tensor tympani and tensor palati muscles. *Ann. Otol. Rhinol. Laryngol.*, 78:792–796.
31. Macbeth, R. (1960): Some thoughts on the eustachian tube. *Proc. R. Soc. Med.*, 53:151–161.
32. McMyn, J.K. (1940): The anatomy of the salpingopharyngeus muscle. *J. Laryngol. Otol.*, 55:1–22.
33. Mitchell, G.A.G. (1954): The autonomic nerve supply of the throat, nose and ear. *J. Laryngol. Otol.*, 68:495–516.
34. Myers, E.N., Beery, Q.L., Bluestone, C.D., Rood, S.R., and Sigler, B.A. (1984): Effect of certain head and neck tumors and their management on the ventilatory function of the eustachian tube. *Ann. Otol. Rhinol. Laryngol.*, 93(Suppl. 114):1–16.
35. Nathanson, S.E., and Jackson, R.T. (1976): Vidian nerve and the eustachian tube. *Ann. Otol. Rhinol. Laryngol.*, 85:83–85.
36. Proctor, B. (1967): Embryology and anatomy of the eustachian tube. *Arch. Otolaryngol.*, 86:503–526.
37. Proctor, B. (1973): Anatomy of the eustachian tube. *Arch. Otolaryngol.*, 97:2–8.
38. Rees-Jones, G.F., and McGibbon, J.E. (1941): Radiological visualization of the eustachian tube. *Lancet*, 241:660–662.
39. Rich, A.R. (1920): A physiological study of the eustachian tube and its related muscles. *Bull. Johns Hopkins Hosp.*, 31:206–214.
40. Rich, A.R. (1920): The innervation of the tensor veli palatini and levator veli palatini muscles. *Bull. Johns Hopkins Hosp.*, 31:305–310.
41. Rood, S.R. (1973): Morphology of m. tensor veli palatini in the five-month human fetus. *Am. J. Anat.*, 138:191–196.
42. Rood, S.R., and Doyle, W.J. (1978): The morphology of the tensor veli palatini, tensor tympani, and dilator tubae muscles. *Ann. Otol. Rhinol. Laryngol.*, 87(2):202–211.
43. Rood, S.R. and Doyle, W.J. (1982): The nasopharyngeal orifice of the auditory tube: implications for tubal dynamics anatomy. *Cleft Palate J.*, 19:119–128.
44. Rosen, L.M. (1970): The morphology of the salpingopharyngeus muscle. Unpublished Master's Thesis, University of Pittsburgh.
45. Ross, M. (1971): Functional anatomy of the tensor palati—its relevance in cleft palate surgery. *Arch. Otolaryngol.*, 93:1–8.
46. Simkins, C. (1943): Functional anatomy of the eustachian tube. *Arch. Otolaryngol.*, 38:476.
47. Speilberg, W. (1927): Visualization of the eustachian tube by roentgen ray. *Arch. Otolaryngol.*, 5:334–340.
48. Takahara, T., Sando, I., Bluestone, C.D., and Myers, E.N. (1986): Lymphoma invading the anterior eustachian tube: temporal bone histopathology of functional tubal obstruction. *Ann. Otol. Rhinol. Laryngol.*

49. Terracol, A., Corone, A., and Guerrier, G. (1949): *La Trompe D'Eustache*. Masson, Paris.
50. Thomsen, K.A. (1957): Studies on the function of the eustachian tube in a series of normal individuals. *Acta Otolaryngol. (Stockh.),* 48:516–529.
51. VanDishoeck, H.A.E. (1947): Resistance measuring of the eustachian tube and the ostium and isthmus valve mechanisms. *Acta Otolaryngol. (Stockh.),* 35:317–326.
52. Wolf, D. (1931): Microscopic anatomy of the eustachian tube. *Ann. Otol. Rhinol. Laryngol.,* 40:1055–1067.
53. Yee, A.L., and Cantekin, E.I. (1986): The effect of changes in systemic oxygen tension on middle ear gas exchange. *Ann. Otol. Rhinol. Laryngol.*
54. Zollner, R. (1942): *Physiologie, pathologie und klinik der ohrtrompete XVI. Die tube und maligne tumoren der nachbarschaft*. Berlin: Springer Verlag.

Immunology of the Ear, edited by J. Bernstein and P. Ogra. Raven Press, New York © 1987.

Immune Functions and Immunopathology of Palatine and Nasopharyngeal Tonsils

Per Brandtzaeg

Laboratory for Immunohistochemistry and Immunopathology, Institute of Pathology, University of Oslo, The National Hospital, Rikshospitalet, 0027 Oslo 1, Norway

TONSILS AS LYMPHOEPITHELIAL ORGANS

Introduction

The lymphoid tissues constituting Waldeyer's ring, including the palatine, lingual, and nasopharyngeal tonsils (adenoids), show an architecture similar to lymph nodes except for the lack of afferent lymphatics that carry antigens to the latter organs. Conversely, the tonsils are particularly designed for direct transport of foreign material from the exterior to the lymphoid cells via epithelial crypts. The tonsils are indeed favorably located to mediate regional immunological protection because they are exposed to both airborne and alimentary antigens. Their development is not antigen-dependent since it starts at about the 14th gestational week, and shortly afterward a specialized crypt epithelium can be found (173).

Altogether, the lymphoid organs of Waldeyer's ring seem to have features in common with both lymph nodes and typical lymphoepithelial structures such as bronchus-associated (BALT) and gut-associated (GALT) lymphoid tissues. However, the latter structures, particularly the Peyer's patches, have been subjected to much more extensive functional studies *in vivo* than the tonsils (7,18).

Antigen Uptake and Presentation

Structural Aspects

The human palatine tonsils (PT) are covered by stratified squamous epithelium that extends into deep and partly branched crypts, of which there are about 10 to 30. These crypts greatly increase the contact surface between environmental influences and lymphoid tissue (Fig. 1). It has been shown experimentally in animals that various substances can be transported via the crypts to the lymphoid follicles where germinal centers are induced as a sign of immunological activation (3,125,181).

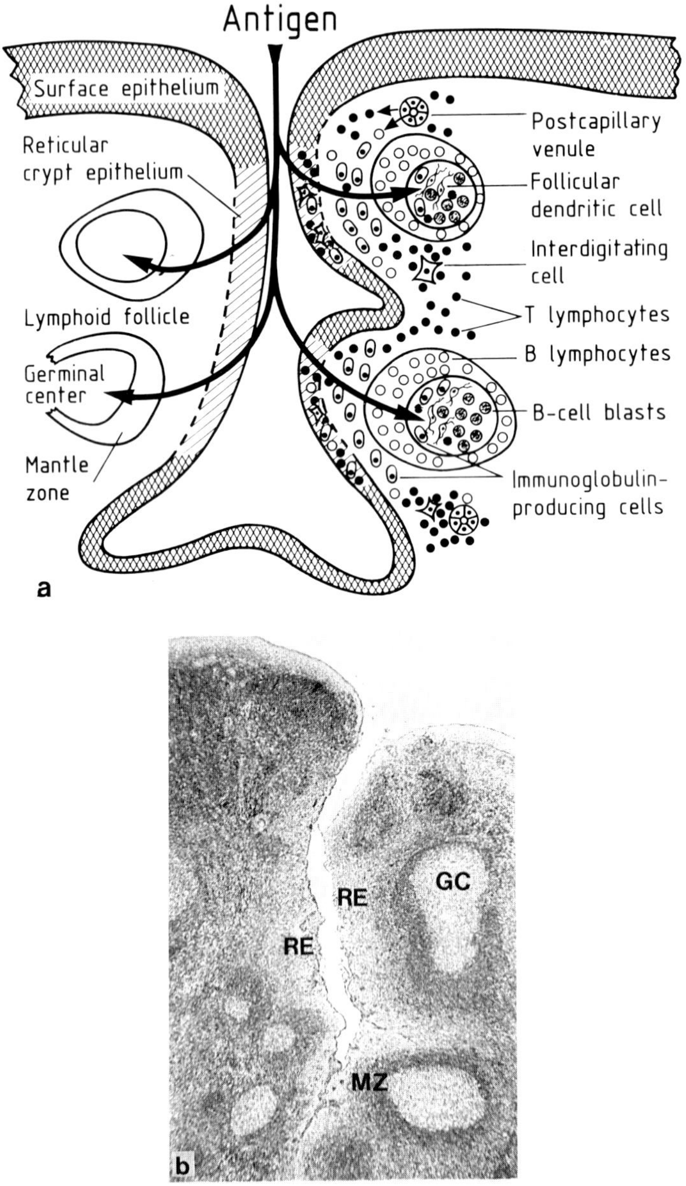

FIG. 1. **(a)** Schematic representation of various tissue elements that are important for the immunological functions of human palatine tonsil (crypt in the center). The principal route of antigen uptake is shown (*heavy arrows*). The migration of B and T lymphocytes into extrafollicular region from postcapillary venule is also shown (*small arrows*). Accessory cells are represented by follicular dendritic cells and interdigitating cells (macrophages not shown). **(b)** Field from section of human palatine tonsil including a crypt partly lined by reticular epithelium (RE). Note secondary lymphoid follicles with germinal center (GC) and mantle zone (MZ). [Hematoxylin-eosin staining ($\times$25).]

Influx of foreign material takes place mainly through the reticular parts of the crypt epithelium (Fig. 1) which rest on a discontinuous basal lamina and contain a system of channels partly covered by antigen-transporting membrane cells (also known as M cells) (68,130). These channels are remarkably extensive in the deeper layers of the epithelium and are infiltrated with lymphocytes, plasma cells, macrophages, and dendritic cells of the interdigitating and Langerhans varieties (67,174). Some of the channels open directly into the crypt lumen, particularly when shedding of superficial epithelial cells is increased due to inflammation (100).

The reticular parts of the crypt epithelium are found corresponding to the dome regions of the underlying lymphoid follicles (Fig. 1) and seem to develop according to topical immunological activity (50,143). The result is facilitation of contact between available antigens, antigen-presenting cells (APC), and lymphocytes. Compared with the relatively large extension of the reticular epithelium in early childhood, there is almost a 60% reduction around puberty and a further decrease later on (Table 1).

It is unknown how antigen is translocated from the reticular epithelium into the lymphoid follicles (Fig. 1). Nevertheless, the highly reactive state of tonsillar lymphoid tissue, even in young healthy children (88), shows that such a transfer does normally take place; the formation of germinal centers is in fact dependent on antigenic stimulation (91).

The surface of the nasopharyngeal tonsil (NPT) is covered mainly by epithelium of the respiratory type, which, however, may be partly replaced by patches of the squamous or intermediate type (55). The crypts of NPT are less conspicuous than those of PT and often appear like vertical furrows (130). The follicle-associated epithelium contains reticular parts infiltrated with mononuclear cells as described above for PT (55). Similar antigen uptake pathways have been indicated structurally in the lingual tonsil (130) and also in the scattered oral tonsils (103). Histomorphometric measurements have shown that the extension of the reticular epithelium is comparable on a relative basis in NPT and PT of young children (88).

TABLE 1. *Relative extension (mean area percentage ± SD) of different lymphoid compartments in palatine tonsils of three age groups*[a]

Lymphoid compartment	Age in years (mean and range) 5 (2–11)	14 (4–25)	60 (30–81)
Germinal center	18.0 ± 5.8	20.5 ± 8.5	17.4 ± 8.7
Mantle zone	15.4 ± 5.2	14.5 ± 4.9	8.4 ± 5.5
Extrafollicular area	50.5 ± 9.7	57.7 ± 8.5	69.6 ± 16.1
Reticular epithelium	16.6 ± 6.9	7.3 ± 2.5	4.6 ± 4.2

[a]Histomorphometric data modified from Brandtzaeg et al. (26) and Korsrud and Brandtzaeg (88).

Cellular and Molecular Aspects

It is generally accepted that molecules encoded by the class II region of the human major histocompatibility complex (MHC) are critical as restricting elements in immune regulation (72,122). These gene products are called Ia antigens in animals—the best known human counterparts being the HLA-DR molecules. Helper T cells (T_h) can only be stimulated by antigens presented to them by accessory cells in the context of class II surface determinants (Fig. 2). HLA-DR and similar molecules thus exert a genetically determined "guidance" function in the immune response to foreign material. Since also B lymphocytes and B blasts express DR, a second possibility for MHC restriction is introduced through T_h-B cell interactions. Class II molecules may, moreover, by themselves represent signals for activation of certain T_h cells (77).

Among the accessory cells, only the macrophages are able to mediate substantial internalization of bound foreign material; after processing it by as yet unknown mechanisms, they present some of the degraded antigenic substances to T_h cells in the context of class II molecules which they generally express (60). However, DR-

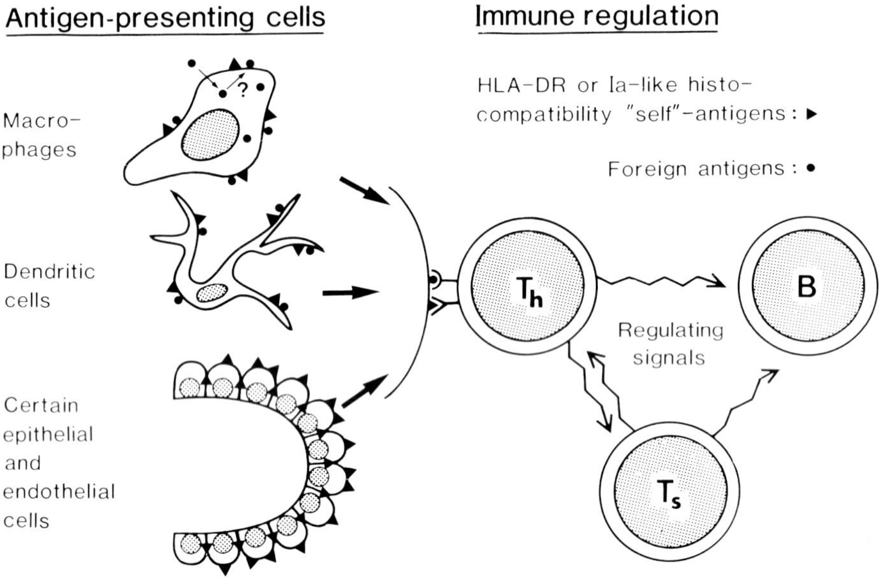

FIG. 2. Schematic representation of HLA-DR-positive antigen-presenting cells, which may be involved in immune regulation both in lymphoepithelial structures and secretory tissues. Most soluble antigens have to be presented to helper T cells (T_h) along with class II MHC determinants such as HLA-DR to elicit efficient B-cell responses. Antigens presented by macrophages are first taken up by these cells (*small arrows*), processed by unknown mechanisms (*question mark*), and then presented on the cell surface in a modified form. Immunoregulatory factors released from activated T_h cells are important not only for proliferation and differentiation of B cells, but also for stimulation of suppressor T cells (T_s), which in various ways modulate the immune response. (From ref. 17.)

positive dendritic histiocytic cells (162), such as interdigitating reticulum cells and Langerhans cells, are apparently functioning even better as APC (Fig. 2). Recent evidence has indicated that also DR-positive epithelial cells (99) and perhaps endothelial cells may present antigens that need no prior processing (Fig. 2).

HLA-DR-expressing cells abound in the reticular areas of the crypt epithelium (Fig. 3). Some are macrophages (33) or dendritic cells in close contact with putative T_h cells (174). The dendritic cells are part of the CD1(OKT6)-positive Langerhans type (108). In addition, the crypt epithelium shows weaker patchy DR expression (Fig. 4a). The positive epithelial cells may partly represent so-called "nurse cells," which were recently identified in suspensions of human PT and NPT (101); they were shown to be similar to "nurse cells" from thymus, being DR positive and containing five to 30 lymphocytes. Because the intraepithelial lymphocytes are of both T- and B-cell varieties (66), the spatial requirement is fulfilled for all cellular interactions involved in immune regulation (Fig. 2) to take place even at the level of the reticular epithelium. Also, the faucial surface epithelium contains DR-positive cells of various morphologies which may participate in antigen presentation (Fig. 4b).

Large pleomorphic mononuclear cells that express HLA-DR likewise abound in the extrafollicular area (Fig. 5b); they may partly represent monocyte-derived macrophages, which can be identified in this compartment by specific monoclonal antibody (Fig. 6a), or dendritic cells (Fig. 6b), which have been tentatively identified as interdigitating cells by electron microscopy (86) and immunohistochemistry

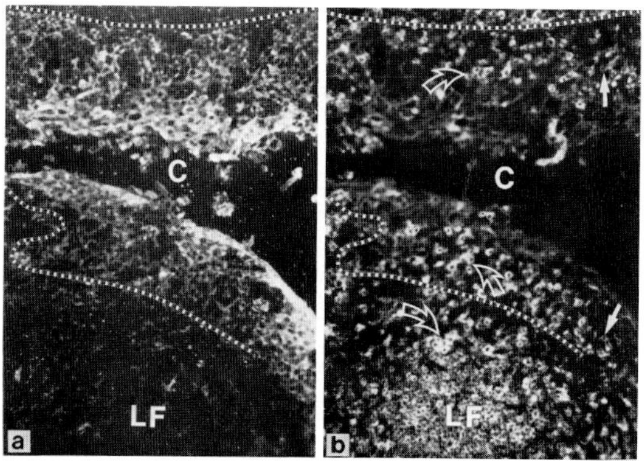

FIG. 3. Paired immunofluorescence staining for L1 antigen [(**a**) rhodamine] and HLA-DR [(**b**) fluorescein] in same field from section of ethanol-fixed palatine tonsil. L1 is a myelomonocytic marker protein that is also present in squamous oral epithelium; its labeling, therefore, outlines reticular crypt (C) epithelium (basement membrane zone indicated by *dashed lines*) in addition to showing macrophages. Note that numerous DR-expressing large pleomorphic mononuclear cells (*open arrows*) and smaller lymphocytes (*solid arrows*) are found both within and beneath the reticular epithelium. Superficial epithelial cells likewise show DR positivity (cf. Fig. 4a). Lymphoid follicle (LF) is abundantly DR positive (×70). (From ref. 17.)

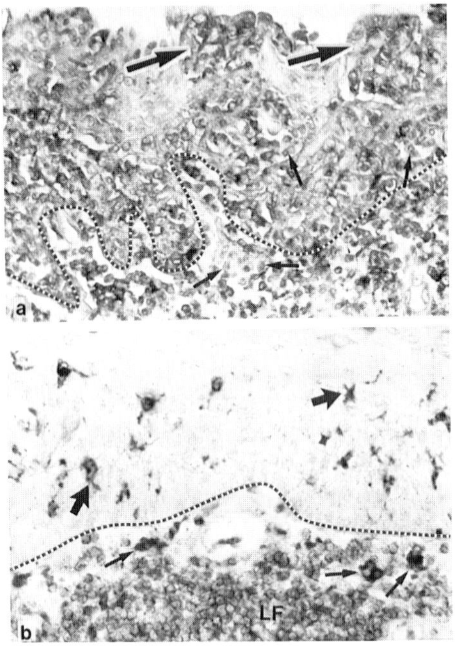

FIG. 4. Immunoenzyme staining for HLA-DR determinants in section of ethanol fixed palatine tonsil. (**a**) A variety of DR-expressing mononuclear cells of different intensity (dark color) are found within and beneath the reticular crypt epithelium (basement membrane zone indicated by *dashed line*). Also, patches of epithelial cells (*large arrows*) are DR positive. Note negative plasma cells (*small arrows*) within and beneath the epithelium. (**b**) Surface epithelium contains DR-positive dendritic cells (*large arrows*), which probably are mainly of Langerhans type. Part of lymphoid follicle (LF) with DR-expressing B lymphocytes and also several large DR-positive accessory cells (*small arrows*) are seen beneath the basement membrane zone (*dashed line*). [Alkaline phosphatase labeling lightly counterstained with hematoxylin (×80).]

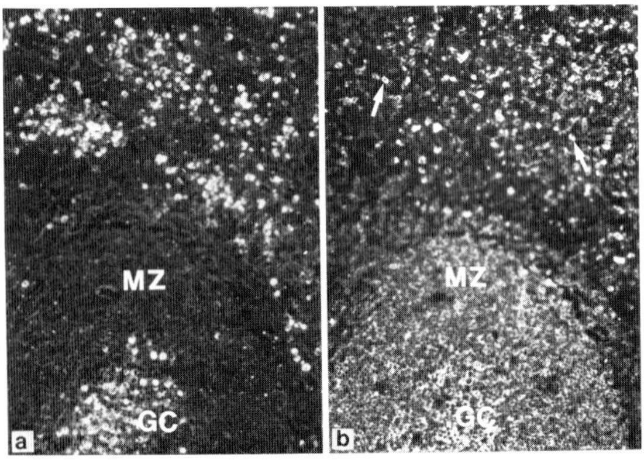

FIG. 5. Paired immunofluorescence staining for Ig [(**a**) rhodamine] and HLA-DR [(**b**) fluorescein] in same field from section of saline-extracted and ethanol-fixed specimen (14,25) of palatine tonsil. Numerous Ig-producing immunocytes are present in germinal center (GC) and extrafollicular area (*top*). B lymphocytes in mantle zone (MZ) are DR positive and germinal-center cells are even more intensely stained, including follicular dendritic cells and many of the Ig-positive blasts. Conversely, Ig-positive plasma cells in extrafollicular area are generally negative for DR; extrafollicular cells showing DR expression (*arrows*) are macrophages, dendritic cells, and lymphocytes (×70).

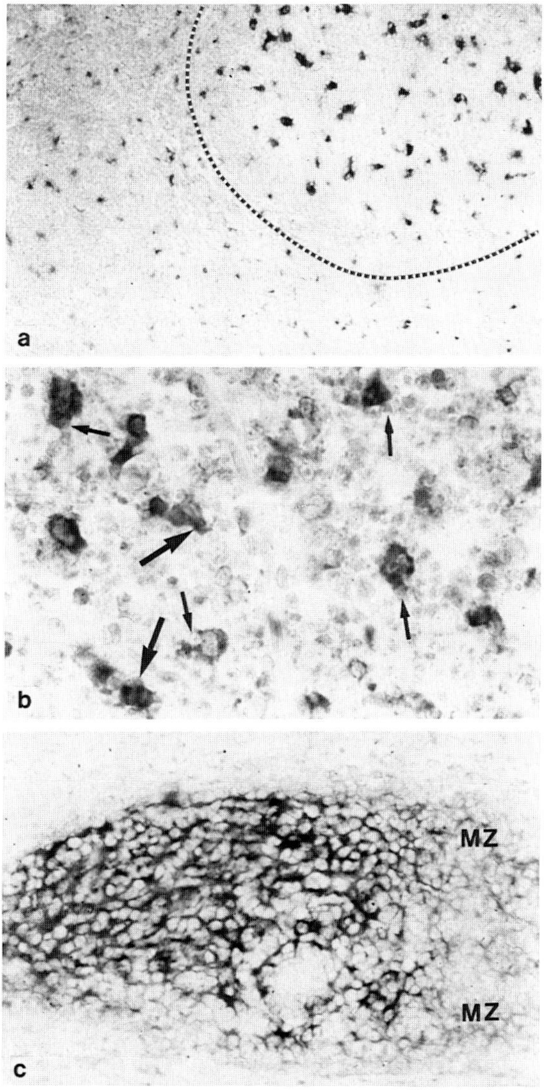

FIG. 6. Immunoenzyme staining in sections of palatine tonsil with monoclonal antibody to (**a**) macrophages, (**b**) HLA-DR, or (**c**) C3b receptor. (a) Large macrophages are distributed within lymphoid follicle (*dashed line*) and smaller ones in extrafollicular area. (b) DR-positive cells in extrafollicular area show dendritic morphology (*large arrows*) and probably represent interdigitating cells. Lymphocytes are found in close contact with these cells (*small arrows*). (c) Germinal center shows strong lacy staining for C3b receptor, signifying the distribution of dendritic follicular cells. B lymphocytes in mantle zone (MZ) are faintly positive. [Alkaline phosphatase labeling lightly counterstained with hematoxylin: (a) ×80; (b) ×220; (c) ×220.]

(74,174). Some of them may in fact be CD1(OKT6)-positive Langerhans cells (168). Both processing and presentation of antigen can therefore take place in the extrafollicular area. The putative interdigitating cells are often closely surrounded by T lymphocytes (48) that are mainly of the CD4 (T4, putative T_h) phenotype (74,174).

Macrophages are also present within the lymphoid follicles (Fig. 6a); but the framework of these structures consists of characteristic follicular dendritic cells (Fig. 1), which, unlike other accessory cells, may not be derived from bone marrow precursors (69). These cells are DR-positive (Fig. 5b) and retain antigens on their surface for long periods in the form of antigen-antibody complexes bound via complement (C3) receptors (63,138) and Ig Fc receptors (64,144). The lacy staining pattern seen for Ig, particularly occurring in the "light zone" of germinal centers and mainly signifying bound IgM, reflects this dendritic trapping mechanism (26,164). A similar pattern is produced by staining with monoclonal antibody specific for the C3b receptor (Fig. 6c).

Because the follicular dendritic cells also express DR molecules (63,68,144,168), the germinal centers represent unique sites for persistent immunological stimulation and generation of memory B cells. It is possible that preformed immune complexes are carried into the lymphoid follicles by migrating B cells (49) that also express C3b receptors (Fig. 6c); but recent evidence indicates that antibodies produced within the germinal centers may, in addition, be responsible for *in situ* formation of immune complexes (169).

Tonsillar B- and T-Cell Populations

Lymphoid Compartments

Lymphoid cells are found in four tonsillar tissue compartments: reticular crypt epithelium, extrafollicular area, mantle zones of lymphoid follicles, and the follicular or germinal centers (Fig. 1). In these compartments, the mechanisms that lead to highly varying proportions of B and T cells and different distribution of APC are poorly understood.

Both B and T lymphocytes arriving from the blood enter the extrafollicular tonsillar area through so-called postcapillary or high-endothelial venules (166). Their extravasation is apparently guided by endothelial surface receptors (30), which in animals have been found to be different in lymph nodes and Peyer's patches (32). In addition, there seems to be different endothelial recognition specificities in BALT and Peyer's patches (167), but nothing is known about the tonsils regarding this.

Most extravasated T cells accumulate alongside the lymphoid follicles (Fig. 7b), and sometimes in additional mats they accumulate deeper in the tissue. These areas are thus comparable to the paracortex or thymus-dependent area of lymph nodes. The T-cell areas vary largely among individual tonsils (66).

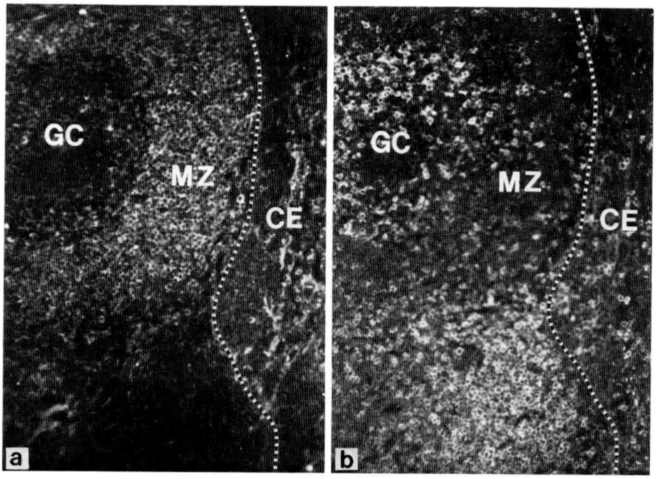

FIG. 7. Paired immunofluorescence staining for IgD [(**a**) rhodamine] and pan-T-cell marker CD5 [(**b**) fluorescein] in same field from section of ethanol-fixed palatine tonsil. Mantle zone (MZ) of lymphoid follicle is densely packed with B lymphocytes expressing membrane IgD, whereas germinal-center (GC) cells are negative or only faintly stained for this isotype. Although most T cells are located extrafollicularly, many do occur within the follicle, particularly in the germinal center. Several T and some B lymphocytes are present in the crypt epithelium (CE), which is indicated by *dashed line* (×85).

The relative extensions of the four lymphoid compartments have been determined by histomorphometric measurements (Table 1). It appears that below the age of 30 years the two compartments constituting the B-cell follicles occupy about one-third of the total tonsillar lymphoid tissue area. The follicles are in a reactive state with extensive germinal centers (secondary follicles) both in PT and NPT, even in young children who have experienced no tonsillar disease (88). In addition, the two other compartments contain B-cell infiltrates of varying density, including immunoglobulin(Ig)-producing immunocytes of various morphologies (centroblasts, immunoblasts, plasmacytoid cells, and mature plasma cells). The plasma cells accumulate mainly in the extrafollicular area between the follicles and the crypts and in the deeper layers of the reticular epithelium (Fig. 8). Davis (40) reported as early as 1912 that plasma cells appear beneath the crypt epithelium 2 to 3 weeks after birth and are present there even at advanced age.

Generation of B Cells

Studies of cell suspensions made from dissociated PT or NPT have indicated that both organs contain an increased proportion of surface Ig-positive B lymphocytes (40–50%) compared with the T-to-B-cell ratio in blood (28,61, 110,141,182). Most of the B lymphocytes detected in such studies have obviously been obtained from the mantle zones and germinal centers of lymphoid follicles.

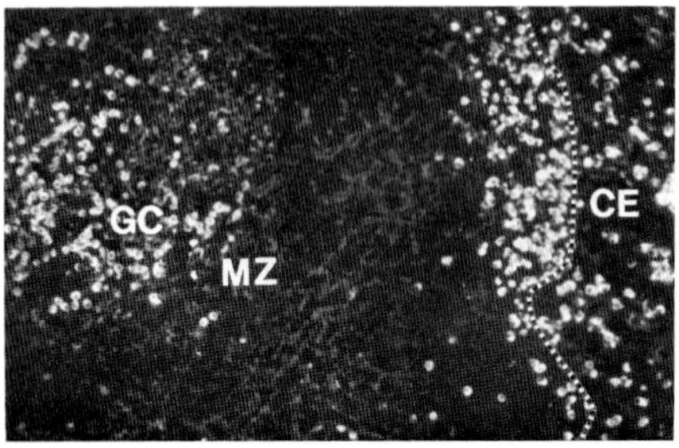

FIG. 8. Immunofluorescence staining of IgG-producing immunocytes in section of saline-extracted and ethanol-fixed specimen (14,25) of palatine tonsil. Many positive cells are present in germinal center (GC) but not in mantle zone (MZ) of lymphoid follicle. Most positive cells occur beneath reticular crypt epithelium (CE) and to some extent within this epithelium (basement membrane zone indicated by *dashed line*) (×70).

The germinal centers represent an antigen-dependent B-cell compartment responsible for both proliferative expansion of memory clones and differentiation to Ig-producing immunocytes (91,126).

In normal tonsils from young children, the average density of Ig-producing immunocytes in the germinal centers amounts to about 70% of that in the extrafollicular areas (88). This fact reflects a remarkable degree of intrafollicular B-cell differentiation, as also pointed out by others on the basis of studies on diseased tonsils removed surgically (37,152).

The most immature germinal-center cells (centroblasts) and the highest proliferative activity occur at the base of the follicles (the "dark zone"), whereas increasing differentiation—resulting in centrocytes, immunoblasts, and plasmacytoid cells—takes place toward the pole (the "light zone") where the mantle zone is developed to a cap (Fig. 1), which generally faces a crypt (37,68,152,165). This observation suggests that increasing maturity of tonsillar B cells is associated with migration within the germinal center from the base to the pole. Experiments in rabbit tonsils have suggested that the follicular proliferative activity contributes both to the lymphocyte caps and to the extrafollicular and intraepithelial B-cell populations (87). It seems likely, moreover, that some of the immunoblasts reach the blood via efferent lymph and become seeded to other tissue sites, although there as yet is no direct evidence of such a migratory pattern for tonsillar lymphoid cells.

Characteristics of Intrafollicular B Cells

The precursors of the germinal-center cells are believed to be mantle lymphocytes, which mostly express both IgD and IgM (91). Surface membrane staining for these isotypes can be seen in the mantle zones of tonsillar lymphoid follicles by immunofluorescence (Fig. 7a) and immunoenzyme methods (26,38,72,155).

When the B cells have entered the germinal center, switching of isotype expression takes place in the course of clonal differentiation; the first step largely involves loss of IgD (68,91), which is absent or barely detectable on most cells in this compartment (Fig. 7a). In contrast to the extrafollicular Ig-producing plasma cells, most intrafollicular B cells seem to express HLA-DR—including the blasts with cytoplasmic Ig. However, because the follicular dendritic cells are DR-positive, it is difficult to identify the various cell types by immunohistochemistry (Fig. 5). Altogether, the abundant intrafollicular DR expression probably serves to modulate local interactions between APC, T cells, and B cells as discussed above.

Work on tonsillar lymphoid cells has mainly been carried out on suspensions. In general agreement with the immunohistochemical observations described above, most of the B lymphocytes have been shown to express IgD and IgM, whereas surface staining for IgA and IgG has produced remarkably discrepant results (41,61,165,170). The reason may be that these isotypes are present on the lymphoid cell surfaces in low concentrations and are perhaps variably bound through Fc receptors rather than being expressed as integral membrane proteins. Various sample proportions obtained from different intrafollicular B-cell populations will also influence the results (165).

In tissue sections, distinct labeling of surface-associated IgA and IgG is obtained for only rare tonsillar cells (66,68,155). This may be so because low membrane concentrations of Ig afford a poor signal-to-noise ratio against unwanted extracellular staining; some retention of IgA—and particularly of IgG—is commonly seen on various tissue elements, including lymphoid cells, even after thorough washing of the specimen (Fig. 8).

Cell sorter analysis of murine Peyer's patch suspensions has demonstrated that most germinal-center cells express very small amounts of surface Ig—being constituted mainly of IgA with some additional IgM or IgG; this pattern contrasts with the prominent IgM and IgD expression seen in the mantle zone (29). Germinal-center cells from murine peripheral lymph nodes were found to express mainly IgM in a primary immune response, whereas IgG was the predominant surface isotype after secondary stimulation (91). Analysis of suspensions of human tonsillar germinal-center cells revealed IgM as the most prominent surface isotype, followed by IgA, IgG, and IgD—in that order (165). Altogether, therefore, tonsillar follicular B cells seem to have phenotypic features in common with counterparts from both Peyer's patches and lymph nodes.

Differentiation of B Cells to Ig-Producing Immunocytes

Before a single cytoplasmic Ig class appears in a B cell, the same isotype is generally expressed on the cell surface either alone or—as a result of phenotypic switching—in combination with another isotype (58,120,133,137). Coincident expression of the same isotype on the surface and in the cytoplasm has been shown also for human tonsillar B cells, although most Ig-producing plasmacytoid cells lack surface Ig (52).

Differentiation to IgG-producing cells in lymph nodes involves phenotypic switching from IgM expression (91); the same process seems to be pronounced in tonsillar germinal centers where 55% to 72% of the immunocytes with cytoplasmic Ig belong to the IgG isotype, whereas only 14% to 25% are IgM producers (Fig. 9). Many of the latter have retained surface membrane expression of IgD along with IgM (52).

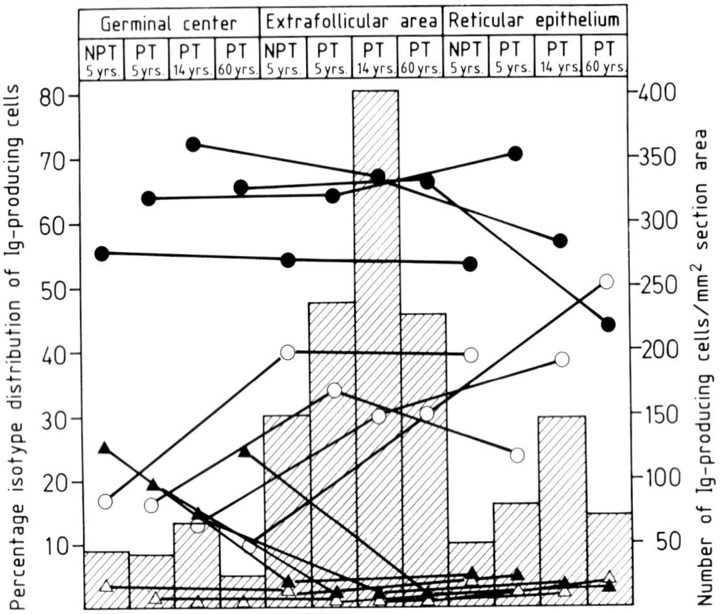

FIG. 9. Percentage distribution of IgG(●)-, IgA(○)-, IgM(▲)-, and IgD(△)-producing immunocytes within three lymphoid compartments of clinically normal nasopharyngeal (NPT) and palatine (PT) tonsils from three age groups (mean age in years; see Table 1 for ranges). Vertical columns indicate average numeric distribution (cells/mm^2 section area) of all Ig-producing immunocytes. Only cells with cytoplasmic staining were included. (Adapted from refs. 26 and 88; reproduced from ref. 17.)

Also, differentiation to IgA-producing immunocytes takes place in the tonsillar follicles as shown by the fact that 13% to 18% of the cells with cytoplasmic Ig belong to this isotype in the germinal centers, with a higher percentage in the extrafollicular area and reticular epithelium (Fig. 9). A recent study indicated that there may be various combinations of multiple isotypes on the surface of tonsillar lymphocytes; in addition to the common dual expression of IgM + IgD, triple expression of IgM + IgD + IgA or IgM + IgG + IgA was often seen (120,170). This finding could reflect that IgD and IgG expression are important intermediate phenotypic characteristics in the differentiation to IgA-producing immunocytes in human tonsils. In contrast to the situation in peripheral blood, there was a numerical correlation between the tonsillar cell surface staining obtained for IgG and IgA (171). This result indicated a particularly close relationship between the expression of these two isotypes during tonsillar B-cell differentiation.

Animal experiments have suggested that isotype-specific T cells may not be crucial for B-cell differentiation in lymphoepithelial structures; constant exposure to environmental antigens may instead stimulate proliferation and phenotypic switching in a vectorial manner according to the order of Ig heavy-chain constant (C_H) genes on the chromosome (31,57). In humans the sequence of Ig expression, including the known subclasses, would then be IgM → IgD → IgG3 → IgG1 → IgA1 → IgG2 → IgG4 → IgE → IgA2 (53). The characteristics of human tonsillar B cells are compatible with such a development.

Distribution and Characteristics of T Cells

Most tonsillar T lymphocytes accumulate alongside and beneath the lymphoid follicles, but, in addition, a considerable number may appear among the B cells in the mantle zones and especially inside the germinal centers (Fig. 7b). Immunohistochemical studies based on monoclonal antibodies to T-cell subsets (Fig. 10) indicate that among the extrafollicular T lymphocytes there are about 70% of the CD4 (T4) phenotype (putative "helper/inducer" subset) and 30% of the CD8 (T8) phenotype (putative "cytotoxic/suppressor" subset), whereas the germinal centers contain a higher proportion of the former variety (45,109,147,155,168,186).

This observation is important in view of the decisive role T_h cells are generally believed to play in B-cell differentiation (Fig. 2). Two functionally different types of T_h cells have been cloned from murine Peyer's patches. One variety induces IgM-positive B lymphocytes to switch directly to IgA expression (78–80). The other variety represents postswitch T_h cells that transform IgA-expressing B cells to IgA-producing immunocytes (82,83). These T lymphocytes were generally found to express Fcα receptors, which may be directly involved in T_h-B cell interactions (85). When such receptors or "IgA-binding factors" are released from T cells in experimental test systems, they may promote or suppress IgA responses depending on the applied concentration (84).

Human T cells with Fcα receptors and the ability to promote IgA responses have been identified (107), but it is not known whether they are present in the tonsils. In addition to postswitch activity of cloned human T cells (104), a recently described neoplastic human T-cell clone was shown to promote switching of B cells from IgM to IgG and IgA expression (105). Such a helper activity is of great interest in view of the characteristics described above for tonsillar B cells. There are probably also T cells with Fcδ receptors, which may regulate IgD responses (34).

Although HLA-DR determinants are mainly found on B lymphocytes, B blasts, and various accessory cells, some of the positive lymphocytes present in the various tonsillar tissue compartments (Figs. 3b and 4) may in fact be T cells that express DR as a sign of activation (42). It is interesting that tonsillar T cells are DR-positive more frequently than those from peripheral blood (56) or peripheral lymph nodes (145). It has been indicated that about 25% of T cells from both human PT and NPT express DR (48), which is similar to the figure (15–20%) reported for class II antigen positivity of T cells in murine Peyer's patches (92).

Activated T cells can, in addition, be identified by a receptor for interleukin 2 (IL2) expressed on their surface. Their activation is in fact highly dependent on IL2, which is a T-cell-derived growth factor. Immunohistochemistry with a mono-

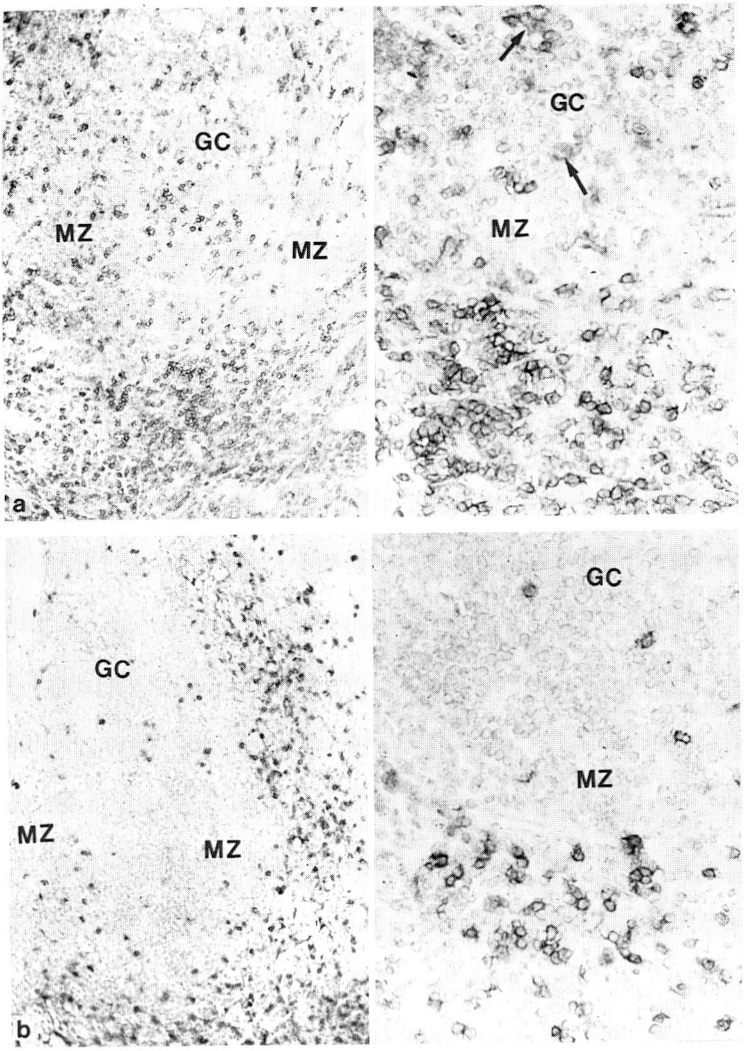

FIG. 10. Immunoenzyme staining of T-cell subsets in adjacent frozen sections of palatine tonsil. (**a**) Monoclonal antibody to CD4 (T4, putative T_h subset) labels cells in extrafollicular region but also within mantle zone (MZ) and germinal center (GC) of lymphoid follicle. Note that this antibody shows weak cross-reactivity with macrophages (*arrows*). (**b**) Monoclonal antibody to CD8 (T8, putative T_s subset) labels mainly cells in extrafollicular region. (Alkaline phosphatase labeling lightly counterstained with hematoxylin: *left panels* ×80; *right panels* ×220.)

clonal antibody (anti-Tac) demonstrated T cells with IL2 receptor both in the follicles and in the extrafollicular areas of human tonsils, mainly in the latter compartment (113). Most of the activated cells were of the CD4 (T4) phenotype (putative T_h subset). Moreover, *in vitro* studies have indicated that IL2-activated T cells are involved in differentiation of tonsillar B cells to plasma cells (119). Most likely, therefore, the striking development of Ig-producing immunocytes in human PT and NPT is at least, in part, T-cell regulated.

Some of the CD4-positive cells in tonsillar germinal centers express the additional phenotype (Leu-7) of natural killer (NK) cells (136). Leu-7-positive small lymphocytes are, in fact, relatively numerous in this compartment (174), but their relation to T cells and NK cells is not clear. In one study, cells with the Leu-7 phenotype were found in smaller numbers in the crypt epithelium where they, by electron microscopy, were identified as large granular lymphocytes (174). Such cells from blood show strong NK activity, whereas the low NK activity found in suspensions of tonsillar lymphocytes could, instead, be ascribed mainly to macrophages (33). The role and nature of tonsillar cells with the Leu-7 marker thus remain unsettled.

IMMUNOLOGICAL FUNCTIONS OF TONSILS

The Humoral Immune System

Ig Production in Normal Tonsils

Only two studies have been carried out to quantify Ig-producing immunocytes in clinically normal human tonsils (Fig. 9). Most such cells were found in the extrafollicular area, but considerable numbers were, in addition, present in the reticular crypt epithelium; the highest immunocyte density (cell number/mm^2) was, in fact, observed in the latter compartment. Immunoblasts and plasmacytoid cells present in germinal centers, moreover, contributed to the local production of Ig, although the follicles varied considerably in this respect. The mantle zones contained so few Ig-producing immunocytes that they could be neglected.

In the youngest age group there was virtually no difference between NPT and PT as to the composition of the Ig-producing cell populations; only a trend toward higher extrafollicular and epithelial immunocyte numbers, with a slightly more pronounced overall predominance of IgG cells, was indicated for PT, whereas the proportion of IgA cells tended to be higher in NPT (Fig. 9). These tendencies might reflect an intenser B-cell stimulation in PT owing to deeper crypts with massive retention of antigens and mitogens. Also, there is some contribution of the secretory IgA immune system in NPT, as discussed below.

A marked predominance of IgG immunocytes agreed with several other studies, which, however, have been carried out on material obtained at tonsillectomy (6); possible reasons for discrepant reports have been discussed elsewhere (26). We found in all age groups that the proportion of IgG cells was similar in the germinal centers and in the extrafollicular area (Fig. 9). By contrast, the IgG-cell ratio decreased with increasing age in the reticular epithelium because of a relatively raised number of IgA-producing immunocytes in that compartment (Fig. 9).

Regardless of age there was a much higher proportion of IgA immunocytes in both the reticular epithelium and extrafollicular area compared with the germinal centers; this shift was accompanied by a comparable reduced proportion of IgM-producing cells (Fig. 9). The latter difference was probably somewhat underestimated because immature germinal-center cells with small amounts of cytoplasmic IgM (164) might, to some extent, have been undetected by immunofluorescence observed against the background of reticular IgM staining of dendritic cells regularly seen in this compartment.

The subclass distribution of IgG- and IgA-producing immunocytes has recently been determined in PT. The IgG1-, IgG2-, IgG3-, and IgG4-cell percentages are approximately 61%, 22%, 16%, and 1%, respectively (106). The IgG1-producing cells predominate both within and outside the lymphoid follicles (Fig. 11a). Very few IgA2-producing cells are usually found in the tonsils (Fig. 11b), the median proportion (and range) of IgA1 immunocytes being 95% (49–97%), which is similar to that in peripheral lymph nodes (81).

The study of Crabbé and Heremans (36) indicated that NPT contains more IgD-producing cells than other lymphoid tissues; this agrees with our observations despite the fact that the proportion of such immunocytes was small in both the germinal centers and other lymphoid compartments (Fig. 9). They tended to be slightly fewer in PT than in NPT, but the individual variations were large. The only tissue sites containing a higher proportion of IgD-producing cells than the tonsils are the glandular areas of the upper respiratory tract, such as the nasal mucosa and the lacrimal glands (15,21).

The presence of IgE-producing cells in human tonsils remains a controversial issue and will be discussed below in relation to allergy. T cells exerting a suppressive effect on IgE synthesis have been identified in dissociated PT (124), and we were unable to detect a significant number of IgE-producing immunocytes in normal specimens of PT and NPT (26,88). The same held true for a recent study of oral tonsils (103). The latter study also reported results for IgG, IgA, and IgM cells similar to those obtained by us in NPT and PT, but failed to detect substantial numbers of IgD cells. This discrepancy might be explained by the fact that it was based on trypsin-treated sections of formalin-fixed tissue, which in our opinion is an unreliable approach for the detection of IgD (14,25).

Specificities of Tonsillar Immune Responses

The immunohistochemical studies discussed above indicated that human tonsils contain the complement of cells necessary to mount a primary antibody response, namely APC, different T-cell subsets, and B cells. This notion has been supported by *in vitro* experiments (179). In addition, tonsils of children immunized with diphtheria toxoid were found to contain memory cells that could produce a secondary antibody response against the same antigen *in vitro* (135).

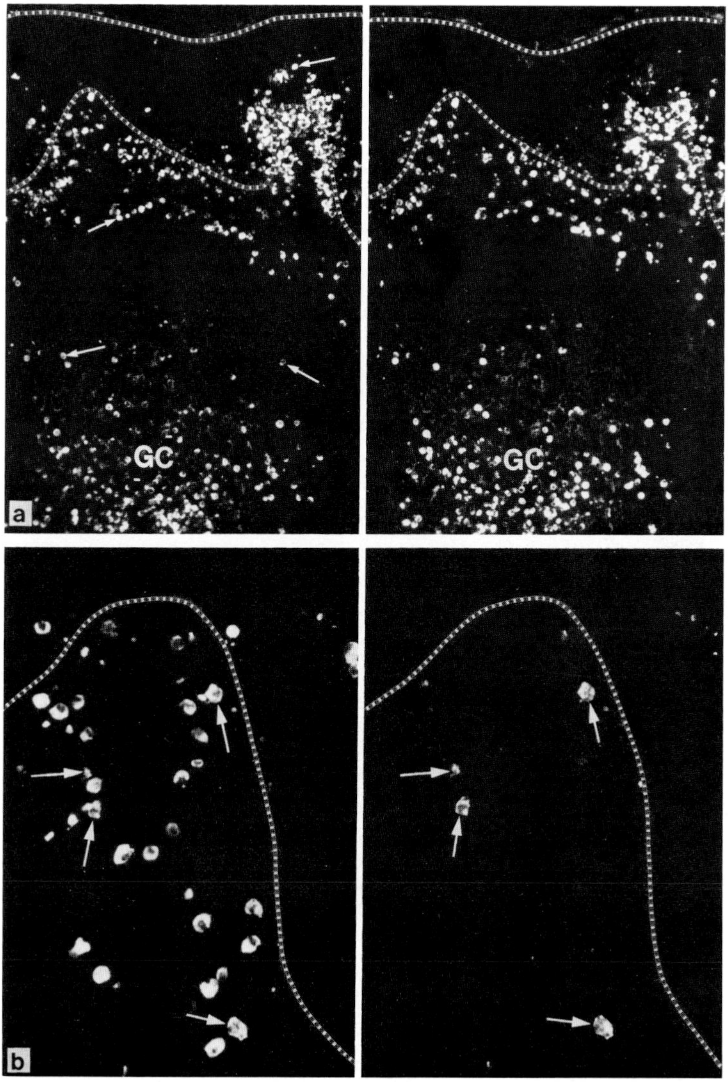

FIG. 11. Paired immunofluorescence staining for Ig subclasses in adjacent sections of saline-extracted and ethanol-fixed specimen (14,25) of palatine tonsil. (**a**) IgG (*left panel*, rhodamine) and IgG1 subclass (*right panel*, fluorescein) shown in same field to document that most IgG-producing cells are of the IgG1 subclass, both in germinal center (GC) of lymphoid follicle and in extrafollicular region, including the reticular parts of crypt epithelium (*dashed line*). Examples of IgG cells of another subclass are shown (*arrows*). (**b**) IgA (*left panel*, rhodamine) and IgA2 subclass (*right panel*, fluorescein) staining in same field from subepithelial area shows that only four of the IgA-producing cells (*arrows*) are of this subclass. [(a) ×85; (b) ×215.]

In the latter study (135) it was shown that the antidiphtheria response gave rise to a marked production of IgG and IgA of unrelated specificities, probably as a result of polyclonal co-stimulation. Similar results have emerged from other experiments (54,140,141). Thus, polyclonal activation of B cells from NPT was successful with bacteria such as *Diplococcus pneumoniae, Hemophilus influenzae,* and hemolytic streptococci group A, whereas lipopolysaccharide from *Escherichia coli* and purified protein derivative (PPD) of tuberculin elicited relatively poor *in vitro* responses. Since the two latter substances are good polyclonal activators for B cells from spleen and mesenteric lymph nodes, it appears that the successful polyclonal activation of adenoid B cells with nasopharyngeal bacteria may, to some extent, be ascribed to concomitant specific immune responses. Moreover, mitogenic effects on tonsillar lymphocytes seem to depend, in part, on interactions between T and B cells and perhaps also on macrophages (41,70,139).

There is, in addition, more direct evidence indicating that the nasopharyngeal bacterial flora stimulates tonsillar lymphocytes *in vivo*. Such cells harvested from patients whose tonsils were colonized by *Staphylococcus aureus* showed a particularly marked spontaneous lymphoproliferative response *in vitro* (44). High *in vivo* background stimulation apparently decreased *in vitro* sensitivity to additional mitogenic or antigenic challenge. This observation could explain why some authors observed a higher level of mitogenic activation and a better immune response to PPD *in vitro* for peripheral blood lymphocytes than for adenoid lymphocytes (110,114). Better responses obtained *in vitro* with lymphocytes from NPT compared to lymphocytes from PT (54) might likewise be explained by a higher degree of *in vivo* activation in the latter organ. Along the same line of reasoning, it was not unexpected that *in vitro* stimulation of adenoid lymphocytes with *H. influenzae* turned out to be successful only when the cells had been obtained from children who apparently were free from immediately preceding nasopharyngeal exposure to the same bacterium (110).

Altogether, therefore, several pieces of direct and indirect evidence indicate that PT and NPT are continuously engaged in immune responses to microorganisms of the nasopharyngeal flora and that, concomitantly with such responses, polyclonal activation of the tonsillar lymphocytes takes place. Both parenteral and oral immunization result in migration of specifically primed lymphocytes to the tonsils (131), but persistent topical exposure to antigens seems to be particularly efficient in inducing tonsillar immune responses. Thus, natural infection or intranasal immunization with live attenuated rubella virus vaccine has been reported to prime tonsillar lymphocytes much better than subcutaneous vaccination (116). Also, natural infection with varicella zoster virus was found to stimulate tonsillar lymphocytes better than lymphocytes in peripheral blood (10).

Production of J Chain and Dimeric IgA

The J chain is a polypeptide that is associated with dimeric IgA and pentameric IgM; it is crucial for the transport of these Ig polymers through secretory epithelium (19). Intra- and extrafollicular tonsillar IgA and IgG immunocytes are remarkably different with regard to J-chain-expressing capacity (Fig. 12). On an average, cytoplasmic J chain is present in almost 40% of the IgG-producing germinal-center cells in normal PT and NPT, whereas only about 2% of the extrafollicular counterparts are positive (80,89). Conversely, the percentage of IgA immunocytes expressing J chain is increased in the extrafollicular region. These findings will be discussed below in relation to tonsillar differentiation of B-cell clones.

Cytoplasmic staining for J chain in tonsillar IgA immunocytes was of heterogeneous intensity and was highly dependent on unfolding of intracellular IgA dimers by exposure to acid urea; without such pretreatment of the tissue sections, only 6% to 9% of the extrafollicular IgA cells were positive (16,89). Moreover, cytoplasmic affinity for free secretory component (SC) *in vitro,* which signifies intracellular dimeric IgA (11,12,16), was obtained for only 20% to 30% of the cells (24). SC is the epithelial receptor protein responsible for transport of J-chain-containing Ig polymers (19).

Taken together, J-chain expression and cytoplasmic SC-binding activity indicated that 20% to 30% of the extrafollicular IgA immunocytes elaborate a mixed product with substantial amounts of dimers whereas the remainders form mainly monomers. This conclusion agrees with the results obtained by Smith et al. (151) in 3-day cultures of tonsillar lymphoid cells. Conversely, Platts-Mills and Ishizaka (135) and Kutteh et al. (94) reported that tonsillar IgA immunocytes cultured for 7 days secreted at least 40% dimers. This figure was probably artifactually high because J-chain expression has been shown to increase progressively up to the 7th day for IgA- and IgG-producing cells from peripheral blood kept in mitogen-stimulated cultures (187).

Mogi (115) stated that SC-binding IgA immunocytes were more frequently found in NPT than in PT, but he reported no data to support this claim. Since his

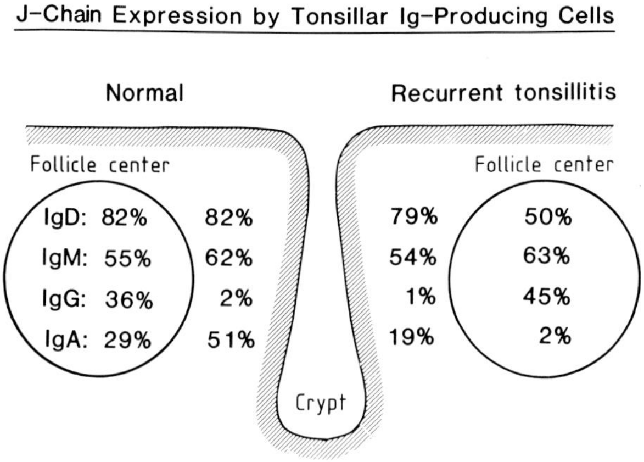

FIG. 12. Schematic representation of average J-chain positivity shown by intra- and extrafollicular Ig-producing immunocytes of various isotypes as indicated. (Adapted from refs. 89 and 90.)

study was not based on paired staining, quantitation of SC affinity in relation to cytoplasmic isotype could not be performed. We have noted that some specimens of NPT contain an extrafollicular IgA-cell population that shows more than 40% cytoplasmic SC binding (Fig. 13). Such high positivity has not been seen in specimens of PT (16,24). However, we found no significant difference between normal PT and NPT in young children with regard to the J-chain positivity of extra- and intrafollicular IgA-producing immunocytes (89).

Immunological Surface Protection

Although a substantial number of immunocytes in PT produce dimeric IgA, no SC is expressed by epithelial elements in this organ except when it contains occasional small salivary glands (11,26,142). PT should therefore not be considered as a secretory organ. Because SC acts as an epithelial receptor for J-chain-containing dimeric IgA and pentameric IgM, their active external translocation takes place only through SC-positive glandular epithelium (19).

Nevertheless, IgG, IgA, and IgM, in that order, are transferred to the surface of PT, particularly into the crypt lumen, by passive intercellular diffusion through the epithelium (26,142). A plexus of thin-walled small blood vessels is present beneath the crypt epithelium, and many capillaries actually lie within its reticular parts (37). An abundance of extravascular Ig (177), dominated by the IgG isotype, is therefore seen in this area (Fig. 14). It can be inferred that antibodies, both from serum and local immunocytes, permeate the crypt epithelium and contribute to local surface protection.

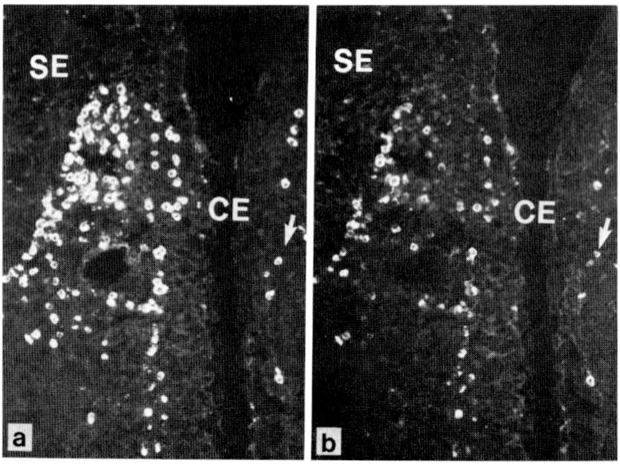

FIG. 13. Immunofluorescence SC-binding test on infiltrate of IgA immunocytes beneath surface (SE) and crypt epithelium (CE) in section of adenoid tissue. Paired staining shows isotype identification [(**a**) fluorescein] and *in vitro* bound SC [(**b**) rhodamine] in same field. With one exception (*arrow*) all SC-positive cells in this field are of the IgA isotype. Note that most of them tend to occur close to the epithelium. [Adapted from ref. 16 (×85).]

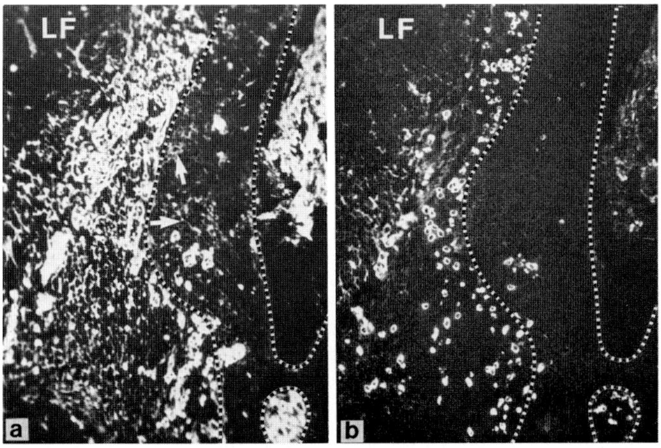

FIG. 14. Immunofluorescence staining for IgG (**a**) and IgA (**b**) in comparable fields from adjacent sections of palatine tonsil. The specimen had been directly fixed in ethanol to preserve diffusible proteins (14,25). Note that large amounts of extracellular IgG tend to mask numerous IgG-producing immunocytes in area between crypt epithelium (outlined by *dashed line*) and lymphoid follicle (LF). Less extracellular IgA is present and most IgA immunocytes are clearly visualized. Traces of intercellular IgG (*arrows*) and some IgG-producing cells occur in reticular crypt epithelium. IgG(and IgA)-positive material is present in crypt lumen on the right ($\times 85$).

By contrast, NPT harbors, to a varying extent, a secretory immune system (88,115); patches of respiratory-type secretory epithelium appearing on the surface and in the crypts of this organ contain SC and IgA in a similar distribution (Fig. 15). This IgA is associated with J chain and is therefore of the secretory type; it often occurs in a granular intracellular pattern along with IgM, signifying their concomitant external translocation (89).

NPT is thus, in part, a secretory immunological organ that contributes directly to the surface protection of the upper respiratory tract. Its output of secretory IgA is most likely of local origin because almost 40% of the extrafollicular IgA immunocytes in NPT are J-chain positive (89) and bind SC *in vitro* (Fig. 13). The IgA cells sometimes accumulate just beneath the SC-positive epithelium (Fig. 15), particularly those with prominent cytoplasmic SC affinity (Fig. 13). Such a spatial interrelationship will conceivably facilitate local secretory immunity.

Relation Between Protection and Pathogenesis of Inflammatory Disease

Wright (184) noted as early as 1906 that inert dust particles of a certain size passed the crypt epithelium of PT, whereas bacteria of the same or even smaller size did not. Such selective exclusion of antigenic material was probably caused mainly by IgG antibodies to the bacteria. IgG antibodies have, in experimental models, been shown to exert specific immune exclusion at epithelial surfaces (156), but increased penetrability for unrelated bystander antigens may develop as

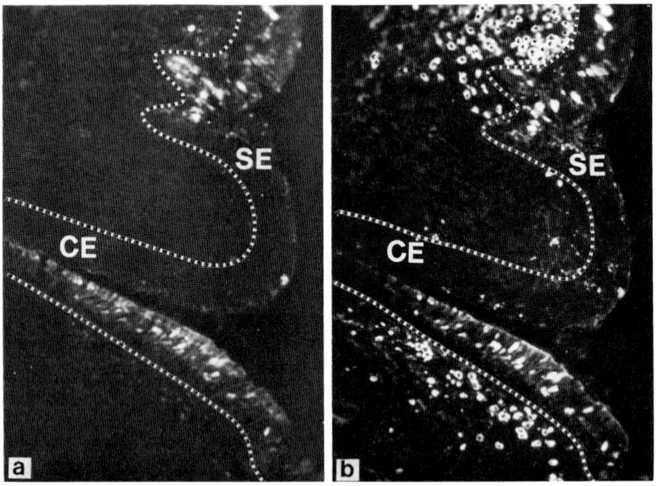

FIG. 15. Paired immunofluorescence staining for SC [(**a**) rhodamine] and IgA [(**b**) fluorescein] in same field from section of directly ethanol-fixed specimen (14,25) of nasopharyngeal tonsil. Surface (SE) and crypt (CE) epithelium are shown (*dashed line*). Note similar distribution of SC and IgA in patches of secretory epithelium. Numerous IgA-producing immunocytes are present beneath these patches (×85).

a side effect (27,97). In this way, immunopathology may evolve locally if IgG-mediated C-dependent protective mechanisms are continuously being maintained in the crypt area.

According to the bacterial-viral etiology of recurrent tonsillitis (RT) proposed by Sprinkle and Veltri (154), relapses are initiated by reactivation of dormant indigenous viruses. One candidate indicated by tonsillar lymphocyte responsiveness is Epstein-Barr virus (185). In view of the above considerations, therefore, it may be postulated that unsuccessful immunological elimination of virus particles results in decreased epithelial barrier function and thereby prepares the ground for a variety of bacteria, including streptococci, *S. aureas, H. influenzae,* and pneumococci. The pathogenesis of RT may thus, in part, have an immunological basis. Moreover, free pneumococcal capsular antigen, taken to reflect immune complexes, has been reported to occur in about 40% of adenoids removed from patients with chronic secretory otitis media (132).

B-Cell Functions Indicated by J-Chain Expression and Antibody Pattern

Generation and Dissemination of Early Memory Clones

Although the immunoregulatory role of surface membrane-associated IgD of B lymphocytes is still obscure, it seems to be important for the propagation of immunological memory (188). The IgD-expressing lymphocytes present in the mantle zones of tonsillar follicles (Fig. 7a) are therefore most likely able to generate memory cells through antigen-driven proliferation. Retained surface IgD is apparently a marker of early memory clones, whereas persistent secondary stimulation seems to result in IgD-negative more mature memory clones with potential for production of antibody of higher affinity (8,65). However, there are controversial opinions with regard to the relationship between IgD expression and clonal affinity maturation (95).

As discussed above, most tonsillar germinal-center cells lack surface IgD, and it is likely that those expressing only IgG largely belong to mature memory clones. Nevertheless, almost 40% of the intrafollicular IgG-producing immunocytes are J-chain positive, which suggests a substantial derivation from early memory clones (13,19). Cells with concomitant production of IgA and J chain are scarce in the germinal centers, whereas about 50% of the relatively numerous extrafollicular IgA immunocytes are J-chain positive (Fig. 12). This observation indicates that extensive isotype switching takes place in an early phase of clonal proliferation and differentiation of tonsillar B cells.

Such a clonal development of tonsillar IgA cells would strengthen the potential of PT and NPT as a putative precursor source for the secretory IgA system, similarly to BALT and GALT. Since a substantial number of tonsillar B cells terminate in the extrafollicular region with concomitant production of IgA and J chain, it seems likely that precursors committed for this phenotype may leave the tonsils and migrate to glandular sites. The observation that *in vitro* secondary stimulation with an alimentary antigen (β-lactoglobulin) resulted mainly in generation of IgA immunocytes from tonsillar lymphoid cells (131) supports the notion that they are integrated with the secretory immune system.

Such an integration is further indicated by a significantly increased number of tonsillar IgA immunocytes producing J-chain-containing dimers in PT of patients with IgA nephropathy (6,46). Moreover, these patients seem to have increased amounts of secretory IgA in their pharyngeal secretions (163). The mesangial deposits of dimeric IgA characteristic of this disease are thought to reflect mucosal IgA responses elicited by infections of the upper respiratory tract; and the patients do have a raised number of circulating B cells that produce dimeric IgA after *in vitro* stimulation (47). However, whether these cells are largely generated in the tonsils or become activated locally after migration into these organs remains to be determined.

Altogether, circumstantial evidence indicates that tonsillar B cells with a potential for J-chain expression may contribute to the secretory immune system in glandular tissues of the upper respiratory tract such as nasal and middle ear mucosa. PT and NPT may indeed contribute significantly to all IgA dimer-producing cell populations of this region and also to the relatively high number of accompanying J-chain-positive IgG and IgD immunocytes (15,21). It is known that B cells, after activation to Ig production, tend to migrate to the blood (118); and the J-chain expression shown by circulating IgG and IgD blasts is similar to that of tonsillar germinal-center cells (13). Moreover, the fact that nasal IgA antibodies show relatively broad specificity (146,176) supports the notion that they are products of B-cell clones in an early phase of maturation.

Expansion of Mature Memory Clones

IgG-committed B cells relatively resistant to T_s effects have been identified in tonsillar suspensions (73). This observation agrees with the fact that more than half of the extrafollicular immunocytes in normal tonsils are of the IgG isotype and lack J chain (89); these cells presumably belong to mature memory clones that have been expanded by proliferation in the tonsillar germinal centers, where about 60% of the IgG-producing immunocytes are J-chain negative (Fig. 12). This fraction most likely gives rise to the extrafollicular J-chain-negative IgG and IgA immunocytes. However, their derivation from J-chain-positive germinal-center cells cannot be excluded because repression of J-chain synthesis has been observed after prolonged stimulation (111).

The J chain is not incorporated into IgG or IgD. In contrast to the situation in IgA and IgM immunocytes, therefore, J chain is not secreted from IgG-producing cells but accumulates intracellularly where it apparently becomes degraded (117); a negative feedback associated with clonal maturation may hence be visualized. Such a mechanism could explain repression of J-chain synthesis in most extrafollicular IgG immunocytes and also in a fraction of the intrafollicular ones since some of the latter are ultrastructurally indistinguishable from mature plasma cells (164). One might expect a similar repression mechanism in IgD-producing cells, but most of the extrafollicular immunocytes of this isotype are J-chain positive (Fig. 12). This fact probably signifies that they are still in an early phase of clonal development. As discussed above, animal experiments have indicated that IgD is expressed by unprimed and early memory B cells but not by the mature ones (9). It is unexpected, however, that almost 40% of the extrafollicular IgM immunocytes lack J chain (Fig. 12). This finding indicates that J-chain repression is unrelated to negative feedback or that a fraction of IgM cells develops by switching from J-chain-negative precursors.

The notion that most tonsillar IgG immunocytes belong to mature memory clones was supported by the antibody response pattern disclosed after secondary stimulation *in vitro;* tonsillar cells obtained from children sensitized parenterally with diphtheria toxoid secreted specific antibody mainly of the IgG class—the IgA class accounted for less than 10%, and the IgM class accounted for less than 1% (135). When the tonsillar cells were obtained from children immunized parenterally with tetanus toxoid, the *in vitro* response resulted mainly in IgG and IgM production, which contrasted strikingly with the predominating secondary IgA response elicited by an alimentary antigen (131). Natural exposure of lymphoepithelial tissues to the latter antigen (β-lactoglobulin) had apparently not afforded sufficiently strong stimulation to induce preferential expansion of corresponding mature memory clones.

ALTERATIONS OF TONSILLAR FUNCTIONS

Age-Associated Changes

On the basis of histological observations of tonsillar lymphoid follicles, Awaya (4) suggested that human PT are functionally most active between the ages 4 and 10 years, with a marked decline after the age of 20 years. Our histomorphometric measurements performed on clinically normal tonsils showed, after the age of 20 years, a significant decrease of the relative area occupied by the follicular mantle zones and an even greater decrease of the reticular crypt epithelium (Table 1). The latter change became apparent at around 14 years of age. In addition, Siegel et al. (149) reported that the number of dendritic accessory cells occurring in the crypt epithelium was largely reduced in adults.

Since the crypt epithelium with its accessory APC is the main route of tonsillar antigen uptake, a relation between its extension of reticulation and the local immunological activity can be expected. We did, in fact, find a progressive increase of the overall numerical density of Ig-producing cells in normal PT up to about the age of 20 years and a marked decrease thereafter (Fig. 16). A similar age-dependent pattern has been reported for tonsillar T cells (148). Nevertheless, the T-to-B-cell ratio seems to be higher in adults than in children (28). Moreover, analysis of tonsillar suspensions has revealed a much smaller fraction of activated B cells in adults than in children (149). Because the tissue weight of PT grows to a maximum in the late teens (148), it seems that PT continues its immunological develop-

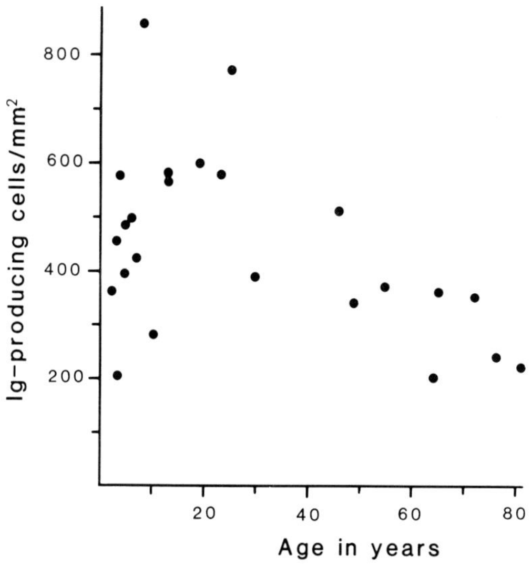

FIG. 16. Scatter diagram of relation (in 24 subjects) between age and overall density of Ig-producing immunocytes (cells/mm^2 section area) in clinically normal palatine tonsils. (Adapted from refs. 26 and 88; reproduced from ref. 17.)

ment until a few years after puberty. Later on, a steady involution takes place, although considerable tonsillar B-cell activity can be seen in clinically healthy PT as late as at 80 years of age (26).

Despite the different densities of Ig-producing cells found in PT of various age groups (Fig. 9), the overall isotype distribution seemed to be fairly independent of age. This held true for all lymphoid compartments, except the reticular epithelium in which the proportion of IgA immunocytes increased from 24% in the younger children to 38% in the older ones, and further increased to 51% in adults (Fig. 9). In the latter age group, moreover, the tonsillar IgA-cell density showed a negative correlation ($r = 0.811$, $p = 0.05$) with the estimated rate of serum IgA synthesis (26). Since IgA is important for immunological homeostasis because of its lack of C-activating properties, regulatory mechanisms may conceivably be reflected in inversely related levels of local and systemic IgA synthesis; local IgA compensation is perhaps particularly marked in the reticular epithelium, where an antiphlogistic effect may be desirable to retard influx of foreign material.

Ishikawa et al. (71) studied both PT and NPT from two groups of children, aged 1 to 4 and 5 to 17 years, respectively. They found a 1.5-fold increase in the overall density of Ig-producing cells in PT from the older group as compared to the younger group; this result agreed well with the 1.7-fold increase noted from 5 to 14 years in Fig. 9. However, the isotype distribution recorded by Ishikawa et al. (71) was quite different from that seen in Fig. 9; they found a slight predominance of IgA cells (40%) in the younger age group and a relatively high overall percentage of IgM cells in both groups (16–21%). The overall age-related increase of Ig-producing cells in NPT was reported to be 2.1-fold—with an even more remarkable change in the IgA-cell percentage than that noted for PT; in the younger group the figure was 58% and in the older group it was 34%. This finding might reflect a more consistent participation of the secretory IgA system in the adenoid B-cell activity at young ages, perhaps due to less extensive metaplastic changes in the covering epithelium. Nevertheless, it is difficult to judge if the study of Ishikawa et al. (71) is representative in terms of immunocyte quantitation since the reported isotype distribution varied substantially from that found in our study of NPT (Fig. 9).

Disease-Associated Changes

Altered Antigen Reception

Histomorphometric comparisons made between normal and diseased tonsillar specimens have revealed only small alterations in the proportions of the four lymphoid compartments (88,160). Both recurrent tonsillitis (RT) and adenoid hyperplasia (AH) lead to a relative increase (1.2- to 1.4-fold) of the extrafollicular area, whereas hyperplastic tonsillitis (HT) and idiopathic tonsillar hyperplasia (ITH) induce virtually no divisional shifts because the individual lymphoid follicles are expanded.

Despite the fact that RT leaves the relative extention of the reticular crypt epithelium fairly unaltered, its antigen-transporting function may be affected in various ways. Maeda et al. (100) reported that shedding of M cells was increased in PT of children—resulting in pores that could allow direct passage of foreign material through the crypt epithelium. Surjan (159) found in older children and adults with RT that the reticular epithelium was largely covered by stratified epithelial cells rather than by M cells and that the remaining M cells had a reduced tubulovesicular transport system. By contrast, M cells were well developed in the crypts of healthy canine PT, and the reticular epithelium likewise seemed to be normal in three young children (3–6 years old) with RT. It is interesting that *in vivo* lymphocyte activation, as suggested by increased nuclear birefringence, was demonstrated only in tonsillar suspensions from these three patients (159). In older children and adults with RT, therefore, lack of appropriate lymphocyte stimulation was tentatively ascribed to alterations in the reticular epithelium.

Altered B-Cell Activity

The possibility that tonsillar disease is associated with reduced activation of the local B-cell system was likewise suggested by our immunohistochemical observations of Ig-producing immunocytes. In patients with RT, the density of such cells in germinal centers and extrafollicular areas was markedly and progressively reduced above the age of about 10 years (Fig. 17). This decrease affected IgG, IgA, and IgM cells fairly equally on a relative basis, so the isotype proportions were virtually unaltered (160). Only the number of IgD immunocytes remained normal or tended to be increased.

The reduced overall activation of the tonsillar B-cell system above 10 years of age (Fig. 17) contrasted with the elevated serum Ig levels in this group of RT patients (160). The latter finding showed that their immune system was, in fact, exposed to an increased antigen burden—presumably of microbial nature (154). A negative correlation ($r = 0.720$, $p < 0.05$) between the estimated rate of synthesis of serum IgA and the tonsillar density of IgA immunocytes indicated a local compensatory mechanism as discussed above in relation to age-associated changes.

Below the age of 10 years, RT affected the tonsillar density of Ig-producing cells to a much lesser degree (Fig. 17). The density rather tended to be increased in the germinal centers, particularly with regard to IgG-producing cells (88). The latter feature suggested intensified B-cell stimulation, in contrast to the situation in older children or adults. Taking the histomorphometric data into account, the decreased extrafollicular immunocyte density in young children might, at least in part, be explained by inflammatory expansion of the tissue volume; but this explanation could not fully account for the markedly reduced tonsillar density of Ig-producing cells associated with RT above the age of 10 years.

HT and ITH, which occur mainly in young children, were found to be associated with tonsillar changes of Ig-producing cells principally like those described for RT (160). Thus, the overall reductions in immunocyte density were compara-

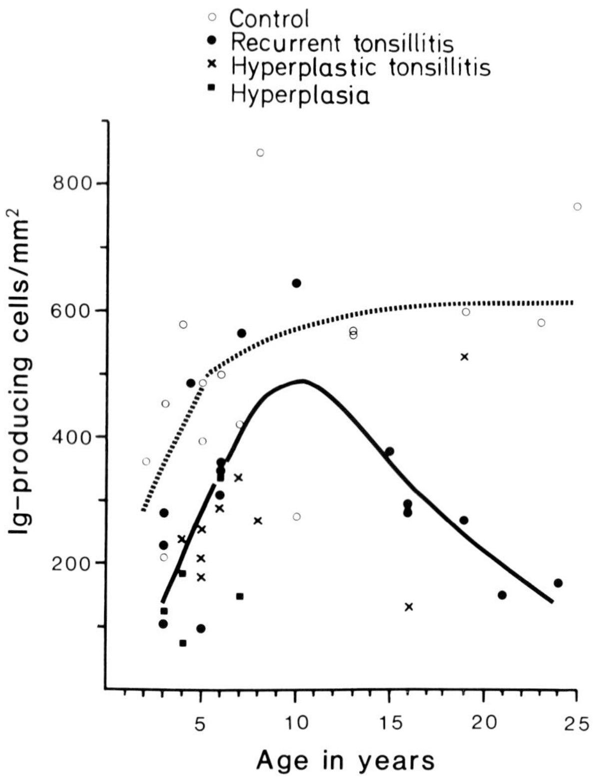

FIG. 17. Scatter diagram of relation between subject age and overall density of Ig-producing immunocytes (cells/mm^2 section area) in palatine tonsils categorized according to clinical state. Dashed and solid curves are arbitrarily drawn to indicate apparent trends for clinically normal controls and recurrent tonsillitis, respectively. (Adapted from refs. 160 and 88; reproduced from ref. 17.)

ble at low age regardless of the category of tonsillar disease (Fig. 17). Sugiyama et al. (157) were likewise unable to show any difference between RT and HT with regard to tonsillar T-cell characteristics. Nevertheless, in contrast to the increased germinal-center activity observed in RT below 10 years of age, the density of Ig-producing cells in this compartment tended to be decreased in HT and was indeed strikingly reduced in ITH. This finding probably reflected that immunological stimulation by microbial antigens is not involved in the pathogenesis of tonsillar hyperplasia to the same extent as in RT.

Maturity of B Cells in Tonsillitis and Adenoid Hyperplasia

In RT of young children, tonsillar B-cell stimulation seems to result mainly in expansion of mature memory clones; this was indicated both by a significant shift to a more marked IgG expression in the germinal centers (88) and by a strikingly reduced J-chain production by intra- and extrafollicular IgA immunocytes (Fig. 12). Cytoplasmic J chain likewise tended to be decreased in intrafollicular IgD immunocytes (90), perhaps reflecting a particular link between IgA and IgD in tonsillar B-cell differentiation as discussed above.

Altogether, an increased burden of microbial antigens in the crypts apparently gives rise to strong stimulation of tonsillar B cells in RT as long as the reticular epithelium is fairly normal. However, exaggerated shedding of M cells probably facilitates direct influx rather than specialized epithelial delivery of antigenic material; the consequence may be altered antigen presentation favoring expansion of mature B-cell clones with decreased J-chain-expressing potential. In addition, regulatory T cells particularly needed for expansion of early B-cell clones are perhaps relatively few in inflamed tonsils. Lack of certain T_h cells has indeed been indicated by studies of suspensions made from diseased PT (5), and an increased proportion of tonsillar cells with the CD8 (putative T_s) phenotype has been noted immunohistochemically in adults with RT (186).

NPT of young children afflicted with AH tended to show an increased density of Ig-producing cells, particularly in the extrafollicular area where the number of IgG immunocytes was significantly raised (88). There was also a significantly increased expression of this isotype in the intrafollicular population of Ig-producing cells. Thus, the enhanced stimulation of the adenoid B-cell system seems to generate both early and late memory clones since J-chain expression was only slightly reduced in germinal-center cells and was virtually unaltered in extrafollicular IgA immunocytes (90).

In contrast to the situation in RT, therefore, the particular immunoregulatory conditions necessary for maintenance of early memory B cells seems to be well preserved in AH. The reason is most likely that the reticular epithelium with its specialized APC is less affected by inflammation in NPT than in PT, although this possibility remains to be studied. Nevertheless, the disproportionate change toward IgG production in AH may be of pathogenetic importance and may perhaps, in part, explain disease persistency through immunopathological mechanisms as discussed in a previous section.

Immunodeficiency

Some studies have indicated that a slight deficiency of serum IgA may underlie RT and predispose to infection, especially with *H. influenzae* (39,43,128). Østergaard (127) claimed, moreover, that in 30% of the patients such a deficiency might be manifested in the tonsils by a complete lack of IgA-producing cells. Also, Nezelof et al. (121) reported absence of tonsillar IgA, IgG, and IgM cells in 17% of young children with HT, despite the concurrent presence of normal Ig levels in serum. If these findings were obtained with representative tissue specimens, they are clearly different from our results, which showed a decreased density but never an absence of Ig-producing cells in diseased PT (Fig. 9).

Allergy

Controversy prevails with regard to the occurrence of IgE-producing immunocytes in diseased tonsils. Since the original report describing a remarkably high number of such cells (161), others have published similar findings (37,96). Conversely, Ishikawa et al. (71) found only a small number of IgE-positive cells, which, however, were observed in 28% of diseased specimens. Østergaard (127) found such cells in PT from 40% of children with RT and claimed that their presence, particularly in conjunction with a slight IgA deficiency, might indicate subsequent development of atopic allergy (129). Moreover, Ali et al. (1,2) reported, on the basis of immunoenzyme staining, that PT and NPT from patients with inhalant allergy contained a strikingly large number of plasma cells with cytoplasmic IgE.

In our immunofluorescence studies, IgE-producing immunocytes were virtually undetectable in diseased PT and NPT (88,160), and a similar observation was made by Pesak (134). Tissue culture studies have likewise failed to reveal tonsillar IgE production (135). We believe that methodological difficulties should be seriously considered in immunohistochemical studies of IgE-producing cells (20). In addition to unwanted staining artifacts, there is the possibility of interpreting IgE-positive mast cells as immunocytes. Feltkamp-Vroom et al. (51) found, in both PT and NPT of an atopic patient, that mast cells were intensely stained for IgE. In a large immunofluorescence study of adenoids from children, Loesel (98) reported that the presence of IgE-positive mast cells afforded a sensitivity of 58% and a specificity of 89% for allergic disease, as defined by traditional criteria. It is possible that such sensitized mast cells may contribute to local immediate type of hypersensitivity reactions.

Loesel (98) also reported that some of the NPT specimens contained IgE-producing plasma cells in large numbers; but this finding needs verification in view of the methodological difficulties mentioned above. As discussed elsewhere (17,18), the mast cells are not necessarily armed by locally produced IgE but may, instead, acquire IgE in regional lymph nodes and subsequently return to the mucosal tissue. It is possible that these armed mast cells may release IgE locally and contribute to IgE antibodies detected in nasopharyngeal secretions. Welliver et al. (180) have speculated that such antibodies to respiratory syncytial virus may intensify infectious disease of the upper airways.

Changing Functions of Palatine Tonsils—a Hypothetical Scheme

The information discussed above allows visualization of certain age- and disease-associated functional changes of PT (Fig. 18). In healthy young children, the tonsillar germinal centers support a significant proliferation of early memory B cells which contribute to the IgD-expressing mantle zone lymphocytes. The expanding clones, in addition, generate precursor cells that partly terminate locally as extrafollicular J-chain-positive IgA immunocytes and partly migrate via the general circulation to secretory sites of the upper respiratory tract.

The J-chain-expressing potential of these early memory clones is mandatory for the formation of IgA dimers, which can combine with epithelial SC and thereby become transported to the exocrine fluids of the upper respiratory tract as secretory IgA. The microenvironmental conditions necessary for tonsillar proliferation of such clones may depend both on antigen presentation by M cells found in the reticular crypt epithelium and on particular subsets of regulatory T cells.

Nevertheless, normal tonsils are, to an even higher degree, involved in generation of mature memory B-cell clones as evidenced by the predominance of extrafollicular J-chain-negative IgG and IgA immunocytes. This activity is disproportionately enhanced in young children afflicted with RT (Fig. 18). A significant consequence is decreased maintenance of those early clones that may contribute to secretory immunity of the upper respiratory tract. The putative role of the tonsils as a precursor source for the secretory immune system is thus jeopardized by tonsillar disease. Further study needs to be done to determine if such a development is reflected by less IgD expression in the mantle zone of tonsillar lymphoid follicles.

The mechanisms underlying this disease-associated shift in tonsillar function are most likely related to immunoregulatory alterations. Increased shedding of M cells

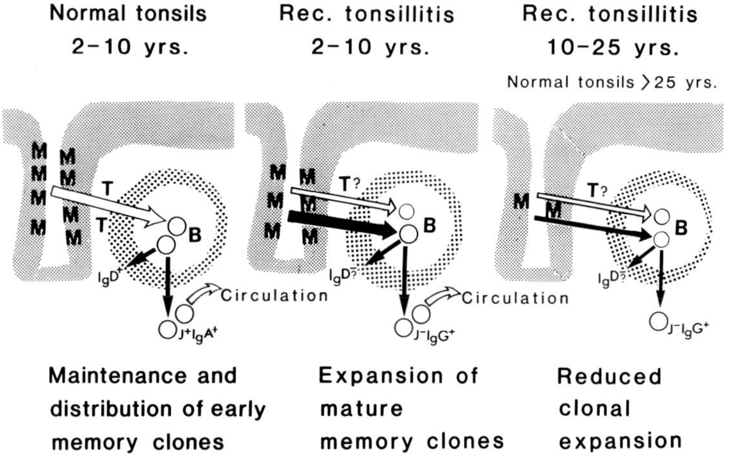

FIG. 18. Hypothetical scheme for age- and disease-associated changes of immunologic functions of palatine tonsils. Tissue elements of particular interest in this scheme are: M cells (M), whose number may decrease in the reticular parts of the crypt epithelium; T lymphocytes (T), whose immunoregulatory functions may become defective owing to lack of certain subsets of helper cells (T?); IgD-bearing (IgD^+) B lymphocytes in mantle zone of lymphoid follicles, which may express less of this isotype (IgD^-?) as a result of disproportionate expansion of mature memory clones; and J-chain-positive IgA-producing (J^+IgA^+) and J-chain-negative IgG-producing (J^-IgG^+) B cells, which, in addition to being retained in the extrafollicular compartment, may become disseminated to the general circulation. Differentiation to the latter phenotype is favored by expansion of mature memory clones. Such a development may be related to reduced antigen presentation by M cells (*graded open large arrows*) and more direct passage of foreign material through crypt epithelium (*graded filled large arrows*) along with changed T-cell functions (T?). At higher age, decreased entrance of antigenic material into the tonsils results in reduced expansion of both early and mature memory B-cell clones. Further details are discussed in the text. (From ref. 17.)

will change the way in which foreign material is presented to be lymphoid tissue, and more direct passage through the reticular epithelium will conceivably result in enhanced engagement of nonepithelial APC. The latter may, through antigen processing and presentation, preferentially stimulate particular T_h cells that favor the expansion of mature, rather than early, B-cell clones.

In older children and adults with RT, expansion of both early and mature memory clones seems to be decreased. This development is indicated by reduced numbers of Ig-producing cells in the intra- and extrafollicular tonsillar compartments and by absence of increased nuclear birefringence of tonsillar lymphocytes. In addition to possible changes in T_h subsets, the underlying mechanism may be the decreased passage of antigens into the tonsils. First, the number of active M cells is largely reduced in RT of these age groups and, second, direct influx of foreign material is probably hampered as the reticular epithelium becomes covered by a stratified and partly keratinized lining. Similar changes occur in clinically normal tonsils above 25 years of age (Fig. 18).

Altogether, inflammatory conditions continuing after the age of about 10 years seem to accelerate the aging process of PT. However, RT may significantly change the immunological competence of PT even before that age. The observed alterations may be irreversible since they were revealed in periods when the patients had been without inflammatory symptoms for at least 4 weeks (88,90,160). Altered immunological function may, in fact, contribute to recurrence of RT, and a vicious cycle may thereby develop. Nevertheless, considerable immunological activity persists in diseased tonsils, so the functional changes cannot by themselves justify surgical removal of these organs.

POSSIBLE CONNECTION BETWEEN TONSILLAR FUNCTION AND IMMUNOLOGICAL DEFENSE

Systemic Defense

The question as to whether removal of the tonsils may compromise immunological protection of the upper respiratory tract—and perhaps produce long-term adverse effects on the immune system in general—is the subject of a continuing debate (178). Numerous epidemiological studies have reported discrepant results with regard to disease susceptibility after tonsillectomy. Thus, the possibility of a causal relation to Hodgkin's disease was refuted by Johnson and Johnson (76), questioned by Gutensohn et al. (62), and considered positively by Vianna et al. (172), but was again refuted by Silingardi et al. (150). With regard to mononucleosis, tonsillectomy seems to afford some protection, probably because a target for Epstein-Barr virus infection is removed (59,158). Conversely, the observation that this operation had been performed in 80% of patients with Hashimoto's disease and in 66% of those with thyrotoxicosis (112) may reflect a role of the tonsils in maintaining immunological homeostasis. It cannot be excluded, however, that a common immunoregulatory defect predisposes for both thyroid and tonsillar disease.

Similar difficulties are encountered with regard to the interpretation of associations between low serum Ig levels and tonsillectomy. In a large study of a female population, Wingerd and Sponzilli (183) found that those with a history of this operation had a significantly reduced gamma globulin fraction in serum. A low serum level of IgA has likewise been reported to be associated with previous tonsillectomy (39,175). Conversely, other studies have shown that patients undergoing tonsillectomy may have a significantly reduced concentration of IgA in serum before this operation (43,128). Nevertheless, two studies have demonstrated directly that tonsillectomy may, in fact, lead to reduced serum Ig levels (75,128).

Defense of the Upper Respiratory Tract

A significant decrease of salivary IgA throughout an observation period of several months was reported in a recent study by Jeschke and Ströder (75). Moreover, in patients with mononucleosis affecting the tonsils, the salivary levels of secretory IgA were found to be markedly reduced (102). These findings are in keeping with the classic report of Ogra (123) on IgA antibodies to poliovirus in nasopharyngeal secretions of children previously immunized perorally with live vaccine; after removal of both PT and NPT, the pre-existing average titers decreased 3- to 4-fold, and in some children no antibody could be detected. Attempts to vaccinate a seronegative group of children who had been subjected to tonsillectomy and adenoidectomy resulted in a delayed and poor nasopharyngeal secretory IgA response.

These immunological observations are in harmony with numerous earlier epidemiological studies demonstrating increased incidence of paralytic poliomyelitis after combined removal of PT and NPT (reviewed by Ogra in ref. 123). Also, it has recently been reported that there is an increased meningococcal carrier rate after tonsillectomy (93). Decreased nasopharyngeal resistance may, in part, be explained by reduced output of secretory IgA directly from NPT. However, the balance of evidence indicates that tonsillar immunological activity reinforces the whole secretory IgA system of the upper respiratory tract; combined tonsillectomy and adenoidectomy may therefore result in a more extensive defect involving the defense of distant mucosae such as that of the middle ear.

Generation of B cells belonging to early memory clones is the basis for a putative tonsillar reinforcement of secretory immunity beyond the epithelial lining of NPT, as discussed above. Some of these cells probably become disseminated to glandular sites of the upper respiratory tract where differentiation takes place mainly to immunocytes producing dimeric IgA.

We have proposed (23) that differentiation to IgA immunocytes of the secretory immune system may follow alternative pathways (Fig. 19). There is much evidence indicating that murine Peyer's patch cells can undergo T_h-cell-regulated switching directly from IgM to IgA expression (78–80); observations on human B cells have suggested that this pathway leads preferentially to IgA2 production (35). Secretory sites seeded mainly with precursors from Peyer's patches and other parts of GALT may hence show preferential accumulation of IgA2 immunocytes, as observed by us for the distal intestinal tract (81). Conversely, antigen- or mitogen-

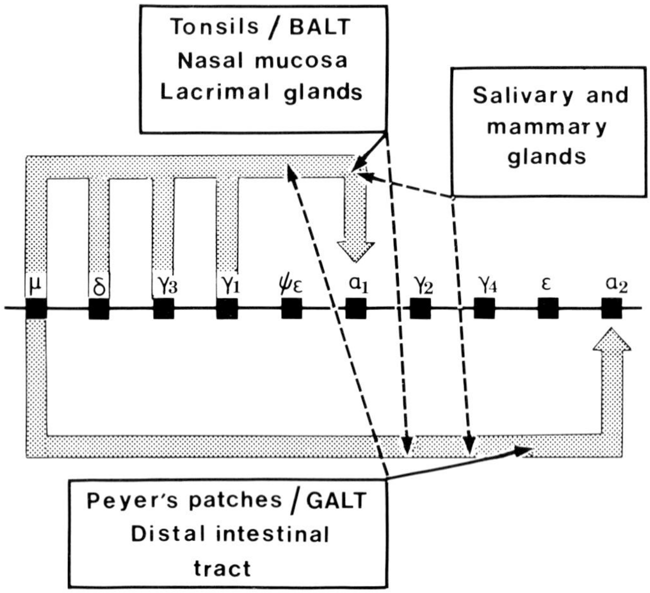

FIG. 19. Putative B-cell switching pathways leading to preferential production of IgA1 or IgA2 in the secretory immune system. This hypothetical scheme is based on the sequence of human Ig constant heavy-chain (C_H) genes (53). It is proposed that sequential switching is preferred in tonsillar tissue and BALT, whereas direct switching from μ to $\alpha 2$ is preferred in GALT. The importance of these two pathways for the development of immunocyte populations in representative types of various secretory tissues is indicated: preferential (*solid arrows*); subsidiary (*broken arrows*). Salivary and mammary glands apparently are in an intermediate position, probably because they are seeded with precursor cells in similar numbers from BALT and GALT. (Adapted from ref. 23.)

driven sequential B-cell switching (31), or differentiation regulated by T_h cells promoting switching from expression of IgM and IgD to IgG and IgA (105), might be expected to lead mainly to IgA1 production. Predominant accumulation of IgG1- and IgA1-producing cells is a common feature of tonsils and nasal mucosa (23,81) and may signify a vectorial link in the regional immunocyte development (Fig. 19).

This scheme fits with our previously proposed dichotomy of the secretory immune system; the J-chain-positive IgD- and IgG-producing cells found in nasal mucosa (15,21) may thus be considered as ''spin-off'' from the sequential differentiation process indicated to be the preferential development in BALT, tonsils, and mucosae of the upper respiratory tract (Fig. 19). It is interesting in this connection that IgD-producing cells seem to be relatively numerous in inflamed middle ear mucosa (153). Salivary and mammary glands probably receive precursor cells in similar numbers from GALT and tonsils/BALT (Fig. 19) and are hence in an intermediate position, both with regard to frequency of IgD immunocytes (15,21) and accumulation of IgA1- and IgA2-producing cells (81).

Although studies in IgA-deficient subjects generally have supported the proposed scheme for B-cell differentiation (21), it has recently appeared that large individual variations probably exist with regard to involvement of the vectorial IgD/IgG-expressing pathway and the direct IgM-expressing pathway in the development of nasal secretory immunity (22). This observation may reflect that GALT in some—but not in all—individuals contribute a substantial fraction of the B cells normally terminating with IgA production in the upper respiratory tract mucosa. Speculations about the possible role of such individual variations for mucosal defense and the clinical condition of the upper airways (22) are schematically depicted in Fig. 20.

Altogether, the putative role of PT and NPT as active immunological organs—generally reinforcing mucosal immunity of the whole upper respiratory tract—should be seriously considered before a child is subjected to tonsillectomy and adenoidectomy. Moreover, the relative role of GALT, BALT, and the tonsils as precursor sources for the secretory immune system must be better defined to aid the development of efficient vaccines and their administration.

ACKNOWLEDGMENTS

Studies in the author's laboratory have been supported by the Norwegian Research Council for Science and the Humanities, the Norwegian Cancer Society, Anders Jahre's Foundation, and the Norwegian Society for Fighting Cancer. Thanks are due to Ms. Hege Eliassen for invaluable help in the preparation of this manuscript, to the Phototechnical Department of the National Hospital for expert assistance with the illustrations, and to Dr. David Y. Mason, University of Oxford, Oxford, England, for some of the reagents used for immunoenzyme staining with alkaline phosphatase.

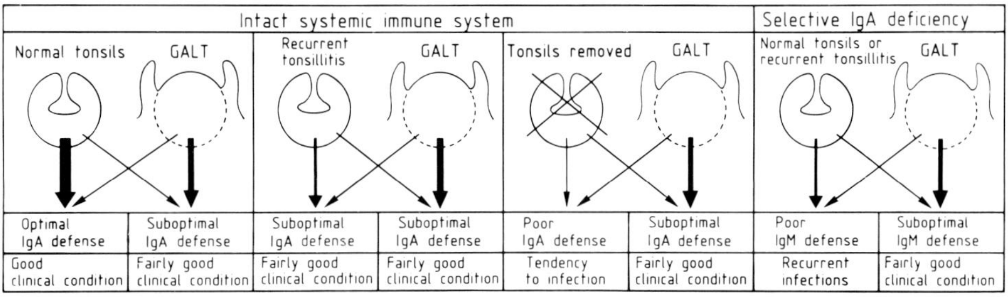

FIG. 20. Schematic depiction of speculations about how the clinical condition of the upper respiratory tract beyond the tonsils may depend on individual variations in the magnitude of the supply to the regional secretory tissues of stimulated B cells (*graded arrows*) derived from tonsils or GALT. It is suggested that in subjects with an intact immune system the secretory antibody defense of this region is better when most stimulated B cells come from the tonsils, whereas in IgA deficiency it is better when most such cells come from GALT because secretory IgA in that case is more likely to be replaced, to some extent, by protective secretory IgM. The same may be the case when the tonsillar source of IgA-producing cells has been removed surgically.

REFERENCES

1. Ali, M., Fayemi, A.O., and Nalebuff, D.J. (1979): Localization of IgE in adenoids and tonsils. *Arch. Otolaryngol.*, 105:695–697.
2. Ali, M., Mesa-Tejada, R., Fayemi, A.O., Nalebuff, D.J., and Connell, J.T. (1979): Localization of IgE in tissues by an immunoperoxidase technique. *Arch. Pathol. Lab. Med.*, 103:274–275.
3. Anderson, J.C. (1974): The response of the tonsil and associated lymph nodes of gnotobiotic piglets to the presence of bacterial antigen in the oral cavity. *J. Anat.*, 117:191–198.
4. Awaya, K. (1969): The aging of the secondary nodules in relation to the postnatal development and involution of the human palatine tonsils. *Acta Haematol. Jap.*, 32:127–134.
5. Baumöhl, Z., Kellerhals, B., Stolp, W., and Lefkovits, I. (1977): Antibody formation by human tonsil cells in vitro. *Clin. Exp. Immunol.*, 28:116–122.
6. Bene, M.C., Faure, G., Hurault de Ligny, B., Kessler, M., and Duheille, J. (1983): Immunoglobulin A nephropathy. Quantitative immunohistomorphometry of the tonsillar plasma cells evidences an inversion of the immunoglobulin A versus immunoglobulin G secreting cell balance. *J. Clin. Invest.*, 71:1342–1347.
7. Bienenstock, J. (1985): Bronchus-associated lymphoid tissue. *Int. Arch. Allergy Appl. Immunol.* 76:62–69.
8. Black, S.J., Tokuhisa, T., Herzenberg, L.A., and Herzenberg, L.A. (1980): Memory B cells at successive stages of differentiation: expression of surface IgD and capacity for self renewal. *Eur. J. Immunol.*, 10:846–851.
9. Black, S.J., Van Der Loo, W., Loken, M.R., and Herzenberg, L.A. (1978): Expression of IgD by murine lymphocytes. Loss of surface IgD indicates maturation of memory B cells. *J. Exp. Med.*, 147:984–996.
10. Bogger-Goren, S., Bernstein, J.M., Gershon, A.A., and Ogra, P.L. (1984): Mucosal cell-mediated immunity to varicella zoster virus: role in protection against disease. *J. Pediatr.*, 105:195–199.
11. Brandtzaeg, P. (1973): Two types of IgA immunocytes in man. *Nature (New Biol. London)*, 243:142–143.
12. Brandtzaeg, P. (1974): Presence of J-chain in human immunocytes containing various immunoglobulin classes. *Nature (London)*, 252:418–420.
13. Brandtzaeg, P. (1976): Studies on J chain and binding site for secretory component in circulating human B cells. II. The cytoplasm. *Clin. Exp. Immunol.*, 25:59–66.
14. Brandtzaeg, P. (1982): Tissue preparation methods for immunohistochemistry. In: *Techniques in Immunocytochemistry*, edited by G.R. Bullock and P. Petrusz, pp. 1–75. Academic Press, London.
15. Brandtzaeg, P. (1983): The secretory immune system of lactating human mammary glands compared with other exocrine glands. *Ann. NY Acad. Sci.*, 409:353–381.
16. Brandtzaeg, P. (1983): Immunohistochemical characterization of intracellular J chain and binding site for secretory component (SC) in human immunoglobulin(Ig)-producing cells. *Molec. Immunol.*, 23:941–966.
17. Brandtzaeg, P. (1984): Immune functions of human nasal mucosa and tonsils in health and disease. In: *Immunology of the Lung and Upper Respiratory Tract*, edited by J. Bienenstock, pp. 28–95. McGraw-Hill, New York.
18. Brandtzaeg, P. (1985): Research in gastrointestinal immunology—state of the art. *Scand. J. Gastroenterol.* (Suppl. 114), 20:137–156.
19. Brandtzaeg, P. (1985): Role of J chain and secretory component in receptor-mediated glandular and hepatic transport of immunoglobulins in man. *Scand. J. Immunol.*, 22:111–146.
20. Brandtzaeg, P., and Baklien, K. (1976): Inconclusive immunohistochemistry of human IgE in mucosal pathology. *Lancet*, 1:1297–1298.
21. Brandtzaeg, P., Gjeruldsen, S.T., Korsrud, F., Baklien, K., Berdal, P., and Ek, J. (1979): The human secretory immune system shows striking heterogeneity with regard to involvement of J chain-positive IgD immunocytes. *J. Immunol.*, 122:503–510.
22. Brandtzaeg, P., Karlsson, G., Hansson, G., Petruson, B., Björkander, J., and Hanson, L.Å. (1987): The chemical condition of IgA-deficient patients is related to the proportion of IgD- and IgM-producing cells in their nasal mucosa. *Clin. Exp. Immunol. (in press)*.
23. Brandtzaeg, P., Kett, K., Rognum, T.O., Söderström, R., Björkander, J., Söderström, T., Pe-

truson, B., and Hanson, L.A. (1986): The distribution of mucosal IgA and IgG subclass-producing immunocytes and alterations in various disorders. *Monogr. Allergy,* 20:174–194.

24. Brandtzaeg, P., and Korsrud, F.R. (1984): Significance of different J chain profiles in human tissues: generation of IgA and IgM with binding site for secretory component is related to the J chain expressing capacity of the total local immunocyte population, including IgG and IgD producing cells, and depends on the clinical state of the tissue. *Clin. Exp. Immunol.*, 58:709–718.
25. Brandtzaeg, P., and Rognum, T.O. (1983): Evaluation of tissue preparation methods and paired immunofluorescence staining for immunocytochemistry of lymphomas. *Histochem. J.*, 15:655–689.
26. Brandtzaeg, P., Surjan, L., and Berdal, P. (1978): Immunoglobulin systems of human tonsils. I. Control subjects of various ages: quantification of Ig-producing cells, tonsillar morphometry, and serum Ig-concentrations. *Clin. Exp. Immunol.*, 31:367–381.
27. Brandtzaeg, P., and Tolo, K. (1977): Mucosal penetrability enhanced by serum-derived antibodies. *Nature (London)*, 266:262–263.
28. Brochier, J., Samarut, C., Bich-Thuy, L.T., and Revillard, J.P. (1978): Study of human T and B lymphocytes with heterologous antisera. IV. Subpopulations in tonsil and adenoid cell suspensions. *Immunology*, 35:827–835.
29. Butcher, E.C., Rouse, R.V., Coffman, R.L., Nottenburg, C.N., Hardy, R.R., and Weissman, I.L. (1982): Surface phenotype of Peyer's patch germinal center cells: implications for the role of germinal centers in B cell differentiation. *J. Immunol.*, 129:2698–2707.
30. Butcher, E.C., Stevens, S.K., Reichert, R.A., Scollay, R.G., and Weissman, I.L. (1982): Lymphocyte-endothelial cell recognition in lymphocyte migration and segregation of mucosal and nonmucosal immunity. In: *Recent Advances in Mucosal Immunity*, edited by W. Strober, L.Å. Hanson, and K.W. Sell, pp. 3–24. Raven Press, New York.
31. Cebra, J.J., Fuhrman, J.A., Horsfall, D.J., and Shahin, R.D. (1982): Natural and deliberate priming of IgA responses to bacterial antigens by the mucosal route. In: *Seminars in Infectious Disease, Vol. 4, Baterial Vaccines*, edited by J.B. Robbins, J.C. Hill, and J.C. Sadoff, pp. 6–12. Thieme-Stratton, New York.
32. Chin, Y.-H., Rasmussen, R., Cakiroglu, A.G., and Woodruff, J.J. (1984): Lymphocyte recognition of lymph node high endothelium. VI. Evidence of distinct structures mediating binding to high endothelial cells of lymph nodes and Peyer's patches. *J. Immunol.*, 133:2961–2965.
33. Christmas, S.E., Allan, G., and Moore, M. (1985): Naturally cytotoxic tonsillar leukocytes: phenotypic characterization of the effector population. *Scand. J. Immunol.*, 22:61–71.
34. Coico, R.F., Xue, B., Wallace, D., Pernis, B., Siskind, G.W., and Thorbecke, G.J. (1985): T cells with receptors for IgD. *Nature (London)*, 316:744–746.
35. Conley, M.E., and Bartelt, M.S. (1984): In vitro regulation of IgA subclass synthesis. II. The source of IgA2 plasma cells. *J. Immunol.*, 133:2312–2316.
36. Crabbé, P.A., and Heremans, J.F. (1967): Distribution in human nasopharyngeal tonsils of plasma cells containing different types of immunoglobulin polypeptide chains. *Lab. Invest.*, 16:112–123.
37. Curran, R.C., and Jones, E.L. (1977): Immunoglobulin-containing cells in human tonsils as demonstrated by immunohistochemistry. *Clin. Exp. Immunol.*, 28:103–115.
38. Curran, R.C., and Jones, E.L. (1978): The lymphoid follicles of the human palatine tonsil. *Clin. Exp. Immunol.*, 31:251–259.
39. D'Amelio, R.D., Palmisano, L., Le Moli, S., Seminara, R., and Aiuti, F. (1982): Serum and salivary IgA levels in normal subjects: comparison between tonsillectomized and nontonsillectomized subjects. *Int. Arch. Allergy Appl. Immunol.*, 68:256–259.
40. Davis, D.J. (1912): On plasma cells in the tonsils. *J. Infect. Dis.*, 10:142–161.
41. Delespesse, G., Duchateau, J., Gausset, P., and Govaerts, A. (1976): In vitro response of subpopulations of human tonsil lymphocytes. I. Cellular collaboration in the proliferative response to PHA and Con A. *J. Immunol.*, 116:437–445.
42. DeWolf, W.C., Schlossman, S.F., and Yunis, E.J. (1979): DRw antisera react with activated T cells. *J. Immunol.*, 122:1780–1784.
43. Donovan, R., and Soothill, J.F. (1973): Immunological studies in children undergoing tonsillectomy. *Clin. Exp. Immunol.*, 14:347–357.
44. Drucker, M.M., Agatsuma, Y., Drucker, I., Neter, E., Bernstein, J., and Ogra, P.L. (1979): Cell-mediated immune response to bacterial products in human tonsils and peripheral blood lymphocytes. *Infect. Immun.*, 23:347–352.
45. Dvoretsky, P., Wood, G.S., Levy, R., and Warnke, R.A. (1982): T-lymphocyte subsets in fol-

licular lymphomas compared with those in non-neoplastic lymph nodes and tonsils. *Hum. Pathol.*, 13:618–625.

46. Egido, J., Blasco, R., Lozano, L., Sancho, J., and Garcia-Hoyo, R. (1984): Immunological abnormalitis in the tonsils of patients with IgA nephropathy: inversion in the ratio of IgA:IgG bearing lymphocytes and increased polymeric IgA synthesis. *Clin. Exp. Immunol.*, 57:101–106.
47. Egido, J., Blasco, R., Sancho, J., Lozano, L., Sanchez-Crespo, M., and Hernando, L. (1982): Increased rates of polymeric IgA synthesis by circulating lymphoid cells in IgA mesangial glomerulonephritis. *Clin. Exp. Immunol.*, 47:309–316.
48. Ennas, M.G., Murru, M.R., Bistrusso, A., Cadeddu, G., Tore, G., and Manconi, P.E. (1984): Lymphocyte subsets in human adenoids and tonsils. Rosette formation, alpha-naphthyl acetate esterase cytochemistry, monoclonal antibodies and peanut lectin reactivity. *Immunol. Lett.*, 8:1–9.
49. Enriquez-Rincon, F., Andrew, E., Parkhouse, R.M.E., and Klaus, G.G.B. (1984): Suppression of follicular trapping of antigen-antibody complexes in mice treated with anti-IgM or anti-IgD antibodies from birth. *Immunology*, 53:713–719.
50. Falk, P., and Mootz, W. (1973): Morphologische Untersuchungen zur Reticulierung des Tonsillenepithels. *Acta Otolaryngol.*, 75:85–103.
51. Feltkamp-Vroom, T.M., Stallman, P.J., Aalberse, R.C., and Reerink-Brongers, E.E. (1975): Immunofluorescence studies on renal tissue, tonsils, adenoids, nasal polyps, and skin of atopic and nonatopic patients, with special reference to IgE. *Clin. Immunol. Immunopathol.*, 4:392–404.
52. Ferrarini, M., Viale, G., Risso, A., and Pernis, B. (1976): A study of the immunoglobulin classes present on the membrane and in the cytoplasm of human tonsil plasma cells. *Eur. J. Immunol.*, 6:562–565.
53. Flanagan, J.G., and Rabbits, T.H. (1982): Arrangement of human immunoglobulin heavy chain constant region genes implies evolutionary duplication of a segment containing γ, ε, and α genes. *Nature (London)*, 300:709–713.
54. Freijd, A., and Rynnel-Dagöö, B. (1982): Aspects on the immunological function of the adenoid tissue. *Acta Otolarynol.* (Suppl.), 386:127–128.
55. Friedmann, I., Michaels, L., Gerwat, J., and Bird, E.S. (1972): The microscopic anatomy of the nasopharyngeal tonsil by light and electron microscopy. *ORL J. Otorhinolaryngol. Relat. Spec.*, 34:195–209.
56. Gazit, E., Mizrahi, Y., Orgad, S., Efter, T., Lewenstein, M., and Ostfeld, E. (1979): HLA, DRW (IA-like) and additional surface antigens expressed on adenoid T and B lymphocytes. *Vox. Sang.*, 37:193–200.
57. Gearhart, P.J., and Cebra, J.J. (1979): Differentiated B lymphocytes. Potential to express particular antibody variable and constant regions depends on site of lymphoid tissue and antigen load. *J. Exp. Med.*, 149:216–227.
58. Gearhart, P.J., and Cebra, J.J. (1981): Most B cells that have switched surface immunoglobulin isotypes generate clones of cells that do not secrete IgM. *J. Immunol.*, 127:1030–1034.
59. Goode, R.L., and Coursey, D.L. (1976): Tonsillectomy and infectious mononucleosis—a possible relationship. *Laryngoscope*, 86:992–995.
60. Guidos, C., Wong, M., and Lee, K.-C. (1984): A comparison of the stimulatory activities of lymphoid dendritic cells and macrophages in T proliferative responses to various antigens. *J. Immunol.*, 133:1179–1184.
61. Gupta, S., Pahwa, R., Siegal, F.P., and Geod, R.A. (1977): Rosette formation with mouse erythrocytes. IV. T, B and third population cells in human tonsils. *Clin. Exp. Immunol.*, 28:347–351.
62. Gutensohn, N., Li, F.P., Johnson, R.E., and Cole, P. (1975): Hodgkin's disease, tonsillectomy and family size. *N. Engl. J. Med.*, 292:22–25.
63. Heinen, E., Lilet-Leclercg, C., Mason, D.Y., Stein, H., Bonvier, J., Radoux, D., Kinet-Denoël, C., and Simar, L.J. (1984): Isolation of follicular dendritic cells from human tonsils and adenoids. II. Immunocytochemical characterization. *Eur. J. Immunol.*, 14:267–273.
64. Heinen, E., Radoux, D., Kinet-Denoël, C., Moeremans, M., De Mey, J., and Simar, L.J. (1985): Isolation of follicular dendritic cells from human tonsils and adenoids. III. Analysis of their Fc receptors. *Immunology*, 54:777–784.
65. Herzenberg, L.A., Black, S.J., Tokuhisa, T., and Herzenberg, L.A. (1980): Memory B cells at successive stages of differentiation. Affinity maturation and the role of IgD receptors. *J. Exp. Med.*, 151:1071–1087.

66. Hoffmann-Fezer, G., Löhrs, U., Rodt, H.V., and Thierfelder, S. (1981): Immunohistochemical identification of T- and B-lymphocytes delineated by the unlabelled antibody enzyme method. III. Topographical and quantitative distribution of T- and B-cells in human palatine tonsils. *Cell Tissue Res.*, 216:361–375.
67. Howie, A.J. (1980): Scanning and transmission electron microscopy on the epithelium of human palatine tonsils. *J. Pathol.*, 130:91–98.
68. Hsu, S.-M., and Jaffe, E.S. (1984): Phenotypic expression of B-lymphocytes. 2. Immunoglobulin expression of germinal center cells. *Am. J. Pathol.*, 114:396–402.
69. Humphrey, J.H., Grennan, D., and Sundaram, V. (1984): The origin of follicular dendritic cells in the mouse and the mechanism of trapping of immune complexes on them. *Eur. J. Immunol.*, 14:859–864.
70. Insel, R.A., and Merler, E. (1977): The necessity for T cell help for human tonsil B cell responses to pokeweed mitogen: induction of DNA synthesis, immunoglobulin, and specific antibody production with a T cell helper factor produced with pokeweed mitogen. *J. Immunol.*, 118:2009–2014.
71. Ishikawa, T., Wicher, K., and Arbesman, C.E. (1972): Distribution of immunoglobulins in palatine and pharyngeal tonsils. *Int. Arch. Allergy Appl. Immunol.*, 43:801–802.
72. Janeway, C.A., Bottomly, K., Babich, J., Conrad, P., Conzen, S., Jones, B., Kaye, J., Katz, M., McVay, L., Murphy, D.B., and Tite, J. (1984): Quantitative variation in Ia antigen expression plays a central role in immune regulation. *Immunol. Today*, 5:99–105.
73. Janossy, G., Gomez de la Concha, E., Luquetti, A., Snajdr, M.J., Waxdal, M.J., and Platts-Mills, T.A.E. (1977): T-cell regulation of immunoglobulin synthesis and proliferation in pokeweed (Pa-1)-stimulated human lymphocyte cultures. *Scand. J. Immunol.*, 6:109–123.
74. Janossy, G., Tidman, N., Selby, W.S., Thomas, J.A., and Granger, S. (1980): Human T lymphocytes of inducer and suppressor type occupy different microenvironments. *Nature (London)*, 287:81–84.
75. Jeschke, R., and Ströder, J. (1980): Verlaufsbeobachtung klinischer und immunologischer Parameter, inbesondere des Speichel-IgA, bei tonsillektomierten Kindern. *Klin. Padiatr.*, 192:51–60.
76. Johnson, S.K., and Johnson, R.E. (1972): Tonsillectomy history in Hodgkin's disease. *N. Engl. J. Med.*, 287:1122–1125.
77. Kawanishi, H., Ozato, K., and Strober, W. (1985): The proliferative response of cloned Peyer's patch switch T cells to syngeneic and allogeneic stimuli. *J. Immunol.*, 134:3586–3591.
78. Kawanishi, H., Saltzman, L.E., and Strober, W. (1982): Characteristics and regulatory function of murine Con A-induced, cloned T cells obtained from Peyer's patches and spleen: mechanisms regulating isotype-specific immunoglobulin production by Peyer's patch B cells. *J. Immunol.*, 129:475–483.
79. Kawanishi, H., Saltzman, L.E., and Strober, W. (1983): Mechanisms regulating IgA class-specific immunoglobulin production in murine gut-associated lymphoid tissues. I. T cells derived from Peyer's patches that switch sIgM B cells to sIgA B cells in vitro. *J. Exp. Med.*, 157:433–450.
80. Kawanishi, H., Saltzman, L.E., and Strober, W. (1983): Mechanisms regulating IgA class-specific immunoglobulin production in murine gut-associated lymphoid tissues. II. Terminal differentiation of postswitch sIgA-bearing Peyer's patch B cells. *J. Exp. Med.*, 158:649–669.
81. Kett, K., Brandtzaeg, P., Radl, J., and Haaijman, J. (1986): Different subclass-distribution of IgA-producing cells in human lymphoid organs and various secretory tissues. *J. Immunol.*, 136:3631–3635.
82. Kiyono, H., Cooper, M.D., Kearney, J.F., Mosteller, L.M., Michalek, S.M., Koopman, W.J., and McGhee, J.R. (1984): Isotype specificity of helper T cell clones. Peyer's patch Th cells preferentially collaborate with mature IgA B cells for IgA responses. *J. Exp. Med.*, 159:798–811.
83. Kiyono, H., McGhee, J.R., Mosteller, L.M., Eldridge, J.H., Koopman, W.J., Kearney, J.F., and Michalek, S.M. (1982): Murine Peyer's patch T cell clones. Characterization of antigen-specific helper T cells for immunoglobulin A responses. *J. Exp. Med.*, 156:1115–1130.
84. Kiyono, H., Mosteller-Barnum, L.M., Pitts, A.M., Williamson, S.I., Michalek, S.M., and McGhee, J.K. (1985): Isotype-specific immunoregulation. IgA-binding factors produced by Fcα receptor-positive T cell hybridomas regulate IgA responses. *J. Exp. Med.*, 161:731–747.
85. Kiyono, H., Phillips, J.O., Colwell, D.E., Michalek, S.M., Koopman, W.J., and McGhee, J.R. (1984): Isotype-specificity of helper T cell clones: Fcα receptors regulate T and B cell collaboration of IgA responses. *J. Immunol.*, 133:1087–1089.

86. Klug, H. (1984): Ultrastructure of interdigitating cells in the human tonsil. *Acta Morphol. Hung.*, 32:113–119.
87. Koburg, E. (1967): Cell production and cell migration in the tonsil. In: *Germinal Centers in Immune Responses*, edited by H. Cottier, N. Odartchenko, R. Schindter, and C.C. Congdon, pp. 176–182. Springer-Verlag, Berlin.
88. Korsrud, F.R., and Brandtzaeg, P. (1980): Immune systems of human nasopharyngeal and palatine tonsils: histomorphometry of lymphoid components and quantification of immunoglobulin-producing cells in health and disease. *Clin. Exp. Immunol.*, 39:361–370.
89. Korsrud, F.R., and Brandtzaeg, P. (1981): Immunohistochemical evaluation of J-chain expression by intra- and extra-follicular immunoglobulin-producing human tonsillar cells. *Scand. J. Immunol.*, 13:271–280.
90. Korsrud, F.R., and Brandtzaeg, P. (1981): Influence of tonsillar disease on the expression of J chain by immunoglobulin-producing cells in human palatine and nasopharyngeal tonsils. *Scand. J. Immunol.*, 13:281–287.
91. Kraal, G., Weissman, I.L., and Butcher, E.C. (1982): Germinal centre B cells: antigen specificity and changes in heavy chain class expression. *Nature (London)*, 298:377–379.
92. Krco, C.J., Challacombe, J., Lafuse, W.P., David, C.S., and Tomasi, T.B. (1981): Expression of Ia antigens by mouse Peyer's patch cells. *Cell. Immunol.*, 57:420–426.
93. Kristiansen, B.-E., Elverland, H., and Hannestad, K. (1984): Increased memingococcal carrier rate after tonsillectomy. *Br. Med. J.*, 288:974.
94. Kutteh, W.H., Prince, S.J., and Mestecky, J. (1982): Tissue origins of human polymeric and monomeric IgA. *J. Immunol.*, 128:990–995.
95. Lafrenz, D., Strober, S., and Vitetta, E. (1981): The relationship between surface immunoglobulin isotype and the immune function of murine B lymphocytes. V. High affinity secondary antibody responses are transferred by both IgD-positive and IgD-negative memory B cells. *J. Immunol.*, 127:867–872.
96. Lamelin, J.P., Thomasset, N., Andre, C., Brockier, J., and Revillard, J.P. (1978): Study of human T and B lymphocytes with heterologous antisera. III. Immunofluorescence studies on tonsil sections. *Immunology*, 35:463–469.
97. Lim, P.L., and Rowley, D. (1982): The effect of antibody on the intestinal absorption of macromolecules and on intestinal permeability in adult mice. *Int. Arch. Allergy Appl. Immunol.*, 68:41–46.
98. Loesel, L.S. (1984): Detection of allergic disease in adenoid tissue. *Am. J. Clin. Pathol.*, 81:170–175.
99. Londei, M., Lamb, J.R., Bottazzo, G.F., and Feldmann, M. (1984): Epithelial cells expressing aberrant MHC class II determinants can present antigen to cloned human T cells. *Nature (London)*, 312:639–641.
100. Maeda, S., Mogi, G., and Oh, M. (1982): Microcrypt extensions of tonsillar crypts. *Ann. Otol. Rhinol. Laryngol.*, 91:1–8.
101. Manconi, P.E., Ennas, M.G., Murru, M.R., Cadeddu, G., Tore, G., and Lantini, S. (1984): Epithelial-like cells containing lymphocytes (nurse cells) in human adenoids and tonsils. *Thymus*, 6:351–357.
102. Marklund, G., Carlsson, B., and Lundberg, C. (1984): Low secretory IgA concentrations in oral secretions during the acute phase of infectious mononucleosis. *Scand. J. Infect. Dis.*, 16:241–246.
103. Matthews, J.B., and Basu, M.K. (1982): Oral tonsils: an immunoperoxidase study. *Int. Arch. Allergy Appl. Immunol.*, 69:21–25.
104. Mayer, L., Fu, S.M., and Kunkel, H.G. (1982): Human T cell hybridomas secreting factors for IgA-specific help, polyclonal B cell activation, and B cell proliferation. *J. Exp. Med.*, 156:1860–1865.
105. Mayer, L., Posnett, D.N., and Kunkel, H.G. (1985): Human malignant T cells capable of inducing an immunoglobulin class switch. *J. Exp. Med.*, 161:134–144.
106. Mayumi, M., Kuritani, T., Kubagawa, and Cooper, M.D. (1983): IgG subclass expression by human B lymphocytes and plasma cells: B lymphocytes precommitted to IgG subclass can be preferentially induced by polyclonal mitogens with T cell help. *J. Immunol.*, 130:671–677.
107. McCaughan, G.W., Adams, E., and Basten, A. (1984): Human antigen-specific IgA responses in blood and secondary lymphoid tissue: an analysis of help and suppression. *J. Immunol.*, 132:1190–1196.
108. McMillan, E.M., Brubaker, D.B., Peters, S., Jackson, I., Beeman, K., Wasik, R., Stoneking,

L.E., and Resler, D.R. (1983): Demonstration of cells bearing the OKT6 determinant in human tonsil and lymph node. *Cancer Immunol. Immunother.*, 15:221–226.
109. McMillan, E.M., Wasik, R., and Everett, M.A. (1981): Identification of T-lymphocytes and T-subsets in human tonsil using monoclonal antibodies and the immunoperoxidase technic. *Am. J. Clin. Pathol.*, 76:737–744.
110. Meistrup-Larsen, K.I., Mogensen, H.H., Helweg-Larsen, K., Permin, H., Andersen, V., Rygaard, J., and Sørensen, H. (1979): Lymphocytes of adenoid tissue. *Acta Otolaryngol.* (Suppl.), 360:204–207.
111. Mestecky, J., Winchester, R.J., Hoffman, T., and Kunkel, H.G. (1977): Parallel synthesis of immunoglobulins and J chain in pokeweed mitogen-stimulated normal cells and in lymphoblastoid cell lines. *J. Exp. Med.*, 145:760–765.
112. Metcalfe-Gibson, C., and Keddie, N. (1978): Spleen size and previous tonsillectomy in autoimmune disease of the thyroid. *Lancet*, 1:944.
113. Miyawaki, T., Ohzeki, S., Ikuta, N., Seki, H., Taga, K., and Taniguchi, N. (1984): Immunohistologic localization and immune phenotypes of lymphocytes expressing Tac antigen in human lymphoid tissues. *J. Immunol.*, 133:2996–3000.
114. Mogensen, H.H., Meistrup-Larsen, K.I., Meistrup-Larsen, U., and Andersen, V. (1980): The in vitro response of lymphocytes from adenoid vegetations and tonsils to PPD. Influence of autologous blood monocytes, T lymphocytes and unseparated lymphocytes. *Acta Pathol. Microbiol. Scand. C*, 88:23–29.
115. Mogi, G. (1977): IgA immunocytes in tonsils. *Acta Otolaryngol.*, 83:505–513.
116. Morag, A., Morag, B., Bernstein, J.M., Beutner, K., and Ogra, P.L. (1975): In vitro correlates of cell-mediated immunity in human tonsils after natural or induced rubella virus infection. *J. Infect. Dis.*, 131:409–416.
117. Mosmann, T.R., Gravel, Y., Williamson, A.R., and Baumal, R. (1978): Modification and fate of J chain in myeloma cells in the presence and absence of polymeric immunoglobulin secretion. *Eur. J. Immunol.*, 8:94–101.
118. Moticka, E.J. (1974): The non-specific stimulation of immunoglobulin secretion following specific stimulation of the immune system. *Immunology*, 27:401–412.
119. Mudde, G.C., Sauerwein, R.W., Vooijs, W.C., Rozemuller, E., Aarden, L.A., and de Gast, G.C. (1985): Tonsil T cells require addition of extra IL-2 for optimal help in pokeweed mitogen induced plasma cell differentiation. *Abstracts of the 7th European Immunology Meeting*, Jerusalem, p. 198.
120. Mudde, G.C., Verberne, C.J.M., and de Gast, G.C. (1984): Human tonsil B lymphocyte function. II. Pokeweed mitogen-induced plasma cell differentiation of B cell subpopulations expressing multiple heavy chain isotypes on their surface. *J. Immunol.*, 133:1896–1901.
121. Nezelof, C., Diebold, N., Meyer, B., and Vialatte, J. (1974): Les infections rhino-pharyngées repetees de l'enfant: leurs liens avec la production immunoglobulinique locale, étudiée en immunofluorescence. *Arch. Fr. Pediatr.*, 31:843–859.
122. Nixon, D.F., Ting, J.P.Y., and Frelinger, J.A. (1982): Ia antigens on non-lymphoid tissues. Their origins and functions. *Immunol. Today*, 3:339–342.
123. Ogra, P.L. (1971): Effect of tonsillectomy and adenoidectomy on nasopharyngeal antibody response to poliovirus. *N. Engl. J. Med.*, 284:59–64.
124. Ohta, K., Manzara, T., Harbeck, R.J., and Kirkpatrick, C.H. (1983): Human tonsillar IgE biosynthesis in vitro. I. Enhancement of IgE and IgG synthesis in the presence of pokeweed mitogen by T-cell irradiation. *J. Allergy Clin. Immunol.*, 71:212–223.
125. Olah, I., Surjan, L., and Törö, I. (1972): Electronmicroscopic observations on the antigen reception in the tonsillar tissue. *Acta Biol. Sci. Hung.*, 23:61–73.
126. Opstelten, D., Stikker, R., van der Heijden, D., and Nieuwenhuis, P. (1980): Germinal centres and the B-cell system. IV. Functional characteristics of rabbit appendix germinal centre (-derived) cells. *Virchows Arch. B*, 34:53–62.
127. Østergaard, P.A. (1975): Presence of immunoglobulin-containing plasma cells in tonsils from tonsillectomized children. *Acta Pathol. Microbiol. Scand. C*, 83:406–412.
128. Østergaard, P.A. (1976): IgA levels and carrier state of *Haemophilus influenzae* and beta-haemolytic streptococci in children undergoing tonsillectomy. *Acta Pathol. Microbiol. Scand. C*, 84:290–298.
129. Østergaard, P.A. (1982): Tonsillar IgE plasma cells predict atopic disease. *Clin. Exp. Immunol.*, 49:163–166.
130. Owen, R.L., and Nemanic, P. (1978): Antigen processing structures of the mammalian intestinal

tract: a SEM study of lymphoepithelial organs. *Scan. Electron Microsc.*, 2:367–378.

131. Paganelli, R., and Levinski, R.J. (1981): Differences in specific antibody responses of human tonsillar cells to an oral and a parenteral antigen. *Scand. J. Immunol.*, 14:353–358.
132. Palva, T., Lehtinen, T., and Virtanen, H. (1983): Immune complexes in the middle ear fluid and adenoid tissue in chronic secretory otitis media. *Acta Otolaryngol.*, 95:539–543.
133. Parkhouse, R.M.E., and Cooper, M.D. (1977): A model for the differentiation of B lymphocytes with implications for the biological role of IgD. *Immunol. Rev.*, 37:105–126.
134. Pesak, V. (1971): The localization of IgA and IgE globulins in the palatine tonsils, nasal mucous membrane and nasal polypi. *Folia Microbiol.*, 16:323–325.
135. Platts-Mills, T.A.E., and Ishizaka, K. (1975): IgG and IgA diphtheria antitoxin responses from human tonsil lymphocytes. *J. Immunol.*, 114:1058–1064.
136. Porwit-Ksiazek, A., Ksiazek, T., and Biberfeld, P. (1983): Leu 7^+ (HNK-1^+) cells. I. Selective compartmentalization of Leu 7^+ cells with different immunophenotypes in lymphatic tissues and blood. *Scand. J. Immunol.*, 18:485–493.
137. Preud'Homme, J.L., Brouet, J.C., and Seligmann, M. (1977): Membrane-bound IgD on human lymphoid cells, with special reference to immunodeficiency and immunoproliferative diseases. *Immunol. Rev.*, 37:127–151.
138. Reynes, M., Aubert, J.P., Cohen, J.H.M., Audonin, J., Tricottet, V., Diebold, J., and Kazatchkine, M.D. (1985): Human follicular dendritic cells express CR1, CR2, and CR3 complement receptor antigens. *J. Immunol.*, 135:2687–2694.
139. Romagnani, S., Maggi, E., Amadori, A., Giudizi, M.G., and Ricci, M. (1977): Co-operation between T and B lymphocytes from human tonsils in the response to mitogens and antigens. *Clin. Exp. Immunol.*, 28:332–340.
140. Rynnel-Dagöö, B. (1978): Polyclonal activation to immunoglobulin secretion in human adenoid lymphocytes induced by bacteria from nasopharynx in vitro. *Clin. Exp. Immunol.*, 34:402–410.
141. Rynnel-Dagöö, B., Möller, E., and Waterfield, E. (1977): Characterization of human adenoid cells using surface and functional markers for lymphocyte subpopulations. *Clin. Exp. Immunol.*, 27:425–431.
142. Schmedtje, J.F., and Batts, A.F. (1973): Immunoglobulins and blood vessels in the tonsillar crypt epithelium. *Ann. Otol. Rhinol. Laryngol.*, 82:359–369.
143. Schmedtje, J.F., Chinea, J.J., and Kletzing, D.W. (1979): Immunologically induced changes in the tonsillar crypt epithelium. *Ann. Otol. Rhinol. Laryngol.*, 88:397–406.
144. Schnizlein, C.T., Kosco, M.H., Szakal, A., and Tew, J.G. (1985): Follicular dendritic cells in suspension: identification, enrichment and initial characterization indicating immune complex trapping and lack of adherence and phagocytic activity. *J. Immunol.*, 134:1360–1368.
145. Seymour, G.J., Greaves, M.F., and Janossy, G. (1980): Identification of cells expressing T and p 28,33 (Ia-like) antigens in sections of human lymphoid tissue. *Clin. Exp. Immunol.*, 39:66–75.
146. Shvartsman, Y.S., Agranovskaya, E.N., and Zykov, M.P. (1977): Formation of secretory and circulating antibodies after immunization with live inactivated influenza virus vaccines. *J. Infect. Dis.*, 135:697–705.
147. Si, L., Roscoe, G., and Whiteside, T.L. (1983): Selective distribution and quantitation of T-lymphocyte subsets in germinal centers of human tonsils. Definition by use of monoclonal antibodies. *Arch. Pathol. Lab. Med.*, 107:228–231.
148. Siegel, G. (1978): Description of age-depending cellular changes in the human tonsil. *ORL J. Otorhinolaryngol. Relat. Spec.*, 40:160–171.
149. Siegel, G., Linse, R., and Macheleidt, S. (1982): Factors of tonsillar involution: age-dependent changes in B-cell activation and Langerhans' cell density. *Arch. Otorhinolaryngol.*, 236:261–269.
150. Silingardi, V., Venezia, L., Tampieri, A., and Gramolini, C. (1982): Tonsillectomy, appendectomy and malignant lymphomas. *Scand. J. Haematol.*, 28:59–64.
151. Smith, R.S., Sherman, N.A., and Newcomb, R.W. (1974): Synthesis and secretion of immunoglobulin, including IgA, by human tonsil and adenoid tissue cultured in vitro. *Int. Arch. Allergy Appl. Immunol.*, 46:785–801.
152. Sordat, B., Moser, R., Gerber, H., and Cottier, H. (1969): Differentiation pathway within germinal centers of human tonsils. *Adv. Exp. Med. Biol.*, 5:73–82.
153. Sorensen, C.H. (1983): Quantitative aspects of IgD and secretory immunoglobulins in middle ear effusions. *Int. J. Pediatr. Otorhinolaryngol.*, 6:247–253.

154. Sprinkle, P.M., and Veltri, R.W. (1976): Recurrent adenotonsillitis: a new concept. *Laryngoscope*, 86:58–63.
155. Stein, H., Bonk, A., Tolksdorf, G., Lennert, K., Rodt, H., and Gerdes, J. (1980): Immunohistologic analysis of the organization of normal lymphoid tissue and non-Hodgkin's lymphomas. *J. Histochem. Cytochem.*, 28:746–760.
156. Stokes, C.R., Sothill, J.F., and Turner, M.W. (1975): Immune exclusion is a function of IgA. *Nature (London)*, 255:745–746.
157. Sugiyama, M., Sakashita, T., Cho, J.S., and Nakai, Y. (1984): Immunological and biochemical properties of tonsillar lymphocytes. *Acta Otolaryngol.* (Suppl.), 416:45–55.
158. Sumaya, C.V., Downey, K., and Ullis, K.C. (1978): Tonsillectomy and infectious mononucleosis. *Am. J. Epidemiol.*, 107:65–70.
159. Surjan, L. (1980): Reduced lymphocyte activation in repeatedly inflamed human tonsils. *Acta Otolaryngol.*, 89:187–194.
160. Surjan, L., Brandtzaeg, P., and Berdal, P. (1978): Immunoglobulin systems of human tonsils. II. Patients with chronic tonsillitis or tonsillar hyperplasia: quantification of Ig-producing cells, tonsillar morphometry and serum Ig concentrations. *Clin. Exp. Immunol.*, 31:382–390.
161. Tada, T., and Ishizaka, K. (1970): Distribution of γ E-forming cells in lymphoid tissues of the human and monkey. *J. Immunol.*, 104:377–387.
162. Tew, J.G., Thorbecke, G.J., and Steinman, R.M. (1982): Dendritic cells in the immune response: characteristics and recommended nomenclature (A report from the Reticuloendothelial Society Committee on Nomenclature). *J. Reticuloendothel. Soc.*, 31:371–380.
163. Tomino, Y., Endoh, M., Kaneshige, H., Nomoto, Y., and Sakai, H. (1983): Increase of IgA in pharyngeal washings from patients with IgA nephropathy. *Am. J. Med. Sci.*, 286:15–21.
164. Tsunoda, R., Terashima, K., Takahashi, K., and Kojima, M. (1978): An ultrastructural study with enzyme-labeled antibody technique on immunoglobulin-containing cells in human tonsils, especially in germinal centers. *Acta Pathol. Jpn.*, 21:53–75.
165. Tsunoda, R., Yaginuma, Y., and Kojima, M. (1980): Immunocytological studies on the constituent cells of the secondary nodules in human tonsils. *Acta Pathol. Jpn.*, 30:33–57.
166. Umetani, Y. (1977): Postcapillary venule in rabbit tonsil and entry of lymphocytes into its epithelium: a scanning and transmission electron microscope study. *Arch. Histol. Jpn.*, 40:77–94.
167. Van der Brugge-Gamelkoorn, G.J., and Kraal, G. (1985): The specificity of the high endothelial venule in bronchus-associated lymphoid tissue (BALT). *J. Immunol.*, 134:3746–3750.
168. Van der Valk, P., van der Loo, E.M., Jansen, J., Daha, M.R., and Meijer, C.J.L.M. (1984): Analysis of lymphoid and dendritic cells in human lymph node, tonsil and spleen. A study using monoclonal and heterologous antibodies. *Virchows Arch. (Cell. Pathol.)*, 45:169–185.
169. Van Rooijen, N., and Kors, N. (1985): Mechanism of follicular trapping: double immunocytochemical evidence for a contribution of locally produced antibodies in follicular trapping of immune complexes. *Immunology*, 55:31–34.
170. Vessière-Louveaux, F.M.Y.R., Hijmans, W., and Schuit, H.R.E. (1980): Presence of multiple isotypes on the surface of human tonsillar lymphocytes. *Eur. J. Immunol.*, 10:186–191.
171. Vessière-Louveaux, F.M.Y.R., Hijmans, W., and Shuit, H.R.E. (1981): Multiple heavy chain isotypes on the membrane of the small B lymphocytes in human blood. *Clin. Exp. Immunol.*, 43:149–156.
172. Vianna, N.J., Lawrence, C.H., Davies, J.N.P., Arbuckle, J., Harris, S., Marani, W., and Wilkinson, J. (1980): Tonsillectomy and childhood Hodgkin's disease. *Lancet*, 11:338–340.
173. Von Gaudecker, B., and Müller-Hermelink, H.K. (1982): The development of the human tonsilla palatina. *Cell Tissue Res.*, 224:579–600.
174. Von Gaudecker, B., Pfingsten, U., Müller-Hermelink, H.K. (1984): Localization and characterization of T-cell subpopulations and natural killer cells (HNK 1^+ cells) in the human tonsilla palatina. An ultrastructural-immunocytochemical study. *Cell Tissue Res.*, 238:135–143.
175. Wagner, V., Wagnerova, M., Wokounova, D., Munzarova, J., Foltynova, J., and Kriz, J. (1977): Levels of immunoglobulins and lysozyme in 10-year-old children from different regions and the conditions of the lymphatic apparatus. I. Condition of tonsils in connection with some immunological parameters and different environment. *J. Hyg. Epidem. Microbiol. Immunol.*, 21:72–83.
176. Waldman, R.H., Wigley, F.M., and Small, P.A. (1970): Specificity of respiratory secretion antibody against influenza virus. *J. Immunol.*, 105:1477–1483.
177. Waldmann, T.A., and Strober, W. (1969): Metabolism of immunoglobulins. *Prog. Allergy*, 13:1–110.

178. Walker, A.R.P., and Segal, I. (1982): Tonsillectomy and appendicectomy—do they prejudice subsequent health? *South Afr. Med. J.*, 61:570.
179. Watanabe, T., Yoshizaki, K., Yagura, T., and Yamura, Y. (1974): In vitro antibody formation by human tonsil lymphocytes. *J. Immunol.*, 113:608–616.
180. Welliver, R.C., Sun, M., Rinaldo, D., and Ogra, P. (1985): Respiratory syncytical virus-specific IgE responses following infection: evidence for a predominantly mucosal response. *Pediatr. Res.*, 19:420–424.
181. Williams, D.M., and Rowland, A.C. (1972): The palatine tonsils of the pig—an afferent route to the lymphoid tissue. *J. Anat.*, 113:131–137.
182. Willson, J.K.V., Zaremba, J.L., Pitts, A.M., and Pretlow, T.G. (1976): A characterization of human tonsillar lymphocytes after separation from other tonsillar cells in an isokinetic gradient of Ficoll in tissue culture medium. *Am. J. Pathol.*, 83:341–358.
183. Wingerd, J., and Sponzilli, E.E. (1977): Concentrations of serum protein fractions in white women: effects of age, weight, smoking, tonsillectomy, and other factors. *Clin. Chem.*, 23:1310–1317.
184. Wright, J. (1906): The difference in the behavior of dust from that of bacteria in the tonsillar crypts. *NY Med. J.*, 83:17–21.
185. Yamanaka, N., and Kataura, A. (1984): Viral infections associated with recurrent tonsillitis. *Acta Otolaryngol.* (Suppl.), 416:30–37.
186. Yamanaka, N., Sambe, S., Harabuchi, Y., and Kataura, A. (1983): Immunohistological study of tonsil. Distribution of T cell subsets. *Acta Otolaryngol.*, 96:509–516.
187. Yasuda, N., Kanoh, T., and Uchino, H. (1981): J chain synthesis in lymphocytes from patients with selective IgA deficiency. *Clin. Exp. Immunol.*, 46:142–148.
188. Zan-Bar, I., Strober, S., and Vitetta, S. (1979): The relationship between surface immunoglobulin isotype and immune function of murine B lymphocytes. IV. Role of IgD-bearing cells in the propagation of immunologic memory. *J. Immunol.*, 123:925–930.

Immunology of the Ear, edited by J. Bernstein
and P. Ogra. Raven Press, New York © 1987.

Respiratory Tract Lymphoid Tissue and Other Effector Cells

Raffaele Scicchitano, Peter Ernst, and John Bienenstock

Host Resistance Programme, Department of Pathology and Intestinal Disease Research Unit, McMaster University Health Sciences Centre, Hamilton, Ontario, Canada L8N 3Z5

The upper respiratory tract, in part, is a mucosal tissue, characterized by the glandular secretions that it secretes onto the epithelial surface. These secretions contain products that are common to mucosal surfaces. One hallmark of these secretions is secretory IgA (sIgA), which is made up of two molecules (a dimer) of serum-type IgA with two additional components, J chain and secretory component (SC). Bienenstock and Befus (25) have recently classified mucosal tissues into several classes based on the presence of IgA in secretions and on the presence of SC in glandular components of mucosal tissue. In this classification (Table 1) the respiratory tract falls into class I—those tissues characterized by the presence of IgA plasma cells capable of producing IgA and a mechanism for its transport into external secretions.

Another component of mucosal tissues is the mucosa-associated lymphoid tissue (MALT), which consists of organized collections of lymphoid tissue found predominantly in the gut and lungs.

However, the distal respiratory tract (namely, terminal bronchioles and lung parenchyma) has fewer features of a mucosal tissue in that (a) sIgA may not be the predominant antibody in secretions and (b) organized collections of lymphoid tissue are less frequent.

There are certain features regarding the immune response in the respiratory tract peculiar to that organ. The humoral immune response in the lungs may demonstrate the predominant characteristics of a mucosal response (characterized by sIgA) or a systemic response (characterized by IgG) or both. Furthermore, the type of response found (mucosal versus systemic) is dependent on which part of the respiratory tract is under study. The response of the upper respiratory tract (nasopharynx, large airways) is most often mucosal, whereas the lower respiratory tract and draining lymph nodes may more correctly be considered part of the systemic immune apparatus. Therefore, the respiratory tract represents an immunologic organ where close interaction between the mucosal and systemic immune systems occurs under normal circumstances.

In its role as a mucosal immunologic organ, the respiratory tract interacts with

TABLE 1. *Categories of tissues that contain secretory IgA or its component parts*[a]

Glands	Tissues
Class I: *Evidence for local predominance of IgA plasma cells and secretory component*	
Salivary	Gastrointestinal tract
Mammary	Upper respiratory tract
Lacrimal	Nose
Prostate	Middle ear
	Gallbladder
	Cervix
	Biliary duct
Class II: *Evidence for local secretory component but no evidence for local IgA plasma cells*	
Skin (sweat glands)	Amnion
Kidney	Fallopian tubes
Urinary bladder	Uterine mucosa
Hepatic parenchymal cells	Thymus
Class III: *No evidence for either local secretory component or local IgA plasma cells*	
Ureter	
Esophagus	
Vagina	
Buccal squamous epithelium	
Gingiva	

[a]From Bienenstock and Befus (25).

other mucosal surfaces, particularly the gut, and forms part of the common mucosal immunologic system. It shares many of the functional and structural characteristics of other mucosal surfaces, particularly the gut.

Many nonspecific factors, including the presence of a glycocalyx and mucociliary transport, aerodynamic-structural characteristics (which determine to a large extent antigen access), surfactant, and the presence of a resident population of phagocytic cells in the lumen of the respiratory tract, act to modify its immune response to a particular inhaled antigen. It should be noted that some naturally inhaled antigen, by virtue of these nonspecific mechanisms, will always be ingested so that the immune response may represent the response at the mucosal surfaces of both gut and lungs.

This review will deal with the functional and structural basis of immunity in the respiratory tract, with particular reference to the mucosal response. It will emphasize similarities and differences between the gut and respiratory tracts as immunologically competent organs and will attempt to identify areas of recent advances and controversy, with particular reference to lung immunity.

LYMPHOID TISSUE OF THE RESPIRATORY TRACT

The lymphoid tissue of the respiratory tract consists of:

1. Organized lymphoid tissue in the wall of the respiratory tract.
2. Lymphocytes loosely arranged in the lamina propria.
3. Lymphocytes within the epithelium.
4. Lymph nodes.
5. Lymphocytes found within the lumen.

The first compartment, bronchus-associated lymphoid tissue (BALT), consists of lymphocytes and accompanying cells organized into aggregates, follicles, or solitary lymphoid nodules (23). In recent years there has been some confusion regarding the terminology used to describe this lymphoid tissue. We have suggested that the term BALT be reserved for such collections of lymphoid tissue with a recognizable relationship to the lumen and covered by specialized lymphoepithelium (see below). In some species—for example, the rat—there are collections of lymphocytes covered by normal epithelium (36,55). These lymphocyte collections are usually found in smaller bronchioles, contain plasma cells but no high endothelial venules (HEV), and therefore differ from typical BALT. Lymphoid aggregates may also be found in the interstitial tissue, alveolar walls, and pleura without a clear relationship to any particular structure, although they may be associated with a central blood vessel giving the appearance of perivascular cuffing (36).

In this review the term BALT is used to refer to aggregates of lymphocytes and accompanying cells which are covered by, and bear a clear relationship to, lymphoepithelium (LE). In our original description (17,18) the term *lymphoid follicle* was used to describe these aggregates. However, in later descriptions (32,137) the term *follicle* has been used to refer to a presumed B-cell area of BALT. However, because the existence of microscopically recognizable B- and T-cell-dependent areas in BALT is still uncertain, unlike Peyer's patches (PP), this term is best avoided.

Lymphocytes are also found arranged loosely throughout the lamina propria of the respiratory tract. A large majority of these are plasma cells, usually of the IgA isotype (160). T cells are also found in the lamina propria, but an exact quantitation of these has not been made.

There is also a large compartment of leukocytes found within the epithelium of the respiratory tract in both mammals and birds (5). In the gut these leukocytes are predominantly T cells (54), but there is little information regarding these cells in the respiratory tract. Another large population of lymphocytes is found within the lumen of the respiratory tract, where, together with the companion macrophages, they are usually referred to as *bronchoalveolar cells*.

In addition to all of the above, the respiratory tract is associated with lymph nodes that appear to be similar in structure and function to those found elsewhere in the body.

INDUCTIVE EVENTS IN RESPIRATORY IMMUNITY

Bronchus-Associated Lymphoid Tissue

In 1971, during a study of immune complex deposition in the rabbit lung, we noted the presence of large lymphoid aggregates in the bronchial wall. In 1973 a more systematic study of this BALT was made (17,18), and its similarity to gut-associated lymphoid tissue (GALT), particularly PP, was noted. Although these observations awakened new interest in BALT, its existence had been documented previously (reviewed by Bienenstock in ref. 23), probably as early as 1867 by Burdon-Sanderson. In 1875 Klein (quoted by Bienenstock in ref. 23) published his description of the anatomy of the lymphocytic tissue of the lung, and his book contains the first drawing of BALT. Furthermore, in this treatise, the observation was made that "these lymphoid follicles in the bronchial wall are therefore in every respect analogous to the lymph follicles found in other mucous membranes, e.g., the tonsil and intestine."

BALT has been described in a variety of species, including rats (17,36,55), rabbits (17,18,137,170), mice (113), and sheep (150) as well as chickens, guinea pigs, and pigs. It has best been characterized in rats and rabbits. In humans, BALT is present and has many of the characteristics described in other species and consists mainly of diffuse collections of subepithelial lymphocytes in the bronchi.

Ontogeny

BALT is not found in neonatal rabbits delivered by cesarean section one day before birth (17). In rats raised in specific pathogen-free conditions, BALT appears after the second week of life; it appears even earlier in conventionalized rats (17). Antigen exposure is not necessary for the development of BALT since it is found in germ-free rats (17) and mice (113) and developed in fetal lungs transplanted subcutaneously into syngeneic adults (113). In this situation, BALT (and GALT) developed as early as 30 days after transplantation and was always present at 60 days. In this case, however, the BALT is primitive, although easily recognized, and possesses a lymphoepithelium. Racz et al. (137) demonstrated in rabbits, immunized with BCG, that there was hyperplasia of BALT. Therefore, the bulk of evidence suggests that BALT arises independently of antigen but that antigenic stimulation leads to hyperplasia and development.

In humans, diffuse lymphoreticular aggregates are seen after birth in the normal lung and are found just below the epithelial surface. They first appear at 1 week of age in the neonate and increase in number thereafter. Larger, confluent aggregates are found in some pathologic states (49,50). Kyriazis and Esterly (100) studied mononuclear cell aggregates in the lungs and intestine of human embryos and fetuses. Lymphoid aggregates were found in the intestine by 14 days gestation, adjacent to the epithelium, and similar but less numerous aggregates were found in the lungs. Meuwissen and Hussain (112) described a series of patients in whom recurrent infections of an unexplained nature occurred. Biopsy of these patients' lungs showed remarkable proliferation of the BALT, in some cases occluding the bronchiolar lumen. This tissue, like BALT elsewhere, had a lymphoepithelium.

Morphology

Macroscopic

Peyer's patches are visible with the naked eye whereas BALT is not, although in several species it may be detected by using a dissecting microscope. In the chicken, BALT is then seen as finger-like projections into the lumen of the trachea. With acetic acid fixation (39), BALT, devoid of the overlying epithelium, is seen as white aggregates. Using this technique, BALT may be demonstrated in rabbits, rats, guinea pigs, chickens, and sheep (17,150). In the latter two species, BALT is demonstrated in the trachea whereas in other species it is generally distributed along the major bronchi in all lung lobes. In the chicken, BALT may also be demonstrated by staining with periodic acid-Schiff because the LE contains no goblet or secretory cells and BALT shows up as areas of negative staining (17). In the rat there are said to be 30 to 50 BALT aggregates per adult (134).

Microscopic

We have already alluded to the morphologic similarities between BALT and GALT. BALT has a similar structure to PP, although it is less readily divisible into distinct functional and anatomic regions. The epithelium overlying BALT has the characteristics of an LE and is heavily infiltrated with lymphocytes (17,18). The epithelial cells are attenuated and characteristically lack cilia and goblet cells. Over the most superficial aspect of the lymphoid aggregate, they may possess scant cytoplasm; scanning electron microscopy confirms the absence of cilia and shows the presence of M (microfold) cells as described in mammalian PP and the bursa of Fabricius (27,28,129,130). The epithelial cell surface over BALT may be folded and irregularly shaped and appears to possess crypts, tunnels, and crevices (20).

The cytoplasm of the lymphoepithelium forms a reticulum within which lymphocyte clusters are found. Such clusters have been described in GALT by Schmedtje (149) and are said to be characteristic of MALT (122), where they have been called "nurse cells." Werkele et al. (179) have described "nurse cells" in the thymus, and in this situation these cells are large, macrophage-like cells that have lymphocytes lying within their cytoplasm. In BALT it is uncertain if the intraepithelial lymphocytes are contained within the cytoplasm of the lymphoepithelial cells, although Bienenstock and Befus (24) have isolated "nurse cells" from mouse PP. Studies to confirm the phenotype of these cell clusters in BALT and PP have yet to be done (see below).

BALT consists of a reticulin framework in which a variety of cells, the majority of which are lymphocytes, are found. Bienenstock et al. (17) described several anatomic regions in BALT, including the dome or "area under the epithelium" (AUE; 134) and the follicle. Germinal centers are not routinely found in normal animals except the chicken (17,134), although they are readily described following antigenic stimulation (137). Even in normal animals the follicle is often bordered by a rim of lymphocytes with darker-staining nuclei (17). Tenner-Racz et al. (170) also described a parafollicular region particularly seen in animals following immunization and they ascribed T-cell function to this area. Lymphoblasts are also found in BALT, usually described as occurring in the periphery (17,134). Plasma cells are scarce in BALT even after immunization (16), although some are generally found at the periphery (17,134,135) but rarely within the follicle itself. Macrophages were first described in BALT by Chamberlain et al. (36) and they are found throughout BALT. Tingible body macrophages, said to be typical of germinal centers, are also found (137). A variety of accessory cells, including follicular dendritic cells (FDC) and interdigitating dendritic cells (IDC), have also been described (134,137). The function of these cells is discussed below.

A variety of blood vessels are found in BALT. High endothelial venules, the preferential site of leukocyte migration, were first described in BALT by Chamberlain et al. (36). These vessels are generally found at the junction of B- and T-dependent areas and can be shown to contain lymphocytes, including lymphoblasts as well as monocytes. Racz et al. (137) demonstrated hyperplasia of HEV in rabbit BALT following immunization with BCG. BALT is said not to possess afferent lymphatics, but efferent lymphatics arise in BALT and generally drain into a large peripheral sinus lymph vessel (55,134) and eventually drain into the lymph vessel that accompanies the artery. In addition, Plesch (134) has described lymphatic-like structures in rat BALT which contain a variety of mononuclear cells but which bear no clear relationship to efferent lymphatics. Arterioles and veins are found in BALT and there is always a nerve with sometimes a small ganglion to be identified (134). Mast cells may be found in BALT (135). Bienenstock and Johnston (20) described basophil-like cells in the BALT of rabbits. These cells contain granules that are smaller and less numerous than those found in mast cells and have indented nuclei with several lobes. They were found inside the follicles, on the luminal surface and in normal bronchoepithelium where they were often found to be in an intercellular location.

It has been suggested that the parafollicular area of BALT is a T-dependent area (137); this is based on the finding of HEV in this area and the presence of IDC, which are said to be characteristic of such areas in lymph nodes and spleen. In BALT, when secondary follicles are present and germinal centers are found, this distinction can be made (135). However, in normal animals in which germinal centers are often absent, no fixed T- or B-cell areas can be determined histologically. In chickens, neonatal thymectomy or bursectomy does not lead to any obvious morphological changes in BALT (19); a similar lack of effect was noted after neonatal thymectomy in rats (17,18,135). Using immunohistochemical techniques with antibody markers for T and B cells, Plesch (135) and Bruge-Gamelkoorn and Kraal (32) have defined areas containing predominantly T or B cells in rat BALT. However, these areas bore no fixed relation to any anatomic structures within

BALT, and where HEV were found, both T and B cells could be discerned. Few T cells can be identified in the AUE. In the guinea pig, similar techniques have demonstrated that the T- and B-cell areas are more constant in their localization, with the B-cell areas located next to the associated artery.

In rabbit BALT, 18% of lymphocytes bore the T-cell marker rabbit thymic lymphocyte antigen (RTLA), a percentage similar to that in PP (145). Fifty percent of cells were identified as bearing surface immunoglobuin (Ig), with equal proportions staining with anti-IgM and anti-IgA and less with anti-IgG. Relatively more IgA-bearing cells were found than in PP. In rats, a similar percentage of cells were B cells (32), but the majority of cells stained with anti-IgM (40%) and anti-IgG (40%), less stained with anti-IgA (15%), and few stained with anti-IgE (5%).

In addition to surface Ig, Plesch (134,135) identified a reticular staining for all immunoglobulin isotypes within the follicle and she suggested that this represented antigen-antibody complexes on the surface of FDC. Few cells in the epithelium stained with T- or B-cell markers (134), but both intraepithelial leukocytes and LE cells bore surface Ia (histocompatibility) antigen, as do the B cells, macrophages, and other accessory cells in the BALT follicle itself (135).

Function

In the previous discussion, evidence that BALT has structural similarities to PP was presented. The discussion that follows presents evidence that these mucosa-associated lymphoid tissues also have functional similarities.

Antigen Uptake

The LE overlying BALT has the same structural appearance as the follicle-associated epithelium (FAE) described in PP, bursa of Fabricius, and the appendix in mammals and birds (27,129,130). Specialized M cells (130) are found within this epithelium, and there is evidence that these cells are sites of preferential uptake of antigen, both particulate and soluble, from the lumen. For example, following the installation of horseradish peroxidase (HRP) into the intestinal lumen of mice, this soluble antigen is taken up into the cytoplasm of M cells by a process of reverse pinocytosis and is soon found in the intercellular spaces of the LE in close proximity to, and within the cytoplasm of, lymphocytes closely associated with M cells (130). In contrast, the antigen is poorly taken up by normal columnar epithelium. Similarly, in the respiratory tract, HRP is preferentially taken up by the LE over BALT (55,170). Furthermore, after antigenic stimulation with BCG there was hyperplasia of the LE and the uptake and transport of HRP was more rapid than in normal animals. It should be emphasized that, in the respiratory tract, absorption of antigen may also occur across intact bronchoepithelium (30). In the intestine, the FAE overlying PP has been identified as the site of entry of reovirus (181), and several observations suggest that BALT is also the site of entry of pathogens into the respiratory tract. For example, following intratracheal immunization of rabbits with BCG, Tenner-Racz et al. (170) found organisms in macrophages in BALT. From older work (reviewed by Bienenstock in ref. 23) it is known that BALT may be the first site in the respiratory tract in which particulate antigens, including bacteria, are found. Therefore, it can be concluded that BALT is a major, but not the only, site for the selective transfer of viruses, bacteria, and soluble materials from the lumen of the respiratory tract into contact with the internal lymphoid environment.

The origin of the M cells in the specialized LE of the respiratory tract is not known. However, in the FAE of the intestine, M cells probably develop from columnar cells in adjoining crypts (14,159), and the end differentiation to M cells occurs in the FAE itself under the influence of lymphokines (Owen, quoted in ref. 23). It is uncertain whether M cells in the LE of BALT are able to act as antigen-processing cells (APC) or whether they merely serve an antigen-uptake function with subsequent processing of antigen by accessory cells in BALT. In view of the need for antigen to be presented in the context of Ia surface antigens, it is noteworthy that the LE cells do bear surface Ia antigens and also express Ia antigen in the cytoplasm, probably synthesizing it themselves. There is virtually no information regarding the mechanism(s) by which cells in BALT may process antigen. Several cell types, which in other sites are able to process and present antigen, are found in BALT. These include macrophages that bear Ia antigens and IDC and FDC that can be shown to have antigen-antibody complexes on their surface (134). Macrophages that bear Ia antigens are also found in the lumen and alveolar walls, and Lipscomb et al. (102) suggested that alveolar macrophages may migrate into BALT and demonstrated that they may present antigen to initiate an immune response. Racz et al. (138) concluded that antigen and bacteria may be transported via macrophages from BALT to other sites such as the draining hilar lymph nodes. When rabbits were immunized with bovine Calmette Guerin (BCG) organisms, macrophage-lymphocyte clusters, typical of early immune responses, were seen in BALT and in adjacent lymphatics, as well as in the subcapsular and medullary sinus of the lymph nodes. Following intrapulmonary immunization of mice with heterologous red blood cells, the main site of antibody formation appears to be the hilar lymph nodes; these nodes are the site in which most antigen is located (173). Following mesenteric adenectomy, large numbers of macrophages and other non-lymphoid cells are found in thoracic duct lymph, suggesting that, in the intestinal tract, these cells may migrate normally from PP to the regional lymph nodes.

Antigen transport in BALT may be bidirectional. Following the intravascular injection of HRP, antigen was noted in BALT under the LE tight junctions and pinocytosis of antigen by LE cells was noted (119). In the intestine, intravascular antigen is transported by the FAE into the intestinal lumen (28).

Immune Responses

The local application of antigen to the upper respiratory tract often leads to an antibody response that is primarily IgA and may occur in the absence of a serum antibody response. In the following section a discussion of the role of BALT in the induction of an immune response is considered. Of necessity, this will also include a discussion of cell traffic and the common mucosal immunologic system.

B Cells

IgA and IgG

Craig and Cebra (40), using allotypic markers and adoptive transfer of PP cells in rabbits, found that this lymphoid tissue is an enriched source of IgA plasma cell precursors. Following antigenic stimulation, these cells, which are characterized by bearing surface IgA, travel via the mesenteric lymph nodes (MLN) and thoracic duct into the general circulation and subsequently relocate to the intestinal lamina propria.

With regard to BALT, the repopulation studies of Rudzik et al. (146,147) also demonstrated that this tissue is an enriched source of IgA precursors. In these experiments, cells derived from the bronchial lamina propria of rabbits, and thought to predominantly reflect the cell population of BALT, were transferred to lethally irradiated recipients and immunoglobulin-containing cells (ICC) in various tissues were examined. It was found that cells derived from BALT were able to repopulate the gut and bronchial mucosa predominantly with IgA-ICC. The converse, using GALT cells, was also true.

The reasons why mucosal lymphoid tissue is an enriched source of IgA precursors are uncertain. Gearhart and Cebra (59) have suggested that it may be because of the local environment and that lymphocyte differentiation leading to a commitment to IgA expression may depend on cell division and occurs during antigen-stimulated clonal expansion. These workers also presented evidence that the IgA precursors in PP represented secondary B cells. Therefore, antigen challenge and exposure to lipopolysaccharides (LPS) might force all B cells in MALT to eventually develop into surface IgA^+ cells if they were exposed sufficiently and often enough to antigen.

The form in which antigen is presented may also be important. For example, there is evidence that, compared to parenteral priming, oral immunization leads to increased numbers of precursors expressing surface IgA in both PP and spleen (58).

Although clonal expansion by antigen appears to play a role in differentiation of IgA precursors, there is now ample evidence for the involvement of immunoregulatory T cells in a site-specific manner in this process. Elson et al. (48) first demonstrated increased numbers of IgA-specific helper T cells in PP. Based on experiments employing both antigen-stimulated and mitogen-induced T-cell clones derived from PP, several subpopulations of T lymphocytes have now been shown to be involved in IgA immunoregulation (93,96). These T-cell clones also bore surface receptors for IgA (RFcα), and there is evidence that such cells may play a role in immunoregulation. Both T and B lymphocytes bearing RFcα are found in most lymphoid tissues, but generally higher numbers are found in GALT (164), and both IgA-specific help (97) and suppression (81) have been demonstrated by cells bearing RFcα. Recent interest has focused on various factors that bind immunoglobulins in an isotype-specific way secreted by these cells. For example, mouse T cells secrete an IgA-binding factor, which provides specific help for IgA responses *in vitro* (98).

A Common Mucosal Immunologic System

Following the rediscovery of BALT, Bienenstock et al. (17,18) suggested that the concept of a separate mucosal immune system (171) be extended to that of a universal immune system. As a result of studies to be reviewed below, this view was expanded to that of a common mucosal immunologic system (107). Earlier studies had shown that B lymphoblasts derived from MLN and thoracic duct lymph (TDL) had a propensity to localize to the intestinal lamina propria, at which site they formed predominantly IgA plasma cells. This observation, initially made by Gowans and Knight (66), has been amply demonstrated in several species (69,70,72,85). Furthermore, this selective localization is a propensity of both T and B lymphoblasts (70,162). In addition, these early studies showed that some of these GALT-derived lymphoblasts localized to other mucosal sites, particularly the lungs. For example, following the intravenous injection of radiolabeled thoracic duct lymphocytes in rats, Hall and Smith (72) found that although the majority of radioactivity was localized to the intestine, some activity was also detected in the lungs; autoradiographic studies revealed labeled cells in the trachea and lung parenchyma. The repopulation studies of Rudzik et al. (146,147), cited earlier, showed that PP or BALT cells were able to repopulate the intestinal and bronchial lamina propria with IgA-producing cells.

Subsequently, the concept of a common mucosal system involving the gut and lungs has been extended to other mucosal sites, including the mammary gland and genitourinary tract. Saif et al. (148) first demonstrated the existence of a gut-mammary axis. Following infection of swine with transmissible gastroenteritis virus, IgA antibodies were detected in milk in titers higher than in serum. Goldblum et al. (63) found antibody-forming cells to gut bacterial antigens in lactating women who were fed nonpathogenic *E. coli*. In similar studies involving oral ingestion of *Streptococcus mutans,* Mestecky et al. (111) detected IgA antibodies in saliva but not serum. Direct evidence for a common mucosal system was provided by studies employing immunofluorescence and/or autoradiography. After oral immunization of mice with ferritin, Weisz-Carrington et al. (178) detected antibody-containing cells (ACC) not only in the intestine but also in the lungs and mammary glands, and the majority of these cells were of the IgA class. McDermott and Bienenstock (107) provided evidence for both the tissue (mucosal versus nonmucosal) and organ specificity of cells derived from MLN and bronchial lymph nodes (BLN). These workers studied the homing patterns of radiolabeled blast cells from MLN, BLN, and peripheral lymph nodes (PLN). They showed that MLN cells not only repopulated the intestine with IgA-ACC but also the lungs, mammary glands, and cervix (108). In the mammary gland (144) and cervix (108), the localization and local proliferation of such cells appear to be under hormonal control. Organ selectivity was demonstrated in that lymphocytes derived from GALT tended to return to the intestine whereas those from the respiratory tract tended to return to the lungs. A similar preference for cells derived from lung efferent lymph to localize to the lungs has been demonstrated in sheep (161).

Surprisingly, the studies of McDermott and Bienenstock (107) showed that IgG cells also exhibited a mucosal selectivity. Some 12 times as many IgG cells derived from BLN returned to the lung, as compared to the number of such cells in the lungs derived from MLN.

The importance of a common mucosal immunologic system, with the gut as a major component, is that immunization strategies may be derived to harness the immune apparatus of the gut; this is to provide immunity at mucosal surfaces, including the middle ear, where lymphoid tissue is poorly developed or readily inaccessible to antigen. We have performed experiments to compare GALT and BALT as a source of IgA-ACC in the respiratory tract. In sheep, a single intraperitoneal injection of antigen in Freund's complete adjuvant leads to an IgA-ACC response in intestinal lymph (10). These cells arise in GALT and relocate via TDL and blood to the intestine, where secondary local immunization leads to clonal expansion and retention (84,85). When animals that had been primed by intratracheal or intraperitoneal administration of ovalbumin were given a secondary intratracheal immunization, the numbers of antiovalbumin ACC in the tracheal and intestinal lamina propria did not differ, but the proportion of IgA-ACC was higher in those animals given intraperitoneal priming. Continuous drainage of efferent intestinal lymph, which denied GALT precursors access to the circulation, abrogated the IgA-ACC, but not the IgG-ACC, response (152).

Following reinfusion of radiolabeled, autologous intestinal efferent lymph cells, the IgA-ACC response in the trachea was restored and the labeled cells could be detected at this site (150). We concluded that in sheep, where BALT is functionally poorly developed, priming of GALT, followed by local secondary immunization, was more effective in producing an IgA-ACC response in the respiratory tract than by local immunization alone.

Recent evidence that circulating polymeric IgA (pIgA) without SC is selectively transported into bile (89) and other external secretions (150,155) has extended the concept of the common mucosal immunologic system.

In the hepatobiliary tract, this transport is mediated by complexing of circulating pIgA to SC that is synthesized by hepatocytes. Of particular relevance are studies demonstrating that circulating IgA, with defined antibody activity (73), as well as IgA-antigen complexes (131) are also transported into bile. It was suggested (87) that all mucosal surfaces possess this ability and that the amount of serum IgA transported into secretions is inversely proportional to the amount of IgA which is synthesized locally by plasma cells and which is able to compete for SC-binding sites. For example, following intravenous injection of radiolabeled dimeric IgA prepared from intestinal lymph (and not containing SC), no activity was detected in intestinal secretions of sheep in keeping with the large number of IgA plasma cells in the intestinal lamina propria. In milk, activity was readily detected in early lactation when low IgA plasma cell numbers were present in the gland, but not during involution when many IgA plasma cells were found (155). In similar experiments, selective transport of circulating IgA into respiratory secretions was demonstrated, although in this case the major portion of IgA in secretions was nevertheless produced locally (153). These studies suggest another mechanism (apart from relocation of IgA-ACC) whereby oral immunization may contribute to immunity at distant mucosal sites since, in many species, much of the circulating IgA is derived from the intestine.

Furthermore, in view of the studies of MacPherson and Steer (105), which showed large numbers of nonlymphoid cells in the TDL of mesenteric adenectomized rats, it is likely that the concept of a common mucosal immunologic system will be extended to include the traffic of APC and probably other inductive and effector cells between mucosal surfaces.

IgE

There is some evidence that MALT may also be a source of IgE precursors. Lymphocytes bearing surface IgE are found in rat BALT (134) and, in mice, Durkin et al. (47) showed that the PP of germfree mice possess large numbers of surface IgE^+ cells. Such cells concomitantly bear IgA, and the relationship between these two immunoglobulins and subsequent isotypic expression is unknown. When these mice are subsequently conventionalized, these surface IgE^+ cells are found in MLN but not in PP, suggesting migration of these cells from PP to MLN following antigenic exposure. Following intestinal priming with tetanus toxoid, some cells expressing surface IgE were found in the lung and/or BALT of mice but not in PP (34). The degree to which these isolated findings reflect immuoregulation by T cells is uncertain. Suppressor T cells for IgE responses have been described in PP (121); following exposure to aerosolized antigen, suppression of IgE synthesis can be shown to occur and suppressor cells can be demonstrated in regional BLN (see below; 154).

Several studies have demonstrated IgE-ACC in mucosal tissues and associated lymph nodes in normal animals (169) and in those following immunization with aerosolized antigen (61) and in response to nematode infection (106). There is some evidence that in the latter situation, most of the IgE synthesis occurs in the regional lymph nodes or TDL (154). However, the nature of IgE-ACC in the intestinal and respiratory lamina propria is uncertain, following the observations of Mayrhofer et al. (106) that, in nematode-infected rats, the majority of these cells in the intestinal lamina propria are mucosal mast cells (MMC). This observation, however, has recently been disputed (101). Although the observation that MMC contain IgE was initially made in nematode infection, the findings by Alhstedt et al. (2)—that, following immunization with aerosolized ovalbumin in mice and rats, there is a pulmonary mastocytosis—suggest that this may not be unique to infected states.

It was suggested previously that IgE may be considered to be a mucosal antibody (21). However, apart from evidence suggesting that some IgE in secretions is locally produced, there is little evidence to support this hypothesis. There is presently no known selective transport mechanism for IgE, and the traffic of IgE precursors and IgE-ACC is uncertain. There is evidence that following exposure to antigen, surface IgE^+ cells are able to migrate to the MLN (47); also, IgE-ACC may be found in TDL following mesenteric adenectomy, suggesting that they may demonstrate traffic similar to IgA precursors.

T Cells

In BALT, T cells constitute 18.4% of lymphocytes (145); this figure compares to 16.6% in PP. T cells with both the helper and suppressor phenotypes have been localized by immunohistochemical techniques in rat BALT (135), and there is now much evidence that T cells play an immunoregulatory role in mucosal tissues. T cells that provide specific help for IgA have been found in PP, and it may be assumed that similar cells will be characterized from BALT (48).

Intimately connected with immune regulation is the phenomenon of systemic hyporesponsiveness (tolerance) whereby important regulatory interactions take place between the mucosal and systemic immune systems.

Systemic unresponsiveness following oral immunization has been shown using a variety of antigens, both soluble (121,143) and particulate (35). Systemic hyporesponsiveness may include both humoral (121,143) and cell-mediated immunity (74) and is antigen-specific. Secretory immunity may exist in the presence of systemic hyporesponsiveness (35). Several mechanisms may be responsible for tolerance induction following oral immunization: these include regulatory T-suppressor cells (35,121,143), circulating immune complexes (4), B-suppressor cells (6), and specific serum antibodies including autoanti-idiotypic antibodies (90); several of these mechanisms may coexist (74,121,143).

Although systemic hyporesponsiveness has been most extensively studied following oral immunization, similar events may follow immunization of the respiratory tract (56).

There is some evidence that the microbial flora in the gut appears to play a role in immunoregulation. For example, germfree LPS-responsive mice demonstrate a heightened IgA response following oral immunization, and this response is markedly reduced following conventionalization owing to the development of T-suppressor cells (95).

Several studies have shown that T lymphoblasts from MLN and TDL will preferentially localize to the intestinal lamina propria, suggesting a similar circulation pathway to that outlined for B lymphoblasts (70,162). In addition, these cells will also localize to the intestinal epithelium; Guy-Grand et al. (71) have suggested that these cells may, in part, be derived from PP. Bienenstock (23) has shown that B lymphoblasts are unable to localize to the intestinal or respiratory epithelium. In experiments involving influenza-specific T-cell clones, it has been shown that these cells exhibit a propensity to localize to the lung, including the respiratory epithelium but not the intestinal lamina propria or epithelium (22).

The mechanisms underlying the selective localization of lymphocytes are uncertain and have been considered by McDermott et al. (109). Of particular interest, Husband and Gowans (84) have demonstrated that blast cells from TDL will localize nonselectively to the intestine but thereafter the ACC response is dependent on antigen for clonal expansion and proliferation.

EFFECTOR CELLS IN THE RESPIRATORY TRACT

The preceding sections have dealt largely with inductive events in respiratory tract immunity, and evidence has been presented that BALT is the source of IgA plasma cells and probably other immunoglobulin precursors. In the following section we discuss effector cells in the respiratory tract.

B Cells

Respiratory tract secretions contain immunoglobulins of all classes, but in the upper respiratory tract, including the nasopharynx, IgA is the most abundant immunoglobulin. In the lower respiratory tract the relative concentration of IgG increases and may exceed that of IgA (118), and IgG may be functionally more important (141). IgM is also found in respiratory tract secretions, but in lower concentrations than IgA and IgG (150); in some species, IgM is not detectable (142).

A major source of IgA found in external secretions is the abundant population of IgA plasma cells located in the lamina propria of mucosal tissues. The distribution of plasma cells in the respiratory tract reflects the immunoglobulin concentrations in secretions. IgA plasma cells are most numerous in the upper respiratory tract, and IgA is the predominant isotype synthesized *in vitro* by this tissue. Substantial synthesis of IgG by the respiratory tract also occurs in keeping with the numerous IgG plasma cells present.

The abundant IgA plasma cells found in the respiratory tract and IgA/IgG concentration ratios higher than those in serum suggested the existence of a selective transport mechanism for the secretion of IgA into external secretions. It is now known that plasma cells in the lamina propria of the intestine and other mucosal sites produce IgA as a polymer, usually a dimer incorporating a J chain. Polymeric IgA then complexes with SC, which is synthesized by epithelial cells and expressed on their basolateral surfaces. The IgA-SC complex is transported through the epithelial cell and is secreted, by a process of reverse pinocytosis, into the lumen where much of it is incorporated into the mucus coat (31). *In vitro* ultrastructural evidence for this process in the respiratory tract has been provided by Goodman et al. (64).

Therefore, the IgA content of mucosal secretions has generally been considered to reflect the activity of IgA plasma cells underlying the epithelium. In view of (a) the finding that circulating IgA is transported into bile by an SC-mediated mechanism and (b) the evidence that most of the IgA in intestinal secretions, at least in rodents, may be derived from this source, this assumption must be questioned. One approach to addressing the question of the origin of immunoglobulins in secretions is to inject radiolabeled immunoglobulins into the circulation and then compare the specific activities of immunoglobulins in regional efferent lymph, secretions, and blood. In sheep, the use of this technique has established that IgA in intestinal secretions is largely produced by plasma cells in the lamina propria (42). Similar experiments have been performed in sheep and have demonstrated that a large proportion of IgA in lung efferent lymph is derived from the circulation (151) and that circulating dimeric IgA but not IgG may be selectively transported into respiratory secretions. However, this component of the total IgA content in respiratory secretions is relatively small in comparison to the locally produced IgA (153). The extent and possible mechanism by which IgA may be transported into external secretions in humans are not known. In humans, most of the circulating IgA is monomeric and is thus poorly able to complex with SC for subsequent transport into secretions (99).

The function of IgA may be summarized as one of "immune exclusion" (167). IgA provides protection against viruses and bacteria at mucosal surfaces, and resistance to reinfection is generally correlated with the induction of sIgA. For example, Fazekas de St. Groth and Donnelly (57) showed that resistance to influenza virus in mice was related to local secretory antibodies and that local antigen was more effective in eliciting these antibodies than parenteral immunization. The production of protective antibodies may be independent of the serum antibody response (123), and when both a systemic and mucosal response are seen, immunity may best be correlated with the local secretory response (158).

IgA is, by virtue of the presence of SC, more resistant to proteolysis, although even without SC, IgA is more resistant to proteolysis than IgG (174). However, although IgA is relatively resistant to enzymic degradation, the pathogenicity of some bacteria (e.g., *Hemophilus influenzae* and *Streptococcus pneumoniae*) may be related to their ability to secrete a protease, specific for IgA (94).

There is some evidence that IgA may also function to reduce inflammation at mucosal surfaces in that it inhibits neutrophil chemotaxis (175) and the binding of antigen to IgG and fails to activate complement (38,68).

Although the role of IgG in mucosal defense has received less attention than IgA, there is a substantial amount of evidence to suggest that it is functionally important. In keeping with both its local synthesis and serum derivation, IgG antibodies may be detected in respiratory secretions after both systemic (82,139) and local intratracheal immunization (139).

In the respiratory tract, IgG exerts a protective effect against microbes and viruses (7,139); the mechanisms whereby it does this include antigen exclusion by immune complex formation (177), agglutination and phagocytosis by macrophages (140), virus neutralization (163), and antibody-dependent cell-mediated cytotoxicity (ADCC; 41).

IgE is the principal reaginic antibody and, by virtue of its ability to bind to the surface of mast cells with subsequent mediator release, plays a central role in allergic reactions. IgE is found in the respiratory secretions in both normal (46) and allergic individuals (133), and there is evidence that much of it is locally produced by plasma cells in the respiratory mucosa, regional lymph nodes, and lumen of the lungs (46,60,133,169) although some of it may be serum-derived (46).

IgM is found in respiratory secretions in low concentrations (142), and the presence of plasma cells producing IgM in the respiratory tract argues for its local synthesis. Very little is known of the functions of IgM in respiratory secretions, and these can only be inferred from those of serum IgM. On this basis it would be expected to agglutinate particulate antigens and activate complement during inflammation. That IgM at mucosal surfaces may play a protective role is suggested by the finding that in IgA-deficient individuals, IgM may assume the role of the major secretory immunoglobulin (31).

T Cells

T cells in the respiratory mucosa have been poorly studied. However, from analogy with the gut, several inferences can be drawn. In the gut, T lymphocytes are found in both the lamina propria and the epithelium. In the epithelium, the majority of cells bear the T-suppressor/cytotoxic phenotype, whereas the majority of T cells in the lamina propria are of the helper phenotype. In addition, 40% of intraepithelial leukocytes (IEL) are granulated and in this regard resemble the granulated leukocytes in peripheral blood, which have been shown to have natural killer (NK) cell activity. Intraepithelial leukocytes and lamina propria T cells have been demonstrated to possess a number of activities including ADCC and cytotoxic and NK activity. Cytotoxic cells with NK characteristics have been documented in the lungs of mice (136,165), and this cytotoxic activity is enhanced by inducers of interferon or by viral infection.

In the respiratory tract, cell-mediated immunity (CMI) has been assessed by the production of lymphokines (usually macrophage inhibition factor, MIF), by the *in vitro* demonstration of antigen-specific T-cell proliferation, or by demonstration of antigen-specific or natural cytotoxicity (cytotoxic T cells or NK cells).

In 1971, Truitt and MacKaness (172) showed that resistance to *Listeria monocytogenes* infection was associated with an influx of mononuclear cells into the lungs. Waldman and Henney (176) demonstrated the production of MIF by bronchoalveolar, but not spleen, cells in guinea pigs following intrapulmonary immunization with soluble antigen. Subcutaneous immunization led to the reverse situation. Nash and Holle (120) confirmed these findings and showed that, after large doses of intrapulmonary antigen, both local and systemic CMI could be elicited. Local and systemic CMI may also be produced by intrapulmonary immunization with bacteria (33).

Antigen-specific T cells following immunization with both soluble and particulate antigen and after viral infections have also been demonstrated in the respiratory tract (15,77). Ennis et al. (53) studied influenza A virus infection in mice and were able to demonstrate antigen-specific cytotoxicity in the lungs as well as the spleen, blood, and PLN. These workers were also able to show *in vitro* antigen-specific T-cell proliferation at a time when cytotoxic T-cell activity could no longer be demonstrated, suggesting the presence of more than one effector population. Yap et al. (183) confirmed these results and, in adoptive transfer experiments, showed that these cytotoxic T cells afforded protection against clinical infection following intranasal challenge with virus. Furthermore, cytotoxicity could be detected in BLN and lungs at a time when no such cytotoxicity was detected in the blood. Cytotoxic T cells have been found in the lungs following a variety of virus infections (37,168), as have their protective effects (110) and following local, systemic, and oral immunization with allogeneic cells (44,86,103).

Other Cells

Bronchoalveolar Cells

Macrophages

The lumen of the respiratory tract contains a resident population of immunoreactive cells consisting predominantly of macrophages and lymphocytes, generally referred to as *bronchoalveolar cells* (BAC). In most species studied, pulmonary alveolar macrophages (PAM) make up the majority of the BAC (109). PAM are phagocytic, adherent cells and form a functionally heterogeneous population (80,109). They display a number of surface receptors for immunoglobulins, including IgG (141), IgE (91) and probably IgA (140). PAM are ultimately derived from the bone marrow (62), although they may also arise by *in situ* proliferation (1).

Lymphocytes

In most species a substantial percentage of BAC are lymphocytes (83). Most of these are T cells and, depending on the species studied, up to 20% or more may bear surface immunoglobulin (109), whereas a variable percentage of species lack both T- and B-cell markers. The origin of bronchoalveolar lymphocytes is uncertain, but there is evidence they may be derived from BALT (18) and also from the circulation in both normal animals (43) and in those following intrapulmonary immunization (51).

Several studies have demonstrated that PAM interact with lymphocytes, although the nature of the interaction is dependent on the species. Lyons and Lipscomb (104) demonstrated that antigen-primed macrophages in guinea pigs supported the *in vitro* proliferation of T cells, similar findings to those of Holt and Batty (79). In contrast, in the rat, PAM suppressed the *in vitro* proliferative response of peripheral blood T cells in response to mitogen stimulation, a response enhanced by peritoneal macrophages (78–80). In the dog, Demenkoff et al. (45) demonstrated PAM suppression of mitogen-induced T-lymphocyte proliferation and provided evidence for the involvement of prostaglandins synthesized by PAM in this process.

Mast cells

Mast cells, basophils, and basophiloid cells are found throughout the respiratory tract, including BALT (20,92,134). In recent years, much interest has focused on the heterogeneity of mast cells based on histochemical and functional characteristics (26). Histochemical heterogeneity was initially described by Enerback (52), based on differences in dye binding following fixation with neutral buffered formalin versus other fixatives such as Mota's lead-acetate or Carnoy's fixative. Formalin inhibits dye binding to atypical or mucosal mast cells (MMC), which differ from connective tissue or peritoneal mast cells. MMC have best been characterized in the rat intestine, particularly following nematode infection (8). Their granules appear less numerous and lack heparin, compared to granules in peritoneal mast cells. They are unresponsive to several secretagogues, including 48/80, bee venom peptide 401, and various endorphins and neurotransmitters. The widely used antiasthmatic preparation, cromoglycate sodium, does not inhibit antigen-mediated release of histamine and other mediators from MMC. In humans, both types of mast cells are found in the intestine (9) but the major type in the lamina propria is the MMC type. In addition, as in nematode-infected rat intestine, mast cells were found in the epithelium and were almost exclusively MMC in type. Therefore, in humans, intestinal mucosal mast cells appear to be functionally similar to their counterpart in the rat. Mast cell heterogeneity in the lung has been studied following bleomycin treatment of rats. Bleomycin-induced pulmonary fibrosis is a condition known to be associated with pulmonary mastocytosis. Following intratracheal instillation of bleomycin, there is an increase in parenchymal mast cells, the majority of which are connective tissue in type, based on histochemical criteria. Functionally, this mast cell also appears to be more like the peritoneal mast cell rather than the mucosal mast cell. There are no significant changes in numbers or types of mast cells in the bronchial mucosa of bleomycin-treated rats (65).

Basophils and mast cells are infrequent in normal nasal mucosa (125,127). In patients with allergic rhinitis the majority of cells with metachromatic granules in nasal secretions were basophils, based on morphological and histochemical characteristics (126), but mast cells were more abundant in the nasal epithelium and underlying tissues. Recently, Otsuka et al. (128) have studied mast cells in nasal scrapings of patients with allergic rhinitis. The major cell type was the MMC, and there was good correlation between the numbers of these cells and symptom scores. The distribution and abundance of mast cell subpopulations in normal nasal mucosa have not been determined. In nasal biopsies, basophils were confined to the epithelium and adjacent lamina propria.

CONCLUSIONS

Evidence for a Local Immune System in the Middle Ear

The normal middle ear mucosa is relatively inaccessible to antigen, and this is reflected in the paucity of immunocompetent cells normally found (88,117,124).

The epithelium consists of basal, secretory, and ciliated cells and in some areas resembles normal respiratory epithelium, namely, pseudostratified, ciliated columnar epithelium (76). However, there is now ample evidence that the middle ear mucosa is a latent immunocompetent organ which, when exposed to viral, bacterial, or other antigens, responds vigorously with a response that has many characteristics of a mucosal immune response (Table 2). This has been best characterized in otitis media with effusion (OME).

In this situation there is marked infiltration of the lamina propria with plasma cells, lymphocytes, and mononuclear cells, including macrophages (12), and often there is metaplasia of the epithelium to a respiratory type with many goblet cells and submucous glands (11). The humoral response is similar to that seen at other mucosal surfaces in that most plasma cells produce IgA (67,114,117,124), the predominant form of which is sIgA (11S), and its secretion is SC-mediated (12,114,115,124). Much, if not all, of the IgA is synthesized locally, as evidenced by the higher IgA/IgG concentration ratios in middle ear effusions (MEE) compared to serum, the presence of specific antiviral and antibacterial antibodies (usually IgA) in MEE (but often their absence in serum), and the *in vitro* demonstration of IgA and SC synthesis by middle ear mucosa (12,124,156,157). IgG plasma cells are also found in the middle ear mucosa, and *in vitro* synthesis of this immunoglobulin by this tissue has been demonstrated (124). The role of IgE in OME is more controversial in that although this immunoglobulin has been demonstrated in MEE (reviewed in ref. 29) and there is evidence for its local synthesis, the demonstration of IgE plasma cells in middle ear mucosa has been inconsistent (116,124,132,156).

In OME, the middle ear mucosa may also mount a CMI response (12), as suggested by the large numbers of lymphocytes and macrophages in both the lamina

TABLE 2. *A comparison of mucosal immunity in the respiratory tract and middle ear mucosa*[a]

Characteristic	Respiratory tract	Middle ear in OME
Ciliated epithelium	Present	Present
Mucus production	Yes	Yes
Predominance of 11S IgA	Yes	Yes
Evidence for local synthesis		
IgA	Yes	Yes
IgG	Yes	Yes
IgE	Yes	Probable
SC	Yes	Yes
SC-mediated transport of IgA	Yes	Yes
Transport circulating IgA into secretions	Yes	Unknown
Cell-mediated immunity	Yes	Yes
Mast cells —heterogeneity	Yes	Unknown

[a]Adapted from Ogra et al. (124).

propria and MEE (182). Of particular interest is the finding that the macrophages may have an immunoregulatory role. Both enhancement and suppression of immunoglobulin synthesis and mitogen-induced lymphocyte proliferation by MEE macrophages have been demonstrated (13,182).

Some recent studies in rats have demonstrated that mast cells are found in both normal and OME middle ear mucosa (3,75,166). These cells are found in a layer in the subepithelial connective tissue, close to the basement membrane, particularly in the pars flaccida, and it has been shown that degranulation of these cells produces an effusion in the attic space of the middle ear (3,180). The pars flaccida in humans is also rich in mast cells (180).

REFERENCES

1. Adamson, I.Y.R., and Bowden, D.H. (1980): Role of monocytes and interstitial cells in the generation of alveolar macrophages. II. Kinetic studies after carbon loading. *Lab. Invest.*, 42:518–524.
2. Ahlstedt, S., Smedegard, G., Nygren, H., and Bjorksten, B. (1983): Immune response in rats immunized with aerosolized antigen. Antibody formation, lymphoblastic response and mast cell and goblet cell development related to bronchial reactivity. *Int. Arch. Allergy Appl. Immunol.*, 43:102–112.
3. Alm, P.E., Bloom, G.D., Hellstrom, S., Salen, B., and Stenfors, L.E. (1982): The release of histamine from the pars flaccida mast cells. One cause of otitis media with effusion? *Acta Otolaryngol.*, 94:517–522.
4. Andre, C., Heremans, J.F., Vaerman, J.P., and Cambiaso, C.L. (1975): A mechanism for the induction of immunological tolerance by antigen feeding: antigen-antibody complexes. *J. Exp. Med.*, 142:1509–1519.
5. Andrew, W., and Burns, M.R. (1974): Leucocytes in the trachea epithelium of the mouse. *J. Morphol.*, 81:317–341.
6. Asherson, G.L., Perera, M.A.C.C., Thomas, W.R., and Zembala, M. (1979): Contact sensitizing agents in the intestinal tract: the production of immunity and unresponsiveness by feeding contact-sensitizing agents and the role of suppressor cells. In *Immunology of Breast Milk*, edited by P.L. Ogra and D. Dayton, pp.9–36. Raven Press, New York.
7. Barber, W.H., and Small, P.A. (1978): Local and systemic immunity to influenza infections in ferrets. *Infect. Immun.*, 21:221–228.
8. Befus, A.D., Pearce, F.L., Gauldie, J., Horsewood, P., and Bienenstock, J. (1982): Mucosal mast cells. I. Isolation and functional characteristics of rat intestinal mast cells. *J. Immunol.* 128:2475–2480.
9. Befus, A.D., Goodacre, R., Dyck, N., and Bienenstock, J. (1985): Mast cell heterogeneity in man. I. Histologic studies of the intestine. *Int. Arch. Allergy Appl. Immunol.*, 76:232–236.
10. Beh, K.J., Husband, A.J., and Lascelles, A.K. (1979): Intestinal response of sheep to intraperitoneal immunisation. *Immunology*, 37:385–388.
11. Bernstein, J.M., and Hayes, E.R. (1971): Middle ear mucosa in health and disease. *Arch. Otolaryngol.*, 94:30–35.
12. Bernstein, J.M., and Ogra, P.L. (1980): Mucosal immune system: implications in otitis media with effusion. *Ann. Otorhinolaryngol.*, 89 (Suppl. 68):326–333.
13. Bernstein, J.M., Yamanaka, T., Cumella, J., and Ogra, P.L. (1984): Characteristics of lymphocyte and macrophage reactivity in otitis media with effusion. *Acta Otolaryngol. (Stockh.)* (Suppl.), 414:131–137.
14. Bhalla, D.K., and Owen, R.L. (1982): Cell renewal and migration in lymphoid follicles of Peyer's patch and caecum—an autoradiographic study in mice. *Gastroenterology*, 82:232–242.
15. Bice, D.E., and Schnizlein, C.T. (1980): Cellular immunity induced by lung immunization of Fischer 344 rats. *Int. Arch. Allergy Appl. Immunol.*, 63:438–445.
16. Bienenstock, J., and Dolezel, J. (1971): Peyer's patches: lack of specific antibody-containing cells after oral and parenteral immunization. *J. Immunol.*, 106:938–945.

17. Bienenstock, J., Johnston, N., and Perey, D.Y.E. (1973): Bronchial lymphoid tissue. I. Morphologic characteristics. *Lab. Invest.*, 28:686–692.
18. Bienenstock, J., Johnston, N., and Perey, D.Y.E. (1973): Bronchial lymphoid tissue. II. Functional characteristics. *Lab. Invest.*, 28:693–698.
19. Bienenstock, J., Rudzik, O., Clancy, R.L., and Perey, D.Y.E. (1974): Bronchial lymphoid tissue. *Adv. Exp. Med. Biol.*, 45:47–56.
20. Bienenstock, J., and Johnston, N. (1976): A morphologic study of rabbit bronchial lymphoid aggregates and lymphoepithelium. *Lab. Invest.*, 35:343–348.
21. Bienenstock, J., and Befus, A.D. (1980): Mucosal immunology. *Immunology*, 41:249–270.
22. Bienenstock, J., Befus, A.D., McDermott, M.R., Mirski, S., Rosenthal, K., and Tagliabue, A. (1983): The mucosal immunologic network: compartmentalization of lymphocytes, natural killer cells, and mast cells. *Ann. NY Acad. Sci.*, 409:164–170.
23. Bienenstock, J. (1984): Bronchus-associated lymphoid tissue. In: *Immunology of the Lung and Upper Respiratory Tract*, edited by J. Bienenstock, pp. 96–118. McGraw-Hill, New York.
24. Bienenstock, J., and Befus, A.D. (1984): Gut- and bronchus-associated lymphoid tissue. *Am. J. Anat.*, 170:437–445.
25. Bienenstock, J., and Befus, A.D. (1985): The gastrointestinal tract as an immune organ. In: *Gastrointestinal Immunity for the Clinician*, edited by R.G. Shorter and J.B. Kirsner, pp. 1–22. Grune and Stratton, Orlando, Fla.
26. Bienenstock, J., Befus, A.D., Denburg, J., Goto, T., Lee, T., Otsuka, H., and Shanahan, F. (1985): Comparative aspects of mast cell heterogeneity in different species and sites. *Int. Arch. Allergy Appl. Immunol.*, 77:126–129.
27. Bockman, D.E., and Cooper, M.D. (1973): Pinocytosis by epithelium associated with lymphoid follicles in the bursa of Fabricius, appendix and Peyer's patches. An electron microscopic study. *Am. J. Anat.*, 136:455–477.
28. Bockman, D.E., and Stevens, W. (1977): Gut-associated lymphoepithelial tissue: bidirectional transport of tracer by specialized epithelial cells associated with lymphoid follicles. *J. Reticuloendothel. Soc.*, 21:245–254.
29. Boedts, D., De Groote, G., and Van Vuchelen, J. (1984): Atopic allergy and otitis media with effusion. *Acta Otolaryngol. (Stockh.)* (Suppl.), 414:108–114.
30. Braley, J.F., Dawson, C.A., Moore, V.C., and Cozzini, B.O. (1978): Absorption of inhaled antigen into the circulation of isolated lungs from normal and immunized rabbits. *J. Clin. Invest.*, 61:1240–1246.
31. Brandtzaeg, P., and Baklien, K. (1977): Intestinal secretion of IgA and IgM: a hypothetical model. *Ciba Found. Symp.*, 46:77–108.
32. Bruge-Gamelkoorn, G.J. van der, and Kraal, G. (1985): The specificity of the high endothelial venule in bronchus-associated lymphoid tissue (BALT). *J. Immunol.*, 134:3746–3750.
33. Cantey, J.R., and Hand, W.L. (1974): Cell-mediated immunity after bacterial infection of the lower respiratory tract. *J. Clin. Invest.*, 54:1125–1134.
34. Cebra, J.J., Cebra, E.R., Clough, E.R., Fuhrman, J.A., Komisar, J.L., Schweitzer, P.A., and Shahin, R.D. (1983): IgA commitment: models for B-cell differentiation and possible roles for T-cells in regulating B-cell development. *Ann. NY Acad. Sci.*, 49:25–38.
35. Challacombe, S.J., and Tomasi, T.B., Jr. (1980): Systemic tolerance and secretory immunity after oral immunization. *J. Exp. Med.*, 152:1459–1472.
36. Chamberlain, D.W., Napajoroonsri, C., and Simon, G.T. (1973): Ultrastructure of the pulmonary lymphoid tissue. *Am. Rev. Respir. Dis.*, 108:621–631.
37. Clancy, R.L., Rawls, W.E., and Jagannaths, S. (1977): Appearance of cytotoxic cells within the bronchus after local infection with herpes simplex virus. *J. Immunol.*, 119:1102–1105.
38. Colten, H.R., and Bienenstock, J. (1974): Lack of C3 activation through classical or alternate pathways by human secretory IgA anti-blood group A antibody. *Adv. Exp. Med. Biol.*, 45:305–308.
39. Cornes, J.S. (1965): Number, size and distribution of Peyer's patches in the human small intestine. I. The development of Peyer's patches. *Gut*, 6:225–229.
40. Craig, S.W., and Cebra, J.J. (1971): Peyer's patches: an enriched source of precursors for IgA-producing immunocytes in the rabbit. *J. Exp. Med.*, 134:188–200.
41. Cranage, M.P., Gardner, P.S., and McIntosh, K. (1981): In vitro cell-dependent lysis of respiratory syncitial virus-infected cells mediated by antibody from lower respiratory secretions. *Clin. Exp. Immunol.*, 43:28–35.
42. Cripps, A.W., Husband, A.J., and Lascelles, A.K. (1974): The origin of immunoglobulins in intestinal secretions of sheep. *Aust. J. Exp. Biol. Med. Sci.*, 52:711–716.

43. Daniele, R.P., Beacham, H., and Gorenberg, D.F. (1977): The bronchoalveolar lymphocyte. Studies on the life history and lymphocyte traffic from blood to the lung. *Cell. Immunol.*, 31:48–54.
44. Davies, M.D.J., and Parrott, D.M.V. (1981): Cytotoxic T cells in small intestine epithelial lamina propria and lung lymphocytes. *Immunology*, 44:367–371.
45. Demenkoff, J.H., Ansfield, M.J., Kaltreider, H.B., and Adam, E. (1980): Alveolar macrophage suppression of canine broncho-alveolar lymphocytes: the role of prostaglandin E_2 in the inhibition of mitogen responses. *J. Immunol.*, 124:1365–1370.
46. Deuschl, H., and Johansson, S.G. (1974): Immunoglobulins in tracheo-bronchial secretion with special reference to IgE. *Clin. Exp. Immunol.*, 16:401–412.
47. Durkin, H.G., Bazin, H., and Waksman, B. (1981): Origin and fate of IgE-bearing lymphocytes. I. Peyer's patches as differentiation site of cells simultaneously bearing IgA and IgE. *J. Exp. Med.*, 154:640–648.
48. Elson, C.O., Heck, J.A., and Strober, W. (1979): T-cell regulation of murine IgA synthesis. *J. Exp. Med.*, 149:632–643.
49. Emery, J.L., and Dinsdale, F. (1973): The post-natal development of lymphoreticular aggregates and lymph nodes in infants' lungs. *J. Clin. Pathol.*, 26:539–545.
50. Emery, J.L., and Dinsdale, F. (1974): Increased incidence of lymphoreticular aggregates in lungs of children found unexpectedly dead. *Arch. Dis. Child.*, 49:107–111.
51. Emeson, G.E., Norin, A.J., and Veith, F.J. (1982): Antigen-induced recruitment of circulating lymphocytes in the lungs and hilar lymph nodes of mice challenged intratracheally with alloantigens. *Am. Rev. Respir. Dis.*, 125:453–459.
52. Enerback, L. (1966): Mast cells in rat gastrointestinal mucosa. Effects of fixation. *Acta Pathol. Microbiol. Scand.*, 66:289–302.
53. Ennis, F.A., Wells, M.A., Butchco, G.M., and Albrecht, P. (1978): Evidence that cytotoxic T cells are part of the host's response to influenza pneumonia. *J. Exp. Med.*, 148:1241–1250.
54. Ferguson, A. (1977): Intra-epithelial lymphocytes of the small intestine. *Gut*, 18:921–937.
55. Fournier, M., Vai, F., Derenne, J.P., and Pariente, R. (1977): Lymphoepithelial nodules in the rat. Morphologic features and uptake and transport of exogenous protein. *Am. Rev. Respir. Dis.*, 116:685–694.
56. Fox, P.C., and Siraganian, R.P. (1981): IgE antibody suppression following aerosol exposure to antigens. *Immunology*, 32:227–234.
57. Fazekas de St. Groth, S., and Donnelly, M. (1950): Studies in experimental immunology. III. Antibody response. *Aust. J. Exp. Biol. Med. Sci.*, 28:45–60.
58. Fuhrman, J.A., and Cebra, J.J. (1981): Special features of the priming process for a secretory IgA response. B cell priming with cholera toxin. *J. Exp. Med.*, 153:534–544.
59. Gearhart, P.J., and Cebra, J.J. (1979): Differentiated B lymphocytes: potential to express particular antibody variable and constant regions depends on site of lymphoid tissue and antigen load. *J. Exp. Med.*, 149:217–227.
60. Gerbrandy, J.F.L., and Bienenstock, J. (1976): Kinetics and localization of IgE tetanus antibody response in mice immunized by intratracheal, intraperitoneal and subcutaneous routes. *Immunology*, 31:913–919.
61. Gershwin, L.J., Osebold, J.W., and Zee, Y.C. (1981): Immunoglobulin-E containing cells in mouse lung following allergen inhalation and ozone exposure. *Int. Arch. Allergy Appl. Immunol.*, 65:266–277.
62. Godleski, J.J., and Brain, J.F. (1972): The origin of alveolar macrophages in mouse radiation chimeras. *J. Exp. Med.*, 136:630–643.
63. Goldblum, R.M., Ahlstedt, S., Carlsson, B., Hanson, L.A., Jodal, U., Lidin-Janson, G., and Sohl-Akerlund, A. (1975): Antibody-forming cells in human colostrum after oral immunization. *Nature*, 257:797–798.
64. Goodman, M.R., Link, D.W., Brown, W.R., and Nakane, P.K. (1981): Ultrastructural evidence of transport of secretory IgA across bronchial epithelium. *Am. Rev. Respir. Dis.*, 123:115–119.
65. Goto, T., Befus, A.D., Low, R., and Bienenstock, J. (1984): Mast cell heterogeneity and hyperplasia in bleomycin-induced pulmonary fibrosis. *Am. Rev. Respir. Dis.*, 130:797–802.
66. Gowans, J., and Knight, E.J. (1964): The route of recirculation of lymphocytes in the rat. *Proc. R. Soc. London (Biol.)*, 159:257–282.
67. Goycoolea, M.M., Paparella, M.M., Juhn, S.K., and Carpenter, A.M. (1980): Cells involved in the middle ear defence system. *Ann. Otorhinolaryngol.* 89(Suppl. 68):121–128.

68. Griffiss, J.M., and Bertram, M.A. (1977): Immunoepidemiology of meningococcal disease in military recruits. II. Blocking of serum bacterial activity by circulating IgA early in the course of invasive disease. *J. Infect. Dis.*, 136:733–739.
69. Griscelli, C., Vassalli, P., and McCluskey, R.T. (1969): The distribution of large dividing lymph node cells in syngeneic recipient rats after intravenous injection. *J. Exp. Med.*, 130:1427–1451.
70. Guy-Grand, D., Griscelli, C., and Vassalli, P. (1974): The gut-associated lymphoid system: nature and properties of large dividing cells. *Eur. J. Immunol.*, 4:435–443.
71. Guy-Grand, D., Griscelli, C., and Vassalli, P. (1978): The mouse gut T lymphocyte, a novel type of T cell. Nature, origin and traffic in mice in normal and graft-versus-host conditions. *J. Exp. Med.* 148:1661–1667.
72. Hall, J.G., and Smith, M.E. (1970): Homing of lymph-borne immunoblasts to the gut. *Nature*, 226:262–263.
73. Hall, J.G., Orlans, E., Reynolds, J., Dean, C., Peppard, J., Gyure, L., and Hobbs, S. (1979): Occurrence of specific antibodies of the IgA class in the bile of rats. *Int. Arch. Allergy Appl. Immunol.*, 59:75–84.
74. Hanson, D.G., and Miller, S.D. (1982): Inhibition of specific immune responses by feeding protein antigens. V. Introduction of the tolerant state in the absence of specific suppressor T cells. *J. Immunol.*, 128:2378–2381.
75. Hellstrom, S., Cerne, A., and Stenfors, L.-E. (1984): The attic space—its development and some species differences. *Acta Otolaryngol. (Stockh.)* (Suppl.), 414:31–33.
76. Hentzer, E. (1984): Ultrastructure of the middle ear mucosa. *Acta Otolaryngol. (Stockh.)* (Suppl.) 414:19–27.
77. Hill, J.O., and Burrell, R. (1979): Cell mediated immunity to soluble and particulate inhaled antigen. *Clin. Exp. Immunol.*, 38:332–341.
78. Holt, P.G. (1979): Alveolar macrophages. II. Inhibition of lymphocyte proliferation by purified macrophages from rat lung. *Immunology*, 37:429–436.
79. Holt, P.G., and Batty, J.E. (1980): Alveolar macrophages. V. Comparative studies on the antigen presentation activity of guinea-pig and rat alveolar macrophages. *Immunology*, 41:361–366.
80. Holt, P.G., Warner, L.A., and Papadimitriou, J.M. (1982): Alveolar macrophages: functional heterogeneity within macrophage populations from rat lung. *Aust. J. Exp. Biol. Med. Sci.*, 60:607–618.
81. Hoover, R.G., and Lynch, R.G. (1983): Isotype-specific suppression of IgA: suppression of IgA responses in BALB/c mice by T cells. *J. Immunol.*, 130:521–523.
82. Howard, C.J., Gourlay, R.N., and Taylor, G. (1979): Immunity to *Mycoplasma bovis* infections of the respiratory tract in calves. *Res. Vet. Sci.*, 28:242–249.
83. Hunninghake, G.W., Gadek, J.E., Kawanami, O., Ferrans, V.J., and Crystal, R.G. (1979): Inflammatory and immune processes in the human lung in health and disease: evaluation by broncho-alveolar lavage. *Am. J. Pathol.*, 97:149–206.
84. Husband, A.J., and Gowans, J.L. (1978): The origin and antigen-dependent distribution of IgA-containing cells in the intestine. *J. Exp. Med.*, 148:1146–1160.
85. Husband, A.J., Beh, K.J., and Lascelles, A.K. (1979): IgA-containing cells in the ruminant intestine following intraperitoneal and local immunization. *Immunology*, 37:597–601.
86. Husband, A., Cripps, A., and Clancy, R. (1983): Generation and migration patterns of intestinal T- and B-lymphocytes in response to local antigen. *Ann. NY Acad. Sci.*, 409:828.
87. Husband, A.J., Dunkley, M.L., Scicchitano, R., and Sheldrake, R.F. (1984): Induction and delivery of mucosal immune responses. *J. Dental Res.*, 63:465–469.
88. Hussl, H., and Lim, D. (1976): Immunofluorescent studies in experimental middle ear effusions. *Ann. Otorhinolaryngol.*, 85:124–129.
89. Jackson, G.D.F., Lemaitre-Coelho, I., Vaerman, J.-P., Bazin, H., and Beckers, A. (1978): Rapid disappearance from serum of intravenously injected rat myeloma IgA and its secretion into bile. *Eur. J. Immunol.*, 8:123–126.
90. Jackson, S., and Mestecky, J. (1981): Oral-parenteral immunization leads to the appearance of IgG-auto-anti-idiotypic cells in mucosal tissues. *Cell. Immunol.* 60:498–502.
91. Joseph, M., Tonnel, A.B., Capron, A., and Voisin, C. (1980): Enzyme release and superoxide anion production by human alveolar macrophages stimulated with immunoglobuln E. *Clin. Exp. Immunol.*, 40:416–422.
92. Kawanami, D., Ferans, V.J., Fulmer, J.D., and Crystal, R.G. (1979): Ultrastructure of pulmonary mast cells in patients with fibrotic lung disorder. *Lab. Invest.*, 40:717–734.

93. Kawanishi, H., Saltzman, L.E., and Strober, W. (1983): Mechanisms regulating IgA-class specific immunoglobulin production in murine gut-associated lymphoid tissues. I. T cells derived from Peyer's patches that switch sIgM B cells to sIgA B cells in vitro. *J. Exp. Med.*, 157:433–450.
94. Kilian, M., Mestecky, J., and Schrohenloher, R.E. (1979): Pathogenic species of the genus *Haemophilus* and *Streptococcus* pneumoniae produce immunoglobulin A protease. *Infect. Immun.*, 26:142–149.
95. Kiyono, H., Babb, J.L., Michalek, S.M., and McGhee, J.R. (1980): Cellular basis for elevated IgA response in C3H-HeJ mice. *J. Immunol.*, 125:732–737.
96. Kiyono, H., McGhee, J.R., Mosteller, L.M., Eldridge, J.H., Koopman, W.J., Kearney, J.F., and Michalek, S.M. (1982): Murine Peyer's patch T cell clones. Characterization of antigen-specific helper T cells for immunoglobulin A responses. *J. Exp. Med.*, 156:1115–1130.
97. Kiyono, H., Phillips, J.O., Colwell, D.E., Michalek, S.M., Koopman, W.J., and McGhee, J.R. (1984): Isotype-specificity of helper T clones: Fcα receptors regulate T and B cell collaboration for IgA responses. *J. Immunol.*, 133:1087–1089.
98. Kiyono, H., Mosteller-Barnum, L.M., Pitts, A.M., Williamson, S.I., Michalek, S.M., and McGhee, J.R. (1985): Isotype specific immunoregulation. IgA-binding factors produced by Fcα receptor-positive T cell hybridomas regulate IgA responses. *J. Exp. Med.*, 161:731–747.
99. Kutteh, W.H., Prince, S.J., and Mestecky, J. (1982): Tissue origins of human polymeric and monomeric IgA. *J. Immunol.*, 128:990–995.
100. Kyriazis, A.A., and Esterly, J.R. (1970): Development of lymphoid tissues in the human embryo and early fetus. *Arch. Pathol.*, 90:348–353.
101. Lindsay, M.C., Blaies, D.B., and Williams, J.F. (1983): *Taenia taeniaeformis*: immunoglobulin-E containing cells in intestinal and lymphatic tissues of infected rats. *Int. J. Parasitol.*, 13:91–99.
102. Lipscomb, M.F., Toews, G.B., Lyons, R., and Uhr, J.W. (1981): Antigen presentation by guinea pig alveolar macrophages. *J. Immunol.*, 126:286–291.
103. Liu, M.C., Ishizaka, K., and Plaut, M. (1982): T lymphocyte responses of murine lung: immunization with alloantigen induces accumulation of cytotoxic and other T lymphocytes in the lung. *J. Immunol.*, 129:2653–2662.
104. Lyons, C.R., and Lipscomb, M.F. (1983): Alveolar macrophages in pulmonary immune responses. I. Role in the initiation of primary immune responses and in selective recruitment of T lymphocytes to the lung. *J. Immunol.*, 130:1113–1119.
105. MacPherson, G.G., and Steer, H.W. (1979): Properties of mononuclear phagocytes derived from the small intestinal wall of rats. In: *Structure and Function of the Immune System*, edited by W. Muller-Bucholtz and H.K. Muller-Hermelink, pp. 433–438. Plenum Press, New York.
106. Mayrhofer, G., Bazin, H., and Gowans, J.L. (1976): Nature of cells binding anti-IgE in rats immunized with *Nippostrongylus brasiliensis:* IgE synthesis in regional nodes and concentration in mucosal mast cells. *Eur. J. Immunol.*, 6:537–545.
107. McDermott, M.R., and Bienenstock, J. (1979): Evidence for a common mucosal immunologic system. I. Migration of B immunoblasts into intestinal, respiratory and genital tissues. *J. Immunol.*, 122:1892–1898.
108. McDermott, M.R., Clark, D.A., and Bienenstock, J. (1980): Evidence for a common mucosal immunologic system. II. Influence of the estrous cycle on B-immunoblast migration into genital and intestinal tissues. *J. Immunol.*, 124:2536–2539.
109. McDermott, M.R., Befus, A.D., and Bienenstock, J. (1982): The structural basis for immunity in the respiratory tract. *Int. Rev. Exp. Pathol.*, 23:47–112.
110. McMichael, A.J., Gotch, F.M., Noble, G.R., and Beare, P.A.S. (1983): Cytotoxic T-cell immunity to influence. *N. Engl. J. Med.*, 309:13–17.
111. Mestecky, J., McGhee, J.R., Arnold, R.R., Michalek, S.M., Prince, S.J., and Babb, J.L. (1978): Selective induction of an immune response in human external secretions by ingestion of bacterial antigen. *J. Clin. Invest.*, 61:731–737.
112. Meuwissen, J.H., and Hussain, M. (1982): Bronchus-associated lymphoid tissue in human lung: correlation of hyperplasia with chronic pulmonary disease. *Clin. Immunol. Immunopathol.*, 23:548–561.
113. Milne, R.W., Bienenstock, J., and Perey, D.Y.E. (1975): The influence of antigenic stimulation on the ontogeny of lymphoid aggregates and immunoglobulin-containing cells in mouse bronchial and intestinal mucosa. *J. Reticuloendothel. Soc.*, 17:361–369.

114. Mogi, G., Honjo, S., Maeda, S., and Yoshida, T. (1973): Secretory immunoglobulin A (sIgA) in middle ear effusions. *Ann. Otorhinolaryngol.*, 82:302–310.
115. Mogi, G., Honjo, S., Maeda, S., Yoshida, T., and Watanabe, N. (1974): Secretory immunoglobulin A (sIgA) in middle ear effusions. *Ann. Otorhinolaryngol.*, 83:92–101.
116. Mogi, G., Maeda, S., Yoshida, T., and Watanabe, N. (1976): Radioimmunoassay of IgE in middle ear effusions. *Acta Otolaryngol.*, 82:26–32.
117. Mogi, G., Maeda, S., and Watanabe, N. (1980): Immunofluorescent study on middle ear mucosa. *Ann. Otol. Rhinol. Laryngol.*, 89 (Suppl. 68):333–338.
118. Morgan, K.L., Hussein, A.M., Newby, T.J., and Bourne, F.J. (1980): Quantification and origin of the immunoglobulins in porcine respiratory tract secretions. *Immunology*, 31:729–736.
119. Myrvick, Q.N., and Ockers, J.R. (1982): Transport of horse-radish peroxidase from the vascular compartment to bronchial-associated lymphoid tissue. *J. Reticuloendothel. Soc.*, 31:267–278.
120. Nash, D.R., and Holle, B. (1973): Local and systemic cellular immune responses in guinea-pigs given antigen parenterally or directly into the lower respiratory tract. *Clin. Exp. Immunol.*, 13:573–583.
121. Ngan, J., and Kind, L.S. (1978): Suppressor T cells for IgE and IgG in Peyer's patches of mice made tolerant by the oral administration of ovalbumin. *J. Immunol.*, 120:861–865.
122. Nieuwenhuis, P. (1971): On the origin and fate of immunologically competent cells. M.D. Thesis, University of Groningen, The Netherlands.
123. Ogra, P.L., and Karzon, D.R. (1969): Poliovirus antibody response in serum and nasal secretions following intranasal innoculation with inactivated poliovirus. *J. Immunol.*, 102:15–23.
124. Ogra, P.L., Bernstein, J.M., Yurchak, A.M., Coppola, P.R., Tomasi, T.B., Jr. (1974): Characteristics of secretory immune system in human middle ear: implications in otitis media. *J. Immunol.*, 112:488–495.
125. Okuda, M., and Otsuka, H. (1977): Basophilic cells in allergic nasal secretions. *Arch. Otorhinolaryngol.*, 214:283–289.
126. Okuda, M., Kawabori, S., Ohtsuka, H. (1978): Electron microscope study of basophilic cells in allergic nasal secretions. *Arch. Otorhinolaryngol.*, 221:215–220.
127. Otsuka, H., and Okuda, M. (1981): Important factors in the nasal manifestation of allergy. *Arch. Otorhinolaryngol.*, 233:227–235.
128. Otsuka, H., Denburg, J., Dolovich, J., Hitch, D., Lapp, P., Rajan, R.S., Bienenstock, J., and Befus, D. (1985): Heterogeneity of metachromatic cells in human nose: significance of mucosal mast cells. (*in press*).
129. Owen, R.L., and Jones, A.L. (1974): Epithelial cell specialization within human Peyer's patches: an ultrastructural study of intestinal lymphoid follicles. *Gastroenterology* 66:189–203.
130. Owen, R.L. (1977): Sequential uptake of horse radish peroxidase by lymphoid follicle epithelium of Peyer's patches in the normal unobstructed mouse intestine: an ultrastructural study. *Gastroenterology*, 37:440–451.
131. Peppard, J.V., Orlans, E., Andrew, E., and Payne, A.W.R. (1982): Elimination into bile of circulating antigen by endogenous IgA in rats. *Immunology*, 45:467–472.
132. Phillips, M.J., Manning, H., Knight, N.J., Abbott, A.L., and Tripp, W.G. (1974): IgE and secretory otitis media. *Lancet*, II:1176–1178.
133. Platts-Mills, T.A.E. (1979): Local production of IgG1, IgA and IgE antibodies in grass pollen hay fever. *J. Immunol.*, 122:2218–2225.
134. Plesch, B.E.C. (1982): Histology and immunochemistry of bronchus associated lymphoid tissue (BALT) in the rat. In: *In Vivo Immunology*, edited by P. Nieuwenhuis, A.A. van de Broek, and M.G. Hanna, Jr., pp. 491–497, Plenum Publishing Corp., New York.
135. Plesch, B.E.C. (1983): Development of bronchus-associated lymphoid tissue (BALT) in the rat, with special reference to T- and B-cells. *Dev. Comp. Immunol.*, 7:179–188.
136. Puccetti, P., Santoni, A., Riccardi, C., and Herberman, R.B. (1980): Cytotoxic effector cells with the characteristics of natural killer cells in the lungs of mice. *Int. J. Cancer*, 25:153–158.
137. Racz, P., Tenner-Racz, K., Myrvik, Q.N., and Fainter, L.K. (1977): Functional architecture of BALT and lymphoepithelium in pulmonary cell-mediated reactions in the rabbit. *J. Reticuloendothelial Soc.*, 22:59–83.
138. Racz, P., Tenner-Racz, K., Myrvick, Q.N. (1978): Sinus reactions in the hilar lymph node complex of rabbits undergoing a pulmonary cell-mediated immune response: sinus macrophage clumping reaction, sinus lymphocytosis and immature sinus histiocytosis. *J. Reticuloendothel. Soc.*, 24:499–525.

140. Reynolds, H.Y., and Thompson, R.E. (1973): Pulmonary host defences. II. Interaction of respiratory antibodies with *Pseudomonas aeruginosa* and alveolar macrophages. *J. Immunol.* 111:369–380.
141. Reynolds, H.Y., Kazmierowski, J.A., and Newball, H.H. (1975): Specificity of opsonic antibodies to enhance phagocytosis of Pseudomonas aeruginosa by human alveolar macrophages. *J. Clin. Invest.*, 56:376–385.
142. Reynolds, H.Y., Merrill, W.M., Amento, E.P., and Naegel, G.P. (1978): Immunoglobulin A in secretions from the lower human respiratory tract. *Adv. Exp. Med. Biol.*, 107:553–564.
143. Richman, L.K., Graeff, A.S., Yarchoan, R., and Strober, W.S. (1981): Simultaneous induction of antigen-specific IgA helper T cells and IgG suppressor T cells in the murine Peyer's patches after protein feeding. *J. Immunol.*, 126:2079–2083.
144. Roux, M.E., McWilliams, M., and Phillips-Quagliata, J.M. (1977): Origin of IgA-secreting plasma cells in the mammary gland. *J. Exp. Med.*, 146:1311–1322.
145. Rudzik, O., Clancy, R.L., Perey, D.Y.E., Bienenstock, J., and Singal, D.P. (1975): The distribution of a rabbit thymic antigen and membrane immunoglobulins in lymphoid tissue, with special reference to mucosal lymphocytes. *J. Immunol.*, 114:1–4.
146. Rudzik, O., Clancy, R.L., Perey, D.Y.E., Day, R.P., and Bienenstock, J. (1975): Repopulation with IgA-containing cells of bronchial and intestinal lamina propria after the transfer of homologous Peyer's patches and bronchial lymphocytes. *J. Immunol.*, 114:1599–1604.
147. Rudzik, O., Perey, D.Y.E., and Bienenstock, J. (1975): Differential IgA repopulation after transfer of autologous and allogeneic rabbit Peyer's patch cells. *J. Immunol.*, 114:40–44.
148. Saif, I., Bohn, E., and Gupta, R. (1972): Isolation of porcine immunoglobulin and determination of the immunoglobulin classes of transmissible gastroenteritis viral antibodies. *Infect. Immun.*, 6:600–609.
149. Schmedtje, J.F. (1966): Fine structure of intracellular lymphocyte clusters in the rabbit appendix epithelium. *Anat. Rec.*, 154:417.
150. Scicchitano, R. (1984): Respiratory tract immunity in sheep and man. Ph.D. Thesis, University of Newcastle, Australia.
151. Scicchitano, R., Husband, A.J., and Cripps, A.W. (1984): Immunoglobulin-containing cells and the origin of immunoglobulins in the respiratory tract of sheep. *Immunology*, 52:529–537.
152. Scicchitano, R., Husband, A.J., and Clancy, R.L. (1984): Contribution of gut immunization to the local immune response in the respiratory tract. *Immunology*, 53:375–384.
153. Scicchitano, R., Husband, A.J., and Sheldrake, R.F. (1986): Selective transport of IgA into respiratory secretions. *Immunology,* 58:315–321.
154. Sedgewick, J.D., and Holt, P.G. (1985): Induction of IgE-secreting cells and isotype-specific suppressor T cells in the respiratory lymph nodes of rats in response to antigen inhalation. *Cell. Immunol.*, 94:182–194.
155. Sheldrake, R.F., Husband, A.J., Watson, D.L., and Cripps, A.W. (1984): Selective transport of serum-derived IgA into mucosal secretions. *J. Immunol.*, 132:363–368.
156. Sloyer, J.L., Jr., Cate, C.C., Howie, V.M., Ploussard, J.H., and Johnston, R.B., Jr. (1975): The immune response to acute otitis media in children. II. Serum and middle ear fluid antibody in otitis media due to *Hemophilus influenzae*. *J. Infect. Dis.*, 132:685–688.
157. Sloyer, J.L., Jr., Howie, V.M., Ploussard, J.H., Bradac, J., Habercorn, M., and Ogra, P.L. (1977): Immune response to acute otitis media in children. III. Implications of viral antibody in middle ear fluid. *J. Immunol.*, 118:248–250.
158. Smith, C.B., Bellanti, J.A., and Chanock, R.M. (1967): Immunoglobulins in serum and nasal secretions following infection with Type I parainfluenza virus and injection of inactivated vaccines. *J. Immunol.*, 99:133–141.
159. Smith, M.W., Jarvis, L.G., and King, I.S. (1980): Cell proliferation in follicle-associated epithelium of mouse Peyer's patch. *Am. J. Anat.*, 159:157–166.
160. Soutar, C.A. (1976): Distribution of plasma cells and other cells containing immunoglobulin in the respiratory tract of normal man and class of immunoglobulin contained therein. *Thorax*, 31:158–166.
161. Spencer, J., Gyure, L.A., and Hall, J.G. (1983): IgA antibodies in the bile of rats. III. The role of intrathoracic lymph nodes and the migration pattern of their blast cells. *Immunology*, 48:687–693.
162. Sprent, J. (1976): Fate of H2-activated T lymphocytes in syngeneic hosts. I. Fate in lymphoid tissues and intestines traced with ^{3}H-thymidine, ^{125}I-deoxyuridine and ^{51}chromium. *Cell. Immunol.*, 21:278–302.

163. Sprino, P.J., and Ristic, M. (1982): Intestinal, pulmonary and serum antibody responses of feeder pigs exposed to transmissible gastroenteritis virus by the oral and oral-intranasal routes of innoculation. *Am. J. Vet. Res.*, 43:255–261.
164. Stafford, H.A., and Fanger, F.W. (1980): Receptors for IgA on rabbit lymphocytes. I. Distribution, specificity and modulation. *J. Immunol.* 125:2461–2466.
165. Stein-Streilein, J., Bennett, M., Mann, D., and Kumar, V. (1983): Natural killer cells in mouse lung: surface phenotype, target preference and response to local influenza virus infection. *J. Immunol.*, 131:2699–2704.
166. Stenfors, L.-E., Bloom, G.D., and Hellstrom, S. (1984): The tympanic membrane. *Acta Otolaryngol. (Stockh.)* (Suppl.), 414:28–30.
167. Stokes, C.R., Soothill, J.F., and Turner, M.W. (1975): Immune exclusion is a function of IgA. *Nature*, 255:745–746.
168. Sun, C.-S., Wyde, P.R., and Knight, V. (1983): Correlation of cytotoxic activity in lungs to recovery of normal and gamma-irradiated cotton rats from respiratory syncitial virus infection. *Am. Rev. Respir. Dis.*, 128:668–672.
169. Tada, T., and Ishizaka, K. (1970): Distribution of gamma E-forming cells in lymphoid tissues of the human and monkey. *J. Immunol.*, 104:377–387.
170. Tenner-Racz, K., Racz, P., Myrvik, Q., Ockers, J.R., and Geister, R. (1979): Uptake and transport of horse radish peroxidase by lymphoepithelium of the bronchus associated lymphoid tissue in normal and Bacillus Calmette-Guerin immunized and challenged rabbits. *Lab. Invest.*, 41:106–115.
171. Tomasi, T.B., Jr., Tan, E.M., Salomon, A., and Prendergast, R.A. (1965): Characteristics of an immune system common to certain external secretions. *J. Exp. Med.*, 121:101–124.
172. Truitt, G.L., and MacKaness, G.B. (1971): Cell-mediated resistance to aerogenic infection of the lung. *Am. Rev. Respir. Dis.*, 104:829–843.
173. Turner, F.N., and Kaltreider, H.B. (1978): Immunology of the lower respiratory tract. III. Concentrations of antigen and of antibody-forming cells in pulmonary and systemic lymphoid tissues of dogs after intrapulmonary or intravenous administration of sheep erythrocytes. *Clin. Exp. Immunol.*, 33:128–135.
174. Underdown, B., and Dorrington, K. (1974): Studies on the structural and conformational basis of relative resistance of serum and secretory immunoglobulin A to proteolysis. *J. Immunol.*, 112:949–959.
175. Van Epps, D.E., and Williams, R.C., Jr. (1976): Suppression of leucocyte chemotaxis by human IgA myeloma components. *J. Exp. Med.*, 144:1227–1242.
176. Waldman, R.H., and Henney, C.S. (1971): Cell-mediated immunity and antibody responses in the respiratory tract after local and systemic immunization. *J. Exp. Med.*, 134:482–489.
177. Walker, W.A., and Isselbacher, K.J. (1972): Intestinal uptake of macromolecules. Effect of oral immunization. *Science* 177:608–610.
178. Weisz-Carrington, P., Roux, M.E., McWilliams, M., Phillips-Quagliata, J.M., and Lamm, M.E. (1979): Oral and isotype distribution of plasma cells producing specific antibody after oral immunization: evidence for a generalized secretory immune system. *J. Immunol.*, 123:1705–1708.
179. Werkele, H., Ketelsen, U.P., and Ernst, M. (1980): Thymic nurse cells. Lymphoepithelial cell complexes in murine thymuses: morphological and serological characteristics. *J. Exp. Med.*, 151:925–944.
180. Widemar, L., Bloom, G.D., Hellstrom, S., and Stenfors, L.-E. (1984): Mast cells in the pars flaccida of the tympanic membrane. *Acta Orolaryngol. (Stockh.)* (Suppl.), 414:115–117.
181. Wolf, J.L., Rubin, D.H., Finberg, R., Kaufman, R.S., Sharpe, A.H., Trier, J.S., and Fields, B.N. (1981): Intestinal M cells—a pathway for entry of reovirus into the host. *Science*, 212:471–472.
182. Yamanaka, T., Bernstein, J.M., Cumella, J., Parker, C., and Ogra, P.L. (1982): Immunologic aspects of otitis media with effusion: characteristics of lymphocyte and macrophage reactivity. *J. Infect. Dis.*, 145:804–810.
183. Yap, K.L., Ada, G.L., and McKenzie, I.F.L. (1978): Transfer of specific cytotoxic T lymphocytes protects mice innoculated with influenza virus. *Nature*, 273:238–239.

Immunology of the Ear, edited by J. Bernstein and P. Ogra. Raven Press, New York © 1987.

Mucosal Immune System and Local Immunity

*James C. Cumella and **Pearay L. Ogra

**Department of Pediatrics, State University of New York at Buffalo, Buffalo, New York 14214, and Division of Infectious Diseases and Allergy, Children's Hospital of Buffalo, Buffalo, New York 14222; and **Departments of Pediatrics and Microbiology, State University of New York at Buffalo, School of Medicine, Buffalo, New York 14214, and Division of Infectious Diseases, Children's Hospital of Buffalo, Buffalo, New York 14222*

Previous studies have established that a well-defined secretory immune system exists in humans. This system has been analyzed in several monographs and reviews (6,8,20,50,81). The secretory immune system refers to the immunocompetent lymphoid tissue found in the external mucosal surfaces of mammals. It includes the gut-associated lymphoid tissue (GALT), the bronchus-associated lymphoid tissue (BALT), and the lymphoid tissue associated with the male and female external genital tract, the conjunctiva, and the mammary glands. A variety of mechanisms have evolved at mucosal surfaces to protect the host from both invasion by pathogens and other environmental macromolecules and subsequent local damage. These include both immune and nonimmune mechanisms. Nonimmune mechanisms include the integrity of the mucous and epithelial barriers of the gastrointestinal and respiratory tracts that help prevent mucosal penetration by viruses, bacteria, allergens, and a variety of other substances to which mucosal surfaces are exposed. Predominant among the immune mechanisms is the occurrence of 11S secretory IgA (sIgA), the major immunoglobulin constituent of the secretory immune system. Variable quantities of secretory IgM (sIgM), IgE, 7S IgA, and IgG are also present. In addition, components of T-cell-mediated immunity are receiving increasing recognition for their regulatory role in B-cell responses and for the recently recognized role in cell-mediated cytotoxicity (12,26).

The mucosal immune system appears (a) to be distinct from the systemic immune system and (b) to have independent regulation of functions through organized collections of lymphoid follicles localized at the mucosal sites (such as the Peyer's patches in the small intestine). A process of systemic traffic and eventual homing of antigen-reactive precursor cells to mucosal sites other than the site of original antigenic stimulation allows for a sharing of immune experiences between different mucosal sites. Considerable information has become available regarding the components of the mucosal defense and the development of the secretory immune system. A brief discussion of these components and their function follows.

ANTIGEN UPTAKE AND PROCESSING

Antigen penetration across mucosal barriers is now known to involve an elaborate system of controls both immunological and nonimmunological. Such mechanisms permit selective uptake of macromolecules that is important in facilitating selective mucosal responses. The mucosal immune response that is generated further inhibits antigen uptake by specific immune exclusion.

The structural anatomy of mucosal surfaces, itself, is an important determinant of antigen exclusion. A multilayered barrier is provided by the surface mucous layer, the *glycocalyx,* which is a columnar epithelial layer joined by tight junctions and an underlying basement membrane. Macromolecules have been found to transgress this barrier intact (antigenically and biologically active). This occurs in very limited amounts by an endocytotic process that is similar to pinocytosis (1,21). The molecules are deposited in the intestinal space at the basal surface of the cells by a reversal of this process. Macrophages and plasma cells in the lamina propria interact with these absorbed antigens as a secondary line of defense against penetration of these antigens into the circulation (21). Certain disease or altered states may allow for increased amounts of macromolecular transport. This can occur in malnutrition, vitamin A deficiency, alcohol ingestion, pancreatic insufficiency, decreased gastric acidity, and allergy (7,85). A breakdown of the epithelial tight junctional complexes is thought to occur in malnutrition and vitamin A deficiency (7,94). Excessive penetration of foreign macromolecules into the circulation may result in precipitating abnormal immunological responses.

In addition to the columnar epithelial cells, the mucosa of external surfaces, notably of the respiratory and gastrointestinal tracts, contain an appreciable proportion of lymphoid cells, intraepithelial lymphocytes (IEL), and mucosal mast cells. The IELs appear to be quite prominent in both respiratory and intestinal mucosa and exist in a proportion of about one IEL for every 10 to 15 epithelial cells. The IELs are usually localized in the basilar areas of the superficial epithelium and bear markers for suppressor-cytotoxic T cells or of natural killer (NK) cells. About 40% of IELs have been found to be granulated and contain sulfated mucopolysaccharides and histamine. Many of these cells have been shown to possess specific receptors for IgE, although the number of such receptors is estimated to be 10 to 15 times lower than those of tissue mast cells. Their precise function has not been clearly defined. Additional information on the cellular population of the bronchial-associated lymphoid system is reviewed in the chapter by Scicchitano et al. (*this volume*).

A specialized antigen transport system exists within the gut and bronchus which allows for the efficient transport of macromolecules directed to organized intestinal and bronchial lymphoid tissue. Immunocompetent B- and T-lymphocyte precursors are present (a) in large numbers in Peyer's patches in the ileum and appendix and (b) in small lymphoid aggregates scattered diffusely throughout the intestinal tract. Similar aggregates of B and T lymphocytes have been observed in the bronchus-associated lymphoid tissue (6). The epithelium covering the surface of these follicles consists, in part, of columnar epithelial cells, goblet cells, and specialized epithelial cells called M cells or follicle-associated epithelium (FAE). The epithelium that covers the dome-like projections of lymphoid tissue are referred to as *dome epithelium*. The FAE cells are unique and are felt to be especially adapted for antigen transport. Unlike absorptive columnar epithelium, which lines most of the intestine, these cells have a poorly developed glycocalyx (37), a paucity of microvilli (17), and lack enzymatic machinery. They also have a relative paucity of lysosomes (56) and lack the apical membrane enzymes (58,59) that characterize absorptive cells. In addition, these cells are in close association with lymphocytes, lymphoblasts, macrophages, and occasionally plasma cells. In addition to transporting antigen to immunoreactive cells, there is evidence that these cells may function in antigen presentation. Ia-like antigens have been found to be present on intestinal (90) and bronchial epithelial cells (63).

Antigen delivery to the precursor immunocompetent cells in the GALT and BALT by FAE is therefore a deliberate process by which selective samples of the environment are taken up and presented to the lymphocytes below the epithelium, for the initial development and subsequent stimulation of the mucosal immune system. This facilitated uptake of antigenic material overlying intestinal and bronchial lymphoid tissue is felt to be important in directing the mucosal immune response. An important component of the mucosal response is the subsequent generation of IgA.

FUNCTIONAL ACTIVITY OF IgA

Secretory IgA antibodies are well adapted for function in the harsh environment of external secretions—a complex mixture of biological fluids often containing proteolytic enzymes, sometimes poor in complement, and variable in pH. Specific antibody activity against a wide variety of bacteria, viruses, dietary proteins, antigens, and other macromolecules have been detected in most external secretions of humans and other animals. The antiviral activity of sIgA has been demonstrated against a number of viral agents, including poliovirus, echovirus, coxsackievirus, and adenovirus. The antibacterial activity of sIgA has been demonstrated against a variety of mucosal pathogens such as *Shigella, Vibrio cholerae, Streptococci,* and *E. coli*. Mucosal antibodies have also been demonstrated against the toxins of bacteria. IgA antibodies probably mediate their protective effect by a number of different mechanisms (see Table 1) that are related to their location (serum or secretion) and the form of the antibody present (monomer or polymer).

There is evidence to suggest that the primary function of sIgA is the specific "immune exclusion" of nonreplicating macromolecules, microbial toxins, and other infectious agents (84). This is a process by which binding sIgA to viable or nonviable antigens or to mucosal cellular receptors prevents access of these antigens across mucosal surfaces. Studies have indicated that the sIgA can block the specific binding sites on the bacterial cell wall, interfering with their adherence to the epithelium (89). Studies by Freter (31) have shown interference in the attachment of *Vibrio cholerae* to the intestinal mucosa by specific secretory antibody.

TABLE 1. *Proposed functions for IgA*

Function	Reference
1. Immune exclusion	
a. Macromolecules	82,84
b. Microbial toxins	83
c. Infectious agents	28,89
2. Clearance of circulating antigen	
a. Low-molecular-weight complexes ($<10^6$) via hepatocytes—secretory component mediated	13,27,86
b. High-molecular-weight complexes ($>10^6$) via Kupffer cells—Fcα receptor mediated	65
3. Inhibition of inflammation	69
4. Antigen priming—Ag delivery to remote external sites—mammary glands	9

The secretory antibodies to cholera enterotoxin prevent binding of the toxin to receptors on the intestinal microvillous membrane (83). Studies by Walker have suggested that secretory antibody interferes with the uptake of nonviable macromolecules introduced directly into the gastrointestinal tract. Using physicochemical analytic procedures, it has been shown that the hydrophilic, antiadhesive properties of sIgA contribute to keeping enteric microbes away from mucosal surfaces (28). There is additional evidence that antibody-antigen complexes formed in the gastrointestinal tract lead to increased production of mucus and enhanced degradation of antigens, thus further reducing the available antigen load for absorption (82). Based on these observations it has been suggested that the secretory antibody may play an important regulatory role in the host immune response by excluding, or at least limiting, exposure to a variety of otherwise harmful antigens from the systemic immune response and from the deeper sites of mucosal immunocompetent lymphoid tissue. Indeed, penetration of FAE by some viruses or bacteria in the absence of specific antibodies may sometimes serve to disseminate and induce disease.

The role of IgA does not appear to be limited to preventing access of antigens into systemic circulation. Another function of IgA is related to the clearance of circulating antigens. Despite the structural and immunological barriers previously described, relatively large amounts of intact or partially degraded macromolecules are absorbed into circulation (86). Recent evidence provided by Brown et al. (13,14) suggests that serum polymeric IgA mediates the transport of antigen as immune complexes through the liver to the bile. He and co-workers demonstrated that antigens absorbed from the intestine can be eliminated into the bile via specific IgA antibodies and can be transported in largely intact molecular forms (14). The mechanism of the transport has been extensively studied in rodents and involves secretory component on the sinusoidal surface of hepatocytes as specific receptors (13,40). Once the IgA binds to secretory component, it is then endocytosed and transported within vesicles (14,48). The vesicle subsequently fuses with the canalicular surface, discharging the sIgA into the bile. This transport mechanism is important for free polymeric IgA and IgA-immune complexes. The hepatic parenchymal cells are therefore extensively involved in the clearance of physiologically absorbed macromolecules against which IgA antibodies have been synthesized. In this way the IgA antibodies serve at two sites, initially as a barrier to prevent absorption and then as a specific clearance mechanism for those antigens that did give access to systemic circulation.

It should be noted that there appears to be a size limit of 10^6 daltons for this hepatobiliary transport (69). Complexes above this size are cleared by nonparenchymal cells since they would not be able to penetrate the fenestrated endothelial lining of the liver sinusoids (69). There is evidence that the clearance of the larger IgA-immune complexes is mediated by a specific rceptor for IgA on Kupffer cells (65). It has been demonstrated that this receptor does not distinguish between monomeric and dimeric IgA molecules (65). The removal of IgA-immune complexes appears to be limited to the liver and does not take place to any significant extent at other secretory sites such as the salivary gland (13). Submucosal plasma cells that produce IgA may compete for secretory component at these sites and limit transport of serum IgA.

Once antigens gain access to circulation they have the capacity to elicit systemic immune responses. The property of IgA to sometimes act as an antiopsonin may represent still another of its important functional roles. By binding to antigenic sites that otherwise might interact with opsonizing, complement fixing, or bactericidal antibodies of the IgM or IgG classes, IgA may serve as a blocking antibody. This may serve a protective effect in the serum when macromolecules from the gut are present to which specific IgA is directed. By preventing phagocytosis and the resulting inflammatory process that can occur with complement activation and the release of active metabolites from phagocytic cells, the specific IgA can thus mediate a noninflammatory clearance of these proteins through the liver.

The removal of IgA-immune complexes from circulation by transport into secretions appears to be restricted primarily to the liver. Delacroix et al. (25) have shown that, in humans, only 1.6% of total salivary polymeric IgA originates from the serum, as compared with 50% from the bile. However, the limited extent to which the transport of IgA-immune complexes does occur at these secretory sites may have important implications aside from the removal of circulating antigen. Several mucosal tissues have little direct contact with antigens such as the uterus. In addition, the mammary glands, which function as extensions of the gut- and bronchus-associated immunocompetent lymphoid tissue, are also quite remote from direct antigen stimulation. Antigen complexes with circulating dimeric IgA may be selectively transported in limited, but sufficient, amounts in these tissues to play a role in directing the antigen priming of the immunocompetent cells that are resident there.

In addition to the mechanisms outlined above, recent evidence suggests that IgA antibodies have the capacity to exert their antiviral and antibacterial effects in yet another way, at least at mucosal surfaces. Large granular lymphocytes, the main effector cells of antibody-dependent cellular cytotoxicity (ADCC) and NK activity against tumor cells in many species, are present in high numbers in the intestinal epithelium and lamina propria. Tagliabue et al. (78) have demonstrated that GALT lymphocytes can exert antibacterial activity against enteric organisms such as *Shi-* as *Shigella*. He and co-workers demonstrated that the ADCC of GALT lymphocytes was specific for IgA antibodies since no activity was observed with the other isotypes that were studied (77). Lymphocytes obtained from other sources, including spleen, thymus, and popliteal lymph nodes, were unable to mediate ADCC with IgA antibodies, but were capable of mediating this activity with IgG antibodies. Another recent report suggests that peripheral blood monocytes are also capable of mediating ADCC with specific IgA antibodies (44). ADCC is now considered to be one of the most efficient immune mechanisms against a broad range of targets, including bacteria, fungi, protozoa, and nematodes. The role of IgA in ADCC may represent an important local defense mechanism at mucosal surfaces and lend support to the concept that cell-mediated responses may also be very important as a first line of defense against mucosal pathogens.

THE REGULATION OF THE MUCOSAL IMMUNE RESPONSE

Mucosal immunity is largely dependent on IgA production. The steps leading to eventual IgA production appear to extensively involve T-B cell collaboration. In GALT and BALT there is evidence that IgA class-specific regulatory T cells are preferentially present and play a major role in determining the development of IgA B cells (75,76,80). Regulatory T cells characteristically express Fc receptors for IgA. Several studies have shown that both class-specific helper and suppressor cells are involved in regulating the IgA response. In humans, helper T cells that bear Fc receptors for IgA have been demonstrated to promote IgA responses. Functionally distinct subsets of these helper cells that induce isotype switching from precursor cells bearing surface IgM to those expressing IgA and another subset that induces terminal differentiation have been defined (38). Fcα-receptor-bearing T-suppressor cells have also been demonstrated to regulate isotype-specific suppression of IgA responses (34). It therefore appears that the Fcα receptor is the major recognition determinant on T cells for isotype-specific help or suppression. The mechanism by which T and B cells collaborate via the Fc receptor is still not defined. Kirzano et al. (42) proposed two possible mechanisms for this collaboration. The first one involves direct contact of the isotype-specific T cell bearing the Fcα receptor with isotype-committed B cells resulting in B-cell activation, differentiation, and IgA synthesis. Another possible mechanism of T-B cell collaboration for an IgA response is that the Fcα-receptor-bearing T cell may release soluble Fcα receptor or immunoglobulin binding factor for IgA that bind to the Fcα determinant on the B-cell surface. This signal would then induce activation of IgA-committed B cells and lead to IgA synthesis.

Further studies have elucidated the nature of T-helper cells involved in the differentiation of IgA lymphoblasts (74). In addition to having the Fcα receptor, these T helper-inducer cells require histocompatability locus-associated (HLA)-class II restriction and appear to be antigen specific and do not support polyclonal responses to other antigens. Kirzano et al. (41) have recently isolated and characterized several T-cell clones from murine Peyer's patches that exhibit antigen-specific helper activity predominately for IgA isotype responses. Accessory cells (macrophages or dendritic cells) that are HLA-DR positive (express Ia antigens) play an essential role in antigen presentation. Studies have shown that polyclonal IgA secretion is inducible in murine B-cells when dendritic cells and helper cells from Peyer's patches provide the inducing stimulus (74).

The major inductive site for IgA responses is the gut- and bronchus-associated lymphoreticular tissue, which contain significant numbers of IgA-committed B cells and T cells that support IgA responses (39). Once the IgA progenitor cells or IgA lymphoblasts are produced following exposure to luminal antigens, they do not immediately mature and secrete immunoglobulin. The events that precede the development of secretory antibody production in mucous membranes are poorly understood. Studies suggest that B lymphoblasts populating the lamina propria are derived from BALT or GALT. It has been proposed that in response to antigenic exposure in the intestine or respiratory tract, the precursor IgA-B cells migrate out of organized lymphoid follicles in GALT, into regional (mesenteric) lymph nodes, and enter peripheral blood circulation via the thoracic duct. During their circulation in the peripheral blood, the antigen-sensitized cell population appears to home, back preferentially to the site of original antigenic challenge (62,63,68). Data also indicate that there is an organ specificity in mucosally derived B-lymphocyte localization dependent on the source of the donor cells. Cells derived from bronchial lymph nodes tend to localize preferentially in the respiratory tract and to a lesser extent in the gut and vice versa (46). However, a significant number of IgA-antigen-sensitized cells from the GALT and the BALT often populate the lamina propria of other mucosal sites. These include the mammary glands and the genital tract. The circuitous route that IgA progenitor cells follow before maturing

TABLE 2. *Factors that influence IgA-B homing*

Factor	Reference
1. Organ specificity—i.e., bronchial lymph-node progenitors tend to localize in lung	46
2. High endothelial venules	15,16
3. HLA (class-II antigens)	23,33
4. Fcα-receptor-bearing T cells	76
5. Lactational hormones	27,87,88

into IgA-secreting plasma cells is referred to as the *IgA cell cycle*. There is now evidence that other mucosal cells also undergo specific migratory patterns in a manner similar to IgA blasts, including IgE-B cell precursors, mucosal mast cells, and mucosal T cells. The final localization pattern of T- and B-cell blasts, however, is different when they reach the intestine with preferential homing of B cells to lamina propria and T cells to either lamina propria or villous epithelium (10,61).

Although the route by which cells traffic and mature in the IgA cell cycle is fairly well understood, the mechanisms of specific lodging of the circulating IgA lymphoblasts into the mucosa where they remain and complete their differentiation into plasma cells is not well understood. Several other factors have been shown to influence IgA–B-cell homing (see Table 2). Evidence has been presented that the organ specificity of lymphocyte migration may be determined largely by selective interaction of circulating lymphocytes with endothelial cells (16). More specifically, the determinants on T and B lymphocytes appear to home to specific receptors situated on specialized postcapillary high endothelial venules (HEV). These selective endothelial interactions appear to affect the preferential distribution of B and T cells to either Peyer's patches or peripheral lymph nodes. It is suggested that endothelial cells in mucosal and peripheral lymphoid tissue express distinctive determinants or factors for lymphocyte recognition and that lymphocyte migration patterns are programmed by lymphocyte surface receptors complementary to these organ-specific endothelial determinants (15).

Other factors have been studied that may influence or control lymphocyte migratory patterns that are observed. Curtis and co-workers (23,24) have performed a number of experiments that suggest that histocompatibility antigens may play an important role in lymphocyte adhesion and eventual position in the tissues. The finding of T cells that have Fc receptors for IgA has led to the alternative speculation that the predominance of an IgA response in a given area may depend on its T-cell content and that T cells may specifically home to mucosal tissues where they then determine the B-cell traffic. Although there is increasing information on the role of helper T cells in the differentiation of IgA lymphoblasts and in clonal expansion of IgA progenitors, their role in cellular homing in the gut- and bronchus-associated lymphoid tissue remains to be determined.

The process of systemic traffic and eventual homing of antigen-reactive precursor cells to mucosal sites other than the site of original antigenic stimulation allows for sharing of immune experiences between different mucosal sites and is fundamental to the concept of a common mucosal immune system. The observations initially made with cells derived from GALT and BALT have now been extended to include the breast, the salivary glands, the lacrimal glands, and the genitourinary tract. Several unique aspects of the relationship between the mucosal immune system and the mammary glands, the so-called enteromammary and bronchomammary axis, deserve a separate discussion.

There is a great deal of evidence that can be found to support the notion that the mammary glands function as an extra mucosal extension of the secretory immune system. The specificity of milk antibodies for intestinal and respiratory tract microbial agents has now been well established. The colonization experiments with *E. coli* 083 in pregnant women carried out by Goldblum et al. (32) have strongly suggested that lymphoid cells in GALT seed mammary glands where they produce IgA antibodies to that microorganism. Montgomery et al. (47) have shown that bronchial as well as gastrointestinal immunization will induce an antibody response in colostrum and milk. Antibodies in milk directed against pathogens associated with the respiratory tract have been identified in humans on a number of occasions (54).

The mechanisms underlying the transport of antigen-activated IgA cells from BALT and GALT to the mammary glands is not well understood. Several different mechanisms may interplay to account for the cell traffic patterns that have thus far been described.

There is substantial evidence to suggest that in the mammary gland, immunoblast traffic appears to be under the control of the endocrine system. The effect of pregnancy and lactation-related hormones on the regulation of immunologic components present in the resting and lactating breast has been examined in several published studies. Weisz-Carrington et al. (87) demonstrated that during pregnancy and early lactation there is an increase in the number of plasma cells in the breast and that by the first week of lactation most are synthesizing IgA. In a study of virgin mice, treatment with gestational hormones resulted in increased content of IgA cells in the mammary glands and the development of the capacity of gut cells to seed mammary tissues. They demonstrated that an extended exposure to estrogen, progesterone, and prolactin was necessary for maximal increments in IgA-producing plasma cells in the breast. Similarly, castrated males exposed to hormones become moderately receptive to mammary gland homing of cells specific for IgA. Testosterone, as would be expected, eliminated female breast reactivity to these cells (88).

In a study on immunoglobulin production in the nonlactating breast, several interesting findings were observed that suggest that the immunologic makeup of the nonlactating breast was also significantly influenced by the hormonal milieu (27). These included alterations in the number of IgA-secreting cells with the menstrual cycle and the observation that the number of IgA-producing cells increased with parity.

The effect of hormones on cell traffic is not limited to the mammary glands. Adoptive transfer experiments in mice with radiolabeled mesenteric lymphoblasts demonstrate that the number of cells entering the cervix and the vagina varies with the stage of estrus (proestrus, estrus, or diestrus) (7). The greatest number of cells were found in proestrus with a marked decline in diestrus. These studies are strongly suggestive of the existence of a homing mechanism for the mammary gland and other sex hormone target tissues for class-specific immunoglobulin-producing cells dependent on specific hormonal milieu. Weisz-Carrington et al. (87) have suggested that sex hormones induce a receptor in target tissues that directs B-cell localization. Hanson et al. (33) have suggested that lactational hormones may induce Ia antigens coded for by the major histocompatibility complex on glandular epithelial cells in the breast; this may be the signal responsible for the migration of circulating committed IgA cells to home to the mammary glands. HLA-DR-like antigens have been identified in colostral and milk fat globules and epithelial cells in the products of human lactation (11,33,79,91).

The role of sex hormones may not be limited to cell homing. There is evidence to suggest that sex hormones play an important modulating role in isotype-specific immunoglobulin responses. The switch of IgM to IgG during the natural course of autoimmune diseases in NZB/NZW F1 mice is strongly influenced by sex hormones (66,67). The levels of IgA and IgG in cervical secretions alter during the menstrual cycle, a period characterized by profound changes in hormonal concentrations (19,20,36,72). A correlation between plasma progesterone and specific isotype response has also been observed. Fluctuations in the levels of anti-*Candida* antibodies correlated with circulating levels of estradiol or progesterone (45). Studies on antibody formation and antigen-induced cell differentiation have demonstrated that IgM production during primary immune response and IgG production during the secondary immune responses are influenced by sex hormones (29). Recently, prolactin receptors have been identified on human T and B lymphocytes (70). Several studies suggest that prolactin also may play a physiological role in humans in the regulation of humoral and cell-mediated immune responses (2–4,30,39).

Preliminary work carried out in our laboratory on the effects of lactational hormones on immune function suggests that these hormones may be directly involved in directing maturation or expansion of IgA-B cells (22). We observed that prolactin, in combination with estrogen and progesterone levels observed at the onset of parturition, has a profound amplifying effect on IgA secretion and synthesis from peripheral blood lymphocytes. The observations suggested that lactational hormones affect IgA-B cell expansion in the absence of other apparent stimuli.

INTESTINAL AND BRONCHIAL LYMPHOID TISSUE IMMUNOLOGICAL REACTIVITY

In general, natural infections acquired via the mucosa of the respiratory or intestinal tracts appear to be the most efficient means of inducing specific antibody responses at the mucosal portal of entry, as well as at other distant mucosal sites. The wild or live vaccine-induced infection with poliovirus via the intestinal mucosa has been clearly shown to result in the development of a specific secretory antibody response in the intestine (52). On the other hand, parenteral immunization with inactivated (killed) poliovirus has been found to result in little or no intestinal antibody response, although a high level of antibody activity can be observed in the serum. Mucosal immunization with killed poliovirus can, however, result in the appearance of a transient secretory antibody response in the nasopharynx or intestinal mucosa, often in the absence of a detectable response in the serum (51).

The intestinal and respiratory origin of antibody activity in other distant mucosal surfaces has been suggested by a number of recent investigations with respiratory syncytial virus (RSV), rotavirus, enterovirus, and rubella virus. Infection with RSV, which under natural settings is limited to the respiratory tract, has been shown to result in the development of specific secretory IgA activity in colostrum and milk, following naturally acquired or experimentally induced respiratory or intestinal exposures (30). It is also of interest to note that naturally acquired reinfection in lactating mothers has been associated with the development of a booster effect on pre-existing colostral antibody activity. The importance of the local availability of antigen to the bronchial or intestinal immunocompetent cells has been clearly demonstrated and is influenced by the type of antigen and the ability of the organism (virus or bacteria) to replicate. For example, natural rubella infection or intranasal immunization with RA 27/3 live attenuated rubella vaccine is regularly associated with the development of rubella-specific IgA response in the respiratory tract. Frequently, subcutaneous immunization with RA 27/3 rubella vaccine is also associated with the development of secretory antibody response (53,55). After parenteral immunization with HPV-77 strain of live attenuated rubella vaccine, the development of IgA antibody response in the nasopharynx is notably absent (53). However, those subjects who excrete significant amounts of virus in the nasopharynx after parenteral immunization with HPV-77 may develop antibody response to rubella in the nasopharynx (53,55).

In order to examine the differential role of bronchial- versus gut-associated lymphoreticular tissue, as well as the nature of the antigen (soluble versus particulate, replicating versus nonreplicating), Peri et al. (61) immunized groups of pregnant rabbits with RSV or bovine serum albumin (BSA) administered intratracheally, intravenously, or by intragastric intubation. The response to RSV was characterized by the regular appearance of IgA anti-RSV in the colostrum, milk, and bronchial and intestinal secretions following either oral or intratracheal immunization but not after intravenous immunization. RSV-specific IgA appeared in colostrum, milk, and serum regardless of the route of immunization. On the other hand, the response to BSA by all three routes of immunization was characterized by the appearance of anti-BSA antibody in the serum, colostrum, and milk but limited to the IgG isotype. No anti-BSA response was observed. The anti-BSA response was unaffected during the observed nursing period and did not exhibit any change in response to BSA ingestion before or during pregnancy or during nursing. These observations suggest that the appearance of IgA antibody response following mucosal immunization is not uniform for different types of antigen. The presence of mammary IgA antibodies in response to RSV and its absence to BSA following respiratory or intestinal immunization suggest that the physical as well as the chemical nature of antigens may be important determinants of the mucosal response. Furthermore, the presence of a replicating organism may be important and may influence the isotype response, by determining the duration of exposure (prolonging antigenic stimulation) at the mucosal surface and helping to foster the proliferation of antibody-producing cells.

The balance between antigen access to lymphoepithelium, the local immune response subsequently evoked, and the natural nonspecific defense mechanisms available at a particular site are all important factors that determine whether the eventual outcome to a specific antigen will result in disease or in immunity.

Antigen penetration of lymphoreticular tissue may serve to initiate protective response by stimulating an immune response. In BALT the FAE has been shown to be the initial site for sampling a variety of microorganisms (64). In the absence of specific antibodies, penetration of these cells by viruses and bacteria may sometimes serve to disseminate and induce disease. Wolf et al. (92,93) demonstrated that the FAE of GALT are the sites where reoviruses penetrate the intestinal epithelium to infect other distant tissues. Several types of bacteria have been found to penetrate the intestinal mucosa via the FAE (18,37,57).

The mounting of a specific mucosal response with the development of sIgA antibodies therefore plays an important regulatory role in the host immune response by excluding a variety of otherwise harmful antigens and pathogens from deeper sites of mucosal immunocompetent lymphoid tissue. These and other observations suggest that mucosal immunity may indeed be an important mechanism for the mucosal containment and possible elimination of many viral and bacterial agents from the respiratory and intestinal mucosa.

IMMUNE REACTIVITY OF THE MIDDLE EAR

The association of immunological reactivity observed in the middle ear with mucosal immune responses would have important implications to the mechanism of protection or pathogenesis of microbial infections in the middle ear. There are data that suggest the existence of a distinct secretory immune system in the middle ear, and that these responses may be related to the lymphoreticular tissue of GALT and BALT (see Table 3).

Anatomically, the middle ear cavity normally contains air and is lined by both

TABLE 3. *Evidence for a secretory immune response in the middle ear*

Evidence	Reference
1. Anatomical—resembles typical respiratory mucosa	71
2. Predominance of IgA—plasma cells in lamina propria	5
3. Presence of IgA and secretory component in MEE (predominant antibody)	5
4. Ratio of IgG to IgA—suggests local secretion and synthesis	35
5. Demonstration of antigen specificity of IgA-Ab in MEE with complete absence of some specificity in serum	5,73

ciliated columnar and cuboidal cells, thus resembling typical respiratory mucosa (71). However, there is a paucity of mucous glands or goblet cells and a noted absence of organized lymphoid tissue. Plasma cells, although sparse, can be found among the cells lining the submucosa. The evidence supporting the middle ear as part of the GALT and BALT is largely based on the presence and development of secretory immunoglobulins in the middle ear. Immunofluorescent staining of the plasma cells in the lamina propria reveal that most of the cells are IgA-secreting plasma cells (5). Studies have demonstrated that over 80% of middle ear effusions contain secretory component, a protein relatively unique to mucosal surfaces and associated with epithelial transport of IgA. Secretory component has been demonstrated in the epithelial cells lining the middle ear and is absent from the lamina propria (5). Further evidence for the local synthesis of IgA comes from analysis of the immunoglobulin content of middle ear effusions. The findings suggested by analyzing the ratio of IgA to IgG in the serum and secretions are suggestive of local secretion (5,35). The observations of particular significance are the presence of specific IgA antibodies in the middle ear, frequently in the absence of antibodies of the same specificity in the serum. Bernstein et al. (5) demonstrated that specific antibody activity in the middle ear against measles, mumps, rubella, and polio was essentially limited to IgA immunoglobulins. In contrast, the activity in the serum was primarily associated with IgG immunoglobulin. In similar studies performed by Sloyer et al. (73), significant titers of specific antiviral IgA antibodies directed against the above viruses were present in the middle ear in the complete absence of antibodies in the serum. These studies suggest that the middle ear is capable of mounting a specific local antibody response independent of the systemic immune system. The mechanism underlying the production of IgA by the middle ear appears to be the local availability of antigen to immunocompetent cells in the middle ear mucosa or to the immunocompetent tissue in the nasopharynx. The predominance of sIgA immunoglobulin in middle ear effusions is consistent with either a process of local synthesis or a process of active transport of serum IgA mediated by secretory component, which, as previously mentioned, is found in many of the epithelial cells lining the middle ear. The finding that most of the plasma cells present in the lamina propria are IgA-secreting plasma cells and the presence of specific IgA antibodies in middle ear effusions in the absence of serum antibody support the notion of local synthesis.

There is, at present, no available evidence that directly supports the contention that the immunocompetent effector cells found in the middle ear are derived from sites distant to the upper respiratory tract. Crucial to the argument of whether or not these cells are derived from GALT or BALT will be the documentation that T and B lymphocytes specific for enteric antigens appear in these secretions following either gastric or lower respiratory exposure to these antigens, as has already been done in establishing the enteromammary and bronchomammary relationships.

In summary, the middle ear cavity possesses many of the attributes associated with the mucosal immune system, including the presence of sIgA, the ability to mount specific antibody responses against a number of bacteria and viruses, and the independence of the responses from the systemic immune system.

REFERENCES

1. Backman, D.E., and Winlorn, W.B. (1966): Light and electron microscopy of intestinal ferritin absorption. *Anat. Rev.*, 155:603.
2. Berazi, I., and Nagy, E. (1981): Immunodeficiency in hypophyrectomized rats: restoration by prolactin. *Fed. Proc.*, 1031.
3. Berazi, I., and Nagy, E. (1982): A possible role of prolactin in adjuvant arthritis. *Arthritis Rheum.*, 591–594.
4. Berazi, I., Nagy, E., Kerag, K., Harrath, E. (1981): Regulation of humoral immunity in rats by pituitary hormones. *Acta Endocrinol. (Copenh.),* 506.
5. Bernstein, J.M., Tomasi, T.B., and Ogra, P.L. (1974): The immunochemistry of middle ear effusions. *Arch. Otolaryngol.*, 99:320–326.
6. Bienenstock, J., Johnston, N., and Perey, D.Y.E. (1973): Bronchial lymphoid tissue. *Lab. Invest.*, 38:693.
7. Bienenstock, J., McDermott, M., and Befus, D. (1979): A common mucosal immune system. In: *Immunology of Breast Milk,* edited by P.L. Ogra and D. Dayton, Raven Press, New York.
8. Bienenstock, J., and Befus, A.D. (1980): Mucosal immunology. *Immunology,* 41:249.
9. Bienenstock, J., and Befus, A.D. (1983): Some thought on the biologic role of immunoglobulin A. *Gastroenterology,* 198:179–185.
10. Bienenstock, J., Befus, D., McDermott, M., Mirski, S., and Rosenthal, K. (1983): Regulation of lymphoblast traffic and localization in mucosal tissues with emphasis on IgA. *Fed. Proc.*, 42:3212.
11. Bienenstock, J. (1984): The lung as an immunologic organ. *Ann. Rev. Med.*, 35:49.
12. Bienenstock, J. (1984): Mucosal barrier functions. *Nutr. Rev.* 42:105.
13. Brown, T.A., Russell, M.W., Kulharz, R., and Mestecky, J. (1983): IgA mediated elimination of antigens by the hepatobiliary route. *Fed. Proc.*, 42:3218.
14. Brown, T.A., Russell, M.W. and Mestecky, J. (1984): Elimination of intestinally absorbed antigen into the bile by IgA. *J. Immunol.*, 132:780.
15. Butcher, E.C., Scallay, R.G., and Weissman, I.L. (1980): Organ specificity of lymphocyte migration mediation by highly selective lymphocyte interaction with organ specific determinants on high endothelial venules. *Eur. J. Immunol.*, 10:556–561.
16. Butcher, E.C., Stevens, S.K., Reichert, R.A., et al. (1982): Lymphocyte endothelial cell recognition in lymphocyte migration and regregation of mucosal and nonmucosal immunity. In: *Recent Advances in Mucosal Immunity,* edited by W. Strober, L.A. Hanson, K.W. Sell, p. 3024, Raven Press, New York.
17. Bye, W.A., Allan, C.H., Madara, J.L., and Trier, J.S. (1983): Natured and immature M cells—morphology and distribution. *Gastroenterology,* 84:1118.
18. Cantey, J.R., and Inman, L.R. (1981): Diarrhea due to escherichia coli strain RDEC-1 in the rabbit: the Peyer's patch as the initial site of attachment and colonization. *J. Infect. Dis.*, 143:440–446.
19. Chipperfield, E., and Evans, B. (1975): Effect of local infection and oral contraception on immunoglobulin levels in cervical mucus. *Infect. Immun.*, 215–221.
20. Coughlan, B.M., and Skinner, G.R. (1977): Concentrations of immunoglobulin in cervical mucus in patients with normal and abnormal cervical cytology. *Br. J. Obstet. Gynaecol.*, 129.
21. Cornell, R., Walker, W.A., and Isselbacher, K.J. (1971): Small intestinal absorption of horseradish peroxidase. *Lab. Invest.*, 25:42.
22. Cumella, J.C., Raymonda, S.M., Ambrus, J., and Ogra, P.L. (1983): Effects of pregnancy associated hormones on B-cell functions. *Soc. Pediatr. Res.*
23. Curtis, A.S.G. (1981): Clues, concepts, and possible answers from other systems. In: *Lymphocyte Circulation. Experimental and Clinical Aspects,* edited by M. DeSoursa, pp. 162–196, John Wiley & Sons, New York.
24. Curtis, A.S., and Davis, M.D. (1981): H2-D antigens released by thymocytes and cell adhesion. *J. Immunogenet.*, 8:367–377.
25. Delacroix, D.L., Hodgson, H.J.F., McPherson, A., Dive, C., and Vaerman, J.P. (1982): Selective transport of polymeric IgA in bile. *J. Clin. Invest.*, 70:230–247.
26. Dhar, R., and Ogra, P.L. (1985): Local immune responses. *Br. Med. Bull.*, 41:28.

27. Drife, J.O., McClelland, D.B., Pryde, A., et al. (1976): Immunoglobulin synthesis in the resting breast. *Br. Med. J.*, 2:503–506.
28. Edebo, L., Hed, J., Kehlstrom, E., et al. (1980): The adhesion of enterobacteria and the effect of antibiotics of different immunoglobulin classes. *Scand. J. Infect. Dis.*, S24:93.
29. Eidinger, D., and Garrett, T. (1972): Studies of the regulation effects of the sex hormones on antibody formation and stem cell differentiation. *J. Exp. Med.*, 136:1098.
30. Fishaut, M., Murphy, D., Neifert, M., McIntosh, K., and Ogra, P.L. (1981): Bronchomammary axis in the immune response to respiratory syncytial virus. *J. Pediatr.*, 99:186–191.
31. Freter, R. (1974): Interactions between mechanisms controling the intestinal microflora. *Am. J. Clin. Nutr.*, 27:1409.
32. Goldblum, R.M., Ahlstedt, S., Carlsson, B., Hanson, A., et al. (1975): Antibody forming cells in human colostrum after oral immunization. *Nature*, 257–797.
33. Hanson, L.A., Carlsson, B., Cruz, J.R., Garcia, B., et al. (1979): Immune response in the mammary gland. In: *Immunology of Breast Milk*, edited by P.L. Ogra and D. Dayton, pp. 145–157, Raven Press, New York.
34. Hoover, R.G., and Lynch, R.G. (1983): Isotype specific suppression of IgA. *J. Immunol.*, 130:521.
35. Howie, V.M., Ploussard, J.H., Sloyer, J.L., and Johnston, R.B. (1973): Immunoglobulins of the middle ear fluid in acute otitis media. *Infect. Immun.*, 7:589–593.
36. Hulka, J.F., and Omran, W.F. (1969): The uterine cervix as a potential local antibody secretor. *Am. J. Obstet. Gynecol.*, 440.
37. Inman, L.R., and Cantey, J.R. (1983): Specific adherence of escherichia coli (strain RDEC-1) to membranous (M) cells of the Peyer's patch in escherichia coli diarrhea in the rabbit. *J. Clin. Invest.*, 71:1–8.
38. Kawanishi, H., Saltzman, L.E., and Strober, W. (1982): Characteristics and regulatory function of murine Con A-induced cloned T cells obtained from Peyer's patches and spleen. *J. Immunol.*, 129:475.
39. Kelly, J.D., and Dineen, J.K. (1973): The suppression of rejection of *Nippostrongylus braseliensis* in Lewis strain rats treated with ovine prolactin. *Immunology*, 24:551.
40. Kirzano, H., McGhee, J.R., Wanneumuehler, M.J., Frangahis, M.V., et al. (1982): In vitro immune responses to T cell dependent antigen by cultures of disassociated murine Peyer's patches. *Proc. Natl. Acad. Sci. USA*, 79:596.
41. Kiyono, H., Cooper, M.D., Kearnez, J.F., et al. (1984): Isotype specificity of helper T cell clones. *J. Exp. Med.*, 159:798–811.
42. Kiyono, H., Phillips, J.O., Calwell, D.E., Michalek, S.M., et al. (1984): Isotype-specificity of helper T cell clones. *J. Immunol.*, 133:1087.
43. Lamm, M.E. (1976): Cellular aspects of immunoglobulin A. *Adv. Immunol.*, 223.
44. Lowell, G.H., Smith, L.F., McLeod Griffis, J., and Brandt, B.L. (1980): IgA-dependent, monocyte mediated antibacterial activity. *J. Exp. Med.*, 152:452.
45. Mathur, S., Mathur, R.S., Gramling, T.S., Landgrebe, S.C., et al. (1978): Sex steroid hormones and antibodies to *Candida albicans*. *Clin. Exp. Immunol.*, 33:79–87.
46. McDermott, M.R., and Bienenstock, J. (1979): Evidence for a common mucosal immunologic system. *J. Immunol.*, 122:1892.
47. Montgomery, P.C., Connelly, K.M., Cohen, C., and Skandera, C.A. (1978): Remote site stimulation of secretory IgA antibodies following bronchial and gastric stimulation. *Adv. Exp. Med. Biol.*, 107:113.
48. Mullock, B.M., Hinton, R.H., Dobrata, M., Peppard, J., and Orlans, E. (1979): Endocytic vesicles in liver carry polymeric IgA from serum to bile. *Biochem. Biophys. Acta*, 587:381–391.
49. Nagy, E., and Berazi, I. (1981): Prolactin and contact sensitivity. *Allergy*, 36:429.
50. Ogra, P.L., Cumella, J.C., and Welliver, R.C. (1984): Immune response to viruses. In: *Immunology of the Lung and Upper Respiratory Tract*, edited by J. Bienenstock, p. 242, McGraw-Hill Book Co., New York.
51. Ogra, P.L., and Karzon, D.T. (1971): Formation and function of poliovirus antibody in different tissues. *Prog. Med. Virol.*, 13:156–193.
52. Ogra, P.L., Karzon, D.T., and Righthood, F., et al. (1968): Immunoglobulin response in serum and secretions after immunization with live and inactivated poliovaccine and natural infection. *N. Engl. J. Med.*, 279:893–900.

53. Ogra, P.L., Kerr-Grant, D., Umana, G., et al. (1971): Antibody response in serum and nasopharynx after naturally acquired and vaccine induced infection with rubella virus. *N. Engl. J. Med.*, 285:1333–1339.
54. Ogra, P.L. Losonsky, G.A., and Fishaut, M. (1983): Colostrum-derived immunity and maternal-neonatal interaction. In: *The Secretory Immune System*, edited by J. McGhee and J. Mestecky, *Ann. NY Acad. Sci.*, 409:81–95.
55. Ogra, P.L., Morag, A., and Tiku, M.L. (1975): Humoral immune response to viral infections. In: *Viral Immunology and Immunopathology*, edited by A.L. Notkins. Academic Press, New York.
56. Owen, R.L., Apple, R.T., Bhalla, D.K. (1981): Cytochemical identification and morphometric analysis of lysosomes in "M" cells and adjacent columnar cells of rat Peyer's patches. *Gastroenterology*, 80:1246.
57. Owen, R.L., Bhalla, D.K., and Apple, R.T. (1982): Migration of Peyer's patch lymphocytes through intact M cells into the intestinal lumen in mice, rats and rabbits. *J. Cell Biol.*, 57:16084.
58. Owen, R.L., and Bhalla, D.K. (1982): Cytochemical characterization of enzyme distribution over M cells surfaces in rat Peyer's patches. *Gastroenterology*, 82:1144.
59. Owen, R.L., and Bhalla, D.K. (1983): Cytochemical analysis of alkaline phosphatase in esterase activities and of lactin-binding and anionic sites in rat and mouse Peyer's patch M cells. *Am. J. Anat.*, 168:199–212.
60. Parrott, D.M.W. (1981): Lymphocyte circulation outside the lymphoid system. In: *Lymphocyte Circulation. Experimental and Clinical Aspects*, edited by M. DeSousa, pp. 99–122, John Wiley & Sons, New York.
61. Peri, B.A., Theodore, C.M., Losonsky, G.A., Fishaut, J.M., Rothberg, R.M., and Ogra, P.L. (1982): Antibody content of rabbit milk and serum following inhalation or ingestion of respiratory syncytial virus and bovine serum albumin. *Clin. Exp. Immunol.*, 48:91–101.
62. Pierce, N.F., and Gowan, J. (1975): Cellular kinetics of the intestinal immune response to cholera toxoid in rats. *J. Exp. Med.*, 1150.
63. Plesch, B.E.C. (1982): Histology and immunohistochemistry of bronchus-associated lymphoid tissue (BALT) in the rat. *J. Adv. Exp. Biol. Med.*, 149:491–497.
64. Racz, P., Tanner-Racy, K., Myrvik, Q.N., and Fainter, L.L. (1977): Functional architecture of bronchial associated lymphoid tissue and lymphoepithelium in pulmonary cell-mediated reactions in the rabbit. *J. Reticulo, Soc.*, 22:59.
65. Rifai, A., and Mannik, M. (1984): Clearance of circulating IgA immune complexes is mediated by a specific receptor on Kupffer cells in mice. *J. Exp. Med.*, 160:125–137.
66. Roubinion, J., Papoion, R., and Tabal, N. (1977): Androgenic hormones modulate autoantibody responses and improve survival in murine lupus. *J. Clin. Invest.*, 59:1066–1070.
67. Roubinion, J., Talal, N., Siiteri, P.K., and Sadakian, J.A. (1979): Sex hormone modulation of autoimmunity in NZB/NZW mice. *Arthritis Rheum.*, 22:1162.
68. Roux, M.E., McWilliams, M., Phillips-Quagliata, J.M., et al. (1977): Origin of IgA secreting plasma cells in the mammary gland. *J. Exp. Med.*, 1311.
69. Russell, M.W., Brown, T.A., Claflin, J.L., Schroer, K., and Mestecky, J. (1983): Immunoglobulin A—mediated hepatobiliary transport constitutes a natural pathway for disposing of bacterial antigens. *Infect. Immun.* 42:1041–1048.
70. Russell, D.H., Kibler, R., Mattrison, L., Larson, D.F., et al. (1985): Prolactin receptors on human T and B lymphocytes. *J. Immunol.*, 134:3027.
71. Sade, J. (1971): Cellular differentiation of the middle ear lining. *Ann. Otol. Rhinol. Laryngol.*, 80:376–384.
72. Schumacher, G.F. (1976): Soluble proteins in cervical mucus. In: *Biology of the Cervix*, edited by Blondare and Mazkissi, p. 201. University of Chicago Press.
73. Sloyer, J.L., Jr., Howie, V.M., Ploussard, J.A., Bradac, J., Habercarn, M., and Ogra, P.L (1977): Immune response to acute otitis media in children. *J. Immunol.*, 118:248–250.
74. Spaulding, P.M., Welliamson, S.I., Koopman, W.J., et al. (1984): Preferential induction of polyclonal IgA secretion by murine Peyer's patch dendritic T cell mixture. *J. Exp. Med.*, 160:941–946.
75. Strober, W. (1982): Regulation of mucosal immune system. *J. Allergy Clin. Immunol.*, 225.
76. Strober, W., Elson, C.O., Graeff, A. and Richman, L.K. (1982): Class specific T cell regulation of mucosal responses. In: *Recent Advances in Mucosal Immunity*, p. 121, Raven Press, New York.

77. Tagliabue, A., Boraschi, D., Villa, L., Keren, D., et al. (1984): IgA-Dependent cell mediated activity against enteropathogenic bacteria. *J. Immunol.* 133:988–992.
78. Tagliabue, A., Nencioni, L., Villa, L., Keren, D.F., Lowell, G.H. and Boraschi, D. (1983): Antibody dependent cell-mediated antibacterial activity of intestinal lymphocytes with secretory IgA. *Nature,* 306:184–186.
79. Thomas, D.W., Yamashita, V., and Sherach, E.M. (1977): The role of Ia antigens in T cell activation. *Immunol. Rev.,* 35:95–120.
80. Tomasi, T.B. (1976): *The Immune System of Secretion.* Prentice–Hall, Englewood Cliffs, N.J.
81. Tomasi, T.B., Jr. (1980): Mechanisms of immune regulation at mucosal surfaces. *Rev. Infect. Dis.,* 5:5794.
82. Walker, W.A. (1976): Host defense mechanisms in the gastrointestinal tract. *Pediatrics,* 57:901.
83. Walker, W.A., and Isselbacker, K.J. (1974): Uptake and transport of macromolecules by the intestine. *Gastroenterology,* 67:531.
84. Walker, W.A., and Isselbacker, K.J. (1977): Intestinal antibodies. *N. Engl. J. Med.,* 297:767.
85. Walker, W.A., and Block, K.J. (1980): Antigen uptake mechanisms: control and pathologic states. In: *The Mucosal Immune System in Health and Disease,* edited by P.L. Ogra and J. Bienenstock, pp. 51–56, Ross Laboratories, Columbus, Ohio.
86. Walker, W.A., and Block, K.J. (1983): Intestinal uptake of macromolecules in vitro and in vivo studies. In: *The Secretory Immune System,* edited by J. McGhee and J. Mestecky, *Ann. NY Acad. Sci.,* 409:593.
87. Weisz-Carrington, P., Roux, M.E., and Lamm, M.E. (1977): Plasma cells and epithelial immunoglobulins in the mouse mammary gland during pregnancy and lactation. *J. Immunol.,* 119:1306.
88. Weisz-Carrington, P., Roux, M.E., McWilliams, M., Phillips-Quagliata, J.M., and Hamm, M.E. (1978): Hormonal induction of the secretory immune system in the mammary gland. *Proc. Natl. Acad. Sci. USA,* 75:2928.
89. Williams, R.C., and Gibbons, R.J. (1972): Inhibition of bacterial adherence by secretory immunoglobulin A. A merchanism of antigen disposal. *Science,* 177:697.
90. Wilman, K.B., Curman, V., Forsum, L., Kloreskag, U., et al. (1978): Occurrence of Ia antigens on tissues of nonlymphoid origin. *Nature,* 276:711–713.
91. Wilman, K., Curman, B., Tragardh, L., Peterson, P.A., et al. (1979): Demonstration of HLA-DR like antigens on milk fat soluble membranes. *Eur. J. Immunol.,* 9:190–195.
92. Wolf, J.L., Rubin, D.H., Finberg, R., Kauffman, R.S., Sharp, A.H., et al. (1981): Intestinal M cells: a pathway for entry of reovirus into the host. *Science,* 212:471.
93. Wolf, J.L., Kauffman, R.S., Finberg, R., Dambrouskas, R., Fields, B.N., et al. (1983): Determinants of reovirus interaction with the intestinal M cells and absorptive cells of murine intestine. *Gastroenterology,* 85:291–300.
94. Worthington, B.S., and Boatman, E.S. (1974): The influence of protein malnutrition on ileal permeability to macromolecules in the rat. *Am. J. Dig. Dis.,* 19:43–55.

Immunology of the Ear, edited by J. Bernstein
and P. Ogra. Raven Press, New York © 1987.

Pharmacologic Mediators of Inflammation

Jeffrey P. Tillinghast and Dean D. Metcalfe

Mast Cell Physiology Section, Laboratory of Clinical Investigation, National Institute of Allergy and Infectious Diseases, National Institutes of Health, Bethesda, Maryland 20205

Inflammation comprises a complex series of events recognized by the classic signs of redness, swelling, heat, pain, and decreased or altered function of the involved tissue. To understand inflammation, one must possess a knowledge of pharmacologic mediators and their properties, functional capabilities, and cells of origin. Such mediators may exist stored in cell granules as "preformed mediators" or are formed by cells during activation. The latter chemicals are often referred to as *generated mediators*. As will be seen, both types of mediators are rarely associated with a specific cell type, although exceptions exist. Nevertheless, the functions of cells involved in inflammation are invariably reflected, in part, by the cell's ability to form specific mediators and to direct their use through selective mechanisms of cellular activation. In order to understand inflammation, one must first understand the pharmacologic mediators of inflammation and the specific signals by which they are selected for use. This chapter will first review such mediators and then discuss them in relationship to mast cells, basophils, eosinophils, neutrophils, monocytes, and macrophages. Lymphokines, biologically active products derived from complement activation, and the specific relationship of inflammatory mediators to middle ear disease will be discussed elsewhere in this volume.

MEDIATORS OF INFLAMMATION

Preformed Mediators

Histamine

Histamine in tissues is generally associated with mast cells, although exceptions exist. For instance, in the gastrointestinal mucosa, histamine is present in mucosal mast cells and in enteroendocrine cells. In rat peritoneal mast cell granules, histamine is estimated to constitute 10% of the dry weight (58), with the amount of histamine per cell estimated to be 7 to 20 pg. Rat mucosal mast cells have 0.1 to 5.5 pg per cell. Histamine is formed by decarboxylation of L-histidine and degraded by deamination with diamine oxidase or by methylation via histamine-*N*-

methyl transferase. The primary excretory products of histamine catabolism are the riboside of imidazole acetic acid and methylimidazole acetic acid.

The biologic effects of histamine are mediated by at least two distinct histamine receptors, now conventionally termed H_1 and H_2 receptors. Drugs that inhibit the pharmacologic effects of histamine are thus termed either H_1 receptor or H_2 receptor antagonists. H_1 receptor antagonists make up the "classic" antihistamines, including ethanolamines, ethylenediamines, alkylamines, piperazines, phenothiazines, and cyproheptadine. The H_2 receptor inhibitors include cimetidine, metiamide, and burimamide. There are also compounds that are selective agonists for H_1 and H_2 receptors. For example, 2-methylhistamine and 2-pyridylethylamine are selective H_1 agonists, and impromidine and dimaprit are H_2 agonists. Following exposure to histamine, a number of local and systemic effects may be seen (Table 1).

Serotonin

Serotonin in mammals is synthesized from dietary tryptophan, which is first hydroxylated to 5-hydroxytryptophan and then decarboxylated to 5-hydroxytryptamine (5-HT). In humans, serotonin is primarily detoxified by oxidative deamination by monoamine oxidase to form 5-hydroxyindoleacetic acid (5-HIAA) or reduction to 5-hydroxytryptophol (5-HTOL). The principal metabolite, 5-HIAA, is excreted in the urine along with much smaller amounts of 5-HTOL, mainly as the glucuronide or sulfate. Serotonin is found in human platelets at a concentration of 0.4 to 0.8 pg per platelet (99). Serotonin is additionally located in the enteroendo-

TABLE 1. *H_1 and H_2, histamine agonists, antagonists, and functions*

H_1	H_2	H_1 and H_2
"Classic" antihistamines (antagonist)	Cimetidine (antagonist)	Vasodilation
2-Methylhistamine (agonist)	Dimaprit, 4-methylhistamine (agonist)	Flush
2-Pyridylethylamine (agonist)	Impromidine (agonist)	Headache
Smooth muscle contraction	Gastric acid secretion	Tachycardia
Increased vascular permeability	Mucous secretion	
Pruritus	Increases in cyclic AMP	
Irritant-receptor stimulation	Inhibition of basophil release	
	Inhibition of lymphokine release	
Prostaglandin generation	Inhibition of neutrophil-enzyme release	
Increase in cyclic GMP	Inhibition of T-lymphocyte-mediated cytotoxicity	

crine cells of the mucosal layer of the gastrointestinal tract and in nervous tissue. There are a number of compounds that antagonize one or more of the effects of serotonin: these include ergot alkaloids; indole antihistamines of the ethylenediamine type, as well as cyproheptadine and phenothiazines; and sympathetic blocking drugs.

The pharmacologic actions of serotonin include the stimulation of smooth muscle and nerves. In humans, serotonin can cause bronchoconstriction in asthmatics; affect blood vessel tone; induce vasoconstriction of renal, meningeal, and pulmonary vasculature; cause vasodilation in skeletal muscles and superficial vessels; increase gastrointestinal motility; stimulate sensory nerves and autonomic ganglia; and produce discharge of catecholamines from the adrenal medulla. Serotonin stimulation of human monocytes increases cyclic guanosine monophosphate (cyclic GMP) with no change in cyclic adenosine monophosphate (cyclic AMP) (89) and induces the production of a monocyte-specific chemotactic factor from human peripheral blood leukocytes (27).

There is little information on the involvement of serotonin in inflammatory responses in humans. Blood serotonin levels were reported elevated during the appearance of cholinergic urticaria (50). Cyproheptadine, a medication with antihistaminic and antiserotonin effects, is useful in some forms of urticaria, an observation sometimes evoked to suggest a role for serotonin in allergic reactions in humans.

Proteoglycans

Proteoglycans are glycoconjugates that consist of a protein core covalently linked to sugar side chains (glycosaminoglycans) of similar size and composition. The class of proteoglycan (chondroitin sulfates, dermatan sulfate, keratan sulfate, heparan sulfate, heparin) is defined by the alternating sugar groups that make up the glycosaminoglycan side chain. With the single exception of keratan sulfate, a uronic acid always alternates with a hexosamine (Table 2). Proteoglycans are polyanions by virtue of negatively charged side groups on the carbohydrate portion of the molecule. This polyanionic character of proteoglycans plays a major role in determining the nature of the interaction between proteoglycans and other materials. Heparin contains more negative charge units than chondroitin sulfates do, principally because of a higher degree of sulfation.

Heparin is generally considered to be derived from mast cells, although heparin-like molecules are also synthesized from endothelial cells. It is obtained commercially from sources rich in mast cells, such as lung or intestine, and the only cell type, when obtained in reasonable purity, known to contain heparin is the mast cell. Interestingly, histochemical data comparing rat connective tissue and mucosal mast cells first demonstrated that not all mast cells, however, contain heparin. A comparison of the metachromatic spectra of both peritoneal and mucosal mast cells stained with toluidine blue O with polyacrylamide films containing various glycos-

TABLE 2. *Glycosaminoglycan characteristics*

Glycosaminoglycan	Disaccharide repeating unit: Hexuronic acid	Disaccharide repeating unit: Hexosamine	*N*-acetyl group	*O*-sulfate group	*N*-sulfate group
Hyaluronic acid	D-Glucuronic acid	D-Glucosamine	+		
Chondroitin 4-sulfate (chondroitin sulfate A)	D-Glucuronic acid	D-Galactosamine	+	+	
Chondroitin 6-sulfate[a] (chondroitin sulfate C)	D-Glucuronic acid	D-Galactosamine	+	+	
Dermatan sulfate (chondroitin sulfate B)	D-Glucuronic acid or L-iduronic acid	D-Glucosamine	+	+	
Heparan sulfate	D-Glucuronic acid or L-iduronic acid	D-Glucosamine	+	+	+
Heparin	D-Glucuronic acid or L-iduronic acid	D-Glucosamine	+	+	++
Keratan sulfate	Galactose[b]	D-Glucosamine	+	+	

[a]Chondroitin 6-sulfate may occur in oversulfated forms. Chondroitin sulfate E is one such form rich in *N*-acetylgalactosamine-4,6-sulfate.
[b]Not a hexuronic acid.

aminoglycans, some in combination with basic protein, revealed the absence of significant amounts of heparin in rodent mucosal mast cells (104). Further, these mucosal mast cells appeared to have glycosaminoglycans with lower sulfation, such as chondroitin sulfates.

The variation in heparin content of mast cells as observed *in vivo* has been confirmed by experiments with cultured cells. It has been established that purified rat peritoneal mast cells and enriched human lung mast cells contain heparin. However, cells ''persisting'' in cultures of mouse bone marrow (P cells) with characteristics of mouse mucosal mast cells but lacking heparin, consistent with the presence of ''heparin-free'' mucosal mast cells, have been reported (100). A similar subclass of mast cells has been described as having an ''oversulfated'' chondroitin sulfate, termed *chondroitin sulfate E,* rather than heparin (79). Chondroitin sulfate has been noted in basophils, neutrophils, eosinophils, lymphocytes, and platelets and probably serves a function similar to heparin in mast cells. Chondroitin sulfate E has also been identified in monocytes.

There is convincing evidence that heparins and, by extension, chondroitin sulfates function as the storage matrix in the cell granule for histamine, enzymes, and chemotactic factors. For example, in the rat mast cell, exposure of the granule to physiologic buffer results in a selective elution of certain constituents, whereas others remain granule bound. Thus, the proteoglycan constituent of the granule offers a unique mechanism by which the local bioavailability of inflammatory mediators may be regulated.

Heparin, following release from the mast cell, influences both fluid-phase and cell-mediated events. In the fluid phase, heparin binds to a number of cationic molecules by virtue of its negative charge. Heparin binds to eosinophil major basic protein with the loss of heparin's anticoagulant activity and the abolition of the capacity of major basic protein to kill parasites (17). Platelet factor 4, a protein released from the platelet α-granule, binds to heparin and neutralizes heparin's anticoagulant activity. Heparin, by charge interactions, may bind to various enzymes and influence their function. This is illustrated by the demonstration of binding between heparin and granulocyte elastase, which results in stimulation of the elastase activity (56). Heparin may alter cell adherence. For example, heparin potentiates fibronectin binding to native collagen. Thus, fibroblasts, normally coated with fibronectin, would be expected to bind to collagen fibrils more easily in the presence of heparin. Heparin has been shown to interact with cell membranes with subsequent displacement of cell-surface-associated components. For example, heparin induces the release of plasminogen activator from rat vascular endothelium (60) and both a triglyceride lipase and a phospholipase into serum in humans after intravenous injection (25). Both heparin and oversulfated chondroitin sulfate inhibit lymphocyte blastogenesis to lectins or antigens (28).

Heparins have long been known to possess anticomplementary activity. In the classic complement pathway, heparin interferes with C1q binding to immune complexes and the interaction of C1s and C4 and C2 (78). The effect of C1 inhibitor on C1 has been reported to be potentiated by heparin. The alternative complement pathway is influenced by heparin. Heparin inhibits cobra-venom-factor-dependent C3 inactivation in serum. The coupling of heparin to zymosan changes the zymosan surface so that it no longer functions as an activator of the alternative complement pathway (52).

Lysosomal Enzymes

Inflammatory cells have been shown to contain a number of enzymes specifically associated with the granule, including arylsulfatase, β-hexosaminidase, β-glucuronidase, β-D-galactosidase, acid phosphatase, superoxide dismutase, peroxidase, and various proteases. In most instances, the enzymes were first associated with the cell granule by histochemical techniques. Such enzymes are present in mast cells, basophils, neutrophils, monocytes, platelets, and eosinophils. (See appropriate section for list of enzymes associated with each cell type.)

Arylsulfatases are present in a number of cells, including eosinophils, platelets, and mast cells. They consist of a family of enzymes with the ability to hydrolyze a variety of aromatic sulfate esters. Both arylsulfatases A and B are glycoproteins, preferentially hydrolyze ρ-nitrocatechol sulfate at an acid pH, and are inhibited by sulfate and phosphate ions. Arylsulfatase A can hydrolyze cerebroside 3-sulfate, seminolipid, and ascorbic acid 2-sulfate. Arylsulfatase B can hydrolyze hexosamine sulfates as well as chondroitin 4-sulfate tetrasaccharide (37). Arylsulfatase is released from human lung mast cells during degranulation (92). The exoglycosidases β-hexosaminidase, β-D-galactosidase, and β-glucuronidase are variably released from mast cells during degranulation. The function of such enzymes is unknown, although their release into the extracellular space might contribute to tissue remodeling.

Proteolytic enzymes have been associated with the inflammatory cells of a number of species. One of the most thoroughly studied of these enzymes is a chymotrypsin-like enzyme, termed *chymase* (or mast cell protease I), which is located in the rat peritoneal mast cell secretory granule (57). This rat mast cell chymase represents at least 15% of the total granule protein, in contrast to β-hexosaminidase, which makes up less than 1%. Purified chymase is inhibited by concentrations of 5-HT comparable with those present in rat mast cells. Chymase activity is partially masked by the combination of chymase with heparin in granules suspended in physiologic buffer (95).

Rat mast cells from the peritoneal cavity, gastrointestinal tract, lung, skin, and muscle contain proteolytic enzymes. In particular, the protease in mucosal or atypical mast cells in the gastrointestinal tract differs from the chymase in rat peritoneal mast cells by immunologic criteria and in amino acid sequence (111). This protease has been termed *mast cell protease II*. This distinct protease holds promise as a marker for rat mucosal mast cells. A trypsin-like enzyme not obvious in rats has been identified in canine and human mast cells.

A number of possible substrates for proteases have been reported. Chymase will degrade both large proteins such as collagen and small peptides such as bradykinin and will inactivate lipoprotein lipase. Proteases will eliminate the staining of proteoglycans in cartilage, suggesting an enzymatic effect (113). In fact, proteases can be shown to cleave the protein core of cartilage. Such observations suggest that inflammatory cell proteases may degrade ground substance and contribute to tissue remodeling (94).

A number of observations have recently been reported relating to tryptic activity in human mast cells. Tryptase has been isolated from human pulmonary mast cells and is able to generate C3a anaphylatoxin from purified human C3, a complement component (91). Enzymatic activities in antigen-challenged lung include kinin-generating activity, prekallikrein-activating activity, and Hageman-factor-cleaving activity. These latter enzymes represent links between the plasma-kinin-generating system and immediate hypersensitivity reactions.

Chemotactic Factors

Following immediate hypersensitivity reactions induced by antigen in the cutaneous tissue of humans, a biphasic reaction has been observed. The first phase consists of an acute vascular response characterized by a wheal and flare occurring within minutes, which subsides within 30 to 60 min. The first phase is followed by "late-phase" responses characterized by erythema, edema, and an induration beginning within 2 hr and lasting for 12 hr; a subset of patients have reactions for 12 to 24 hr. Histologically, the late-phase reaction is characterized by a prominent neutrophil, eosinophil, basophil, and mononuclear cell infiltrate whereas the 24- to 48-hr reaction involves a mononuclear cell infiltrate. A number of chemotactic factors generated or released from mast cells in this reaction have been identified which may account for these infiltrates. Preformed chemotactic factors reported include histamine, neutrophil chemotactic factor (NCF), and eosinophil chemotactic factors of anaphylaxis of the tetrapeptide and oligopeptide types. Complement activation leads to the generation of potent chemotactic molecules. Additional chemotactic factors generated in inflammatory reactions are lipid in nature, and will be discussed under the section on generated mediators.

Two tetrapeptides, Ala-Gly-Ser-Glu and Val-Gly-Ser-Glu, differing only in their *N*-terminal amino acid, have been identified as the active substances in the eosinophil chemotactic factor of anaphylaxis (ECF-A) (32). ECF-A is selectively chemotactic for eosinophils and has been associated with both rat and human mast cells. An "intermediate" molecular weight (oligopeptide: MW 1,500–2,500) eosinophil chemotactic factor, associated with rat mast cell granules and released by immunologic challenge of rat peritoneal mast cells, has also been described (15). Histamine has been reported to be chemotactic (3).

Neutrophil chemotactic factors have been described in the venous effluents of cold-challenged arms of patients with idiopathic cold urticaria (108) and in the serum of ragweed-sensitive subjects following bronchial provocation challenge using antigen (5). This factor has a molecular weight of 750,000, is preferentially chemotactic for neutrophils, and will deactivate both neutrophils and eosinophils. In this example, deactivation refers to the failure of leukocytes to migrate along a concentration gradient of a chemotactic stimulus as a result of a previous interaction with an active chemotactic factor.

A mast-cell-granule-derived chemotactic factor that will attract neutrophils and mononuclear cells in a pattern reminiscent of the late-phase allergic reaction when injected into rat skin has been described (103). This factor, termed *the inflammatory factor of anaphylaxis* (IF-A), appears to be a protein with a molecular weight of 1,350 and consists of 13 amino acids.

Generated Mediators

A large number of lipid-derived mediators are generated during an inflammatory reaction. The large majority of these newly formed products are metabolites of arachidonic acid, a polyunsaturated fatty acid present in cell membranes. Arachidonic acid is metabolized through two separate pathways: (a) the cyclooxygenase pathway to prostaglandins and thromboxanes and (b) the lipoxygenase pathway. The major products of the lipoxygenase pathway are the leukotrienes.

Prostaglandins and Thromboxanes

Prostaglandins were initially observed as components of seminal plasma having the capacity to influence the tone of uterine smooth muscle. Subsequently, components in human seminal plasma and sheep vesicular gland extracts capable of causing hypotension and smooth muscle constriction were described and termed *prostaglandins* (PG) (107). The first isolation of prostaglandin in crystalline form was in 1957 (9). Prostaglandins are described as oxidized derivatives of the hypothetical molecule prostanoic acid, a C_{20} unsaturated acid. The alphabetical nomenclature of the prostaglandins is based on the nature of the oxidative pattern of the five-membered cyclopentane ring structure of prostanoic acid, whereas the subscript numeral after the letter indicates the degree of unsaturation (Fig. 1). In the F series, the symbol α denotes that the hydroxyl at C-9 is below the plane of the ring, whereas β indicates its position above the ring. The structure of thromboxane A_2 is distinct in that an oxygen molecule is incorporated into the oxane ring structure. PGI_2 is chemically described as Δ^7-6-keto-PGF_1.

Prostaglandins may be formed by almost every mammalian tissue and, in general, appear to be in greater quantity following stimulation than can actually be detected by simple extraction. Stimulation results in the release of arachidonic acid from phospholipids by phospholipase A_2. Archidonic acid is converted to the endoperoxides PGG_2 and PGH_2 by a membrane-associated cyclooxygenase. The endoperoxide intermediates are biologically active, but have a short half-life and are acted upon by a series of enzymes to form prostaglandins I_2, F_2, D_2, and E_2, as well as thromboxanes, and hydroxyheptadecatrienoic acid (HHT). Prostaglandins appear to be rapidly degraded following their synthesis and release. PGE_2 and

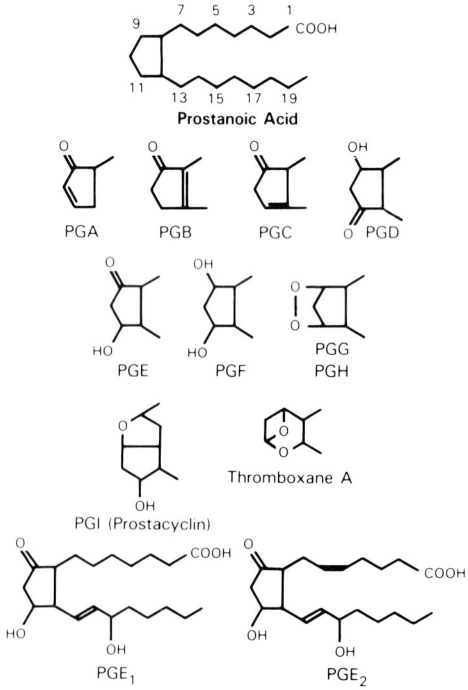

FIG. 1. Nomenclature of cyclooxygenase derivatives of arachidonic acid.

$PGF_{2\alpha}$, when injected intravenously, are rapidly removed from the circulation during one passage through the lung. The first and most important enzyme in the degradation of prostaglandins is 15-OH-prostaglandin dehydrogenase. This ubiquitous enzyme is responsible for the oxidation of the allylic alcohol group at the C-15 position. This oxidation is generally followed by reduction of the C-13 double bond by a 13-PG reductase.

The mast cell is capable both of generating prostaglandins itself (81) and of recruiting prostaglandin generation by action of mast cell granule constituents upon surrounding tissues. In rat mast cells, degranulation results primarily in the production of PGD_2 and PGI_2. The evidence for mast-cell-mediated recruitment of prostaglandin generation is taken from the observations that (a) the mast-cell-dependent reaction in whole tissue generates a number of prostaglandins and (b) certain mast cell mediators themselves, when added to fresh tissue, result in prostaglandin formation.

Other cellular inflammatory effector elements show great differences in their ability to make prostaglandins (11,35,39,75). Lymphocytes make small amounts of PGE_2, with neutrophils, monocytes, and macrophages making large amounts of this prostaglandin metabolite. In addition, monocytes and macrophages make substantial amounts of $PGF_{2\alpha}$.

Thromboxane synthetase forms thromboxane A_2 from PGH_2. It has a very short half-life ($T_{1/2}$ 30 sec), spontaneously degrading to thromboxane B_2 by the addition of water. Thromboxane B_2 is the metabolite most often measured when one is interested in thromboxane metabolism. Platelets, macrophages, and monocytes produce thromboxane A_2. Selected biologic effects of thromboxanes and prostaglandins are listed in Table 3.

Leukotrienes

The biologic activity of these agents was first demonstrated in 1938 to 1940 when perfusates from dog lungs treated with cobra venom (26,49) induced characteristic contractions of guinea pig jejunum with a slow onset of response. The substance was called *slow-reacting substance* (SRS). It was not until 1979 that the structure was reported (40). Since that time, the pathway leading to SRS from arachidonic acid has been elucidated (Fig. 2). Arachidonic acid is metabolized by three lipoxygenase enzymes. Each of these enzymes converts arachidonic acid into biologically active compounds. The 5-lipoxygenase pathway forms 5-hydroperoxyeicosatetraenoic acid (5-HPETE), which is subsequently converted into the leukotrienes, the best known of which is SRS. SRS is actually composed of three fatty acid products of the 5-lipoxygenase pathway: LTC_4, LTD_4, and LTE_4 (LT stands for "leukotriene"). LTC_4 is the initial SRS leukotriene produced (105) and is derived from LTA_4 by the enzymatic addition of glutathione. Once LTC_4 is formed, it is released into the extracellular milieu and converted to LTD_4 and LTE_4 by the release of glutamic acid and glycine, respectively (76).

TABLE 3. *Selected biologic activities of arachidonate metabolites*

Metabolite	Abbreviation	Activities
Prostacyclin	PGI_2	Inhibition of platelet aggregation
Prostaglandin E_2	PGE_2	Inhibition of lymphocyte mitogenesis, lymphokine production, cytotoxicity, and antibody production; stimulation of nondirected neutrophil migration (chemokinesis); induction of fever, erythema, and increased vascular permeability; and inhibition of histamine release, potentiation of edema and pain produced by other mediators
Prostaglandin $F_{2\alpha}$	$PGF_{2\alpha}$	Bronchoconstriction
Prostaglandin D_2	PGD_2	Chemokinesis; bronchoconstriction
Thromboxane A_2	TxA_2	Bronchoconstriction; platelet aggregation
5-Hydroperoxyeicosatetraenoic acid	5-HPETE	Chemotaxis; chemokinesis
5-Hydroxyeicosatetraenoic acid	5-HETE	Chemotaxis; chemokinesis
12-Hydroperoxyeicosatetraenoic acid	12-HPETE	Inhibition of platelet aggregation
Leukotriene B_4	LTB_4	Neutrophil chemotaxis
Leukotriene C_4	LTC_4	Potent bronchoconstrictor (greater in small airways than in large ones); increased vascular permeability with constriction
Leukotriene D_4	LTD_4	Very potent bronchoconstrictor (greater in small airways than in large ones); increased vascular permeability
Leukotriene E_4	LTE_4	Bronchoconstrictor; increased vascular permeability

Sources of leukotrienes include alveolar blood and peritoneal monocytes as well as neutrophils, eosinophils, basophils and mast cells (22,48,93). Leukotriene production may be stimulated by immunologic as well as nonimmunologic mechanisms. These include serum-activated zymozan, cobra venom, immune complexes, and aggregated immunoglobulin. In addition to the smooth muscle contracting activity, many other biologic activities of leukotrienes have been documented (Table 3) (88). Leukotrienes have also been shown to exert sustained effects on Purkinje nerve cell activity (14). These molecules also have effects on chemotaxis and granule enzyme release from neutrophils.

LTB_4 is derived from LTA_4 by the enzymatic addition of H_2O. This compound was first identified in polymorphonuclear leukocytes. LTB_4 has been shown to have potent chemotactic activity, enhance lysosomal enzyme release (33), and augment superoxide anion production (98). LTB_4 has also been implicated in modifying lymphocyte function by inducing specific suppressor lymphocytes (84) and augmenting human natural cytotoxic cell activity (85).

The HETES are formed by all three pathways of lipoxygenase metabolism. They are, by weight, the most prevalent products of the 5-lipoxygenase pathway

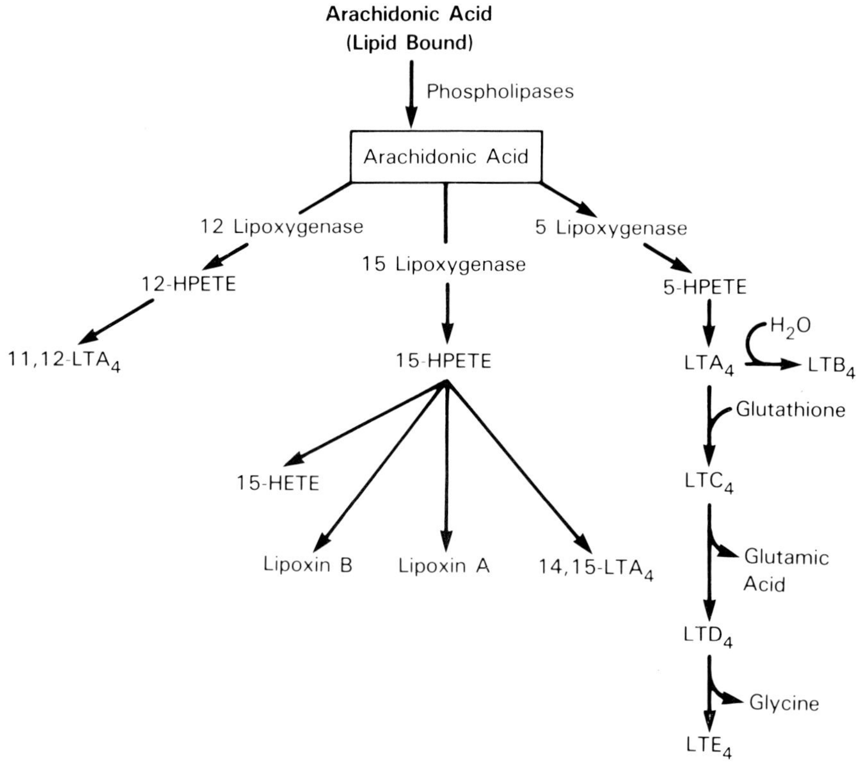

FIG. 2. Lipoxygenase pathway.

in leukocytes and mast cells. These compounds have significant activity on chemotaxis and granule release activity. They are, however, less potent than SRS or LTB_4 (102).

Recently, new products of the 15-lipoxygenase pathway, termed *lipoxins,* have been isolated (96,97). These compounds, isolated from human leukocytes, produce a rapid and sustained generation of superoxide when added to purified human neutrophils. In addition, degranulation was induced without causing aggregation. Lipoxin A is as potent as LTB_4, but less potent than LTB_4 at inducing degranulation.

Platelet-Activating Factor

Platelet-activating factor (PAF) is a basophil-derived mediator in the rabbit and can be released from mixed leukocytes. Rabbit PAF is a lipid mediator with the chemical structure acetyl-glyceryl-ether-phosphorylcholine (AGEPC) (23). PAF will aggregate and degranulate platelets, induce wheal and flare reactions in human skin, increase lung resistance, and lead to systemic hypotension, suggesting a role for this mediator in systemic anaphylaxis.

Bradykinin and Related Kinins

Kinins are small-molecular-weight basic peptides produced by a cascade of reactions initiated by Hageman factor. This factor also activates factor 11 in the clotting system and plasminogen in the fibrinolytic system. Hageman factor generates kallikrein from prekallikrein, an inactive precursor molecule. Kininogens, divided into low- and high-molecular-weight forms, provide the substrates for kallikrein and are converted to kinins. These peptides appear to be involved in the inflammatory response and have been shown to produce an inflammatory reaction if injected in several animal species. Bradykinin, one of the most active kinins, is almost as potent as histamine when vascular permeability is examined. A possible outline for the involvement of all three systems is shown in Fig. 3 (80).

Inflammatory Cells

Mast Cells and Basophils

Mast cells and basophils release their contents after stimulation of a cell surface receptor. In type I reactions this involves IgE receptor activation (20) (see section on secretion). In addition, mast cells have receptors for IgG and C3b which are also capable of initiating degranulation (65). Upon activation, both mast cells and basophils produce superoxide, a hydrogen peroxide, and generate metabolites of arachidonic acid, as has been discussed (81).

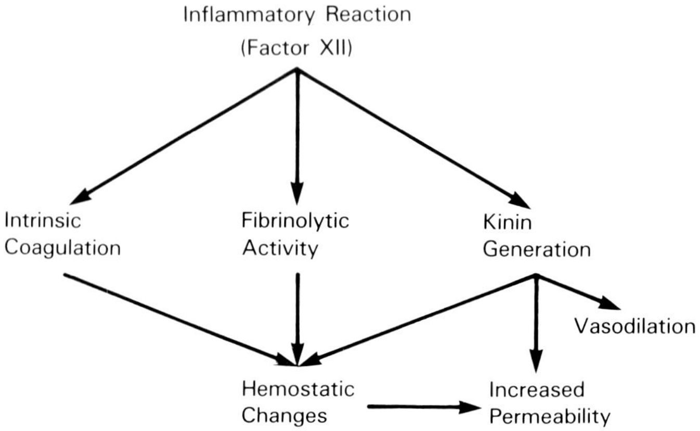

FIG. 3. Kinin generation in inflammation.

Basophils can be differentiated from mast cells by morphology and location (Table 4). Basophils are polymorphonuclear cells comprising 0.3% of nucleated cells in bone marrow and 0.5% to 1% of the circulating leukocytes. They are considered to be derived from bone marrow, a conclusion that is supported by their close resemblance to polymorphonuclear leukocytes. Mast cells, in contrast, have an uncertain origin. Recently, the application of *in vitro* techniques to growth of both mast cells and basophils has resulted in new information concerning the origin of mast cells and specific factors that encourage the proliferation of defined populations of mast cells and basophils. These data suggest that mast cell proliferation may be dependent on thymus-derived lymphocytes (T lymphocytes). In this regard it should be emphasized that the heterogeneity of mast cells has been reported frequently in the last few years, particularly by the laboratory of Enerback in Goteborg, Sweden (see the chapter by Scicchitano et al., *this volume*). Several authors suggest that mucosal mast cells are morphologically different than connective tissue mast cells, possess less heparin, have a different proteoglycan in the granules, and may be stimulated by different agents than connective tissue mast cells. Finally, mucosal mast cells may not be significantly altered by certain drugs that are known to inhibit the release of mediators from connective tissue mast cells (79,100,111).

Basophils rarely occur in extravascular sites other than bone marrow. However, there is recent evidence that basophils may be the most important inflammatory cell on the surface of the nasal mucosa in allergic rhinitis during the allergy season. This information is more specifically addressed in the chapter by Scicchitano et al. (*this volume*).

Basophil granules stain with metachromatic dyes to a lesser degree than mast cell granules. The granule itself is composed of dense particles appearing in a matrix of less density. The cytoplasm of mature basophils additionally contains abundant glycogen deposits, a small Golgi apparatus, a few mitochondria, ribosomes, and strands of rough endoplasmic reticulum. The plasma membrane has variable numbers of short folds and processes and may occasionally exhibit elongated folds.

TABLE 4. *Characteristic morphologic features differentiating basophils from mast cells*

Cell type	Location	Nucleus	Granule size (μm)	Cell surface
Basophils	Bone marrow, vascular compartment	Lobulated	1.2	Short folds and processes
Mast cells	Bone marrow, extravascular compartment	Round to oval	0.1–0.4	Elongated plasmalemmal projection

Mast cells in humans are located predominantly in connective tissue and adjacent to blood vessels, nerves, glandular ducts, and in association with lymphoid tissue. The skin and gastrointestinal mucosa are among the organ systems rich in mast cells. Normal human skin contains, on the average, 7,000 mast cells per cubic millimeter, whereas human duodenal mucosa contains approximately 20,000 mast cells per cubic millimeter. The half-life of normal human mast cells is unknown, but studies of mast cells in rat skin suggest that these cells may live weeks to months (54). Mast cells are 10 to 30 μm in diameter and are generally ovoid or irregularly elongated in tissue. The nucleus is often eccentric and reminiscent of the plasma cell. Mast cells have the usual array of subcellular organelles. The characteristic feature of mast cells is a cytoplasm filled with numerous granules that stain with metachromatic dyes.

Granule morphology varies from species to species and among mast cell populations at different tissue sites in the same species. Such morphologic variation is, in part, used to define subpopulations of mast cells. This is best illustrated by first reviewing mast cell granule morphology in the rat, the species studied in greatest detail with respect to mast cells, and comparing those findings with the more limited morphologic studies of human mast cells. Thus in the rat, the connective tissue or typical mast cell found in such tissue as the dermis, serosa, and intestinal submucosa has a 12.6-μm diameter in suspension and contains granules that are 0.2 to 0.4 μm in diameter. These mast cell granules are homogeneous by electron microscopy and stain intensely with a variety of metachromatic dyes, the most commonly used of which is toluidine blue. During degranulation after cell activation, these granules swell and are extruded into the external environment. In the rat at least one, and perhaps two, other mast cell populations may be distinguished based on granule characteristics. The first of these is the mucosal or atypical mast cell found primarily in the gastrointestinal tract. These mast cells are atypical in comparison to other mast cells because they contain granules that stain less intensely with metachromatic dyes and because the granules themselves appear smaller and more amorphous. The second candidate for a distinct population of mast cells remains controversial. Within the gastrointestinal epithelium of the rat, cells can be found that contain large granules or globules that stain weakly with metachromatic dyes. Such cells have been termed *globule leukocytes* or *intraepithelial mast cells*. In the rat, it has been suggested that globule leukocytes are derived from mucosal mast cells that migrate into the epithelium and partially discharge their granules.

Human mast cells differ from rat mast cells in that they exhibit two types of granules. The first granule contains crystalline contents with three patterns—scrolls, gratings, and lattices—that can coexist within the same granule. The second granule has a homogeneous, amorphous appearance (49). During mast cell activation, amorphous contents become crystalline, presumably as the granule prepares for discharge of mediators into the surrounding extracellular fluid. Later, a fibrillar residue remains in the granule lumen, some of which is lost to the outside.

The interaction of antigen with cell-bound IgE antibodies results in dimerization and initiates a degranulation reaction that is complete within 1 to 2 min at 37°C. The reaction is temperature dependent, being inhibited at temperatures below 12°C and prevented by pretreatment of the cells at 45°C. *In vitro* the reaction requires the presence of calcium.

A number of compounds induce noncytotoxic degranulation of mast cells *in vivo* and *in vitro*. Commonly employed nonimmunologic mast-cell-degranulating agents include concanavalin A; dextran; compound 48/80; anaphylatoxins C3a, C4a, and C5a; calcium ionophore A23187; and ATP. Concanavalin A and dextran appear to activate the mast cell by the same sequence of events as antigen activation and appear to cross-link IgE antibodies on the cell surface. Compound 48/80 bypasses the requirement for extracellular calcium by mobilizing intracellular calcium. The calcium ionophore A23187 shunts calcium across the cell membrane, thereby initiating degranulation (45). The characteristics of mast-cell-degranulating agents are summarized in Table 5. It should be apparent that there are a number of biologically distinct, chemically discrete, mechanistically diverse compounds able to initiate degranulation. This suggests multiple potential mechanisms by which mast cell degranulation can occur *in vivo*.

A number of biochemical events have been noted to occur when mast cells are stimulated to degranulate (Table 6). The exact temporal sequence of events involved remains speculative, but is sure to involve changes in phospholipid composition of the membrane and influx of calcium. The first recognizable event is activation of a membrane-associated diisopropylfluorophosphate-sensitive serine esterase (43). This is followed by transient activation of adenylate cyclase and membrane-associated methyltransferases. Phosphotidylethanolamine is methylated, in the presence of *S*-adenosyl-β methionine, to phosphatidyl monoethylanolamine and then phosphatidylcholine. The phosphatidylcholine is translocated from the cytoplasmic side to the extracellular side of the membrane (36,43,46).

In addition, a receptor-mediated hydrolysis occurs, mediated by phosphatidylinositol phosphodiesterase (phospholipase C), with phosphoinositide being converted to two second messengers, inositol trisphosphate and diacylglycerol. The diacylglycerol can then activate protein kinase C, and the inositol trisphosphate mobilizes intracellular calcium. Diacylglycerol may also be important in membrane fusion as well as being a source of arachidonic acid, which is necessary for the formation of prostaglandins and leukotrienes.

Recently, a metalloendoprotease has been shown to be required in secretion in a step that appears to act after the increase in intracellular calcium. This enzyme appears to be localized in the plasma membrane. From the above, a possible scenario for the events resulting in activation and secretion of mast cells can be hypothesized. Activation of mast cells through its IgE receptors promotes phospholipid metabolism, resulting in the liberation of arachidonic acid, diacylglycerol, and inositol trisphosphate. This results in the formation of fusogenic substances and alterations in membrane fluidity, which may facilitate entry of extracellular

TABLE 5. *Characteristics of mast cell secretion induced by several secretagogues*

	Requirements				
	Ca^{2+}	Energy	Activation of serine esterase	Time course (min)	Phosphatidylserine enhancement
Antigen-IgE	+	+	+	1–2	+
Antigen-IgG_a	+	+	+	1–2	+
Concanavalin A	+	+	+	6	+
Dextran	+	+	+	1	+
Compound 48/80	±	+	±	1	–
C3a, C4a, C5a	+	+	?	30–60	+
ATP	+	+	?	1–2	–
Lysosomal granule proteins	+	+	+	1–2	?
Polymyxin B	+	+	+	1	–
Calcium ionophore A23187	+	+	–	1–5	–

TABLE 6. *Events in mast cell secretion*

Biochemical	Morphological
Activation of serine esterase	Pore formation
Calcium movement	Granule swelling
Energy utilization	Microfilament organization
C-kinase activation	Cistern formation
Phospholipid turnover	Granule dissolution
Diacylglycerol formation	
Arachidonic acid metabolism	
Microtubule assembly	
Actomyosin activation	
Cyclic nucleotide formation	
Cyclic AMP utilization	
Cyclic-AMP-dependent protein kinase activation	
Cyclic-AMP-independent protein kinase activation	
Metalloprotease activation	

calcium as well as mobilization of intracellular calcium. Concurrently, stimulation of adenylate cyclase would activate cyclic-AMP-dependent protein kinases and diacylglycerol would activate protein kinase C, cyclic-AMP-independent kinase. This would result in the phosphorylation of proteins involved in controlling the release reaction.

Monocytes and Macrophages

Mononuclear phagocytes are bone-marrow-derived cells believed to arise from a common progenitor, namely, the colony-forming unit, neutrophil-monocyte (CFU-NM) (34,64,70). This CFU-NM gives rise to all the various tissue mononuclear cells, which include tissue macrophages, Kupffer cells, alveolar macrophages, dermal Langerhans cells, microglial cells of the brain, and osteoclasts (19,44).

Macrophages usually become prominent at sites of inflammation after 8 to 12 hr and are characterized by their high phagocytic activity (73,90), long life, specific interaction with lymphocytes (86), promotion of antigen-specific responses, and by the production of monokines and complement components (70) which have the capacity to affect other cell types. Macrophages are similar to neutrophils because they have high phagocytic capacity and considerable motility as well as the ability to form toxic oxygen metabolites and synthesize an array of hydrolytic enzymes. They differ, however, in the capacity to differentiate *in situ* (having a long life span during which they exhibit sustained responses to external stimuli) and in the ability to reuse phagolysosomes.

Monocytes, during their differentiation to tissue macrophages, undergo a number of morphological and biochemical alterations. As the monocyte differentiates, it increases dramatically in size, becoming 5 to 10 times as large, with a concomitant increase in the number of lysosomes. The morphologic events are accompanied by considerable changes in the enzymatic activities, with azurophilic peroxidase granules being lost and lysosome-containing hydrolytic enzymes becoming prominent (69). In addition, the monocyte-to-macrophage change is accompanied by a marked increase in the number of receptors for complement and immunoglobulin.

These membrane receptors play a prominent role in monocyte-macrophage activation. Receptors have been identified for immunoglobulins IgG, IgA, IgE, with the IgG_1 and IgG_3 subclasses being involved in promoting phagocytosis (55,63). The C3b receptor does not appear to stimulate phagocytosis, but rather increases the efficiency of IgG-mediated phagocytosis (38). The macrophage-lymphocyte interactions are probably mediated through MHC II antigens on the cell membrane, allowing antigen presentation to T lymphocytes (72).

Macrophages and monocytes, in response to receptor stimulation, make and release a diverse group of products (70) (Table 7). These include monokines, an example of which is interleukin-1 (IL-1) (endogenous pyrogen). IL-1 has the capability of activating lymphocytes. Numerous other monokines have been described which affect microvasculature, granulocytes, erythrocytes, and megakaryocytes (83).

Proteolytic enzymes are made and released by activated macrophages. In contrast to neutrophils, macrophages can markedly increase the quantity of these enzymes on activation (31). In addition to myeloperoxidase, elastase, collagenase,

TABLE 7. *Macrophage products*

Enzymes
Lysozyme
Neutral proteases, e.g., angiotensin-converting enzyme
Arginase
Acid hydrolases
Complement components
C_1
C_4
C_2
C_3
C_5
Factor B
Factor D
Properdin
C3b inactivator
BIH
Lipid mediators
Prostaglandins—PGE_2, $PGF_{2\alpha}$, TXA
Leukotrienes—LTC_4, LTD_4, LTE_4, + HETEs
Platelet-activating factor
IL-I (endogenous pyrogen)
Oxygen metabolites
Superoxide
H_2O_2
Inhibitors
α_2 macroglobulin
Plasmin inhibitor
Monokines

and plasmogen activator, macrophages contain angiotensin-converting enzyme, which is increased in some granulomatous diseases. This enzyme is involved in the enzymatic conversion of angiotensin I to angiotensin II and the inactivation of bradykinin. Macrophages are also active in the production of lipid mediators such as PGE_2, thromboxane A_2, LTB_4, LTC_4, 5-HETE, and 15-HETE (HETE stands for hydroxyeicosatetraenoic acid). Many of these molecules undoubtly are involved in the *in vitro* activity of macrophages (61). (See the section on prostaglandins and thromboxanes and the section on leukotrienes.)

Neutrophils

Neutrophils, like monocytes, are derived from a pluripotent bone marrow precursor cell that gives rise to CFU-NM (21,77). The exact molecular mechanisms by which these cells differentiate, as well as the regulation of differentiation, are partly understood. Such processes probably are dependent on one or many of the humoral substances that have been described, such as colony-stimulating factor or granulopoietin (16,82). Differentiation itself involves dramatic biochemical and morphologic changes. Myeloblasts are the earliest recognizable cell granulocyte and are characterized as large cells with dense basophilic cytoplasm. Granules first appear in the late promyelocyte stage.

Neutrophils contain two populations of granules, termed *specific granules* and *azurophilic granules*. Many of the biochemical changes during differentiation can be accounted for by the appearance of the granules. The azurophilic or primary granules contain the lysosomal enzymes and appear first. The specific or secondary granules appear during the myelocyte stage and contain alkaline phosphatase as well as other enzymes also contained in the azurophilic granule.

Neutrophils are short-lived cells. Once they leave the bone marrow they have a half-life ($T_{1/2}$) of approximately 6.7 hr. This $T_{1/2}$ is doubled after the administration of glucocorticoids (10). In addition to being short-lived, neutrophils are also characterized by: (a) availability in large numbers (total body polymorphonuclear leukocyte count, 2.5×10^9 cells/kg), (b) responsiveness to chemotactic stimuli, (c) motility, (d) high phagocytic capacity and (e) large number of oxidative metabolites and digestive enzymes.

Neutrophils are the major cellular elements in most forms of acute inflammation. They have the capacity to be stimulated through surface receptor activation and have been shown to have receptors for F-Met-leu-phe (FMLP), C5a, C3a, leukotriene B4, C3b, and IgG (71). Stimulation at the neutrophil surface results in a series of events called the *respiratory burst*. This is characterized by a marked increase in metabolic activity and the generation of toxic oxygen metabolites such as the superoxide anion (6,62), which degenerates to hydrogen peroxide.

Activation of the neutrophil also results in the generation of arachidonic acid metabolites, with the major products being PGE_2, 5-HETE, LTB_4, LTC_4, and thromboxane A_2 (12,13). Among these compounds, PGE_2 is a major mediator of the inflammatory process leading to edema and erythema (68). 5-HETE has been shown to have chemotactic activity and to cause the release of lysozyme from neutrophils (102).

Discharge of granules during phagocytosis, ingestion, or cell death results in the release of a panoply of enzymes which gives the cell the capability to degrade proteins, nucleic acids, carbohydrates, and lipids (Table 8). These products can obviously have deleterious effects on cellular elements and are sure to be involved in the cell destruction that occurs during acute inflammation (24).

The azurophilic granules also contain small-molecular-weight (4,000–8,000) cationic polypeptides with trypsin-like activity, which have the ability to potentiate the release of vasoactive amines from mast cells and platelets. These molecules also can produce irreversible platelet activation and may affect clotting through intrinsic anticoagulant activity or their ability to neutralize heparin through charge interactions (47,87,106). The neutrophil also contains products that have the potential to limit the inflammatory reaction. They contain C5a-inactivating activity,

TABLE 8. *Neutrophil granule contents*

Azurophil (primary) granules
Hydrolases including cathepsins A, D, E (acid proteases)
α-Furosidase
5′-Nucleotidase
β-Galactosidase
Arylsulfatase
α-Mannosidase
N-Acetyl β-glucosamininidase
β-Glucuronidase
Acid β-glycerophosphatase
Neutral proteases including cathepsin G, elastase, and collagenase
Cationic proteins
Myeloperoxidase
Lysozyme
Specific (secondary) granules
Lactoferrin
Alkaline phosphatase
Vitamin-B_{12}-binding protein
Lysozyme
Collagenase

an inhibitor of histamine release, and a histaminase that oxidizes extracellular histamine (53,112,114).

Eosinophil

The eosinophil is a poorly understood bone-marrow-derived cell, first recognized by Paul Ehrlich in 1879. The cell can first be identified morphologically in the promyelocyte stage of development, when its unique granules arise (59). Differentiation follows the same stages as the neutrophil and occurs in the marrow (42). The proliferation and maturation of these blood elements also appear to be under the control of soluble mediators called *eosinophil-releasing factor* and *eosinophilopoietin* (67).

Morphologically these cells are characterized by prominent granules that stain heavily with acidic dyes such as eosin. Eosinophils contain around 200 granules consisting of large major granules and smaller granules (7). The large granules contain the electron-dense crystalloid core, which is composed mainly of eosinophil major basic protein (74). Eosinophil major basic protein is basic protein with 11 arginine residues per molecule. In addition, it has multiple cysteine residues, allowing covalent formation of aggregates of molecules (30). The function of this protein is unknown, but there is some evidence that it may be involved in parasite killing (17). Many of the neuropathic and cytotoxic effects of the hypereosinophilic syndrome have also been attributed to eosinophilic major basic protein (29).

The eosinophil, like the neutrophil and the macrophage, contains a broad range of enzymes involved in particle digestion and microbial killing. In addition, the esoinophil may play a prominent role in modulating the inflammatory response because of the presence of enzymes capable of inactivating certain inflammatory mediators. These enzymes include a histaminase, kininase, phospholipase D, and lysophospholipase. Extracts of eosinophils have been reported to block the inflammatory effect of mediators such as histamine if the extract was injected just prior to the mediator injection (4).

Response to external stimuli is again mediated through surface membrane receptors. Eosinophils contain receptors for IgG, IgE, and complement which can cause activation and release of granular contents (51) and promote adherence to parasites. Interestingly, mast cell products appear to enhance this response (18), thus suggesting some interaction between mast cells and eosinophils in parasite killing.

Stimulation of eosinophils, in addition to releasing preformed mediators, also leads to generation of superoxide. Eosinophils are particularly long-lived cells with a well-developed Golgi apparatus and numerous ribosomes capable of sustaining prolonged activation and with the capacity to resynthesize granule components (48).

Eosinophils also have the ability to generate various lipid mediators. They have been shown to synthesize PGE_2, HETEs, LTB_4, LTC_4, LTD_4, and LTE_4. These eosinophil mediators contribute to hypersensitivity reactions. Eosinophils uniquely also form Charcot Leydin crystals, thin hexagonal bipyramids that appear to be composed of the enzyme lysophospholipase (110). These crystals are seen in situations characterized by large infiltrations of eosinophils, including the nasal discharge of patients with allergic rhinitis and the sputum of asthmatics.

SUMMARY

Cellular and chemical mediators certainly are involved in the pathogenesis of acute infectious lesions of the ear, including viral and bacterial otitis media. A knowledge of cells and their mediators is critical to the understanding of the basic processes involved. For example, the mechanisms for effusion formation in otitis media are not totally clear. However, recent evidence has suggested mast cell involvement. Blockage of eustachian tubes can lead to fluid accumulation within the middle ear cavity (101), with the first fluid developing in a space near the pars flaccida. Histologic studies (2,109) have shown the pars flaccida to be rich in mast cells. Further, both rat and the human middle ear effusions have elevated levels of histamine (1,8). Experimentally, instillation of compound 48/80, a potent mast cell activator, into the external auditory canal of rats results in the production of otitis media, with fluid rich in histamine. It therefore could be argued that mast cells and their chemical mediators play a prominent role in the pathogenesis of middle ear effusions. The specific role of inflammatory cells and their mediators in this and other diseases of the ear will be discussed throughout this volume.

ACKNOWLEDGMENT

The authors would like to thank Shirley Starnes for her help in the preparation of this manuscript.

REFERENCES

1. Alm, P.E., Bloom, G., Hellstrom, S., Salin, B., and Stenfors, L.-E. (1982): The release of histamine from the pars flaccida mast cells, one cause of otitis media with effusion? *Acta Otolaryngol.*, 94:517–552.
2. Alm, P.E., Bloom, G.D., Hellstrom, S., Stenfors, L.-E., and Widemar, L. (1983): Mast cells in the pars flaccida in the tympanic membrane. A quantitative, morphological and biochemical study in the rat. *Experientia*, 39:287–289.
3. Archer, R.K. (1956): The eosinophil response in the horse to intramedullary and intradermal injections of histamine, ACTH, and cortisone. *J. Pathol. Bacteriol.*, 72:87–94.
4. Archer, R.K. (1959): Eosinophil leukocytes and their reactions to histamine and 5-hydroxytryptamine. *J. Pathol. Bacteriol.*, 78:95–103.
5. Atkins, P.G., Norman, M., Weiner, H., and Zweiman, B. (1977): Release of neutrophil chemotactic activity during immediate hypersensitivity reactions in humans. *Ann. Intern. Med.*, 86:415–418.
6. Babior, B.M. (1978): Oxygen dependent microbial killing by phagocytes. *N. Engl. J. Med.*, 298:659–668.
7. Bainton, P.F., and Farquhar, M.G. (1970): Segregation and packaging of granule enzymes in eosinophilic leukocytes. *J. Cell Biol.*, 45:54–73.
8. Berger, G., Hawke, W.M., Proops, D.W., Ranadive, N.S., and Wong, D. (1978): Histamine levels in middle ear effusions. In: *Recent Advances in Otitis Media with Effusion*, edited by D.J. Lim, C.D. Bluestone, J.O. Klein, J.D. Nelson, pp. 195–198, B.C. Decker, Philadelphia.
9. Bergstrom, S., and Sjovall, J. (1957): The isolation of prostaglandin. *Acta Chem. Scand.*, 11:1906–1911.
10. Bishop, C.R., Athens, J.W., Boggs, D.R., Warner, H.R., Cartwright, G.E., and Wintrobe, M.M. (1968): Leukokinetic studies. XIII: a non-steady-state kinetic evaluation of the mechanism of cortisone-induced granulocytosis. *J. Clin. Invest.*, 47:249–260.
11. Bockman, R.S. (1981): Prostaglandin production by human blood monocytes and mouse peritoneal macrophages: synthesis dependent on culture condition. *Prostaglandins*, 21:9–30.
12. Borgeat, P., Hanburg, M., and Samuelsson, B. (1976): Transformation of arachidonic acid and homo-γ-linolenic acid by polymorphonuclear leukocytes. Monohydroxy acids from novel lipoxygenase. *J. Biol. Chem.*, 251:7816–7820.
13. Borgeat, P., and Samuelsson, B. (1979): Arachidonic acid metabolism in polymorphonuclear leukocytes: effects of ionophore A23187. *Proc. Natl. Acad. Sci. USA*, 76:2148–2152.
14. Borgeat, P., and Samuelsson, B. (1979): Transformation of arachidonic acid by rabbit polymorphonuclear leukocytes. Formation of novel dehydroxyeicosatetraenoic acid. *J. Biol. Chem.*, 254:2643–2646.
15. Boswell, R.N., Austen, K.F., and Goetzl, E.J. (1978): Intermediate molecular weight eosinophil chemotactic factors in rat peritoneal mast cells: immunologic release, granule association and demonstration of structural heterogeneity. *J. Immunol.*, 120:16–20.
16. Brennan, J.K., Lichtman, M.A., DiPersio, J.F., and Abboud, C.N. (1980): Chemical mediators of granulopoiesis: a review. *Exp. Hematol.*, 8:441–464.
17. Butterworth, H.E., Wassom, D.L., Gleich, G.J., Loegering, D.A., and David, J.R. (1979): Damage to schistosomula of *Schistosoma mansoni* induced directly by eosinophil major basic protein. *J. Immunol.*, 122:221–229.
18. Capron, M., Ronsseaux, J., Mazingrie, C., Bazin, H., and Capron, A. (1978): Rat mast cell-eosinophil interaction in antibody-dependent eosinophil cytotoxicity to *Schistosoma mansoni* schistosomula. *J. Immunol.*, 121:2518–2525.
19. Carr, I. (1978): The biology of macrophages. *Clin. Invest. Med.*, 1:59–67.
20. Coombs, R.R.A., and Gill, P.G.H. (1968): Classification of allergic reactions responsible for

clinical hypersensitivity and disease. In: *Clinical Aspects of Immunology,* 2nd ed., edited by R.G.H. Gill and R.R.A. Coombs, pp. 575–596. F.A. Davis Co., Philadelphia.
21. Cronkite, E.P., and Fliedner, T.M. (1964): Granulocytopoiesis. *N. Engl. J. Med.,* 270:1347–1352.
22. Czarnetzki, B.M., Konig, W., and Lichtenstein, L. (1976): Eosinophil chemotactic factor. I. Release from polymorphonuclear leukocytes by calcium ionophore A23187. *J. Immunol.,* 117:229–234.
23. Demopoulos, C.H., Pinckard, R.N., and Hanahan, D.J. (1979): Platelet activating factor (PAF): evidence for 1-*O*-alkyl-2-acetyl-*sn*-glyceryl-3-phosphorylcholene as the active component (a new class of lipid chemical mediators). *J. Biol. Chem.,* 254:9355–9358.
24. Edelson, P.J. and Cohn, Z.A. (1973): Peroxidase-mediated cell cytotoxicity. *J. Exp. Med.,* 138:318–323.
25. Ehnholm, C., Shaw, W., Greten, H., and Brown, W.V. (1975): Purification from human plasma of heparin-released lipase with activity against triglyceride and phospholipids. *J. Biol. Chem.,* 250:6756–6761.
26. Feldberg, W., and Kellaway, C.H. (1983): Liberation of histamine and formation of lysocithin-like substances by cobra venom. *J. Physiol.,* 94:187–226.
27. Foon, K.A., Wahl, S.M., Oppenheim, J.J., and Rosentreich, D.L. (1976): Serotonin-induced production of a monocyte chemotactic factor by human peripheral blood leukocytes. *J. Immunol.,* 117:1545–1552.
28. Frieri, M., and Metcalfe, D.D. (1983): Analysis of the effect of mast cell granules on lymphocyte blastogenesis in the absence and presence of mitogens: identification of heparin as a granule-associated suppressor factor. *J. Immunol.,* 131:1942–1948.
29. Gleich, G.J., Frigas, E., Loegering, D.A., et al. (1979): Cytotoxic properties of the eosinophil major basic protein. *J. Immunol.,* 123:2925–2927.
30. Gleich, G.J., Loegering, D.A., Kueppers, F., Bajaj, J., and Mann, K. (1974): Physiochemical and biologic properties of the major basic protein from guinea pig eosinophil granules. *J. Exp. Med.,* 140:313–332.
31. Goetzl, E.J. (1980): Mediators of immune hypersensitivity derived from arachidonic acid. *N. Engl. J. Med.,* 303:822–825.
32. Goetzl, E.J., and Austen, K.F. (1975): Purification and synthesis of eosinophilotactic tetrapeptides of human lung tissue: identification as eosinophil chemotactic factor of anaphylaxis. *Proc. Natl. Acad. Sci. USA,* 72:4123–4127.
33. Goetzl, E.J., and Pickett, W.C. (1980): The human PMN leukocyte chemotactic activity of complex hydroxy-eicostatetraenoic acids (HETEs). *J. Immunol.,* 125:1789–1791.
34. Golde, D.W., and Cline, M.J. (1974): Regulation of granulopoiesis. *J. Engl. J. Med.,* 291:1388–1395.
35. Goldyne, M.E., and Stobo, J.D. (1979): Synthesis of prostaglandins by subpopulations of human peripheral blood monocytes. *Prostaglandins,* 18:687–695.
36. Gomperts, B.D. (1983): Involvement of guanine nucleotide-binding protein in the gating of CA^{+2} by receptors. *Nature,* 306:64–66.
37. Gorham, S.D., and Cantz, M. (1978): Arylsulfatase B, an exo-sulphatase for chondroitin 4-sulphate tetrasaccharide. *Hoppe-Seyler's Z. Physiol. Chem.,* 359:1811–1814.
38. Griffin, F.M., Jr., and Griff, J.A. (1980): Augmentation of macrophage complement receptor function in vitro. *J. Immunol.,* 125:844–849.
39. Hanburg, M., and Samuelsson, B. (1974): Prostaglandin endoperoxides. Novel transformation of arachidonic acid in human platelets. *Proc. Natl. Acad. Sci. USA,* 71:3400–3404.
40. Hammarstrom, S. (1983): Leukotrienes. *Ann. Rev. Biochem.,* 52:355–377.
41. Hammarstrom, S., Murphy, R.C., Samuelsson, B., Clark, D.A., Mioskowski, C., and Corey, E.J. (1979): Structure of leukotriene C. Identification of the amino acid part. *Biochem. Biophys. Res. Commun.,* 91:1266–1272.
42. Herion, J.C., Glasser, R.M., Walker, R.I., and Palmer, J.G. (1970): Eosinophil kinetics in two patients with eosinophilia. *Blood,* 36:361–370.
43. Hirata, F., and Axelrod, J. (1978): Enzymatic synthesis and rapid translocation of phosphatidyl choline by two methyl transferases in erythrocyte membranes. *Proc. Natl. Acad. Sci. USA,* 75:2348–2352.
44. Hocking, W.G., and Golde, D.W. (1979): The pulmonary-alveolar macrophage. *N. Engl. J. Med.,* 301:580–587.
45. Ishizaka, T. (1982): Biochemical analysis of triggering signals induced by bridging of IgE receptors. *Fed. Proc.,* 41:17–21.

46. Ishizaka, T., Hirata, F., Ishizaka, K., and Axelrod, J. (1980): Stimulation of phospholipid methylation, Ca^{+2} influx, and histamine release by binding of IgE receptors in rat mast cells. *Proc. Natl. Acad. Sci. USA,* 77:1903–1906.
47. Janoff, A., Schaefer, S., Scherer, J., and Bean, M.A. (1965): Mediators of inflammation in leukocyte lysosomes. II. Mechanism of action of lysosomal cationic protein upon vascular permeability in the rat. *J. Exp. Med.,* 122:841–851.
48. Jorg, A., Henderson, W.R., Murphy, R.C., and Klebanoff, S.J. (1982): Leukotriene generation by eosinophils. *J. Exp. Med.,* 155:390–402.
49. Jorpes, J.E., Holmgren, H., and Wilander, O. (1937): Uber das vorkommen von heparin in den gefabwanden und in den augen. *Z. Mikrosk. Anat. Forsch.,* 42:279–282.
50. Kaplan, A.P., Gray, L., Shaff, R.E., Horakova, Z., and Beaven, M.A. (1975): In vivo studies of mediator release in cold urticaria and cholinergic urticaria. *J. Allergy Clin. Immunol.,* 55:394–402.
51. Kay, A.B., and Anwar, A.R.E. (1980): Eosinophil surface receptors. In: *The Eosinophil in Health and Disease,* edited by A.A.F. Mahmoud and K.F. Austen, pp. 207–230. Grune and Stratton, New York.
52. Kazatchkine, M.D., Fearon, D.T., Silbert, J.E., and Austen, K.F. (1979): Surface associated heparin inhibits zymosan-induced activation of the human alternative pathway by augmenting the regulatory action of the control proteins on particle bound C3b. *J. Exp. Med.,* 150:1202–1215.
53. Kelly, M.T., and White, A. (1974): An inhibitor of histamine release from human leukocytes. *J. Clin. Invest.,* 53:1341–1350.
54. Kiernan, J.A. (1979): Production and life span of cutaneous mast cells in young rats. *J. Anat.,* 128:225–238.
55. Kurlander, R.J., and Baker, J. (1982): The binding of human immunoglobulins, GI monomer and small covalently crosslinked polymers of immunoglobulin GI to human peripheral blood monocytes and polymorphonuclear leukocytes. *J. Clin. Invest.,* 69:1–8.
56. Lonky, S.A., Marsh, J., and Wohl, H. (1978): Stimulation of human granulocyte elastase by platelet factor 4 and heparin. *Biochem. Biophys. Res. Commun.,* 85:1113–1118.
57. Lagunoff, D., Phillips, M.T., Iseri, O.A., and Benditt, E.P. (1964): Isolation and preliminary characterization of rat mast cell granules. *Lab. Invest.,* 13:1331–1344.
58. Lagunoff, D., and Pritzl, P. (1976): Characterization of rat mast cell granule proteins. *Arch. Biochem. Biophys.,* 173:553–563.
59. Mahmoud, A.A.F., Stone, M.K., and Kellermeyer, R.W. (1977): Eosinophilopoietin: a circulating low molecular weight peptide-like substance which stimulates the production of eosinophils in mice. *J. Clin. Invest.,* 60:675–682.
60. Markwardt, F., and Klocking, H.P. (1977): Heparin-induced release of plasminogen activator. *Haemostasis,* 6:370–374.
61. McCarthy, J.B., Wahl, S.M., Reese, J.C., Olsen, C.E., Sandberg, A.L., and Wahl, L.M. (1980): Mediation of macrophage collagenase production by 3′-5′ cyclic adenosine monophosphate. *J. Immunol.,* 124:2405–2409.
62. McPhail, L.C., Henson, P.M., and Johnson, R.B., Jr. (1981): Respiratory burst enzyme in human neutrophils. *J. Clin. Invest.,* 67:710–716.
63. Meleurca, F.M., Zeiger, R.S., Mellon, M.H., O'Connor, R.D., and Spielgelberg, H.L. (1981): Increased peripheral blood monocytes with Fc receptors for IgE in patients with severe allergic disorders. *J. Immunol.,* 126:1592–1595.
64. Metcalf, D. (1971): Transformation of granulocytes to macrophages in bone marrow colonies *in vitro. J. Cell Physiol.,* 77:277–280.
65. Metcalfe, D.D., Kaliner, M., and Donlon, M.A. (1981): The mast cell. *Crit. Rev. Immunol.,* 3:23–74.
66. Metcalfe, D.D., Lewis, R.A., Silbert, J.E., Rosenberg, R.D., Wasserman, S.I., and Austen, K.F. (1979): Isolation and characterization of heparin from human lung. *J. Clin. Invest.,* 64:1537–1543.
67. Miller, A.M., and McGarry, M.P. (1976): A diffusible stimulator of eosinophopoiesis produced by lymphoid cells as demonstrated with diffusion chambers. *Blood,* 48:293–300.
68. Moncada, S., Ferreira, S. H., and Vane, J. R. (1973): Prostaglandins, aspirin drugs, and the oedema of inflammation. *Nature,* 246:217–219.
69. Nakagawara, A., Nalkan, C.F., and Cohn, Z.A. (1981): Hydrogen peroxide metabolism in human monocytes during differentiation in vitro. *J. Clin. Invest.,* 68:1243–1252.
70. Nathan, C.F., Murry, H.W., and Cohn, Z. (1980): Current concepts: the macrophage as an effector cell. *N. Engl. J. Med.,* 303:622–626.

71. Newman, S.L., and Johnston, R.B. (1979): Role of binding through C3b and IgG in polymorphonuclear neutrophil function: studies with trypsin generated C3b. *Immunol.*, 23:1839–1846.
72. Niederhuber, J.E., and Shreffler, D.C. (1977): Anti-Ia serum blocking of macrophage function in the *in vitro* humoral response. *Transplant. Proc.*, 9:875–879.
73. Oren, R., Farnham, A., Saito, K., Milofsky, E., and Karnovsky, M. (1983): Metabolic patterns in three types of phagocytizing cells. *J. Cell Biol.*, 17:487–501.
74. Ottesen, E.A., and Cohen, S.G. (1979): The eosinophil, eosinophilia and eosinophil-related disorders. In: *Allergy: Principles and Practice*, edited by E. Middleton, C.E. Reed, and E.F. Ellis, pp. 584–632. C.V. Mosby, St. Louis.
75. Pawlowski, N.A., Scott, W.A., Andreach, M., and Cohn, Z.A. (1982): Uptake and metabolism of monohydroxyeicosatetraenoic acids by macrophages. *J. Exp. Med.*, 155:1653–1664.
76. Parker, C.W., Huber, M.M., and Falkenhiem, S.F. (1980): Sequential conversion of the glutathionyl side chain of slow reacting substance to cysteinyl-glycine and cysteine in rat basophilic leukemia cells stimulated with A23187. *Prostaglandins*, 20:863–880.
77. Quesenberry, P., and Levitt, L. (1979): Hematopoietic stem cells. *N. Engl. J. Med.*, 301:755–759.
78. Raepple, E., Hans-Ulrich, H., and Loos, M. (1976): Mode of interaction of different polyanions with the first (C1), the second (C_2) and the fourth (C_4) component of complement. I. Effect on fluid phase C1 and on C1 bound to EA or EAC4. *Immunochemistry*, 13:251–255.
79. Razin, E., Stevens, R.L., Akiyama, F., Schmid, K., and Austen, K.F. (1982): Culture from mouse bone marrow of a subclass of mast cells possessing a distinct chondroitin sulfate proteoglycan with glycosaminoglycans rich in *N*-acetylgalactosamine 4,6-disulfate. *J. Biol. Chem.*, 257:7229–7236.
80. Regali, D., and Barake, J. (1980): Pharmacology of bradykinin and related kinins. *Pharmacol. Rev.*, 32:1–46.
81. Roberts, L.J., Lewis, R.A., Oates, J.A., and Austen, K.F. (1979): Prostaglandin, thromboxane and 12-hydroxy-5,8-10,14 eicostatetraenoic acid production by ionophore-stimulated rat serosal mast cells. *Biochem. Biophys. Acta*, 575:285–292.
82. Robinson, W.A., and Mangalik, A. (1975): The kinetics and regulation of granulopoiesis. *Semin. Hematol.*, 12:7–25.
83. Rocklin, R.E., Bendlzen, K., and Greineder, D. (1980): Mediators of immunity: lymphokines and monokines. *Adv. Immunol.*, 29:55–136.
84. Rola-Pleszczynski, M., Borgeat, P., and Serois, P. (1982): Leukotriene B_4 induces human suppressor lymphocytes. *Biochem. Biophys. Res. Commun.*, 108:1531–1537.
85. Rola-Pleszczynski, M., Gagnon, L., and Serois, P. (1983): Leukotriene B_4 augments human natural cytotoxic cell activity. *Biochem. Biophys. Res. Commun.*, 113:531–537.
86. Rosenthal, A.S. (1980): Regulation of the immune response: Role of the microphage. *N. Engl. J. Med.*, 303:1153–1161.
87. Saba, H.I., Roberts, H.R., and Herion, J.C. (1967): The anticoagulant activity of lysosomal cationic proteins from polymorphonuclear leukocytes. *J. Clin. Invest.*, 46:580–589.
88. Samuelsson, B. (1983): Leukotrienes: mediators of immediate hypersensitivity reactions and inflammation. *Science*, 220:568–575.
89. Sandler, J.A., Clyman, R.I., Manganiello, V.C., and Vaughan, M. (1975): The effect of serotonin (5-hydroxytryptophan) and derivatives of guanosine 3′,5′-monophosphate in human monocytes. *J. Clin. Invest.*, 55:431–435.
90. Sbarra, A.J., and Karnovsky, M.L. (1959): The biochemical basis of phagocytosis. I. Metabolic changes during the injection of particles by polymorphonuclear leukocytes. *J. Biol. Chem.*, 234:1355–1362.
91. Schwartz, L.B., Kawahara, M.S., Hugli, T.E., Fearson, D.T., and Austen, K.F. (1983): Generation of C3a anaphylatoxin from human C3 by human mast cell tryptase. *J. Immunol.*, 130:1891–1895.
92. Schwartz, L.B., Lewis, R.A., Seldin, D., and Austen, K.F. (1981): Acid hydrolases and tryptase from secretory granules of dispersed human lung mast cells. *J. Immunol.*, 126:1290–1294.
93. Scott, W.A., Pawlowski, N.A., Murray, H.W., Andreach, M., Zrike, J., and Cohn, Z.A. (1981): Regulation of arachidonic acid metabolism by macrophage activation. *J. Exp. Med.*, 155:1148–1160.
94. Seppa, H. (1980): On the role of the chymotrypsin-like protease of .at mast cells in inflammatory vasopermeability and fibrinolysis. *Inflammation*, 4:1–8.
95. Seppa, H., Vaananen, K., and Korhonen, K. (1979): Effect of mast cell chymase of rat skin on intercellular matrix: a histochemical study. *Acta Histochem.*, 64:64–70.

96. Serhan, C.N., Hamberg, M., and Samuelsson, B. (1984): Trihydroxytetraenes: a novel series of compounds from arachidonic acid in human leukocytes. *Biochem. Biophys. Res. Commun.*, 118:943–949.
97. Serhan, C.N., Hamberg, M., and Samuelsson, B. (1984): Lipoxins: novel series of biologically active compounds formed from arachidonic acid in human leukocytes. *Proc. Natl. Acad. Sci. USA*, 81:5355–5359.
98. Serhan, C.N., Raden, A., Smolen, J.E., Korchak, H., Samuelsson, B., and Weissman, G. (1982): Leukotriene B4 is a complete secretagogue in human neutrophils: a kinetic analysis. *Biochem. Biophys. Res. Commun.*, 107:1006–1012.
99. Sjoerdsma, A. (1959): Serotonin. *N. Engl. J. Med.*, 261:181–188.
100. Sredni, B., Friedman, M.M., Bland, C.E., and Metcalfe, D.D. (1983): Ultrastructural, biochemical, and functional characteristics of histamine containing cells cloned from mouse bone marrow: tentative identification as mucosal mast cells. *J. Immunol.*, 131:915–922.
101. Stenfors, L.E., Carlsoo, B., and Winblad, B. (1981): Structural and healing capacity of the rat tympanic membrane after eustachian tube occlusion. *Acta Otolaryngol.*, 91:75–84.
102. Stenson, W., and Parker, C.W. (1980): Mono-hydroxyeicosatetraenoic acids (HETEs) induce degranulation of human neutrophils. *J. Immunol.*, 124:2100–2104.
103. Tannenbaum, S., Oertel, H., Henderson, W., and Kaliner, M. (1980): The biologic activity of mast cell granules. I. Elicitation of inflammatory responses in rat skin. *J. Immunol.*, 125:325–335.
104. Tas, J., and Berndsen, R.G. (1977): Does heparin occur in mucosal mast cells of the rat small intestine? *J. Histochem., Cytochem.*, 25:1058–1062.
105. Vanderhoek, T.Y., Bryant, R.W., and Bailez, J.M. (1980): 15 hydroxy 5,8,11,13 eicostatetraenoic acid: a potent and selective inhibitor of platelet lipoxygenase. *J. Biol. Chem.*, 255:5996–5999.
106. Vinge, P., and Olson, I. (1975): Cationic proteins of human granulocytes. VI. Effects of complement system and mediation of chemotactic activity. *J. Immunol.*, 115:1505–1508.
107. Von Euler, U.S. (1934): A depressor substance in seminal fluid. *J. Soc. Chem. Ind. (London)*, 52:1056–1057.
108. Wasserman, S.I., Soter, N.A., Center, D.M., and Austen, K.F. (1977). Cold urticaria recognition and characterization of a neutrophil chemotactic factor which appears in serum during experimental cold challenge. *J. Clin. Invest.*, 60:189–196.
109. Widemar, L., Bloom, G.D., Hellstrom, S., and Stenfors, L.-E. (1984): Mast cells in the pars flaccida of the tympanic membrane. *Acta Otolaryngol.* (Suppl.), 414:115–117.
110. Willer, P.F., Bach, D., and Austen, K.F. (1982): The human eosinophil lysophospholipase: the sole protein component of Charcot-Leydin crystals. *J. Immunol.*, 128:1346–1349.
111. Woodbury, R.G., and Neurath, H. (1978): Purification of an atypical mast cell protease and its level in developing rats. *Biochemistry*, 17:4298–4304.
112. Wright, D.G., and Gallin, J.I. (1977): A functional differentiation of human neutrophil granules: generation of C5a by a specific (secondary) granule product and inactivation of C5a by an azurophilic (primary) granule product. *J. Immunol.*, 119:1968–1976.
113. Yurt, R.W., and Austen, K.F. (1977): Preparative purification of the rat mast cell chymase. Characterization and interaction with granule components. *J. Exp. Med.*, 146:1405–1419.
114. Zeiger, R.S., Twarog, F.J., and Cotton, H.R. (1976): An inhibitor of histaminase release from human leukocytes. *J. Exp. Med.*, 144:1049–1061.

Immunology of the Ear, edited by J. Bernstein and P. Ogra. Raven Press, New York © 1987.

Immunobiology of Tympanoplasty

*Jan E. Veldman and **Wim Kuijpers

**Department of Otorhinolaryngology, University of Utrecht, 3500 CG Utrecht, The Netherlands; and **Department of Otorhinolaryngology, University of Nijmegen, 6525 EX Nijmegen, The Netherlands*

Although the fundamental techniques of modern reconstructive middle ear surgery in chronic suppurative otitis media began only 30 years ago (45,84,85), it has been recognized for many centuries that hearing impairment could be the result of a defective sound conducting system (5). Modern tympanoplasty procedures were introduced to restore hearing and promote healing after total excision of disease from the middle ear and mastoid. Prior to this pioneering work, ear surgery had been previously performed to eradicate chronic infection and cholesteatoma with the prevention of intracranial complications.

The tympanoplasty era in otological microsurgery resulted also in the use of a large variety of biological tissues for the reconstruction of the tympanic membrane and/or ossicular chain. New techniques with new grafts have been introduced over the past few decades. Within recent years, many of these techniques were followed by reports of disappointing long-term results.

In 1959, Betow (9) used an unpreserved allograft to repair a perforation and noted graft resorption and necrosis within a few weeks post-operatively. It was presumed that this graft necrosis was the result of an immunological rejection phenomenon. A high incidence of perforations in tympanic membrane allografts—even after storage at low temperature in antibiotic solutions—was later reported by others (18,66). However, preoperative tissue preservation by various fixatives or by lyophilization (*vide infra*) augmented the graft take rate considerably without these complications (37,43,65).

The improvement in short- and long-term results of allograft-tympanoplasty has been particularly attributed to refinements in surgical techniques and to the introduction of various methods of preoperative tissue preservation, although rejection of an allograft remains a source of surgical frustration. There is a scarcity of fundamental information in the otological data on the immunobiological behavior of the used materials.

Clinically, allograft-tympanoplasty has mainly been performed on a trial-and-error basis.

In this chapter, special emphasis will be given to the cellular biology and transplantation immunology of tympanoplasty, both in patients and in animal experimental models.

CELL BIOLOGY OF TYMPANOPLSTY

Leading otologists have come to realize that no single operation can be used for the surgical treatment of chronic suppurative otitis media. The two opposing demands of tympanoplasty, namely, radical and complete removal of disease on the one hand, and reconstruction of the sound-conducting system on the other hand, posed a major problem. A healthy, ventilated middle ear cavity covered with mucoperiosteum and an intact healthy tympanic membrane are of course the ideal starting positions for ossicular reconstruction. Through staged tympanoplasty, this may be obtained (4).

Myringoplasty

The first attempts to eliminate the injurious consequences of a persisting perforation of the tympanic membrane on hearing acuity date back to the seventeenth century (5). It was initially performed with the use of a prosthesis and afterward was done by etching the rims of the perforation with chemical caustics. Comprehensive reviews on this subject have been published by Schrimpf (58) and Storrs (70). With the introduction of tympanoplasty, external body skin was used for myringoplasty. However, its usefulness was questioned shortly thereafter, since inflammation and excessive desquamation frequently occurred. This was attributed to the change in environmental conditions. Nadel and Horvath (46) demonstrated that the temperature and humidity near the tympanic membrane were much higher than in the retroauricular region from which the grafts usually originate. The problems caused by the change in environmental conditions explain the far better results obtained with the deep part of the meatal skin (62). The discouraging experience with external body skin encouraged the search for new materials and a large variety of autogeneic grafts of mesodermal origin, such as fascia (23,67), vein (60), perichondrium (19), and fat (54). These are still successfully being used. Simultaneously, also allogeneic grafts, such as perichondrium (28), pericardium (47), dura (1), tympanic membranes (40), and even xenografts (29), were introduced. Presently, it can be concluded from numerous clinical studies that successful healing of a persistent perforation in the tympanic membrane can be achieved with a large variety of fresh autologous and preserved allogeneic grafts of mesodermal origin.

How does one explain the role of these largely differing grafts in the healing process? Traumatically induced perforations of the tympanic membrane can heal spontaneously, whereas perforations as the result of chronic suppurative otitis media usually do not. It can be assumed that a traumatically perforated tympanic membrane has a much better healing potential than the membrane in which a perforation persists after chronic middle ear disease. Support for this assumption can be derived from the fact that in the latter case the membrane, which is generally partly atrophic, poorly vascularized, and scarred, rarely heals completely after surgical or "chemical" removal of the scar tissue at the edges of the perforation. In this way, a nearly comparable situation may be assumed to be created as in the membrane with a fresh, traumatically produced perforation. The healing tendency is, however, completely different. Although small perforations sometimes close by this procedure, covering of the perforation with a graft has been proven necessary in order to obtain complete healing of larger perforations.

Clinical observations and experimental studies have augmented our insight into the role of these tissue grafts in such a healing process (41,53). The function of a graft can be assumed to be twofold. Firstly, it functions as a scaffold and a guide for the migrating epithelium from the residual part of the membrane (Fig. 1). Proof for this assumption can be derived from the observation that spontaneous healing of a traumatically induced subtotal perforation results in a nearly flat membrane without the natural conical form. However, when a tympanic membrane allograft is used, the newly formed membrane regains its natural shape. Secondly, the graft becomes infiltrated by mesenchymal cells and capillaries and a condensation of fibrous elements is formed immediately below the migrating epithelium and mucosa. Owing to the vascularization of the graft, the epithelium migrating along the grafts gets the opportunity to proliferate, as could be experimentally demonstrated through [^{3}H]thymidine labeling (53) (Fig. 2a). At this stage the bridging of the perforation is not dependent anymore on a cell migration from distant proliferative areas, as is the case when no graft is used. These cell proliferation centers are mainly concentrated in the highly vascularized regions on the tympanic membrane. The fibrous tissue growth into the graft contributes to the formation of a new lamina propria (Fig. 2b). In spontaneously healed (nongrafted) perforations, this middle layer is frequently absent. According to this mechanism, the successful healing obtained with fresh and preserved grafts from different origin can be explained.

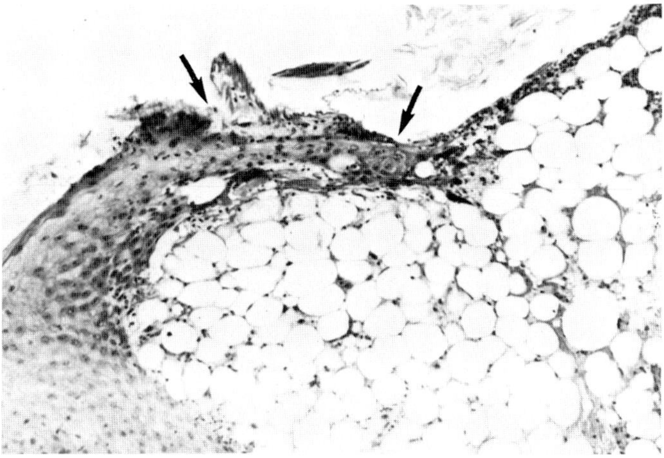

FIG. 1. Migration of a thin sheet of epithelium *(arrows)* along a fat graft, 7 days after a traumatically produced perforation in the cat (hematoxylin and eosin, ×150). (From ref. 53.)

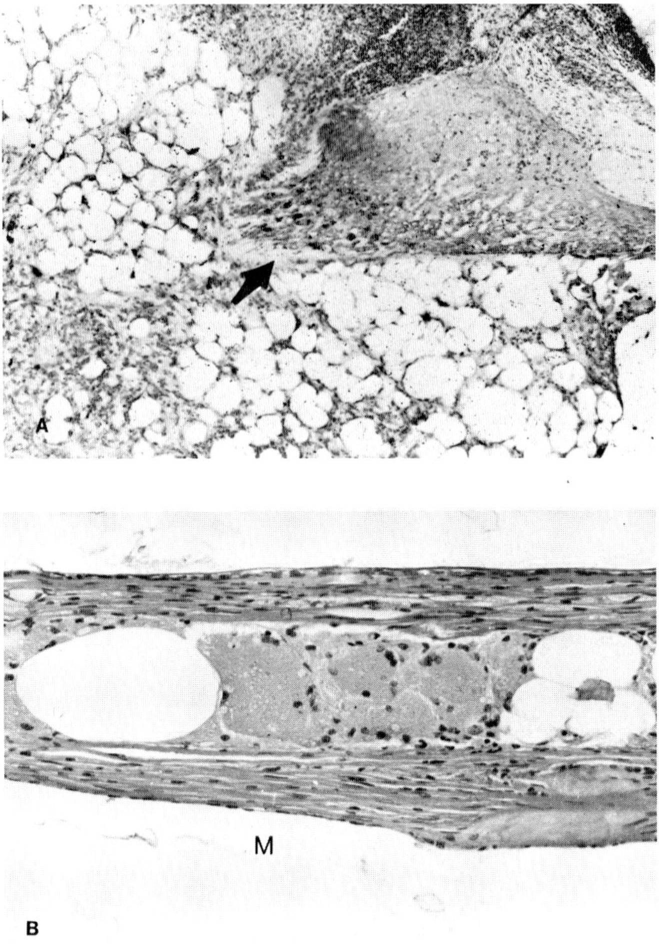

FIG. 2. Autoradiography of a traumatically induced perforation in the mouse tympanic membrane 7 days after myringoplasty with autologous fat. **(a)** [^{3}H]thymidine-labeled epithelial cells, migrating along the graft *(arrow)*. Note labeled fibroblasts in the graft itself (methylgreen-pyronine, ×130). **(b)** Five months after myringoplasty with fat graft in the cat. Note residual fat cells enclosed between subepithelial and submucosal connective tissue. (M) Middle ear space (hematoxylin and eosin, ×150). (From ref. 53.)

The vitality of the graft appears to be of no importance. Autolytic enzymes will be destroyed with some of the currently used preservation methods. Since any graft has to remain intact until the various tissue components of the original tympanic membrane have bridged the gap, preserved grafts can even be considered superior to fresh autografts, since autolysis resulting in graft perforation is more likely to occur. After healing, the membrane gradually grows thinner. Graft remnants may persist for years.

Ossiculoplasty

During the first decade of modern tympanoplasty, restoration of the damaged ossicular chain was mainly performed by alloplastic columellas made of polyethylene, stainless steel, or Teflon. However, many of these procedures soon were abandoned because of displacement or extrusion. In the early seventies, the development of porous implants, proplast, and plastipore led to the introduction of a new class of ossicular chain replacement prostheses (25,61). Since these materials allow the ingrowth of host tissue, they seem to cope well with the problems of displacement and extrusion. However, although the initial results were promising, long-term observations revealed an increasing number of failures (11,21,33,68). More recently, the use of a new family of alloplastic materials, the ceramics (aluminum oxide, glass ceramics, calcium phosphate ceramics) has been advocated for ossicular reconstruction (21). Although their biocompatibility is well established, their durability as ossicular replacement prostheses has yet to be proven.

Because of disappointing results with alloplastic grafts in the early sixties, many surgeons started to use biological grafts. These grafts included fresh autologous cortical bone chips, sculptured in different forms (87). This technique has never been generally accepted, presumably because of the possibility of bone resorption (8,50,52).

Far better results were obtained with fresh autologous tragal cartilage (27) and preserved allogeneic cartilage from the nasal septum (3). Although occasionally the replacement by fibrous tissue of these grafts has been observed, they appear not to be subject to extensive long-term resorption (7,32,71).

Transposition of the incus to renew contact between stapes head and malleus, when the long process of the incus was missing, was introduced by Zöllner (86) and Hall and Rytzner (22). Since then, the use of intact and remodeled ossicles has become very popular and is still considered as one of the most reliable methods for ossicular reconstruction. Histological studies of transposed autologous ossicles demonstrate that the gross structure of the grafts is retained, while a largely varying part consists of living bone (31,74) (Fig. 3a). These observations fit in with the data obtained from experimental studies. In a controlled study on the rat, it appeared that autografted incuses suffer a partial cell death during the first week. A few days after transplantation, bone remodeling was observed—especially marked in the outer part of the ossicle. This course of events was shown to be highly dependent on the time lag between removal and repositioning (Fig. 3b). Bone remodeling never resulted in complete remodeling of the incus. After 2 years, a major portion of the ossicle still consisted of dead bone.

The use of allogeneic ossicles was advocated by House et al. (26) for those cases where the incus was missing, or to avoid the risk of using diseased ossicles. Thereafter, the use of preserved allogeneic ossicles became very popular. The encouraging results obtained with preserved allogeneic tympanic membranes and ossicles resulted in the use of tympano-ossicular monoblock implants, being the ideal physiological reconstruction of the sound-conducting system (41,76). Different methods of preservation have been applied. Although all of these procedures have

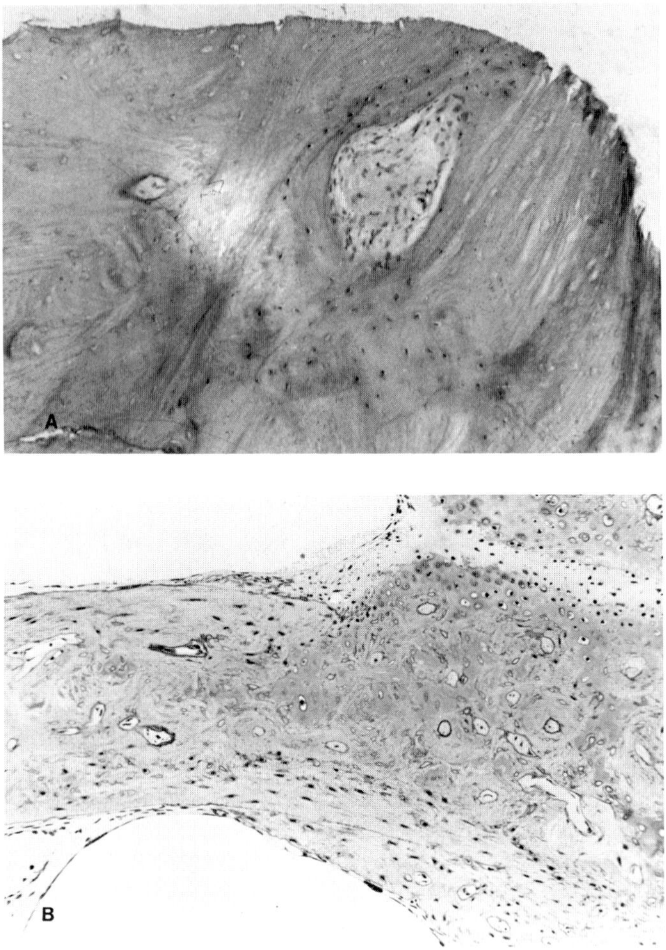

FIG. 3. **(a)** Sculptured autologous incus, removed 1 year after surgery. Human specimen. Note limited area of vital bone (hematoxylin and eosin, ×200). **(b)** Long process of incus (rat; autograft), 6 months after transplantation in the middle ear. Vital bone is confirmed to the outer side (toluidine blue, ×200).

in common that microorganisms are killed, they largely differ in their effects on the mechanical properties and the mode of preservation of the different tissue components of the grafts (35).

At the present time, one can conclude that there is no apparent difference in the functional results obtained between autologous and allogeneic ossicles.

Transplantation of preserved ossicles in experimental animals demonstrated that the reaction of the middle ear toward these grafts did not fundamentally differ from that of fresh autografts (Fig. 4a and b). Within 2 weeks the graft was covered by a mucoperiosteal lining, while small blood vessels were growing into the Haver-

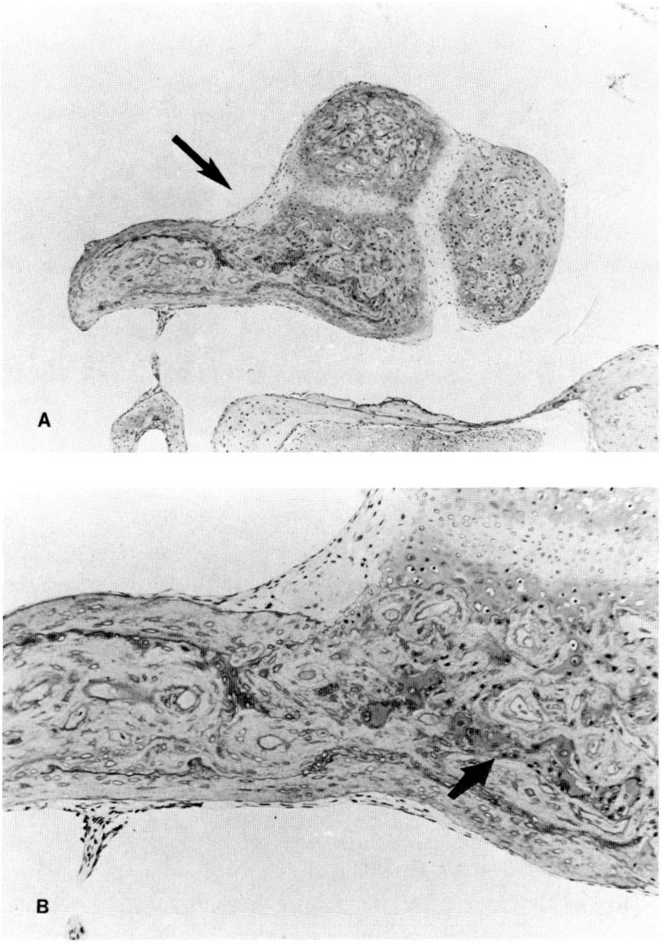

FIG. 4. **(a)** Allograft incus (rat) *(arrow),* formaldehyde preserved, 2 months after transplantation in the middle ear (toluidine blue, ×70). **(b)** Detail of incus allograft in (a). Normal mucoperiosteum layer, absence of new bone formation, and presence of formaldehyde-preserved osteocytes *(arrow)* (toluidine blue, ×200).

sian canals. After several months a limited amount of new bone was formed, especially in the central part of the ossicle, but the main part remained avital. Since the periosteal cells are killed by the preservation procedure and new bone formation depends on the mode of preservation (75), this bone formation is likely to be related to the integrity of the bone morphogenetic protein. This substance has been shown to stimulate undifferentiated cells into bone forming cells (73). No signs of resorption were observed in this experimental study, whose observation period lasted 2 years.

Specimens obtained from revision surgery revealed a large variation in microscopic structure. Among these are intact ossicles showing a varying degree of bone resorption, often without distinct signs of inflammation (35,59,72) (Fig. 5a). Although revitalization of the graft appears to occur, it is without any doubt that large parts of the ossicles remain avital, making its ultimate fate sometimes questionable (Fig. 5b).

From animal experiments it has been shown that preserved ossicles are subject to resorption after ectopic transplantation, whereas fresh autologous ossicles are not. Possibly the poor contact of the graft with host tissue in the middle ear together with the typical nature of the ossicular bone, lacking clear signs of remodeling in the adult state, might be presumed to favor the integrity of these grafts for a prolonged period of time.

IMMUNOBIOLOGY OF ALLOGRAFT-TYMPANOPLASTY

An intriguing observation in allograft-tympanoplasty is the apparent absence of a serious interference of the immunological reflex, although there is substantial evidence that the various tissue preservation methods do not destroy the antigenic properties of the grafts (16,81,83).

The complexity of transplantation immunology necessitates presentation of the following background information.

Histocomptibility Antigens and Transplantation

Many factors determine the immunogenicity of histocompatibility antigens and the ultimate fate of a tissue allograft. This includes the type of tissue transplanted and the method and the site of transplantation. Immunological rejection occurs as a consequence of incompatibility for antigens of the major histocompatibility complex. These antigens on the target organ are called *transplantation antigens,* which in humans are HLA (human leukocyte antigens) and ABO (blood group antigens). Both antigenic systems are present on all nucleated cells.

Two classes of HLA antigens are distinguished: Class I, consisting of HLA-A,B,C antigens present on all nucleated cell membranes; and Class II, consisting of HLA-D(R) antigens, present only on B cells, macrophages, and activated T cells. Prevention of the transplantation reaction can be directed on the induction phase, i.e., matching for HLA antigens, or blocking of the effector phase by medical treatment. What is the significance of such knowledge for allograft-tympanoplasty, since grafting is in a majority of cases quite successful? How can the absence of overt immune reactions to otologic grafts be explained?

Is it a lack of graft or an altered immunogenicity thereof, or do these tissues enjoy a prolonged or indefinite survival, because the middle ear complex is a site of immunological privilege? Over the years, attempts both in experimental and

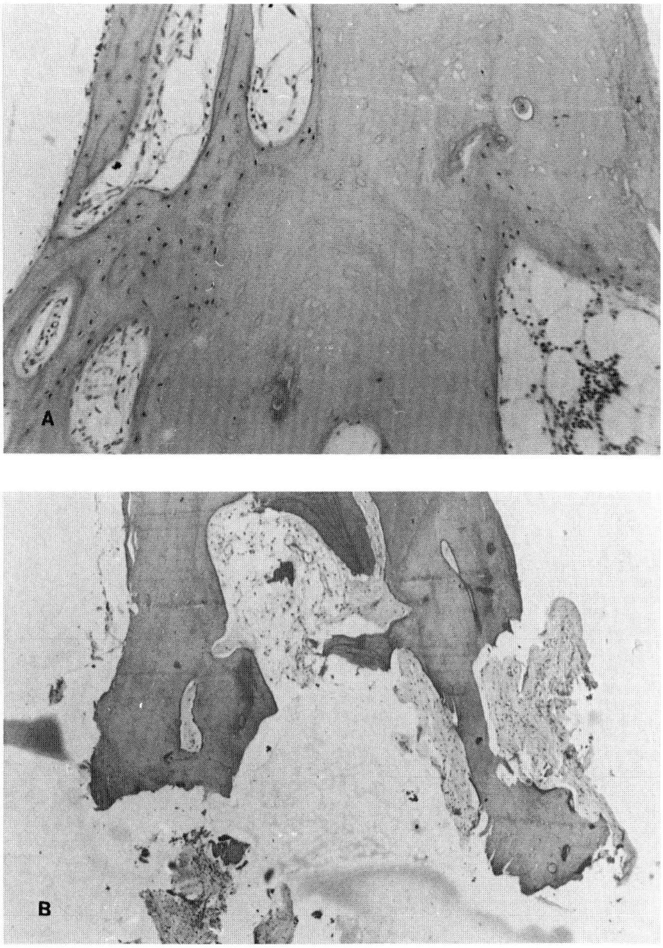

FIG. 5. Cialit-preserved allograft incus, removed 1 year after transplantation during revision surgery. Human specimen. **(a)** Partial revitalization and large marrow spaces (hematoxylin and eosin, ×200). **(b)** Extensive areas of avital bone and bone resorption (hematoxylin and eosin, ×150).

clinical otological transplantation research have been made to answer some of these questions.

In general, an extremely efficient and very well developed protective immune system recognizes the allograft and mobilizes its cellular defenses to destroy the invader. The diversity of antigenicity within a species is remarkable. To most surgeons involved in transplantation these histocompatibility antigens are a source of great frustration. The otologist appears to be an exception.

Lymphocytes, Lymphoid Cell Traffic, and Immune Responses

Cells, rather than humoral antibodies, are necessary for a primary allograft reaction under normal conditions. Allografts enclosed within millipore chambers will not be rejected as long as the pores are not large enough to allow host cells to reach the graft (2). Mitchison (44) had already provided evidence earlier that transplantation immunity could be transferred with cells rather than serum. Billingham et al. (10) demonstrated that the best adoptive transfer could be obtained with lymph nodes draining the graft directly. Histological analyses of these nodes revealed strong immunoblast reactions of T and B cells (78,79,82).

During the past two decades the morphology of lymphoid tissue has been clarified in terms of population dynamics and migration streams. It has been generally recognized that the lymphocyte population of peripheral lymphoid tissue is not static, but instead is one that is continuously exchanged. Mature cells within the lymphoid system have, in addition, the capacity to arrange themselves in clear-cut microenvironments of peripheral lymphoid organs (48,82).

The existence of a pool of recirculating lymphocytes has been definitely demonstrated by Gowans (20). This basic observation was confirmed by the marked decrease of lymphocyte output by the cannulated thoracic duct in rats after a few days of drainage. The collected lymph was returned without cells, and its restoration to normal values was observed when the cells were reinjected intravenously.

Imunologically, elimination of the T-cell population has been found to result in long-lasting immunological unresponsiveness regarding transplantation immunity.

Immune reactions in lymphoid tissue are considered to comprise three antigen-induced processes: the plasma cell reactions representing antibody formation, cellular immunity reactions leading to cell-mediated immunity (as the allograft reaction), and the germinal center reaction. This latter process has been shown to be a source of "memory cells," i.e., the plasma cell precursors of secondary response antibody formation, as well as a site of generation and amplification of antibody-forming cell precursors in general (49). Their ultimate bone marrow origin is established beyond doubt.

These immune reactions occur, in general, simultaneously following the majority of antigenic stimuli. The bias of the response may be toward the cellular or humoral side, depending on the type of antigenic stimulus. Foreign proteins may elicit heavy cellular as well as humoral immunity reactions. The same holds for vital tissue grafts, although the rejection of an allograft is particularly a consequence of the cellular immunity component. Whereas memory cells recirculate after a first challenge, these reactions accelerate even after a second challenge with the same antigen (secondary response or second set—transplantation—reaction). Extensive structural analyses of plasma cell and cellular immunity reactions as well as immunohistophysiological research of the population dynamics of T and B cells have demonstrated that the site of initiation of these complex immunoblast reactions is topographically restricted in the microarchitecture of peripheral lymphoid tissue (78–80).

Histological analyses of lymph nodes, draining the site of tissue grafting, reveal strong immunoblast reactions in two distinct areas of the regional lymph node: a cellular immune response with a progeny of small lymphoid cells in the paracortical area as well as a humoral immune response, initiated in the outer cortex. These immune responses are followed in approximately 4 days after antigen administration by a germinal center reaction. The lymphoid end cells of the cellular immunity reactions are primarily responsible for specificity when dealing with a transplantation response.

This basic knowledge of lymph node histophysiology has now been used in various experiments to analyze the antigenicity of an otologic allograft (see next section).

IMMUNE RESPONSES IN ALLOGRAFT-TYMPANOPLASTY

The reported success rate in tympanoplasty with preserved allogeneic tympanic membranes and tympano-ossicular block grafts (9,38,42,64) compares favorably with the good results of viable corneal transplants in keratoplasty. These two areas of allograft surgery make it almost unique in the field of clinical tissue and organ transplantation. However, by analogy to keratoplasty in ophthalmology, tympanic membrane graft failures also do occur. When failure occurs in allograft-tympanoplasty, it is particularly attributed to deficits in operative techniques, secondary infection, or a recurrence of middle ear disease. Important imunobiological factors leading to graft failure have usually not been taken into account. In order to explain the apparent inability of a recipient to recognize the presence of an allogeneic preserved tympanic or tympano-ossicular block graft, the idea has been suggested that the middle ear is a privileged site. Furthermore, it has been suggested by various authors that tissue antigens are not expressed anymore or are at least extremely diminished after preservation (17,41).

The concurrence of several of the above factors leads either to success or to failure.

Animal Models

Tissue grafts have been repeatedly transplanted to a variety of anatomically unnatural sites of genetically incompatible recipients. The longevity enjoyed by allografts in some of these sites have given rise to the concept that some of these sites may be "immunologically privileged," or favored in the sense that grafts transplanted to them are in some way partially or fully exempted from the normal rigors imposed by their histocompatibility status. It has also been found, often empirically, that a few tissues survive transplantation to allogeneic hosts under conditions in which grafts of nearly all other tissues of similar genetic makeup would suffer prompt rejection: immunologically privileged tissues. Cartilage, for instance, is considered to be a privileged tissue (6).

There is little clinical or experimental evidence to assume that the middle ear, mastoid cavity, and/or external ear canal belong to this first category. The privileged status of cartilage is ascribed to quarantining properties of its matrix, which is thought to have a capacity comparable to that of a cell-impermeable millipore membrane (24). Chondrocytes isolated from cartilage are immunogenic and display normal susceptibility to transplantation immunity. The conjecture that tympanic membrane, external ear skin—even de-epithelialized—or ossicles, after various preservation procedures, would belong to this category of privileged tissue as an explanation for successful allograft-tympanoplasty is not valid. Experimental analyses of the immunogenicity of these grafts clearly demonstrate that at least a part of the original histocompatible antigens remain after using the currently applied preservatives (15,16,83). Reconsidering the existence of an afferent and efferent loop of the immune response in the middle ear complex, the following experimental data are strong arguments against the middle ear being a privileged site. In rats, vital xenogenous incuses, transplanted into the middle ear, are rejected during a primary response (35). Although allogeneic incuses are accepted for observation periods for up to 2 years, they are definitely rejected within 2 to 3 weeks during a secondary immune response, i.e., when the recipients have been presensitized for donor alloantigens (30,83).

The presence of an afferent loop of cellular immune reactivity in the middle ear has further been confirmed in an experimental model, employing a contact sensitizer (oxazolone). Excellent delayed-type reactions could be elicited in the abdominal skin of guinea pigs and rabbits after prior application of this chemical sensitizer to the middle ear mucosal lining (81). The presence of a normal immunological (transplantation) reflex in the middle ear has recently further been confirmed by Frootko et al. (14) and Ryan et al. (56). Both histologically and immunologically there is no doubt that an intact immune mechanism exists in the middle ear complex.

In rats and rabbits, allogeneic tympanic membrane grafts—both fresh and preserved—can elicit a strong cellular and humoral immune response, when implanted ectopically. Histologically, draining lymph nodes showed, in a time sequence study, immunoblast reactions in both the outer cortex (B-cell response) and the paracortical area (T-cell response) (83). These reactions were even more vigorous in second set experiments, when ectopic graft implantation was preceded by a split skin graft of the same antigenic makeup. Since skin and otological (tympanic membrane or incus) grafts were derived from the same donor animal, such strong B- and T-cell reactions during second set responses indicate that tissue preservation keeps part of the original tissue histocompatibility antigens intact. Control studies with fresh or preserved autologous grafts failed to elicit any immunological reaction in draining lymph nodes. Orthotopical transplantation of both fresh and preserved allografts showed hardly any immunological reaction during the first set of transplantation experiments, but showed clear graft rejection (accumulation of mononuclear cells, scattered plasma cells, and graft resorption) during the second set (83). Although it is impossible to quantitate the provoked reactions, the impression gained from these histological studies was that the immunoblast reaction toward fresh and formaldehyde-preserved grafts was more vigorous than toward alcohol and Cialit-preserved tissue. However, histological studies of preserved allogeneic tympano-ossicular grafts obtained both after revision surgery and after animal experiments seem to favor the concept that no immunological interference occurs.

Based on these observations, it has been suggested that the recipient is either unable to recognize the donor antigens or that the tissue antigens are no longer expressed by the preservation procedures (17,41). The apparent inability of the middle ear to respond in an appropriate manner to foreign tissue antigens might be supported by the observation that fresh allogeneic ossicles, transplanted in the middle ear of the rat, are tolerated for observation periods of more than 2 years without clear signs of graft rejection (Fig. 6a and b), whereas ectopical transplan-

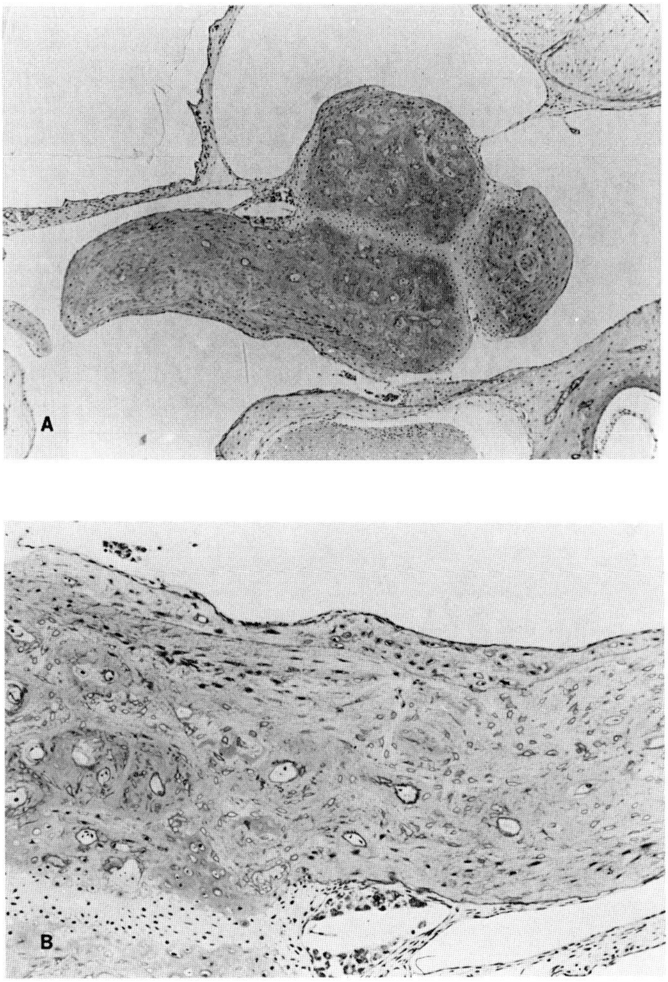

FIG. 6. (a) Allograft incus (rat), nonpreserved, 5 months after transplantation in the middle ear (toluidine blue, ×70). **(b)** Detail of (a): Incus is covered with normal mucoperiosteum. Avital bone. Local bone neogenesis at the outer sites (toluidine blue, ×200).

tation evoked a vigorous transplantation reaction (34). The heavy monocellular reaction elicited by an orthotopically transplanted xenograft incus suggests again the presence of an appropriate functioning immune system in the middle ear (35). This has been further substantiated by experiments in which a contact sensitizer, allogenic lymphocytes, and allogeneic skin grafts, when brought into the middle ear, resulted in a distinct immunization (15,55,69,81). Also, the assumption that the tissue antigens are no longer expressed by the preservation procedures is not a valid explanation for the virtual absence of immunological interference in allograft tympanoplasty.

As stated above, preserved tympano-ossicular grafts failed to show any sign of graft rejection after orthotopical transplantation in experimental animals. However, the persistence of tissue antigens after storage in alcohol, formaldehyde, or Cialit was unequivocally demonstrated by means of ectopical transplantation in the leg muscle, where a heavy monocellular reaction and graft resorption were observed (Fig. 7) (35,75). Comparable observations have been reported by Kastenbauer and Hochstrasser (30).

HLA and Human Otological Grafts

Using monoclonal antibodies to various HLA antigens, Frootko (16) recently investigated the effects of various preservatives (Table 1) on the original Class I and II transplantation antigen makeup in tympanomeatal and dura mater allografts. Unpreserved and freeze-dried tympanomeatal and dura mater grafts were found to express both classes of tissue antigens. In both types of graft transplantation, anti-

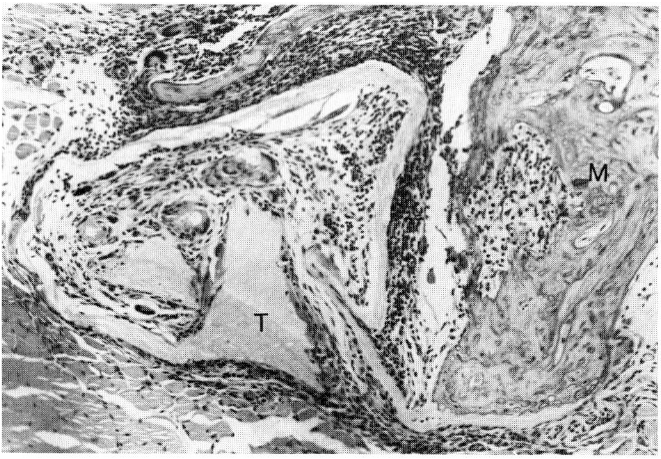

FIG. 7. Formaldehyde-preserved tympano (T)-malleolar (M) allograft (rat), 2 months after ectopical transplantation in the leg muscle. Bone resorption and mononuclear cell infiltrate (hematoxylin and eosin, ×130).

TABLE 1. *Preservation techniques for otologic allografts*

1. Ethyl alcohol (70%)
2. Aqueous Cialit (0.02%), i.e., sodium 2-ethylmercurothiobenz oxazole-5-carboxylate
3. Buffered formaldehyde fixation (4%) and buffered formaldehyde preservation (0.5%)
4. Buffered formaldehyde fixation (4%) and aqueous Cialit preservation (0.05%)
5. Buffered glutaraldehyde fixation (0.5%) and aqueous Cialit preservation (0.02%)
6. Lyophilization and γ-sterilization or ethylene oxide gas sterilization

gens were partially destroyed (or modified?) after Cialit preservation. Using the other preservation methods, HLA antigens were not demonstrable anymore.

In a prospective clinical trial with eight patients, tympano-ossicular monoblock grafts or tympanic membrane allografts (formaldehyde/Cialit-preserved) of unknown HLA composition were transplanted. Antileukocyte (cytotoxic and agglutinating) antibodies were then determined prior to surgery and 3 to 6 months after surgery in the eight different recipients (Table 2).

Immunofluorescence studies of the tympanic membranes of patients A and H (graft "rejected" ?) failed to show cytoplasmic fluorescence for any of the immunoglobulin classes. Hardly any B cells could be found by immunohistochemical methods; however, T cells, identified by a membrane fluorescence technique with a specific human T-lymphocyte antiserum were present throughout the graft, suggesting that immunologically a rejection process could have been responsible for the poor clinical results. Antileukocyte antibody titers were negative in all eight recipients (36).

In a series of 40 allogeneic dura mater myringoplasties, Frootko (16) determined the donor-specific lymphocytotoxic antibody response in these patients. Only five of his patients developed *de novo* these antibodies 2 to 4 weeks after tissue grafting. Prior to surgery they tested negatively. The preservation technique used (see

TABLE 2. *Antibody formation after allograft-tympanoplasty*

Patient	Sex	Age (years)	Tympanoplasty	Result[a]	AB[b] a	AB[b] b
A	M	32	TMO	Rejected[c]	–	–
B	F	56	TM (2x)	Intact	–	–
C	M	56	TMO	Intact	–	–
D	F	34	TMO	Intact	–	–
E	M	21	TMO	Intact	–	–
F	F	44	TMO	Perforation	–	–
G	M	51	TMO	Intact	–	–
H	F	23	TMO	Rejected[c]	–	–

[a]Short-term results (after 6–12 months).
[b]AB a,b, antileukocyte antibody titer prior to (a) and 3–6 months after (b) transplantation; TMO, tympano-ossicular block; TM, tympanic membrane.
[c]Histopathology and tissue immunofluorescence of TM performed.

Table 1) made no difference with regard to the clinical behavior of the grafts (15% perforated between the 3rd and 11th postoperative week) or with regard to the development of postgraft antibodies. In this patient group, 85% of subtotal perforations were successfully repaired, although graft and recipient were certainly mismatched for Class I and II antigens.

Similar conclusions in another series of 10 patients were noted in the laboratory of the authors in patients receiving lyophilized-tissue-typed dura mater allografts. Donor and recipient were HLA mismatched by purpose. Specific anti-HLA antibodies toward the donor Class I and II antigens could not be detected in any of these patients, neither prior to, nor 1 to 3 months after, surgery. Tissue typing and serological data are given in Table 3; surgical procedures and anatomical results are listed in Table 4.

IMMUNOPATHOLOGY OF HUMAN MIDDLE EAR IMPLANTS

Although the cause of failure in tympanoplasty with preserved allogeneic tympano-ossicular grafts is not very well documented, histopathological studies of

TABLE 3. *Transplantation immunology: Dura-tissue typed*[a,b]

Name	Recipient	HLA-AB[c] 0	1	3	Donor	Comment
J.P.	A1,A9,B8,B37,DR3	–	–	–	81030	—
A.K.	A3,A29,B12,B40, CW3,DRW6,DR7	–	–	–	81085	—
A.de Gr.	A2,B15,B40,CW3, DRW6,DR7	–	–	–	81030	—
A.v.d.Z.	A1,AW30,B13,B40, CW3,DRW6,DRW10	–	–	–	81085	—
C.B.	A2,A3,B7,BW16, DR2,DRW8	+(1/30)		–	81030	A9,B15,CW3,DR4, DRW6
S.C.	A1,A9,B8,B15,DR1, DR5	–	–	–	81085	—
F.B.	A1,A28,B8,BW22, DR1,DR5	+(1/30)	+(2/30)	nd	81085	A29,B12,B7
G.N.	A2,B13,BW22,CW3, DR2,DR7	–	–	+(1/30)	81030	A11,BW35,BW21
H.de Gr.	A1,A2,B15,B17, CW3,DRW6,DR7	–	–	–	81041[d]	—
R.P.W.	A2,AW30,B7,B12, CW5,DR2,DR7	–	–	–	81085	—

[a]Adapted from ref. 13.
[b]Donor code 81030—A1,A3,B8,B17,BW4,BW6,DR3,DR7; Donor code 81085—A1,B12,BW14,BW6,BW40,CW3.
[c](HLA-AB) HLA antibodies prior to 0, 1, and 3 months after tympanoplasty, as tested with *30 typed donors;* (nd) no data.
[d]Donor code 81041—tissue typing unsuccessful.

TABLE 4. *Tympanoplasty: Dura-tissue typed*[a]

Name	Date of birth	Date of surgery	Type of surgery	Dura[b]	Result[c]
J.P.	01-03-1932	16-11-1981	Mod. Rad.[d]	81030	+ +
A.K.	27-08-1924	23-11-1981	Mod. Rad.	81085	+ +
A.de Gr.	05-07-1955	10-02-1982	Mod. Rad.	81030	+ +
A.v.d.Z.	09-09-1962	17-02-1982	Mod. Rad.	81085	+ +
C.B.	13-12-1922	19-02-1982	Myringoplasty	81030	+
S.C.	27-01-1960	10-03-1982	Mod. Rad.	81085	+ +
F.B.	16-09-1957	07-04-1982	Myringoplasty	81085	−
G.N.	21-07-1930	14-04-1982	Myringoplasty	81030	+ +
H.de Gr.	08-03-1925	24-05-1982	Myringoplasty	81042	+ +
R.P.W.	13-03-1962	18-06-1982	CAT	81085	+ +

[a]Adapted from ref. 13.
[b]For donor code's tissue see Table 3.
[c]At 12 months or more after surgery.
[d]Mod. Rad., modified radical: mastoid cavity covered with dura; tympanic membrane reconstructed with dura.

some failed preserved grafts unmistakably reveal signs of a transplantation reaction. The postoperative course of the patients from whom these grafts were obtained culminated in a nonspecific myringitis, starting between 2 and 12 months after surgery. The tympanic membranes were hyperemic, thickened, and often slightly moist. The inflammation did not respond well to treatment with antibiotics. Histological examination of the tympanic membrane revealed hyperplastic epithelium, occasionally with local discontinuities and roots of epithelial cells penetrating into the lamina propria (Fig. 8a). The largely thickened lamina propria was composed of connective tissue of varying density with many small vessels, capillaries, and scattered plasma cells. Accumulations of small lymphocytes were found perivascularly and in the neighborhood of graft remnants (36,83) (Fig. 8b). The vessels often appeared to be obliterated. In some of the removed monoblock implants, the ossicular part of the implant showed a fibrous encapsulation with perivascular accumulations of small lymphocytes (Fig. 9a and b). The major part of the bone appeared to be avital, with a varying degree of bone resorption.

Further evidence for the existence of an allograft rejection could be obtained through immunofluorescence studies of two tympanic membranes removed during revision surgery (cf. Table 2 and Fig. 9a and b).

PROCUREMENT, TISSUE PRESERVATION, AND OTOLOGICAL TISSUE BANKS

Allograft-tympanoplasty has to be preceded by procurement of the otological graft. Temporal bone cores are removed from the refrigerated cadaver within 24 hr after death. Only temporal bones uninvolved with neoplasms or infection are selected. Temporal bone cores or ossicles are removed from the cadaver under clean, aseptic conditions. Cores can be stored, prior to dissection, at 4°C in the

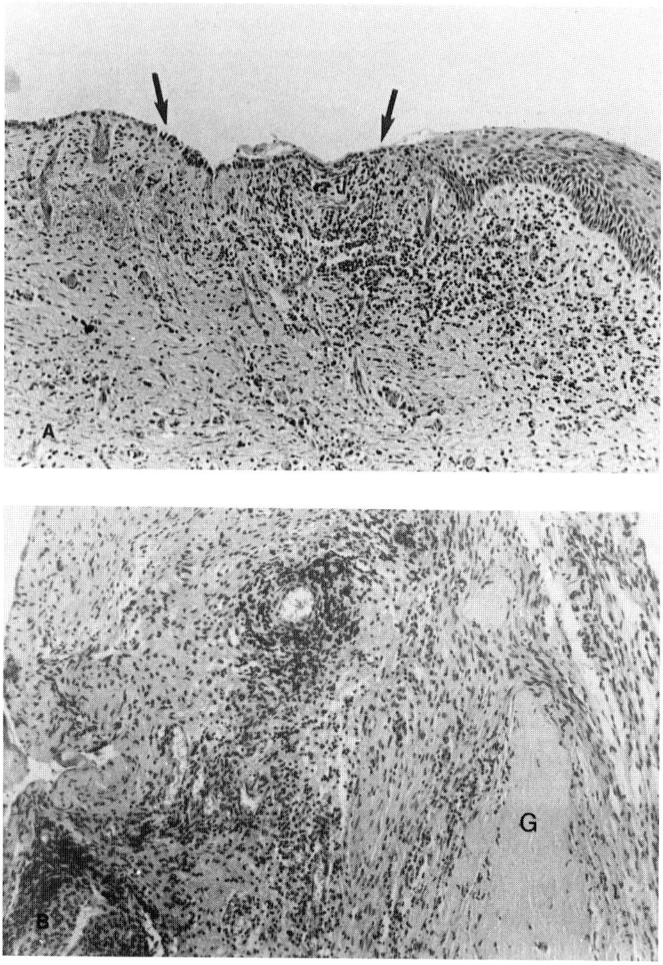

FIG. 8. Cialit-preserved tympanic membrane allograft, removed 1 year after transplantation because of persistent myringitis. Human specimen. **(a)** Hyperplastic epithelium with local interruptions *(arrows)* (hematoxylin and eosin, ×70). **(b)** Lamina propria thickened with mononuclear cell infiltrate. (G) Graft remnant (hematoxylin and eosin, ×150).

refrigerator. After dissection, tissue processing is performed. The preservations and sterilization methods currently used for otological grafts are indicated in Table 1. The more practical problem of procurement and providing otological allografts led to the organization of Ear Tissue Banks and the establishment of a distribution system (regional or national). Smith (63), at the Northern California Transplant Bank, was one of the first to form a practical banking organization. Similar ear tissue banks were later developed in various countries. For medicolegal reasons many of them are only functioning for internal use.

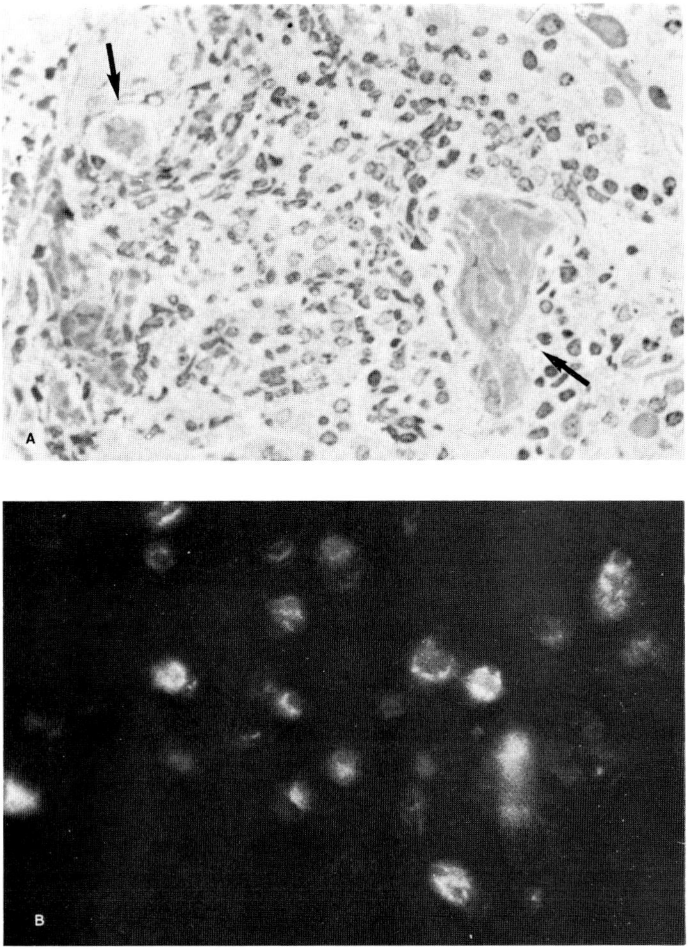

FIG. 9. Cialit-preserved human tympanic membrane allograft, removed ±5 months after transplantation because of persistent myringitis. **(a)** Note perivascular mononuclear cell infiltrate in lamina propria *(arrows)* (basic fuchsin-methylene blue, ×600). (From ref. 83.) **(b)** Same specimen of "rejected" allograft. T-cell membrane fluorescence (×1,500). (From ref. 83.)

DISCUSSION AND CONSIDERATIONS

Successful reconstruction of the sound-transformer mechanism can be achieved with the use of various fresh and preserved biological materials. This approach seems superior to the use of all kinds of alloplasts. In myringoplasty the grafted tissues contribute in various ways to the healing process. First, the graft functions as a scaffold for the various tissue components, which start to proliferate from the residual part of the tympanic membrane. Second, the graft, becoming vascularized and infiltrated by mesenchymal cells, offers the epithelium migrating along the graft the opportunity to proliferate. Furthermore, the mesenchymal cells contribute to the formation of a new middle layer. An important requirement of the grafted tissues is to keep the perforation closed until the proliferating tissues have bridged the gap. The healing process appears not to be dependent on the vitality of the graft.

In ossicular reconstruction the ossicular and cartilaginous grafts function initially as an avital sound conducting system. Subsequently the ossicles may become revitalized to a varying extent, although the histological evidence exists that the major part of the ossicle(s) is still avital after many years. Apart from the incidentally observed resorption in a small percentage of the recovered ossicles, it can be stated that the middle ear reacts in a different way to avital ossicular grafts than other parts of the body do. However, this process may only be retarded. The balance between tissue resorption and possible further revitalization of the grafts will ultimately determine the fate of this borrowed sound conducting system.

Our understanding of the role of immunity in middle ear disease is hampered by a paucity of information concerning immune responses at this site. Information on the immunological status of allografts in the middle ear has been only fragmentary. Immune responses are considered to be an important factor in the pathogenesis of otitis media with effusion (39), tympanosclerosis (56,57), and successful allograft-tympanoplasty (81). In the human the lymphatics of the middle ear have never been clearly demonstrated. Lymphoid cell traffic rules regarding the middle ear mucosa under various pathological conditions are still unknown. In various experimental immunology models it could, however, be proven that the middle ear of guinea pigs, rats, and rabbits has both an afferent and efferent limb of the humoral and cellular immune response (16,55,69,74,76,81,87). By extrapolation, one may assume that the human situation is identical.

The presented controlled animal experiments and clinical pathology data of graft failures make the assumption that there is a lack of proven antigenicity of preserved otological grafts (13,16,83). Poliquin's data (51) on the antigenicity of guinea pig unpreserved tympanic membrane confirm our experimental immunological observations with vital and preserved otological grafts. The currently used preservatives of allografts (formaldehyde, alcohol, or Cialit) do not destroy the tissue histocompatibility antigens, although they might affect the concentration and antigen type. Persistence of the original histocompatibility antigens after tissue preservation—also when Cialit was used—could be proven in our second set of transplantation experiments. Sensitization through prior skin grafting results in a pool of recirculating B and T lymphocytes with a specific immunological memory for the tissue antigens of that species. Triggering these memory cells of the circulation through local lymph node X-irradiation results in two accomplishments: immunological background activity in that node dies out and "virgin" memory cells (B and T) repopulate that node (Figs. 10 and 11). If a preserved allograft from the same donor as the skin allograft is implanted in a vascular bed draining a regional lymph node, a vigorous immune response (plasma-cell, cellular-immunity, and

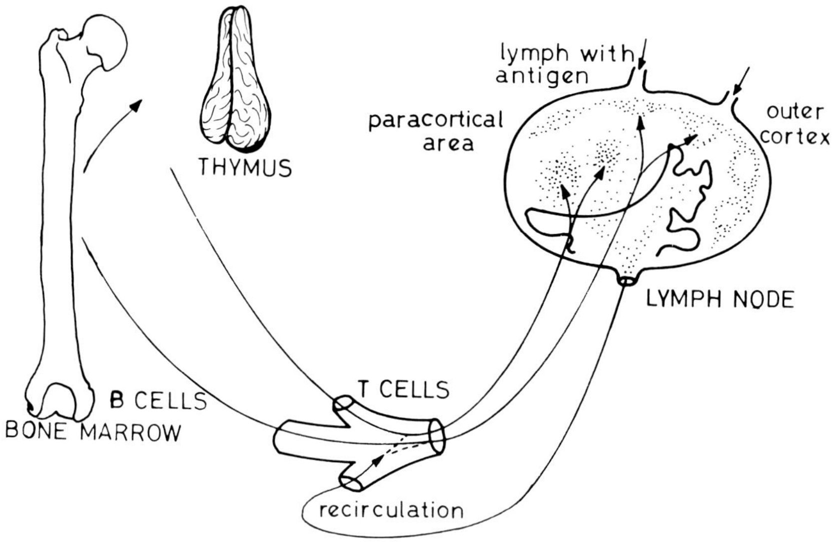

FIG. 10. Recirculation pathway of B and T lymphocytes toward lymph node. Note influx areas *(arrows)* after local lymph-node X-irradiation.

germinal-center reactions) is elicited. The only explanation for this observation is that a considerable amount of the original tissue histocompatibility antigens are still present in the allograft after preservation. This occurs after any of the preservatives are used (83).

These experimental data seem to be in conflict with Frootko's observations (16) using anti-HLA monoclonal antibodies. However, preservation, or rather tissue fixation, probably prevents further detection of HLA antigens with this technique because of membrane receptor modification.

The immunological reflex functions adequately in the middle ear compartment. Thus there is at this stage no solid argument for the concept of a privileged site in the middle ear.

Apart from elimination of any foreign agent through an immune response, we know now a variety of mechanisms whereby exposure of lymphocytes to antigen can produce a state of specifically diminished responsiveness. According to Burnet's clonal selection theory (12), natural tolerance to an autoantigen is a result of elimination of lymphoid cell clones that recognize "self." Tolerance to these "self" tissue components is generally considered to be the result of clonal elimination of both T and B lymphocytes. When dealing with low antigen concentrations, this immunotolerance is usually believed to be the result of T-cell tolerance. B-cell reactivity in terms of production of blocking antibodies might also play an active role in this tolerance phenomenon. To induce a state of immunological unresponsiveness, the following mechanisms are thought to operate: (a) clone inactivation or elimination induced by appropriate antigen administration; (b) active sup-

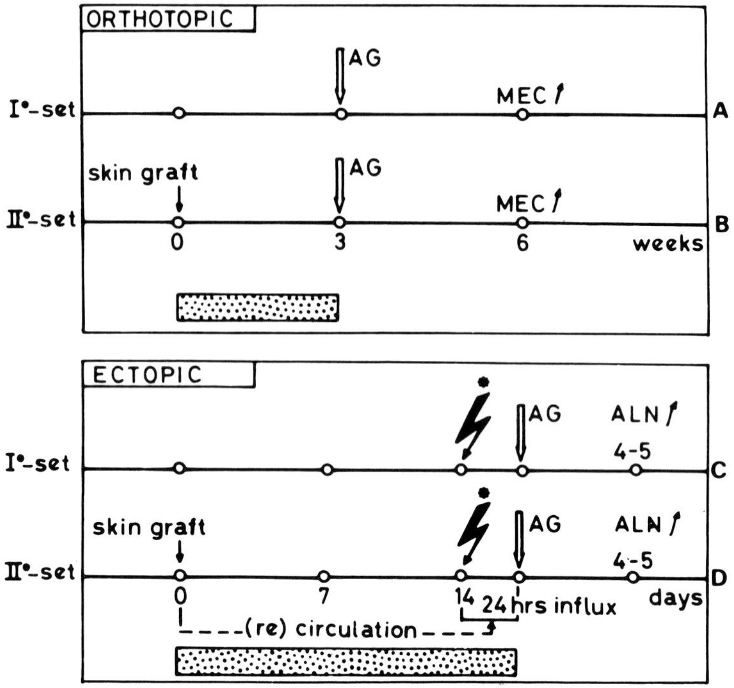

FIG. 11. Experimental design of allograft immunogenicity analyses in animal models (rats and rabbits). (AG) Allografts, i.e., tympanic membrane, external ear canal skin, or incus; (MEC) middle ear compartment; (ALN) axillary lymph node; *(zigzagged arrow)* local lymph node X-irradiation (750 rads); *(dotted areas)* sensitization period. *(Asterisks above zigzagged arrows)* rabbits only; *(diagonal arrows)* specimen removed for histology. (From ref. 83.)

pression by B or T lymphocytes; and (c) blockade by an antibody, an antigen, or a hapten. One may wonder whether these experimentally known circumstances that facilitate the induction of a state of immunotolerance do also operate in clinical allograft-tympanoplasty. No evidence militates against such an extrapolation. It would be a solid explanation for success in middle ear transplantation. Furthermore, there are different situations that have been experimentally applied to induce tolerance and determine the form of antigen and the rate and route of administration. Immunization with killed cells instead of intact cells for instance, which is also done in tissue preservation or lyophilization, favors enhancement over graft rejection. A combination of altering and diminishing antigenicity through preservation of the allograft, as well as its low antigenicity and the particular site of implantation, may favor a situation that is responsible for tolerance induction in allograft-tympanoplasty.

The fact that after several months a primarily successful grafting finally ends up in a graft failure is not in direct conflict with this concept of tolerogenesis in otologic tissue grafting. A delayed rejection phenomenon is a well-known occurrence in clinical and experimental transplantations. It is often thought to be the consequence of an assumed breakthrough in tolerance. Why this occurs in certain cases is virtually unknown. It is also unpredictable as to when it will occur; this will continue to be the situation as long as no surveillance better than clinical judgment after surgery is available.

The apparent absence of an overt immune response to preserved allogeneic grafts used for middle ear reconstructions is unrivaled in all other fields of clinical transplantation. It remains surprising that the success of most allograft-tympanoplasties is achieved on a surgeon's trial-and-error basis and in the presence of a great deal of ignorance about immune reactivity.

Natural materials remain to be better tolerated in the middle ear than any alloplast, as judged in longer follow-up studies (68). Whether the continuous search for improved alloplastic material and microsurgical methods will finally add to further progress in reconstruction of the sound transformer mechanism remains to be determined.

REFERENCES

1. Albrite, J.P., and Leigh, B.G. (1966): Dural homograft myringoplasty. *Laryngoscope,* 76:1687.
2. Algire, G.H., Weaver, J.H., and Prehn, R.T. (1957): Studies on tissue homotransplantation in mice, using diffusion chamber methods. *Ann. NY Acad. Sci.,* 64:1009.
3. Altenau, M.M., and Sheehy, J.L. (1978): Tympanoplasty: cartilage prostheses—a report of 564 cases. *Laryngoscope,* 88:895–904.
4. Austin, D.F. (1969): Types and indications of staging. *Arch. Otolaryngol.,* 89:235–242.
5. Banzer, M. (1640): Disputatio de auditione laesa. Cited by Schuknecht, H.F., and Dunlap, A.M. (1947). *Laryngoscope,* 57:479.
6. Barker, C.F., and Billingham, R.E. (1973): Immunologically privileged sites and tissues. In: *Corneal Graft Failures,* Ciba Foundation Symposium No. 15, pp. 79–104. Excerpta Medica–North Holland, Amsterdam/New York.
7. Belal, A., Linthicum, F.H., and Odnert, S. (1981): Fate of cartilage autografts for ossiculoplasty, an electron-microscopic study. *Clin. Otolaryngol.,* 6:231.
8. Berkovits, R.N.P., Kruithof, C., Bos, C.E., and van der Berg, J. (1978): Reconstruction of the ossicular chain with an autologous bone cylinder, produced with a hollow drill. *J. Laryngol. Otol.,* 92:969–978.
9. Betow, C. (1982): Twenty years of experience with homografts in ear surgery. *J. Laryngol. Otol.* (Suppl. 5).
10. Billingham, R.E., Brent, L., and Medawar, P.B. (1954): Quantative studies on tissue transplantation immunity. II. The origin, strength and duration of actively and adoptively acquired immunity. *Proc. R. Soc. Lond. (Biol.),* 143:58–80.
11. Brackmann, D.E., and Sheehy, J.L. (1979): Tympanoplasty: TORP's and PORP's. *Laryngoscope,* 89:108.
12. Burnet, F.M. (1959): *The Clonal Selection Theory of Acquired Immunity.* Cambridge University Press, Cambridge.
13. De Gast, G.C., and Veldman, J.E. (1985): Human histocompatibility antigens and transplantation in otology. In: *Immunobiology, Autoimmunity and Transplantation in Otorhinolaryngology,* edited by J.E. Veldman, B.F. McCabe, E.H. Huizing, and N. Mygind, pp. 161–163. Kugler Publications, Amsterdam/Berkeley.
14. Frootko, N.J., Ting, A., and Fabre, J.W. (1982): Allograft dura mater myringoplasty (abstract). *Clin. Otolaryngol.,* 2:134.
15. Frootko, N. (1984): Allograft rejection in the middle ear of the rat. MSC Thesis, Oxford.
16. Frootko, N.J. (1985): Immune responses in allograft tympanoplasty. In: *Immunobiology, Auto-*

immunity, and Transplantation in Otorhinolaryngology, edited by J.E. Veldman, B.F. McCabe, E.H. Huizing with N. Mygind, pp. 171–176, Kugler Publications, Amsterdam/Berkeley.
17. Gagnon, N.B., Piche, J., Larochelle, D., and Williams, M. (1979): Homografts of the middle ear: privileged site or privileged tissue. *Arch. Otolaryngol.,* 105:35–38.
18. Glasscock, M.E., House, W.F., and Graham, M. (1972): Homograft transplants to the middle ear. A follow up report. *Laryngoscope,* 82:868–881.
19. Goodhill, V., Harris, I., and Brockman, S.J. (1964): Tympanoplasty with perichondral graft. *Arch. Otolaryngol.,* 79:131–137.
20. Gowans, J.L. (1959): The recirculation of lymphocytes from blood to lymph in the rat. *J. Physiol.,* 146:54.
21. Grote, J.J. (editor) (1984): *Biomaterials in Otology.* M. Nijhoff Publications, The Hague.
22. Hall, A., and Rytzner, C. (1957): Stapedectomy and autotransplantation of ossicles. *Acta Otolaryngol. (Stockh.),* 47:318–324.
23. Heermann, J. (1962): Experiences with free grafts of fascia connective tissue for tympanoplasties and for obliterating of radical cavities. Cartilage bridge from the stapes to the lower margin of the drum. *Z. Laryngol. Rhinol. Otol.,* 41:141.
24. Heyner, S. (1969): Significance of intercellular matrix in survival of cartilage allografts. *Transplantations,* 8:666.
25. Homsey, C.A., Kent, J.N., and Hinds, E.C. (1973): Materials for oral implantation. Biological and functional criteria. *J. Am. Dent. Assoc.,* 86:817.
26. House, W.F., Patterson, M.E., and Linthicum, F.H. (1966): Incus homografts in chronic ear surgery. *Arch. Otolaryngol.,* 84:148–153.
27. Jansen, C. (1962): Stapesersatz durch Knorpel. *Acta Otolaryngol. (Stockh.),* 54:262.
28. Jansen, C. (1963): Cartilage tympanoplasty. *Laryngoscope,* 73:1288–1302.
29. Jansen, C. (1973): Heterologous tympanoplasty. *Trans. Am. Acad. Ophthal. Otolaryngol.,* 77:111.
30. Kastenbauer, E., and Hochstrasser, K. (1973): Der Einfluss des Konservierungsmittel Cialit auf die Proteinloslichkeit und die Antigenitat von allogenen und xenogenen Gehorknochelchen und Trommelfelltransplantaten. *Arch. Otorhinolaryngol.,* 203:225.
31. Kerr, A.G., and Smyth, G.D.L. (1971): The fate of transplanted ossicles. *J. Laryngol. Otol.,* 85:337–347.
32. Kerr, A.G., Byren, J.E.T. and Smyth, G.D.L. (1973): Cartilage homografts in the middle ear. A long-term histological study. *J. Laryngol. Otol.,* 87:1193–1199.
33. Kerr, A.G. (1984): Six years of experience with plastipore. *Clin. Otolaryngol.,* 9:361.
34. Kuijpers, W., and Van den Broek, P. (1972): Fundamental aspects of incus transplantation. *Laryngoscope,* 82:2174–2185.
35. Kuijpers, W., and Van den Broek, P. (1975): Biological considerations for the use of homograft tympanic membranes and ossicles. *Acta Otolaryngol. (Stockh.),* 80:283–293.
36. Kuijpers, W., and Veldman, J.E. (1984): Transplantation in otolaryngology. In: *Immunobiology of the Head and Neck,* edited by J.F. Poliquin, A.F. Ryan, J.R.Harris, Chapter 12, pp. 277–323. College Hill Press, San Diego, Cal.
37. Lesinski, S.G. (1982): Complications of homograft tympanoplasty. *Otolaryngol. Clin. North Am.,* 15:795–811.
38. Lesinski, S.G. (1983): Homograft tympanoplasty in perspective. A long-term clinical-histologic study of formalin-fixed tympanic membranes used for the reconstruction of 125 severely damaged middle ears. *Laryngoscope* (Suppl.), 32:93.
39. Lim, D.J., Bluestone, C.D., Klein J.O., and Nelson, J.D. (editors) (1984): *Recent advances in otitis media with effusion.* B.C. Decker, Philadelphia/Toronto.
40. Marquet, J. (1966): Reconstructive microsurgery of the eardrum by means of a tympanic membrane homograft. *Acta Otolaryngol. (Stockh.),* 62:459–464.
41. Marquet, J., Schepens, P., and Kuijpers, W. (1973): Experiences with tympanic transplants. *Arch. Otolaryngol.,* 97:58.
42. Marquet, J. (1976): Ten years experience in tympanoplasty using homologous implants. *J. Laryngol. Otol.,* 90:897–905.
43. Marquet, J. (1977): Twelve years experience with homograft tympanoplasty. *Otolaryngol. Clin. North Am.,* 3, 10:581–593.
44. Mitchison, N.A. (1953): Passive transfer of transplantation immunity. *Nature,* 171:267.
45. Moritz, W. (1952): Plastiche Eingriffe am Mittelohr zur Wiederherstellung der Innenohr-Schalleitung. *Z. Laryngol. Rhinol. Otol.,* 31:338–351.

46. Nadel, E.R., and Horvath, S.M. (1970): Comparison of tympanic membrane and deep body temperature in man. *Life Science*, 9:869.
47. Nickel, A.L. (1963): The use of homologous vein grafts in otolaryngology. *Laryngoscope*, 73:919.
48. Nieuwenhuis, P., and Veldman, J.E. (1985): Histophysiology of the lymphoid system: an overview of cells and structures involved in immune reactions. In: *Immunobiology, Autoimmunity and Transplantation in Otorhinolaryngology*, edited by J.E. Veldman, B.F. McCabe, E.H. Huizing, and N. Mygind, pp. 3–9. Kugler Publications, Amsterdam/Berkeley.
49. Opstelten, D., Stikker, R., Van der Heyden, D., et al. (1980): Germinal centres and the B-cell system. IV. Functional characteristics of rabbit appendix germinal centre(-derived) cells. *Virchows Arch. (Cell Pathol.)*, 34:53.
50. Plester, D., and Steinbach, E. (1977): Histologic fate of tympanic membrane and ossicle homografts. *Otolaryngol. Clin. North Am.*, 10:3:487–500.
51. Poliquin, M.D., Ryan A.F., Bone, R. and Catanzaro, A. (1979): Immunocompetence of the guinea pig's middle ear. *J. Otolaryngol.*, 8:385–389.
52. Pulec, J.L., and Sheehy, J.L. (1973): Tympanoplasty: ossicular chain reconstruction. *Laryngoscope*, 83:448–465.
53. Reijnen, C.J.H., and Kuijpers, W. (1971): The healing pattern of the drum membrane. *Acta Otolaryngol. (Stockh.)* (Suppl. 287).
54. Ringenberg, J.C. (1962): Fat graft tympanoplasty. *Laryngoscope*, 72:188–192.
55. Ryan, A.F., Hartman, M.T., Cleveland, P.H., and Catanzaro, A. (1982): Humoral and cell mediated immunity in peripheral blood following introduction of antigen into the middle ear. *Ann. Otolaryngol. Chir. Cervicofac.*, 91:70–75.
56. Ryan, A.F., Harris, J.F., and Schiff, M. (1985): Experimental immunology and diseases of the ear. In: *Immunobiology, Autoimmunity and Transplantation in Otorhinolaryngology*, edited by J.E. Veldman, B.F. McCabe, E.H. Huizing, and N. Mygind, pp. 85–92. Kugler Publications, Amsterdam/Berkeley.
57. Schiff, M, Poliquin, J.F., Catanzaro, A., and Ryan, A.F. (1980): Tympanosclerosis: a theory of pathogenesis. *Ann. Otolaryngol. Chir. Cervicofac.*, 89 (Suppl. 70).
58. Schrimpf, W.J. (1954): Repair of tympanic membrane perforations with human amniotic membrane. *Ann. Otolaryngol. Chir. Cervicofac.*, 63:102.
59. Schuknecht, H.F. and Shi, S.R. (1985): Surgical pathology of middle ear implants. *Laryngoscope*, 95:249.
60. Shea, J. (1961): Vein graft closure of eardrum perforations. *J. Laryngol. Otol.*, 74:358.
61. Shea, J.J. (1976): Plastipore total ossicular replacement prosthesis. *Laryngoscope*, 86:239–240.
62. Sheehy, J.L. (1964): Tympanic grafting: early and long-term results. *Laryngoscope*, 74:985.
63. Smith, M.F.W. (1972): An otologic tissue bank. *Trans. Am. Acad. Ophthal. Otolaryngol.*, 76:134–141.
64. Smith, M.F.W., and Ballantyne, J. (1975): The results of an international questionnaire in otologic homografts. *Trans Am. Acad. Ophthal. Otolaryngol.*, 80:71.
65. Smith, M.F.W., and McElveen, J.T. (1982): Lyophilised partial ossicular replacement allografts. *Ann. Otolaryngol. Chir. Cervicofac.*, 91:538–540.
66. Smyth, G.D.L., and Kerr, A.G. (1969): Tympanic membrane homografts. *J. Laryngol. Otol.*, 83:1061–1066.
67. Smyth, G.D.L. (1976): Tympanic reconstruction. Fifteen year report on tympanoplasty. Part II. *J. Laryngol. Otol.*, 90:713–741.
68. Smyth, G.D.L. (1983): TORP's. How have they fared after five years. *J. Laryngol. Otol.*, 97:991.
69. Stewart, I.A., and Heslop, B.F. (1979): The immunological status of allografts in the middle ear. *Acta Otolaryngol. (Stockh.)*, 87:539–544.
70. Storrs, L. (1966): Myringoplasty. *Laryngoscope*, 76:185.
71. Strauss, P., and Schreiter, K. (1979): Konservierte menschliche Knorpelimplantate und Korpereigene vitale Transplantate in Nase und Mittelohr. *Laryngol. Rhinol. Otol. Stuttg.*, 53:201.
72. Strauss, P., and Ickler, P. (1980): Knochenneubildung und Knochenabbau konservierter menschlicher Amboss im Mittelohr. *Laryngol. Rhinol. Otol. Stuttg.*, 59:298.
73. Urist, M.R., Silvermann, B.F., Buring, K., et al. (1967): The bone induction principle. *Clin. Orthop.*, 53:243.
74. Van den Broek, P. and Kuijpers, W. (1967): Incus autografts and homografts in rats. *Arch. Otolaryngol.*, 86:287–293.

75. Van den Broek, P. and Kuijpers, W. (1974): The effect of preservation on the behaviour of homologous ossicular grafts. *Acta Otolaryngol. (Stockh.),* 77:335.
76. Van den Broek, P., and Kuijpers, W. (1976): The preserved tympano-ossicular homograft. *J. Laryngol. Otol.,* 90:907.
77. Van Furth, R. (1985): The role of mononuclear phagocytes in otolaryngology. In: *Immunobiology, Autoimmunity and Transplantation in Otorhinolaryngology,* edited by J.E. Veldman, B.F. McCabe, E.H. Huizing, and N. Mygind, pp. 33–44. Kugler Publications, Amsterdam/Berkeley.
78. Veldman, J.E. (1970): *Histophysiology and Electronmicroscopy of the Immune Response. Parts I and II.* Ph.D. Thesis, Groningen. Dijkstra-Niemeyer, Groningen, The Netherlands.
79. Veldman, J.E., and Keuning, F.J. (1978a): Histophysiology of cellular immunity reactions in B cell deprived rabbits. An X-irradiation model for delineation of an isolated T cell system. *Virchows Arch. (Cell Pathol.),* 28:203.
80. Veldman, J.E., Kuijpers, W., and Overbosch, H.C. (1978b): Middle ear implantation: its place in the immunohistophysiology of lymphoid tissue. Review. *Clin. Otolaryngol.,* 3:93.
81. Veldman, J.E., Boezeman, A.J., Overbosch, H.C., Sedee, G.A., Borst-Eilers, E., Kuijpers, W, Van den Broek, P., and Feltkamp-Vroom, T.M. (1979): Middle ear transplantation: a new concept in clinical otology. In: *Advances in Experimental Medicine and Biology, Vol. 114, Function and structure of the immune system,* edited by H.K. Muller-Hermelink, pp. 357–362, Plenum Press, New York.
82. Veldman, J.E., and Kaiserling, E. (1980): Interdigitating cells. Chapter 10. In: *The reticulo-endothelial system. Vol. 1. Structure in Relation to Function,* edited by I. Carr and W.Th. Deams, pp. 318–416, Plenum Press, New York.
83. Veldman, J.E., and Kuijpers, W. (1981): Antigenicity of tympano-ossicular homografts of the middle ear: analyses of immune responses to viable and preserved grafts in animal models. *Otolaryngol. Head Neck Surg.,* 89:142–152.
84. Wullstein, H. (1953): Die Tympanoplastik als gehorverbesserende Operation bei Otitis media chronica und ihre Resultate. *Proc. Fifth Int. Cong. O.R.L. (Amsterdam),* 104–118.
85. Zöllner, F. (1953): Horverbesserende Eingriffe am Schalleitungsapparat. *Proc. Fifth Int. Cong. O.R.L. (Amsterdam),* 119–126.
86. Zöllner, F. (1955): The principles of plastic surgery of the sound-conducting apparatus. *J. Laryngol. Otol.,* 69:637–652.
87. Zöllner, F. (1960): Technik der Formung einer Columella aus Knochen. *Z. Laryngol. Rhinol. Otol.,* 39:536–540.

Immunology of the Ear, edited by J. Bernstein
and P. Ogra. Raven Press, New York © 1987.

The Effect of Eustachian Tube Obstruction on Middle Ear Mucosal Transformation

Wim Kuijpers and J. M. H. van der Beek

Department of Otorhinolaryngology, University of Nijmegen, N1-6500 HB Nijmegen, The Netherlands

It is generally known that the integrity of the middle ear mucosa is highly dependent on the functional patency of the eustachian tube (see the chapter by Bluestone, *this volume*). Malfunction or obstruction of the eustachian tube is assumed to be a major predisposing factor to otitis media with effusion (OME). This disease, occurring mainly in children between the ages of 2 and 10 years, is characterized by an accumulation of fluid. This fluid ranges from a thin serous to a heavy thick mucous consistency, without clear signs of acute infection. In most cases, OME is a self-limiting disease that largely depends on the ability of the middle ear to reaerate itself. This is directly related to the function of the eustachian tube. In some patients, however, this disease runs a very protracted course and can lead to severe structural changes, including tympanosclerosis, atelectasis, and cholesteatoma.

It is still unknown how tubal dysfunction or obstruction is involved in the pathogenesis and maintenance of this disease. The oldest theory on the genesis of this fluid is the "hydrops *ex vacuo*" theory, which is associated with the names of Politzer and Zaufall (76,77,109). This theory suggests that complete mechanical blockage of the eustachian tube results in a negative pressure in the middle ear cavity owing to gas absorption and subsequently leads to mucosal edema and a transudation of serum into the middle ear cavity. Although many clinical and experimental observations have confirmed this course of events after eustachian tube obstruction, the theory has been the subject of many debates. Even contemporaries of Politzer believed that infection of the middle ear was also an important positive factor in the genesis of this disease. Although it is customary to ascribe the hydrops *ex vacuo* theory to Politzer, he also pointed to the role of infection.

Several clinical observations contradicted the transudation theory as the only explanation for OME. The fluid was not always serous, but frequently had a cloudy white color with a viscid tenacious character; this could not be explained on a transudation origin alone. Secondly, the eustachian tube was not completely blocked in many cases. These observations suggested an exudative genesis of the fluid. Although identification of bacteria in the middle ear fluid could be an argument in favor of the exudation theory, most authors were not able to culture microorganisms from the middle ear fluid or were able to do so only in a small number of cases (14,23,57,90). Later studies with more advanced culturing techniques revealed positive cultures varying between 25% and 75% (7,28,40,46,58,91,95) although no clear relationship between positive cultures and the nature of the effusion—serous or mucous—could be established (28,56). The discrepancy of the results of OME bacteriology may be attributed to the bacteriostatic and bactericidal properties of the middle ear effusion itself. This fluid has been shown to contain lysozyme, lysosomal enzymes, and immunoglobulins, which partially originate from the local immune defense system of the middle ear mucosa (8,38,39, 49,58,65,66,69,94,107). The bacteriological findings, the presence of different inflammatory cells, the data on the etiology, and the natural course and therapy of OME strongly suggest several etiological factors that together may contribute to the pathogenesis of this disease.

Finally, it is generally accepted that both tubal dysfunction and inflammation of the middle ear mucosa are the most important factors in the genesis and/or prolongation of OME, but it is still unknown in what way and to what extent these two factors individually contribute to the pathological changes observed in the middle ear mucosa.

In this chapter the reported data from both clinical and experimental studies on the effect of eustachian tube obstruction on the middle ear mucosa will be discussed. Since morphology and physiology of the tubotympanum have been discussed extensively in the chapter by Bluestone *(this volume),* only the most relevant data will be reported in the first part of this chapter.

MORPHOLOGICAL AND FUNCTIONAL ASPECTS OF THE TUBOTYMPANUM

The middle ear and eustachian tube develop from outpouching of the pharyngeal endoderm, the tubotympanic recess. Thus, the epithelial lining of both structures is of endodermal origin. Since the first histological studies on temporal bones, there has been controversy concerning the character of the normal lining of the middle ear. Most textbooks on otolaryngology have suggested the histology of middle ear epithelium to be a flat to cubic one-layered epithelium. This epithelium was considered to be devoid of cilia and goblet cells, except in the region of the tympanic orifice of the eustachian tube and a limited area of the hypotympanum. This opinion has drastically changed during the last 20 years and it is now recognized that the middle ear epithelium is more complex. In the early sixties, Senturia (92) described the existence of a ''respiratory epithelium'' in the dog, which was composed of a pseudostratified ciliated columnar epithelium passing into the flat epithelium of the bulla. A comprehensive morphological study on the middle ear epithelium in a great number of human temporal bones has been reported (86). A large part of the mucosa is covered with ciliated cells interspersed with goblet cells, forming distinct and consistent tracts extending from different sites in the middle ear cavity to the tympanic orifice of the eustachian tube. This has been confirmed by others (30,45). Comparable observations on the presence of ciliated cells and their arrangement in tracts have also been reported in the middle ear of experimental animals (Fig. 1) (43). The typical arrangement of the ciliated cells and their continuity with the ciliated epithelium of the eustachian tube suggest the existence of a mucociliary transport system for cleaning the middle ear cavity. The functioning of such a system has been convincingly demonstrated (50,51,87).

By far, the largest part of the mastoid cells is covered by a flat one-layered squamous epithelium. Secretory cells are a normal constituent of the ciliated areas, but also part of the squamous epithelium appeared to contain secretory cells, normally only detectable by transmission electron microscopy (Fig. 2) (33,45,48).

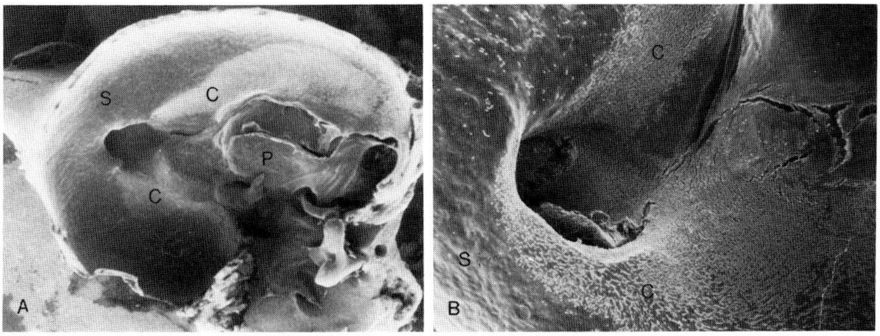

FIG. 1. Scanning electron micrographs of the middle ear cavity of the rat, demonstrating areas with ciliated (C) and squamous epithelium (S). **A:** Survey. **B:** Entrance of ciliated tracts into the eustachian tube orifice. (P) Promontory.

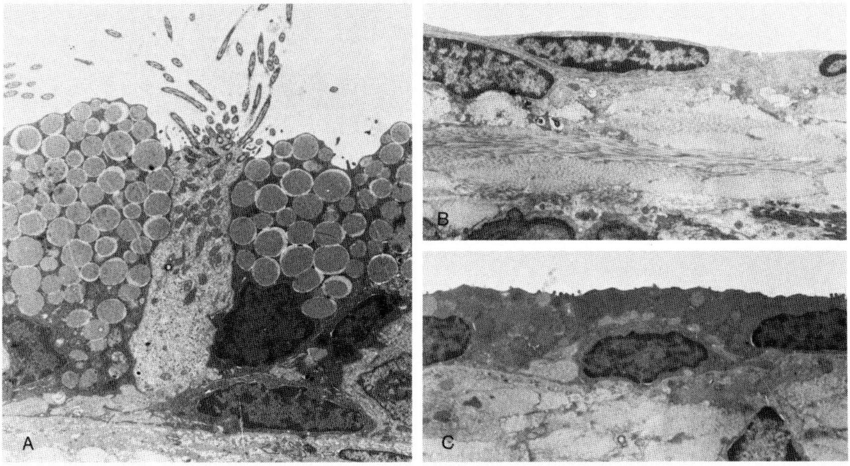

FIG. 2. TEM of middle ear epithelium: **A:** Ciliated epithelium with goblet cells. **B:** Flattened squamous epithelium. **C:** Flattened squamous epithelium with secretory granules.

Although there is still controversy with regard to the presence of subepithelial glands in the normal middle ear, the comprehensive developmental studies of Akaan-Penttilä (1) and Tos (99–104) on human temporal bones indicate that they are normally absent, but can easily be induced by infective processes. With respect to the nature of the secretory products, there is no certainty concerning the nature of the secretory products and there is no certainty concerning their precise chemical composition, but morphological, histochemical, and autoradiographical studies suggest the production of different secretory products (5,37,49). In addition to their contribution to the mucous blanket, necessary for the functioning of the mucociliary transport system, the secretory cells can be assumed to be involved in the production of enzymes as part of the local defense system (38,54,69,73). Also, the capability of the epithelium to phagocytose foreign proteins from the middle ear cavity can be considered to contribute to the mucosal defense (52). The lamina propria of the middle ear mucosa is rather thin and varies in thickness at different sites. It contains blood and lymph capillaries, while frequently scattered lymphocytes, mast cells, and plasma cells can be observed. Summarizing these data, the normal middle ear epithelium can be considered as a modified respiratory epithelium. The major part of the eustachian tube is lined with pseudostratified ciliated epithelium interspersed with numerous goblet cells. It is continuous with the ciliated epithelium of the middle ear and that of the nasopharynx. A minor part of the epithelial lining, especially pronounced near the pharyngeal opening, consists of flat squamous cells. In contrast to the middle ear, the mucosa of the eustachian tube is supplied by large subepithelial glands (51,53,55). They are of the mixed type, and they open up mainly in the lower part of the tube by ducts of varying length (Fig. 3). The eustachian tube fulfills three main functions in order to maintain functional integrity of the middle ear: ventilating of the middle ear cavity, clearance of secretions and debris from the middle ear toward the nasopharynx by means of the mucociliary transport system, and protection of the middle ear from

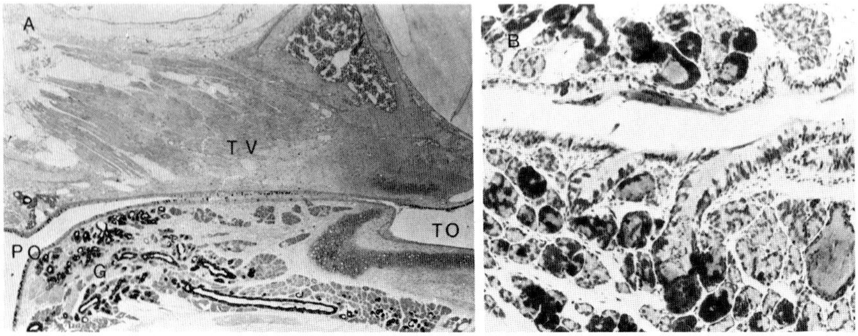

FIG. 3. A: Micrograph of the eustachian tube of the rat. (G) Area with subepithelial glands; (PO) pharyngeal orifice; (TO) tympanic orifice; (TV) tensor veli palatini muscle. **B:** Lower part of the eustachian tube with subepithelial glands and secretory ducts.

nasopharyngeal secretions (15). (These functions are elaborated in Bluestone's chapter, *this volume*.) The tube is in a collapsed state most of the time. It opens intermittently by the contraction of the tensor veli palatini muscle, during swallowing and yawning, in maintaining ambient pressure in the middle ear (18,36). It has been suggested that secretory products from the epithelial lining of the eustachian tube, and probably also from the middle ear, facilitate the opening of the tubes by reducing surface tension analogous to the surface tension lowering substance in the lung (13,27,51). Indirect evidence for the functional significance of such surface-active agents can be derived from the experiments performed by Rapport et al. (82). They observed in the guinea pig that a much higher pressure was required to open the tube after rinsing the lumen with saline. The chemical nature of this substance remains to be elucidated.

HISTOPATHOLOGY IN SECRETORY OTITIS MEDIA

Generally, there are no essential differences in the histopathological findings of the middle ear mucosa in OME reported by various authors (6,24,26,47, 72,91,110). These studies show that the mucosa is largely swollen by hyperemia and edema, while finger-like mucosal folds often extend into the lumen. The lamina propria contains an increased amount of rather loose connective tissue often with a varying number of lymphocytes, macrophages, plasma cells, and sometimes polymorphonuclear cells. Lymphocytes are occasionally found as subepithelial follicle-like aggregations. the most conspicuous observation is the large increase in the number of goblet cells, and mucous cysts and mucus-producing glands or gland-like structures are also frequently described. These phenomena are often more marked in the ears having mucous content than in those with serous content (31,32,47,75,91). A great deal of our present knowledge on changes occurring in the secretory activity of the middle ear epithelium in OME is derived from the studies of Tos and Bak-Pedersen (3,103,105). These authors, using whole mount specimens, quantified the secretory activity at various stages of the disease. With this technique they established a marked increase in the number of goblet cells. Whereas in normal children about 175 goblet cells/mm^2 were present, in children with serous otitis media (SOM) the number of goblet cells appeared to vary between 2,800 and 14,500/mm^2 (mean density 8,000 cells/mm^2). Moreover, extensive gland formation was found. These glands were suggested to develop analogous to the normal embryogenesis of glands. Furthermore, they suggested a positive correlation between the number of secretory elements and the severity of the disease (102). During the healing process a decrease in the number of goblet cells, as well as a gradual degeneration of the glands, could be established, although even after normalization of the aeration of the middle ear cavity, the secretory activity was still higher than in the normal ear (101). This has also been reported by Karja et al. (42). In addition to the transformation of the epithelium into a highly secretory active epithelium, some authors mentioned the presence of islands of stratified squamous epithelium, some of which produce keratin (6,74). This observation is of great interest, especially with respect to the development of cholesteatoma, suggested to be one of the late sequelae of OME.

EXPERIMENTAL OBSTRUCTION OF THE EUSTACHIAN TUBE

To obtain further evidence for the theory that eustachian tube obstruction is the main underlying factor in the development of OME, it is understandable that many experimental studies have been performed with the objective of interfacing with tubal function by creating a dysfunction or complete obstruction. This was attempted by blocking the pharyngeal or tympanal opening by means of a plug (4,39,60,89), by ligation (2,34,35,78), by submucosal injection of various substances to narrow the lumen (20,39,80,83), by electrocauterization (25,46,84,88), and by interference with the function of the tensor veli palatini muscle (17,19,22,79,97). However, the major part of these studies was restricted to short observation periods and to the study of limited areas of the middle ear mucosa. Moreover, some observations are largely complicated by the absence of rigid criteria to exclude spontaneous recanalization or interference through infection. Apart from these imperfections, these studies have nevertheless contributed to our understanding of the effect of tubal obstruction on the middle ear structures. A critical evaluation of these experimental studies demonstrates that successful tubal occlusion invariably resulted in the development of an underpressure, sometimes of more than 100 mm H_2O, within 24 hr, followed by an increasing accumulation of a serous or seromucous fluid. This fluid could change into a seropurulent, purulent, or mucopurulent form. The effusions always contained high numbers of inflammatory cells. In those cases where bacterial culturing was performed, positive cultures were obtained from the majority of the effusions (84,93).

Histopathological studies of the middle ear mucosa showed edema, hypertrophy, and metaplasia of the epithelium and an increase in the number of secretory and ciliated cells. The mucosa was infiltrated to a varying extent by polymorphonuclear cells, macrophages, plasma cells, and lymphocytes. Both bone resorption and bone apposition were observed. The scarce long-term observations revealed a largely thickened mucosa, sometimes obliterating a considerable part of the middle ear cavity, infiltrated by inflammatory cells and sometimes containing cholesterol granuloma. Clinical studies have shown the presence of a functional rather than a mechanical obstruction in some patients with OME. Therefore, experiments in which a functional disturbance of the opening mechanism was induced by interfering with the eustachian tube opening muscles can be supposed to be of clinical relevance. These studies showed the development of a serous middle ear effusion which was dependent on the severity and duration of the impairment in tubal function. Unfortunately, they are all short-term observations and no histological data are available. With the use of this technique, an interesting observation was made by Catekin et al. (17). They found that after inducing eustachian tube dysfunction by transection of the tensor veli palatini muscle, *S. pneumoniae* bacteria introduced into the nasopharynx caused an acute otitis to develop. Comparable findings were obtained by Meyerhoff et al. (63) after applying a slight negative pressure in the middle ear cleft. In chinchillas, middle ear deflation in the presence of nasopharyngeal colonization with *S. pneumoniae* resulted in an acute otitis in 60% of the cases.

In summary, these investigations convincingly demonstrate that both mechanical and functional obstruction of the eustachian tube can evoke an underpressure in the middle ear cavity, resulting in the entry of a transudate into the middle ear. Shortly thereafter, this ''serous otitis'' passes in nearly all cases into an infective middle ear disease. Underaeration of the middle ear seems to involve a higher susceptibility for the development of an infective middle ear disease. The histopathological picture appears to be very similar to that reported for patients with OME.

THE ROLE OF INFECTION IN EXPERIMENTAL EUSTACHIAN TUBE OBSTRUCTION

Since the reported data on experimental eustachian tube obstruction in nearly all cases are complicated by supervening infection, we attempted to elucidate the role of this complicating factor in a controlled longitudinal study in the rat (5,16, 43,44). For this purpose, three groups of rats were used: One group was contaminated with *Mycoplasma pneumoniae;* the second group consisted of specific-pathogen-free rats, harboring only nonpathogenic symbionts; and the third group consisted of completely germ-free rats. The eustachian tube was obstructed in its extratympanic course by electrocauterization.

Eustachian tube obstruction induced the accumulation of a serum-like fluid during the first postoperative days. Subsequently about 90% of the group contaminated with *M. pneumoniae* developed an infective middle ear disease. Culturing revealed the presence of a high population of *M. pneumoniae* and often also various other microorganisms. Mycoplasmas could also be cultured from the nasopharynx and from the unoperated ear, although these ears failed to show any sign of an infective middle ear disease. Comparable observations were made in the group of specific-pathogen-free animals, although a smaller percentage developed an infective middle ear disease. In this group the causal agent was classified as a nonpathogenic symbiont.

The major number of the infected ears remained otoscopically unaltered during an observation period of up to 2 years, but a small number recovered spontaneously after a short infective period and became serous again. Histopathological studies revealed that the natural course of the induced infection was rather divergent. Generally, no clear-cut relation was found between the course of the infection and the types of bacteria cultured, although a destructive process with lysis of the bone was more often observed in the group contaminated with *M. pneumoniae*. The mucosa was greatly thickened and heavily infiltrated by inflammatory cells. The areas with ciliated/secretory cells were often found to be tremendously expanded (Fig. 4), and accumulations of secretory cells acting as glands were another common finding. After prolonged infection, intraepithelial glands appeared to be developed notably in the originally ciliated areas (Fig. 5). The infective process frequently resulted in a partial or nearly total fibrosis of the middle ear cleft. It starts as a local or more generalized proliferation of fibroblasts from the lamina propria after disruption of the epithelial lining (Fig. 6). By this process the original squamous epithelium becomes completely embedded in the fibrous tissue. These epithelial cysts sometimes showed extensive secretory activity (Figs. 7 and 8). This fibrosis is reminiscent of adhesive processes believed to result from chronic

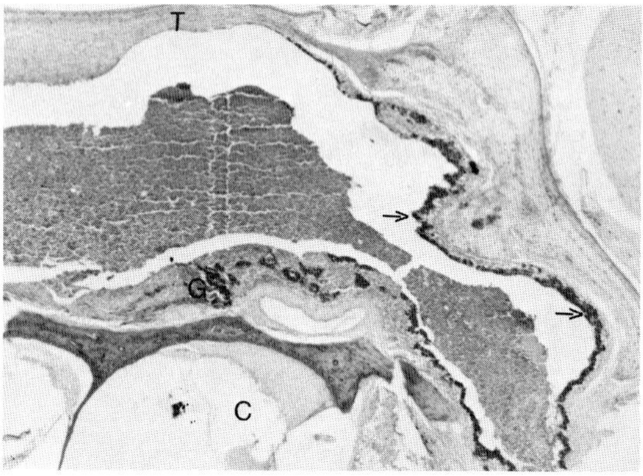

FIG. 4. Micrograph of the rat middle ear 2 months after eustachian tube obstruction. The ear became infected 4 days after obstruction. The mucosa is severely thickened and shows a tremendous expansion of secretory cells (*arrows*). (C) Cochlea; (G) gland-like structures; (T) tympanic membrane.

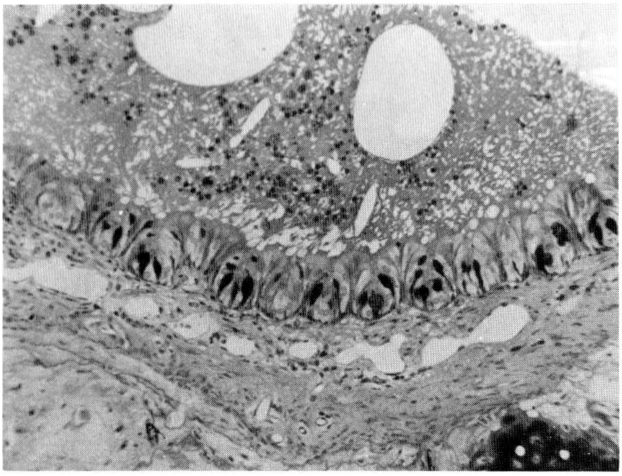

FIG. 5. Intraepithelial gland formation in the originally ciliated area, 6 months after eustachian tube obstruction. The ear developed an infective middle ear disease 1 week after obstruction.

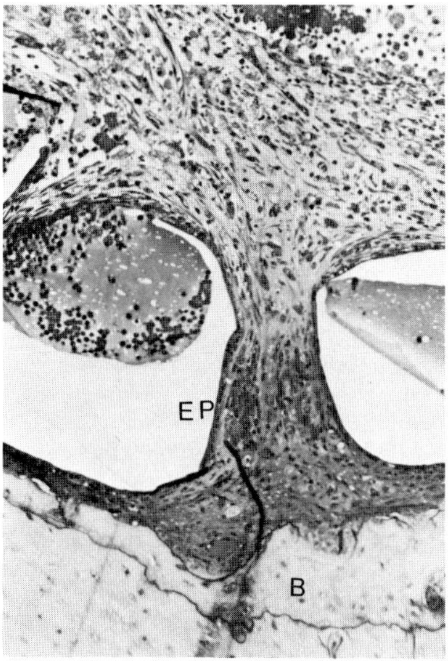

FIG. 6. Proliferation of fibroblasts from the mucosa into the middle ear cavity, 2 weeks after eustachian tube obstruction. The ear developed an infective middle ear disease 1 week after obstruction. (B) bulla; (EP) epithelial lined cyst.

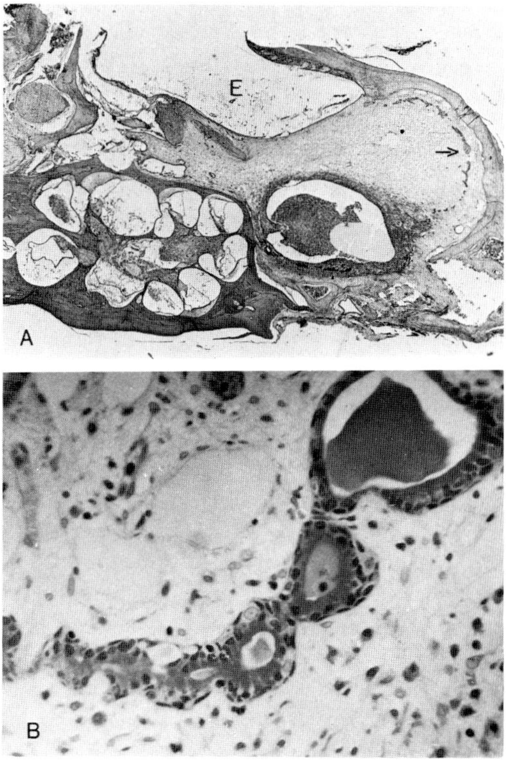

FIG. 7. **A:** Fibrosis of the middle ear cavity, 5 weeks after eustachian tube obstruction. The ear had been serous for 1 week and thereafter became infected. (E) External meatus; (*arrow*) epithelial cysts embedded in fibrous tissue. **B:** Higher magnification of epithelial cysts lined with secretory cells.

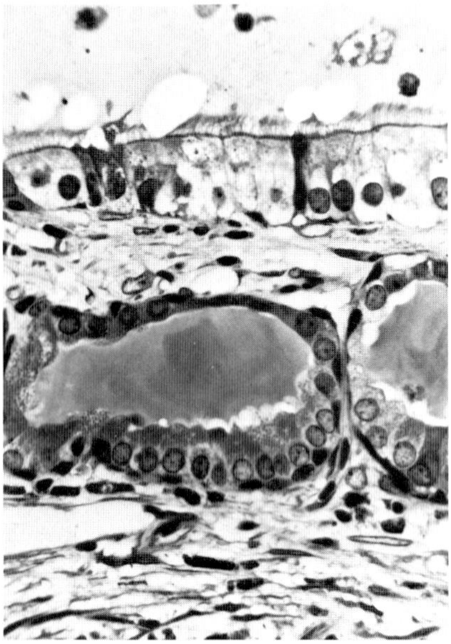

FIG. 8. Epithelial cysts lined with secretory cells, situated below ciliated epithelium, 20 months after eustachian tube obstruction. The ear became infected after a serous period of 1 week.

OME. After longer survival times the bone of the middle ear was largely thickened and ectopic bone and cholesterol granuloma were frequently observed (Fig. 9). Ears that recovered after a limited infective period and became serous again revealed a disturbance of the original arrangment of the ciliated and squamous epithelium. In addition to the originally ciliated tracts, which were often largely broadened, isolated islands of ciliated cells interspersed with secretory cells were present in the squamous area (Fig. 10). All those ears revealed (a) a varying degree of fibrosis in the form of polyps, or (b) an obliteration of a varying part of the middle ear cleft (Figs. 10 and 11). The epithelial cysts originating from the original squamous epithelium, embedded in this fibrous tissue, were often filled with a periodic acid-Schiff (PAS)-positive secretion, whereas some of the lining cells contained secretory granules (Fig. 11). The infection-induced changes appeared to persist for an observation period of more than 8 months after recovery from infection.

The obtained data led us to conclude that obstruction of the normal clearance pathway of the middle ear, together with the favorable nutritional conditions for bacterial growth in the transudated serum-like fluid, can be assumed to favor pathogenic behavior of bacteria that can either be present in the middle ear or enter it from the nasopharynx through the severely damaged eustachian tube during the early postoperative period. In the large majority of the obstructed ears this infection failed to heal. This supervening infection can lead to transformation of the squamous epithelium into secretory/ciliated epithelium and to a varying degree of fibrosis. The sequelae of this infection can persist for a long period after healing.

This investigation shows that the presence of microorganisms in the upper air-

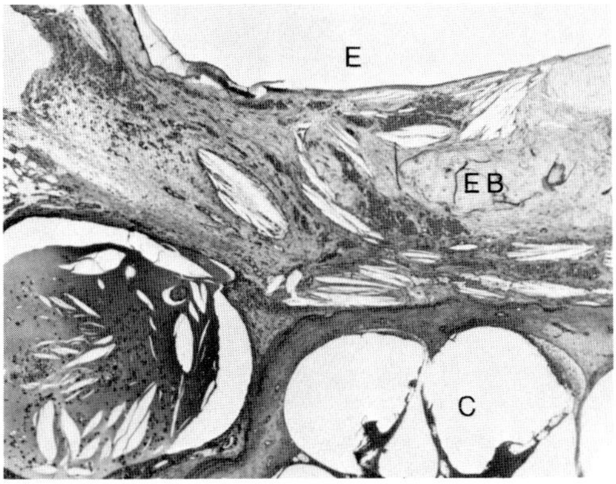

FIG. 9. Fibrosis of the middle ear cavity, 18 months after eustachian tube obstruction. The ear became infected after a serous period of 1 week. The fibrous tissue contains cholesterol clefts and ectopic bone (EB). (C) Cochlea; (E) external meatus.

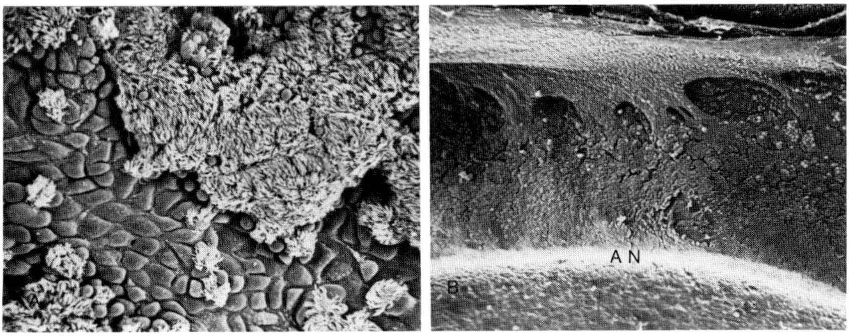

FIG. 10. SEM of squamous epithelium. The ear developed a transient infection 1 week after eustachian tube obstruction. The animal was killed 2 months after recovery. **A:** The original flat squamous epithelium is locally transformed into ciliated epithelium with scattered secretory cells. **B:** Mucosal protrusion near the tympanic annulus (AN).

ways is a serious disturbing factor when attempting to perform a reliable study of the isolated effect of tubal occlusion on the middle ear mucosa. It inevitably leads to infection of the middle ear in the majority of the cases. Such a complicating factor could be prevented by the use of germfree animals, which would guarantee the absence of microorganisms at the moment of tubal occlusion. These animals could be studied during an observation period of up to 2 years without any sign of infection. The first effects of eustachian tube obstruction consisted of an edematous reaction due to dilation of the mucosal vessels and transudation of serum into the intercellular spaces. This process led to a typical cobblestone appearance of the surface of the squamous epithelium on scanning electron microscope micrographs. Sections showed severe arcading and bulging of individual cells (Fig. 12). This

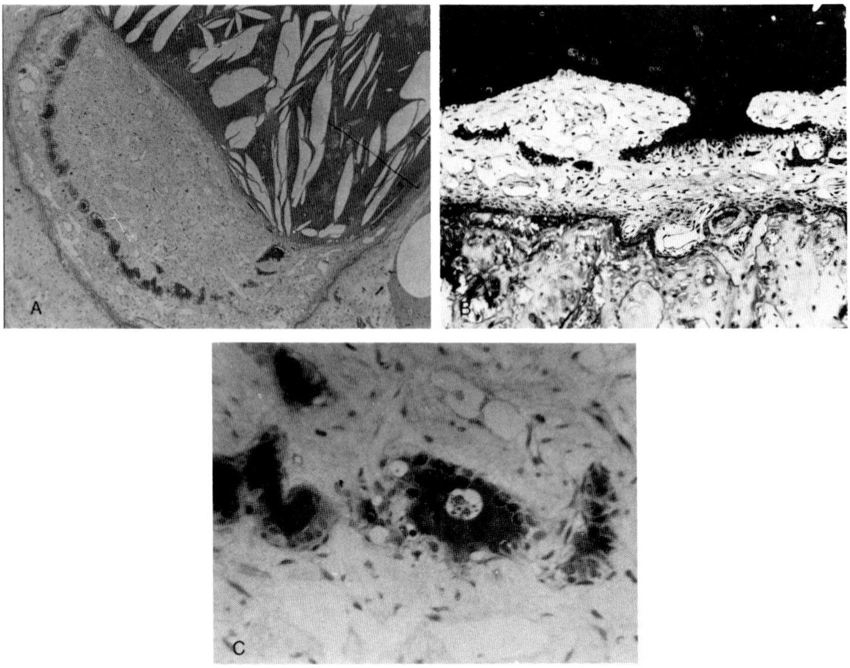

FIG. 11. Micrographs of ears that developed a transient infection after eustachian tube obstruction (serous 2 weeks, infected 1 week, serous 5 months). **A:** Partial obliteration of middle ear cavity with fibrous tissue containing many epithelial cysts filled with a PAS-positive secretion at the site of the originally squamous epithelial lining. The middle ear cavity is filled with fluid containing numerous cholesterol clefts. **B:** Thickened mucosa with polypous protrusions. **C:** Detail from epithelial cysts partly lined with secretory cells.

irregularity of the epithelial surface persisted during an observation period of up to 2 years. After 1 week the middle ear cavity was completely filled with a serum-like fluid containing erythrocytes and some phagocytotic cells. Electrophoresis revealed the same protein pattern as the paired serum. In the lamina propria the first signs of fibrosis leading to a more dense stroma could be seen 1 week after obstruction. At the same time there was an increase in the periosteal activity at the luminal side of the bone of the bulla. This process, resulting in the apposition of bone, appeared to be arrested after about 2 months (Fig. 13) (16). With progression of time the simple squamous epithelium gradually transformed into a two-layered stratified epithelium. Some cells revealed squamous metaplasia as judged from the presence of tonofilaments, although this never resulted in the formation of keratinizing epithelium. The columnar epithelium in the ciliated areas showed basal cell hyperplasia.

After 2 weeks, large clear cells scattered throughout the epithelium and protrusion into the lumen became visible. They subsequently became detached and were found as free-floating cells with signs of degeneration in the middle ear fluid. This

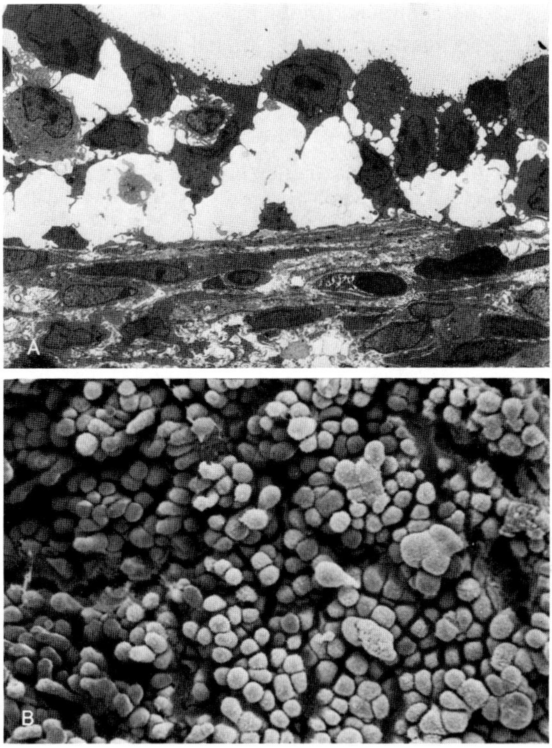

FIG. 12. **Top:** Severe arcading of squamous epithelium by intercellular fluid accumulation, 3 weeks after eustachian tube obstruction. **Bottom:** SEM 2 weeks after eustachian tube obstruction, showing cobblestone-like appearance of the squamous epithelium.

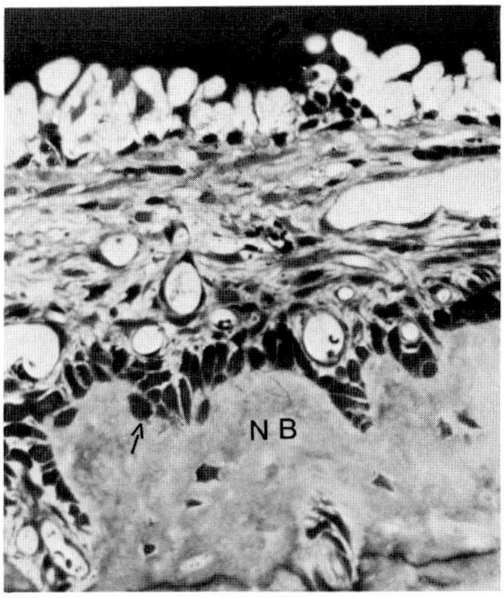

FIG. 13. Bulging epithelial cells and intraepithelial fluid accumulation, 6 weeks after eustachian tube obstruction. Note the active periosteum (*arrow*) and the new bone formed (NB).

process of desquamation continued throughout the whole observation period (Fig. 14). The induced abnormalities in the epithelial lining observed during the first few weeks after occlusion were also common findings in the animals that survived longer, although these abnormalities could differ from site to site and from one ear to another. Those animals that were killed after more than 1 year revealed an increasing number of interdigitations in the basal and lateral cell wall and an increased number of microvilli on the apical cell surface (Figs. 15 and 16). This suggests an increased involvement of the epithelium in fluid transport. The cyto-

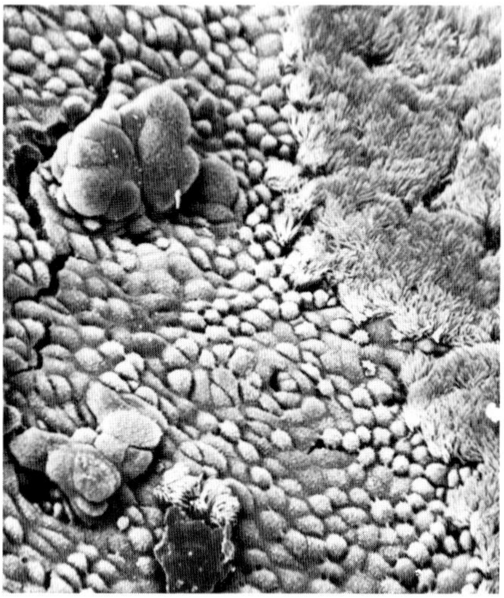

FIG. 14. SEM of middle ear epithelium revealing desquamating cells of the squamous epithelium, 10 weeks after eustachian tube obstruction.

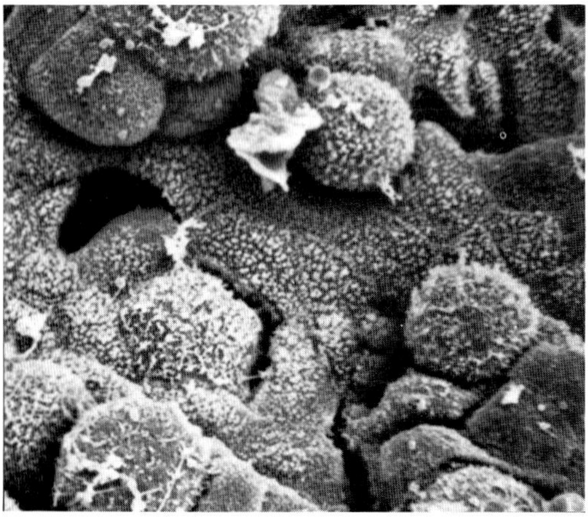

FIG. 15. SEM of squamous epithelium with numerous microvilli, 20 months after eustachian tube obstruction.

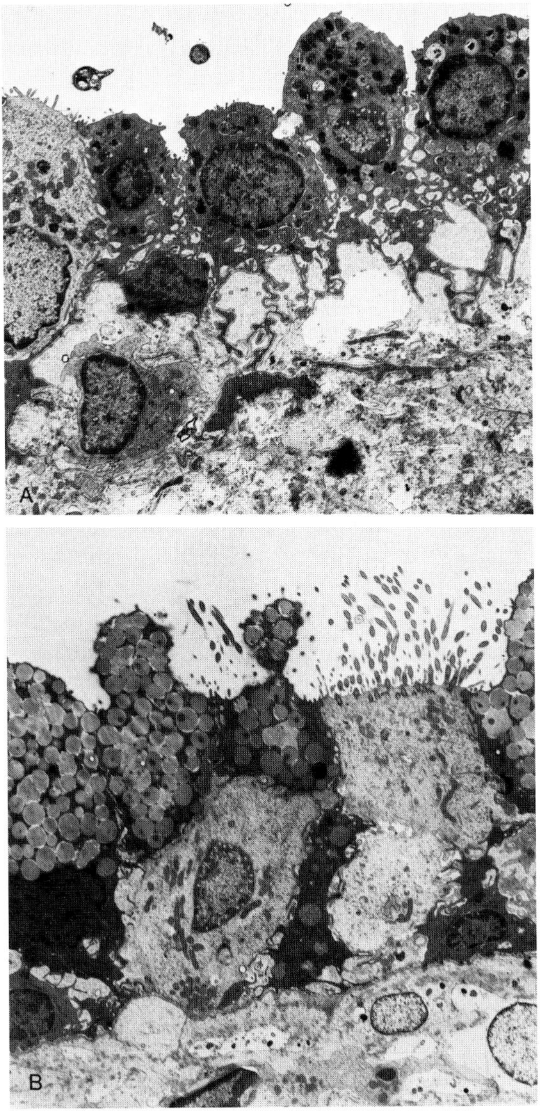

FIG. 16. TEM of squamous (**A**) and ciliated epithelium with goblet cells (**B**) 2 years after eustachian tube obstruction. The squamous epithelium reveals intercellular fluid accumulation and numerous infoldings of basal and lateral cell walls. The cytoplasm contains siderosome-like structures and multivesiculated bodies. The ciliated/secretory epithelium is virtually unaffected.

plasm contained a large number of lysosomes and many electron dense inclusions, presumably siderosomes (Fig. 16). The ciliated/secretory epithelium remained virtually unaffected throughout the observation period (Fig. 16), and no significant alterations in the number of secretory cells could be established. The lamina propria of the tympanic membrane developed comprehensive changes. After 2 months, depositions of an amorphous calciferous substance were seen. This process, which was also incidentally observed in other parts of the mucosa, gradually progressed and after 2 years the tympanic membrane had a nearly total chalky appearance (Fig. 17). With respect to the accumulated fluid in the middle ear, a slight increase in the viscosity and affinity for PAS staining was established with progression of time. Cholesterol clefts appeared in this fluid within 2 weeks and remained present in varying numbers intermingled with phagocytotic cells during an observation period of 2 years (Fig. 18). These data are fundamentally different from those made after tubal obstruction with supervening infection and prove that tubal obstruction per se does not result in a transformation of the epithelium into a highly secretory active epithelium as suggested by some authors (2,106). Therefore, the similarity between the changes found in the infected ears and those encountered in the middle ear mucosa of patients with OME strongly suggests that they cannot be attributed to eustachian tube dysfunction but rather to a supervening infective process.

Some observations on the isolated effect of tubal occlusion deserve special attention in connection with human middle ear pathology. The squamous metaplasia, although never resulting in keratinizing epithelium, is interesting because of the suggested relationship between OME and the origin of cholesteatoma. Further-

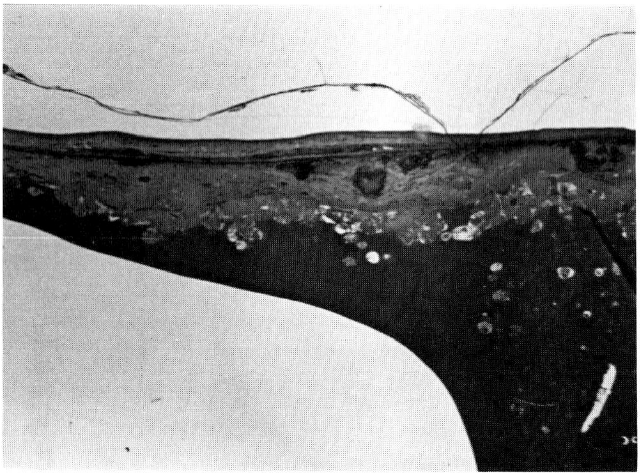

FIG. 17. Largely thickened tympanic membrane with calciferous deposits, 6 months after eustachian tube obstruction.

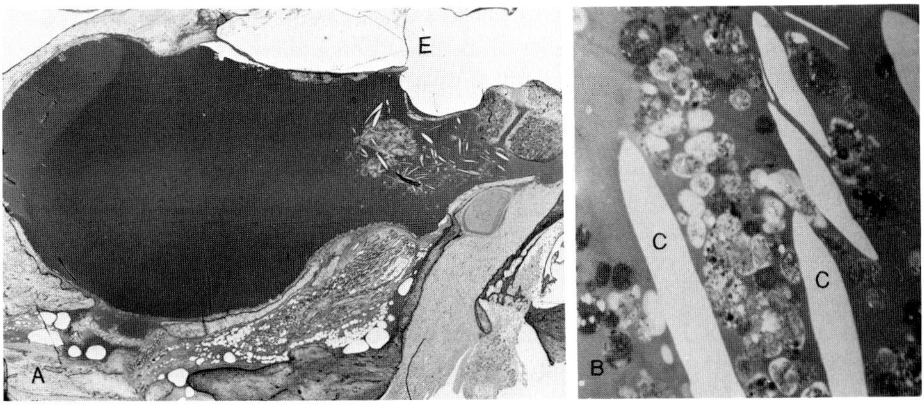

FIG. 18. **A:** Middle ear cavity filled with fluid, containing locally cholesterol clefts, 20 months after eustachian tube obstruction. (E) external meatus. **B:** Area with cholesterol clefts (C) surrounded by numerous phagocytotic cells.

more, this study demonstrates that new bone formation, accumulation of cholesterol, and tympanosclerosis, often ascribed to the effect of infective processes, can be elicited by tubal occlusion without the interference of infection.

MUCOSAL DAMAGE BY IMMUNE INJURY

From the experimental studies described in the previous section, it becomes obvious that bacteria can produce an inflammatory reaction of the middle ear mucosa by direct toxicity, resulting in a large variety of changes. In addition, recent experimental studies indicate that also nonviable bacteria (71) and bacterial endotoxin (47,64) are capable of inducing severe inflammatory changes in the middle ear mucosa.

During the last decade, an indirect involvement of bacterial antigens by means of eliciting nonspecific immune responses, thus causing mucosal inflammation by IgE-mediated hypersensitivity, delayed-type hypersensitivity, or immune complex-mediated complement activation, has been proposed as possible underlying mechanisms for OME. These mechanisms are described in detail in other chapters in this volume and will be only briefly mentioned here.

IgE-Mediated Hypersensitivity

The role of allergy or IgE-mediated hypersensitivity in the pathogenesis of OME is a controversial one. The percentage of instances in which allergy is thought to be responsible for the accumulation of fluid in the middle ear varies widely and is highly dependent on the criteria used for establishing allergy. Those authors who believe that allergy is a major contributing factor in the etiology of OME base their opinion mainly on clinical observations of an atopic constitution, positive family history, signs of nasal allergy, or the beneficial effects of antiallergic drugs (21,29,62,81,108). However, this is not supported by the IgE levels in the middle ear fluid. They are not elevated except when the serum level is elevated (9,67,73). Moreover, eosinophils in middle ear effusions have been reported to be scarce or completely absent (59,73). An important contribution to this discussion has been given by Bernstein (12). He observed that from an unselected group of children with OME, about 35% had an allergic rhinitis, but only 25% of this latter group, i.e., 8% of the total population studied, had IgE levels that were significantly higher in the effusion than in the serum, suggesting a local production of IgE in the middle ear mucosa. These observations indicate that (a) in a very small percentage of children with OME, the middle ear may be the target organ and (b) IgE-mediated hypersensitivity may be the underlying cause for the mucosal inflammation.

The effects on the middle ear mucosa may be assumed to be essentially the same as in other parts of the upper respiratory tract during allergy, as described by Terrahe (98). He established mucosal edema and increased secretory activity.

Allergy might also be involved in an indirect way in the pathogenesis of OME, when the eustachian tube functions as a target organ. The induced swelling of the eustachian tube mucosa will then lead to tubal obstruction, followed by an underpressure in the middle ear cavity and transudation of serum.

Delayed-Type Hypersensitivity

In addition to immediate-type hypersensitivity, mucosal injury resulting from delayed-type hypersensitivity has been postulated to play a role in etiology and progression of the inflammatory disease of the middle ear (11). Although the predominant presence of lymphocytes and macrophages as well as a marked perivascular accumulation of mononuclear cells, observed in some mucosal specimens, can be considered as strong arguments in favor of this hypothesis, substantial proof is still lacking.

Immune Complex Injury

Analysis of the middle ear fluid in OME has shown that components necessary for immune complex injury can be identified in middle ear effusions. This includes the identification of bacteria (7,28,40,58), locally produced immunoglobulins

(70), and inflammatory mediators as components of the complement cascade (60,61). These observations have led to the assumption that OME might be an immune complex disease mediated by complement (96).

Immune complexes are composed from bacterial antigens and antibodies. Their significance is that they can activate the complement system with the production of many inflammatory products resulting from damage of the basement membrane. Immune complexes in OME have been demonstrated by various authors (61,96), and evidence was also found for complement activation (10,61). That immune complexes can cause inflammatory changes in the middle ear of an experimental animal was demonstrated by Mravec et al. (68). The significance of complement in the development of experimentally induced immune mediated middle ear effusions was established by Ryan and co-workers (84,85). They observed that decomplementation of the animals resulted in a marked, but not complete, reduction of the immune-mediated effusion. Although these experimental studies give experimental support for the involvement of complement activation in experimental immune-mediated ear effusions, final proof that immune complexes are an important underlying factor in OME is not yet available.

According to Bernstein (12) the presence of immune complexes can be explained as the result of the physiological elimination of antigen from the middle ear, whereas the observed activation need not necessarily be performed by immune complexes, since many other protein molecules, present in middle ear effusions, can activate the complement system in a nonspecific way; this can be responsible for the maintenance of the inflammatory process in the middle ear mucosa.

One can only guess as to the possible effects of immune injury on the middle ear mucosa. As in the case of direct bacterial toxicity, the release of inflammatory mediators will cause tissue damage to a varying extent. The middle ear mucosa will respond by an increased secretory activity and fibrous tissue proliferation, which can be considered as part of the local defense system. Especially when normal drainage of the middle ear fails to be restored and antigenic stimulus continues, or new antigenic determinants are formed, severe and irreversible damage can be expected.

SUMMARY AND CONCLUSIONS

The eustachian tube has an important function with respect to the protection of the middle ear cavity by draining secretions and cellular debris and by maintaining equality of pressure across the tympanic membrane.

Functional or mechanical obstruction of the eustachian tube, frequently encountered in children, is generally assumed to be a crucial factor in the development and prolongation of OME. Although many etiological factors can be held responsible for abnormal eustachian tube function, there is increasing evidence that the anatomical immaturity of the eustachian tube together with upper respiratory tract infection are two important predisposing factors for eustachian tube obstruction in childhood.

Notably, experimental studies on both germ-carrying and germfree animals have deepened our insight into the contribution of eustachian tube dysfunction to the observed histopathological changes in the middle ear mucosa in patients with OME. Both functional and mechanical obstruction of the tube appeared to evoke an underpressure in the middle ear cavity, followed by a transudation of a serum-like fluid from the submucosal vessels.

In germ-carrying animals this serous phase was nearly always followed by infection of the middle ear mucosa. The effects of these induced infections were rather divergent and are likely related to the kind and virulence of the causal microorganisms. Sometimes a destructive course could be observed with tissue destruction, including osteolysis, but usually the disease process was much milder and in some ears even a spontaneous clearing of the infection occurred after a short period.

In most cases a transformation of the squamous epithelium into a highly secretory active epithelium was observed, and often partial or nearly total fibrosis of the middle ear cleft was established. In this fibrous tissue, gland-like structures, islands of ectopic bone, and cholesterol granuloma were common findings after prolonged survival. These findings strongly suggest that mechanical or functional obstruction of the eustachian tube can stimulate the pathogenic behavior of microorganisms that can enter the middle ear from the nasopharynx during induced tubal dysfunction. The infective process usually continues for a long period since the normal clearance pathway is blocked. Moreover, when spontaneous clearing of the infective process occurs, the sequelae appeared to persist for a long period, although no aggravation of the infection-induced mucosal transformation was found when eustachian tube obstruction persisted after recovery from the infective process.

The isolated effect of eustachian tube obstruction on the middle ear mucosa could only be studied in a reliable way with the use of germfree animals, where supervening infection could be successfully excluded. The induced changes are mainly characterized by a basal cell hyperplasia and stratification of the epithelium, while no change in the number and location of the secretory cells was found. The accumulated fluid retained its serous character for up to 2 years. Remarkably, new bone formation, accumulation of cholesterol, tympanosclerosis, and signs of squamous metaplasia—usually attributed to infective processes—were found to occur in induced sterile OME.

These observations convincingly demonstrate that eustachian tube obstruction without supervening infection does not result in a transformation of the middle ear epithelium into a highly secretory active epithelium. The striking resemblance between the observed changes in the mucosa of experimentally induced eustachian tube obstruction with supervening infection and those described in the mucosa of patients with OME favors the major role of infection in the transformation of the mucosa.

In addition to this established direct effect of bacteria on the middle ear mucosa, an alternative mode of bacterial involvement in OME has been proposed. According to this hypothesis, bacterial antigens are assumed to elicit nonspecific immune responses, resulting in mucosal inflammation. However, although all ingredients have been shown to be present in some effusions, immunopathogenesis and OME still remain to be determined.

It can be concluded that since there is no direct relationship between eustachian tube obstruction and the mucosal transformation in OME, obstruction or malfunctioning can be assumed to contribute to the maintenance of the inflammation by retention of inflammatory products and/or facilitating the entrance of bacteria and antigens from the nasopharynx into the middle ear.

REFERENCES

1. Akaan-Penttilä, E. (1982): Middle ear mucosa in newborn infants. *Acta Otolaryngol.*, 93:251.
2. Arnold, W., and Vosteen, K.H. (1975): Die Reaktion der Mittelohrschleimhaut bei Tubenverschluss. *Acta Otolaryngol.* (Suppl.), 330:48.
3. Bak-Pedersen, K., and Tos, M. (1973): Density of mucous glands in various chronic middle ear diseases. *Acta Otolaryngol.*, 75:273.
4. Beck, K. (1920): Über Mittelohrveränderungen bei experimenteller Läsion der Tube. *Z. Ohrenheilk.*, 78:83.
5. Beek, J.M.H. van der, and Kuijpers, W. (1984): The mucoperiosteum of the middle ear in experimentally induced otitis media. *Acta Otolaryngol.* (Suppl.), 414:71.
6. Bendek, G.A. (1963): Histopathology of transudatory-secretory otitis media. *Arch. Otolaryngol.*, 78:49.
7. Bernstein, J.M., and Hayes, E.R. (1971): Middle ear mucosa in health and disease. *Arch. Otolaryngol.*, 94:30.
8. Bernstein, J.M., Hayes, E.R., Ishikawa, T., Tomasi, T.B., and Herd, J.K. (1972): Secretory otitis media; a histopathologic and immunochemical report. *Trans. Am. Acad. Ophthalmol. Otol.*, 76:1305.
9. Bernstein, J.M., and Reisman, R. (1974): The role of acute hypersensitivity in secretory otitis media. *Trans. Am. Acad. Ophthalmol. Otol.*, 78:120.
10. Bernstein, J.M. (1976): Biological mediators of inflammation in middle ear effusions. *Ann. Otol. Rhinol. Laryngol.*, 85 (Suppl. 25):90.
11. Bernstein, J.M. (1979): Immune mechanisms in otitis media with effusion. In: *Secretory Otitis Media and Its Sequelae,* edited by J. Sadé, pp. 154–170. Churchill Livingstone, New York.
12. Bernstein, J.M. (1984): Observations on immune mechanisms in otitis media with effusion. *Int. J. Pediatr. Otorhinolaryngol.*, 8:125.
13. Birken, E.A., and Brookler, K.H. (1972): Surface tension lowering substance of the canine eustachian tube. *Ann. Otol. Rhinol. Laryngol.*, 81:268.
14. Blegvad, N.R. (1931): Faut il maintenir "l-occlusion de la trompe" comme une maladie indépendante? *Acta Otolaryngol.*, 16:429.
15. Bluestone, C.D. (1983): Eustachian tube function; physiology, pathophysiology, and role of allergy in pathogenesis of otitis media. *J. Allerg. Clin. Immunol.*, 72:242.
16. Broek, P. van den, Beek, J.M.H. van der, and Kuijpers, W. (1983): Effect of tubal occlusion on bone formation in the middle ear of the rat. ORL *J. Otorhinolaryngol. Relat. Spec.*, 45:87.
17. Cantekin, E.I., Bluestone, C.D., Saez, C.A., Doyle, W.J., and Philips, D.C. (1977): Normal and abnormal middle ear ventilation. *Ann. Otol. Rhinol. Laryngol.*, 86 (Suppl. 41):1.

18. Cantekin, E.I., Doyle, W.J., Reichert, T.J., Philips, D.C., and Bluestone, C.D. (1979): Dilation of the eustachian tube by electrical stimulation of the mandibular nerve. *Ann. Otol. Rhinol. Laryngol.*, 88:40.
19. Cantekin, E.I., Philips, D.C., Doyle, W.J., Bluestone, C.D., and Kimes, K.K. (1980): Effect of surgical alterations of the tensor veli palatini muscle on eustachian tube function. *Ann. Otol. Rhinol. Laryngol.*, 89 (Suppl. 68):47.
20. Claus, G. (1930): Experimentelle Studien über den Verschluss der Tuba Eustachii beim Hunde. *Z. H.N.O. Heilk.*, 26:143.
21. Clemis, J.D., Shambaugh, G.E., and Derlacki, E.L. (1966): Withdrawal reactions in chronic food addiction as related to chronic secretory otitis media. *Ann. Otol. Rhinol. Laryngol.*, 75:793.
22. Doyle, W.J. (1984): Functional eustachian tube obstruction and otitis media in a primate model. *Acta Otolaryngol.*, (Suppl.), 414:52.
23. Forschner, L. (1925): Über den sogenannten sekretorischen Mittelohrkatarh. *Z. H.N.O. Heilk.*, 12:477.
24. Friedman, I. (1963): The pathology of secretory otitis media. *Proc. R. Soc. Med.*, 56:695.
25. Goycoolea, M.V., Paparella, M.M., Carpenter, A.M., and Juhn, S.K. (1979): A longitudinal study of cellular changes in experimental otitis media. *Otolaryngol. Head Neck Surg.*, 87:685.
26. Gundersen, T. and Glück, E. (1972): The middle ear mucosa in serous otitis media. *Arch. Otolaryngol.*, 96:40.
27. Hagan, E. (1977): Surface tension lowering substance in eustachian tube function. *Laryngoscope*, 87:1033.
28. Healy, G.B., and Teele, D.W. (1977): The microbiology of chronic middle ear effusions in children. *Laryngoscope*, 87:1472.
29. Heisse, J.W. (1963): Secretory otitis media. Treatment with depomethylprednisolone. *Laryngoscope*, 73:54.
30. Hentzer, E. (1970): Histologic studies of the normal mucosa in the middle ear, mastoid process and eustachian tube. *Ann. Otol. Rhinol. Laryngol.*, 79:825.
31. Hentzer, E. (1972): Ultrastructure of the middle ear mucosa in secretory otitis media. I. Serous effusion. *Acta Otolaryngol.*, 73:394.
32. Hentzer, E. (1972): Ultrastructure of the middle ear mucosa in secretory otitis media. II. Mucous effusion. *Acta Otolaryngol.*, 73:467.
33. Hentzer, E. (1976): Ultrastructure of the middle ear mucosa. *Ann. Otol. Rhinol. Laryngol.*, 85 (Suppl. 25):30.
34. Holmgren, G. (1934): Recherches experimentales sur les fonctions de la trompe d'eustache. *Acta Otolaryngol.*, 20:381.
35. Holmgren, G. (1940): Experimental tubar occlusion. *Acta Otolaryngol.*, 28:587.
36. Honjo, I., Okazaki, N., and Kumazawa, T. (1979): Experimental study of the eustachian tube function with regard to its related muscles. *Acta Otolaryngol.*, 87:84.
37. Hussl, B., and Lim, D.J. (1969): Secretory cells in the middle ear mucosa of the guinea pig. *Arch. Otolaryngol.*, 89:33.
38. Hussl, B., and Lim, D.J. (1974): Experimental middle ear effusions: an immuno-fluorescent study. *Ann. Otol. Rhinol. Laryngol.*, 83:332.
39. Juhn, S.K., Huff, J.S., and Paparella, M.M. (1971): Biochemical analysis of middle ear effusions. *Ann. Otol. Rhinol. Laryngol.*, 80:347.
40. Juhn, S.K., Paparella, M.M., Kim, L.S., Goycoolea, M.V., and Giebink, S. (1977): Pathogenesis of otitis media. *Ann. Otol. Rhinol. Laryngol.*, 86:481.
41. Juhn, S.K. (1982): Studies on middle ear effusions. *Laryngoscope*, 92:287.
42. Karja, J., Jokinen, K., and Seppala, A. (1977): Temporal bone findings in the late stage of secretory otitis media. *J. Laryngol. Otol.*, 91:127.
43. Kuijpers, W., Beek, J.M.H. van der, and Wilart, E.C.T. (1979): The effect of experimental tubal obstruction on the middle ear. *Acta Otolaryngol.*, 87:345.
44. Kuijpers, W., and Beek, J.M.H. van der (1984): The mucoperiosteum of the middle ear in experimentally induced sterile otitis media. *Acta Otolaryngol.* (Suppl), 414:71.
45. Lim, D.J., and Hussl, B. (1969): Human middle ear epithelium. *Arch. Otolaryngol.*, 89:835.
46. Lim, D.J., and Hussl, B. (1970): Tympanic mucosa after tubal obstruction. *Arch. Otolaryngol.*, 91:585.
47. Lim, D.J., and Birck, H. (1971): Ultrastructural pathology of the middle ear mucosa in serous otitis media. *Ann. Otol. Rhinol. Laryngol.*, 80:838.

48. Lim, D.J., and Shimada, T. (1971): Secretory activity of normal middle ear epithelium. *Ann. Otol. Rhinol. Laryngol.*, 80:319.
49. Lim, D.J., Viall, J., Birck, H., and St. Pierre, R. (1972): The morphological basis for understanding middle ear effusions. *Laryngoscope*, 82:1625.
50. Lim, D.J., Shimada, T., and Yoder, M. (1973): Distribution of mucus-secreting cells in normal middle ear mucosa. *Arch. Otolaryngol.*, 98:2.
51. Lim, D.J. (1974): Functional morphology of the lining membrane of the middle ear and eustachian tube. *Ann. Otol. Rhinol. Laryngol.*, 83:5.
52. Lim, D.J., and Hussl, B. (1976): Macromolecular transport by the middle ear and its lymphatic system. *Acta Otolaryngol.*, 80:19.
53. Lim, D.J. (1976): Functional morphology of the mucosa of the middle ear and eustachian tube. *Ann. Otol. Rhinol. Laryngol.*, 85 (Suppl. 25):36.
54. Lim, D.J., Liu, Y.S., and Birck, H. (1976): Secretory lysozyme of the human middle ear mucosa; immunocytochemical localization. *Ann. Otol. Rhinol. Laryngol.*, 85:50.
55. Lim, D.J. (1979): Normal and pathological mucosa of the middle ear and eustachian tube. *Clin. Otolaryngol.*, 4:213.
56. Lim, D.J. (1979): Microbiology and cytology of otitis media with effusion. In: *Secretory Otitis Media and Its Sequelae*, edited by J. Sadé, pp. 125–143. Churchill Livingstone, New York.
57. Löwy, K. (1938): Zur Pathologie des sekretorischen Mittelohrkatarrhs. *Monatsschr. Ohrenheilk.*, 72:40.
58. Liu, Y.S., Lim, D.J., Lang, R.W., and Birck, H. (1975): Chronic middle ear effusions. *Arch. Otolaryngol.*, 101:278.
59. Lupovich, P., and Harkins, M. (1972): The pathophysiology of effusions in otitis media. *Laryngoscope*, 82:1647.
60. Main, Th.S., Shimada, T., and Lim, D.J. (1970): Experimental cholesterol granuloma. *Arch. Otolryngol.*, 91:356.
61. Maxim, D.E., Veltri, R.W., and Sprinkle, P.M. (1977): Chronic serous otitis media. An immune complex disease. *Trans. Am. Acad. Ophthalmol. Otol.*, 84:234.
62. McGovern, J.P., Haywood, Th.J., and Fernandez, A.A. (1967): Allergy and secretory otitis media. *J. Am. Med. Assoc.*, 200:134.
63. Meyerhoff, W.I., Giebink, G.S., and Shea, D. (1981): Pneumococcal otitis media following middle ear deflation. *Ann. Otol. Rhinol. Laryngol.*, 90:72.
64. Meyerhoff, W.L., and Giebink, G.S. (1982): Pathology and microbiology of otitis media. *Laryngoscope*, 92:273.
65. Mogi, G., Yoshida, T., Honjo, S., and Maeda, S. (1973): Middle ear effusions. Quantitative analysis of immunoglobulins. *Ann. Otol. Rhinol. Laryngol.*, 82:196.
66. Mogi, G., Honjo, S., Maeda, S., Yoshida, T., and Watanabe, N. (1974): Quantitative determination of secretory immunoglobulin A (S Iga) in middle ear effusions. *Ann Otol. Rhinol. Laryngol.*, 83:239.
67. Mogi, G., Honjo, S., Maeda, S., Yoshida, T., and Watanabe, N. (1974): Immunoglobulin E (IgE) in middle ear effusions. *Ann. Otol. Rhinol. Laryngol.*, 83:393.
68. Mravec, J., Lewis, D.M., and Lim, D.J. (1978): Experimental otitis media with effusion. An immune complex mediated response. *Trans. Am. Acad. Ophthalmol. Otol.*, 86:258.
69. Ogra, P.L., Bernstein, J.M., Yurchak, A.M., Coppola, P.R., and Tomasi, Th.B. (1974): Characteristics of secretory immunesystem in human middle ear; implications in otitis media. *J. Immunol.*, 112:488.
70. Ogra, P.L., and Bernstein, J.M. (1985): Mucosal defense system. In: *Immunobiology, Autoimmunity, Transplantation in Otorhinolaryngology*, edited by J.E. Veldman, B.F. McCabe, E.H. Huizing and N. Mygind, pp. 27–31. Kugler Publications, Amsterdam.
71. Okazaki, N., DeMaria, T.F., Briggs, B.R., and Lim, D.J. (1984): Experimental otitis media with effusion induced by nonviable *Hemophilus influenzae*. *Am. J. Otolaryngol.*, 5:80.
72. Palva, T., Karma, P., Palva, A., and Kärjä, J. (1975): Middle ear mucosa and chronic ear disease. *Arch. Otolaryngol.*, 101:380.
73. Palva, T., Holopainen, E., and Karma, P. (1976): Protein and cellular pattern of glue ear secretion. *Ann. Otol. Rhinol. Laryngol.*, 85 (Suppl. 25):103.
74. Paparella, M.M. (1964): Enzyme studies in serous otitis media. *Arch. Otolaryngol.*, 79:393.
75. Paparella, M.M., Juhn, S.K., Hiraide, F., and Kaneko, Y. (1970): Cellular events involved in middle ear fluid production. *Ann. Otol. Rhinol. Laryngol.*, 67:440.

76. Politzer, A. (1867): Diagnose und Therapie der Ansammlung seröser Flüssigkeit in der Trommelhöhle. *Wien. Med. Wochenschr.*, 17:244.
77. Politzer, A. (1883): *Diseases of the Ear,* edited by J.P. Cassels. Lea's Son and Co., Philadelphia.
78. Proud, G.O., and Odoi, H. (1970): Effects of eustachian tube ligation. *Ann. Otol. Rhinol. Laryngol.*, 79:30.
79. Proud, G.O., Odoi, H., and Toledo, P.S. (1971): Bullar pressure changes in eustachian tube dysfunction. *Ann. Otol. Rhinol. Laryngol.*, 80:835.
80. Rankin, J.D., and Karnody, C.S. (1970): Serous otitis media—an experimental model. *Arch. Otolaryngol.*, 92:14.
81. Rapp, D.J., and Fahey, D.J. (1975): Allergy and chronic otitis media. *Pediatr. Clin. North Am.*, 22:259.
82. Rapport, Ph.N., Lim, D.J., and Weiss, H.S. (1976): Evidence of surface active agent in the eustachian tube. *Ann. Otol. Rhinol. Laryngol.*, 85 (Suppl. 25):169.
83. Reiner, C., and Pulec, J.L. (1969): Experimental production of serous otitis media. *Ann. Otol. Rhinol. Laryngol.*, 78:880.
84. Ryan, A.F., Cleveland, P.H., Hartman, M.T. and Catanzaro, A. (1982): Humoral and cell-mediated immunity in peripheral blood following introduction of antigen into the middle ear. *Ann. Otol. Rhinol. Laryngol.*, 91:70.
85. Ryan, A.F. and Vogel, C.W. (1984): Complement deprivation by cobra venom factor: effect on immune-mediated middle ear effusion and inflammation. In: *Recent Advances in Otitis Media with Effusion,* edited by D.J. Lim, C.D. Bluestone, and J.D. Nelson, pp. 166–168. B.C. Decker, Philadelphia.
86. Sadé, J. (1966): Middle ear mucosa. *Arch. Otolaryngol.*, 84:137.
87. Sadé, J. (1967): Ciliary activity and middle ear clearance. *Arch. Otolaryngol.*, 86:128.
88. Sala, O., and De Stefani, G. (1963): Modifications caused by the occlusion of the tube on the mucosa of the middle ear, their prevention by corticosteroids. *Laryngoscope,* 73:320.
89. Salen, B., Hellström, S., and Stenfors, L.E. (1984): Experimentally induced otitis media with effusion. *Acta Otolaryngol.* (Suppl.) 414:67.
90. Scheibe, A. (1892): Zur Pathogenese der Transudatbildung im Mittelohr bei Tubenverschluss. *Z. Ohrenheilk.*, 23:62.
91. Senturia, B.H., Gessert, G.F., Carr, Ch.D., and Baumann, E.S. (1958): Studies concerned with tubotympanitis. *Ann. Otol. Rhinol. Laryngol.*, 67:440.
92. Senturia, B.H., Carr, Ch.D., and Ahlvin, R.C. (1962): Middle ear effusions: pathologic changes of the mucoperiosteum in the experimental animal. *Ann. Otol. Rhinol. Laryngol.*, 71:632.
93. Senturia, B.H., Carr, Ch.D., and Rosenblit, B. (1962): Middle ear effusions produced experimentally in dogs. *Acta Otolaryngol.*, 54:383.
94. Siirala, U. (1957): The problem of sterile otitis media. *Pract. Otorhinolaryngol.*, 19:159.
95. Silverstein, H., Miller, G.F., and Lindeman, R.C. (1966): Eustachian tube dysfunction as a cause for chronic secretory otitis in children. *Laryngoscope,* 76:259.
96. Sprinkle, P.M., and Veltri, R.W. (1976): Secretory otitis media: an immune complex disease. *Ann. Otol. Rhinol. Laryngol.*, 85 (Suppl. 25): 135.
97. Stenfors, L.E., Hellström, S., Salen, B. and Söderberg, O. (1984): Appearance of effusion material in the attic space correlated with an impaired eustachian tube function. In: *Recent Advances in Otitis Media with Effusion,* edited by D.J. Lim, C.D. Bluestone, J.O. Klein, and J.D. Nelson, pp. 233–237. B.C. Decker, Philadelphia.
98. Terrahé, K. (1970): *Die Drüsen des respiratorischen Nasenschleimhaut.* Gustav Fischer Verlag, Stuttgart.
99. Tos, M. (1970): Development of mucous glands in the human eustachian tube. *Acta Otolaryngol.*, 70:340.
100. Tos, M. (1971): Goblet cells in the human fetal eustachian tube. *Arch. Otolaryngol.*, 93:365.
101. Tos, M. and Bak-Pedersen, K. (1972): The pathogenesis of chronic secretory otitis media. *Arch. Otolaryngol.*, 95:511.
102. Tos, M., and Bak-Pedersen, K. (1973): Density of mucous glands in a biopsy material of chronic secretory otitis media. *Acta Otolaryngol.*, 75:55.
103. Tos, M., and Bak-Pedersen, K. (1975): Density of goblet cells in chronic secretory otitis media: findings in a biopsy material. *Laryngoscope,* 85:377.

104. Tos, M. and Bak-Pedersen, K. (1976): Goblet cell population in the normal middle ear and eustachian tube of children and adults. *Ann. Otol. Rhinol. Laryngol.*, 85 (Suppl. 25):44.
105. Tos, M., and Bak-Pedersen, K. (1976): Secretory otitis. Histopathology and goblet cell density in the eustachian tube and middle ear in children. *J. Laryngol. Otol.*, 90:475.
106. Tos, M. (1981): Experimental tubal obstruction. Changes in the middle ear mucosa elucidated by quantitative histology. *Acta Otolaryngol.*, 92:51.
107. Veltri, R.W., and Sprinkle, Ph.M. (1973): Serous otitis media. *Ann. Otol. Rhinol. Laryngol.*, 82:297.
108. Weekes, D.J. (1958): Secretory otitis media and nasal allergy. *Arch. Otolaryngol.*, 68:78.
109. Zaufall, E. (1870): Über das Vorkommen seröser Flüssigkeit in der Paukenhöhöhle (otitis media serosa). *Arch. Ohrenheilk.*, 5:38.
110. Zechner, G. (1976): Die Reaktionsformen der Mittelohrschleimhaut. *Acta Otolaryngol.*, 81:78.

Immunology of the Ear, edited by J. Bernstein
and P. Ogra. Raven Press, New York © 1987.

Bacteriology of Otitis Media

*Tasnee Chonmaitree and **Virgil M. Howie

**Division of Infectious Diseases and **Division of Ambulatory Pediatrics, University of Texas Medical Branch, Galveston, Texas 77550*

Selection of appropriate antimicrobial therapy for otitis media (OM) requires identification of its causative agents. Since the early 1900s, this information has been provided by bacterial culture of middle ear fluids (MEFs) obtained by needle aspiration, even though approximately 30% of patients with acute OM and a higher percentage of patients with chronic OM have no bacteria isolated from MEFs (62,91). Recently, studies using other microbiologic tests, such as anaerobic bacterial culture, chlamydial and viral cultures, and bacterial and viral antigen detection, have been used to test MEFs from patients for whom standard aerobic bacterial cultures were negative. The results from these additional tests provide a better understanding of the microbiology of OM. This chapter reviews the bacteriology of various types of OM, with an emphasis on the literature published since 1970.

ACUTE OTITIS MEDIA

Summary of Bacteriological Data

Numerous studies of the bacteriology of acute OM have been reported since the beginning of this century. Although the criteria for patient enrollment, detailed microbiological procedures, and definitions of pathogenic organisms vary, the results have been remarkably consistent in demonstrating the importance of *Streptococcus pneumoniae* and *Haemophilus influenzae* as pathogens (61,91). Table 1 summarizes data on the bacteriology of acute OM in infants and children (0–14 years of age) compiled from 10 studies published between 1970 and 1986 from diverse geographic locations.

Acute Otitis Media in Infants Less than 6 Weeks of Age

In the OM literature, different pathogens have been reported in various population groups among neonates and young infants. Table 2 summarizes data from studies examining the bacteriology of OM in infants less than 6 weeks of age.

TABLE 1. *Bacteriology of acute otitis media: compilation of 10 studies (3,163 cases) published between 1970 and 1985*[a]

Author, year (reference)	No. of cases	Percent of cases showing specific bacteria							
		S. pneu.	H. infl.	Branh.	S. aur.	Str. A	Others[b]	Mixed[c]	NG
Howie et al., 1970 (40)	858	34	20	8[d]	0[e]	3	2	4	30
Howie and Ploussard, 1971 (43)	280	36	23	0[f]	0[e]	1	0	3	38
Howie et al., 1974 (45)	157	35	31	0[f]	0[e]	2	4	0	28
Brook, 1979 (17)	186	24	18	0	3	5	32[g]	5	14
Shurin et al., 1980 (94)	132	37	20	6	2	2	1	5	29
Schwartz, 1981 (91)	1,092	28	31	0	2	2	5[h]	0	31
Shurin et al., 1983 (96)	145	25	17	16	1	1	0	7	34
Fujita et al., 1983 (32)	100	24	18	2	11	5	2	12	26
Marchant et al., 1984 (74)	129	25	19	13	0	1	0	9	33
Chonmaitree et al., 1986 (21)	84	20	20	5	4	0	21[i]	14	15
	Mean (%)	30	24	4	1	2	5	3	30

[a]S. pneu., *Streptococcus pneumoniae;* H. infl., *Haemophilus influenzae;* Branh., *Neisseria/Branhamella;* S. aur., *Staphylococcus aureus;* Str. A, group A β-streptococcus; NG, no growth or nonpathogens (*S. epidermidis*, α-streptococcus, diphtheroids, *Bacillus* sp., and *Candida* sp.).
[b]Others: Gram-negative bacilli, group B streptococcus, *N. meningitides, H. parainfluenzae,* and viruses.
[c]Mixed: Two or more listed pathogenic bacteria.
[d]Pure culture only.
[e]In these studies, *S. aureus* was considered a nonpathogen.
[f]In these studies, *Neisseria* was considered a nonpathogen.
[g]Including anaerobic bacteria; no sterilization of external ear canal performed.
[h]Including *Neisseria*.
[i]Fifteen bacteria and virus, two virus alone, one *Proteus mirabilis*.

TABLE 2. *Bacteriology of otitis media in infants younger than 6 weeks*[a]

Author, year (reference)	Location	No. of cases[b]	Percent of cases showing specific bacteria									
			S. pneu.	H. infl.	S. aur.	Strep. A.	Strep. B.	Branh.	G-rods[c]	G-rods +[d]	Mixed[e]	NG
Bland, 1972 (11)	Hawaii	21	5	5	14	0	0	0	38	19	0	19
Tetzlaff et al., 1977 (109)	Dallas	42	24	17	0	2	2	0	17	2	7	33
Shurin et al., 1978 (93)	Boston and Huntsville	70	13	11	4	1	3	11	4	1	9	41
	Mean (%)		15	12	5	2	2	6	14	5	7	35

[a]S. pneu., *Streptococcus pneumoniae;* H. infl., *Haemophilus influenzae;* S. aur., *Staphylococcus aureus;* Strep. A, group A β-hemolytic streptococci; Strep. B, group B streptococci; Branh., *Neisseria/Branhamella;* NG, no growth and nonpathogens.

[b]Total number of cases is 133.

[c]Including *Escherichia coli, Klebsiella pneumoniae, Proteus mirabilis, Enterobacter aerogenes,* and *Pseudomonas aeruginosa*.

[d]Gram-negative bacilli plus other listed pathogens.

[e]Two or more pathogens, not including Gram-negative bacilli.

In 1971, Bland (11) reported from Hawaii that enteric gram-negative bacilli and *Staphylococcus aureus* were important pathogens in this age group. A subsequent study from Dallas revealed a much lower incidence of enteric bacilli and regarded *S. aureus* as a nonpathogen, since the organism was never found in pure culture (109). Shurin et al. (93), reporting from Boston and Alabama, showed a relatively higher number of cases caused by *S. pneumoniae* and *H. influenzae,* which these authors judged to be the most important causes of OM in this age group, a result similar to those reported for older infants. Other studies suggest that the subset of infants whose OM is caused by gram-negative enteric bacilli is likely to consist of younger infants in neonatal intensive care units who have prolonged nasotracheal intubation (6,7). Older infants living at home are more likely to have the common respiratory pathogens.

Streptococcus pneumoniae

Streptococcus pneumoniae is the most common agent in all age groups and accounts for 20% to 37% of cases of acute OM (Table 1). Studies using rapid pneumococcal antigen detection such as latex agglutination, counterimmunoelectrophoresis, or radioimmunoassay suggest that *S. pneumoniae* may be responsible for up to 60% of cases of acute OM (66,73). Pneumococcal antigen was detected in 15% to 25% of MEFs that yielded no organism by standard aerobic cultures. Repeated cultures in patients treated with placebo also showed an increase in *S. pneumoniae* isolations (42).

Data from serotypes of *S. pneumoniae* isolated from MEFs of children with acute OM are shown in Table 3. Serotypes 3, 6, 14, 18, 19, and 23 account for two-thirds of the pneumococcal otitis episodes. Another 10 serotypes, 1, 4, 7 to 11, 15, 23, and 35 account for an additional 30%. Only 6% to 7% of cases of pneumococcal OM were caused by other serotypes (3,28,35,53,62). Because the majority of the common serotypes causing OM are included in pneumococcal polysaccharide vaccines, these vaccines have been used to prevent recurrent OM. Octavalent vaccine, the vaccine composed of purified, capsular polysaccharide antigens of eight serotypes (Danish 1, 3, 6, 7, 14, 18, 19, and 23), was studied. The vaccine was given to children at 6 to 21 months of age who had had at least one episode of OM before the age of 10 months, in order to prevent recurrent OM (47,48,104). When compared to tests of the control vaccine (containing serotypes 2,4,5,8,9,12,25), use of the octavalent vaccine correlated with a lowered incidence of recurrent OM, especially among black children. This octavalent vaccine, however, was never licensed for clinical use. The first available pneumococcal polysaccharide vaccine, the 14-valent polysaccharide vaccine, was first licensed in 1977. This vaccine contained antigens of Danish serotypes 1 to 4, 6A, 7F, 8, 9N, 12F, 14, 18C, 19F, 23F, and 25. A study from Sweden showed that the vaccine was effective in prevention of recurrent OM in children 2 to 5 years of age, but had no effect on children under 2 years of age (84). The current pneumococcal vaccine, which was licensed in 1983 and replaced the previous vaccine, contains antigens to 23 serotypes: 1 to 5, 6B, 7F, 8, 9N, 9V, 10A, 11A, 12F, 14, 15B,

TABLE 3. *Serotypes of* S. pneumoniae *isolated from middle ear fluids of children with acute otitis media*[a]

Serotype[b]	Number of strains	Percentage
1	38	2.0
3	161	8.6
4	65	3.5
6	220	11.8
7	44	2.4
8	28	1.5
9	55	3.0
10	27	1.4
11	35	1.9
14	196	10.5
15	60	3.2
18	109	5.8
19	429	23.0
22	33	1.8
23	232	12.4
35	20	1.1
Others	115	6.2
Totals	1,867	100

[a]Data compiled from refs. 3,28,35,53, modified from ref. 62.
[b]Danish classification; all types mentioned except type 35 are in 23-valent pneumococcal polysaccharide vaccine.

17F, 18C, 19A, 19F, 20, 22F, 23F, and 33F (1). A study of the current 23-valent pneumococcal vaccine for prevention of recurrent otitis media is presently being performed by one of us (Howie and co-workers).

Haemophilus influenzae

Approximately one-fourth of MEFs from children with acute OM reveals *H. influenzae*. The incidence increases in OM, which is unresponsive to initial antibiotic therapy (105,108) or associated with purulent conjunctivitis (conjunctivitis-otitis syndrome) (12,13). Although it is generally believed that *H. influenzae* does not commonly cause infection in children older than 5 years of age, several studies have documented the importance of the organism in OM in that age group (40,87,89). Nonencapsulated, nontypable strains of *H. influenzae* account for 85% to 90% of the cases that test positive for this organism; the remaining 10% to 15% of cases appear to be caused mainly by the encapsulated type b organism (55,91,92), although other encapsulated types (a,c to f) have been reported (51). The emergence of β-lactamase-positive, ampicillin-resistant *H. influenzae* was recognized in 1973. Since then, the incidence of ampicillin-resistant *H. influenzae* in OM has been increasing (Table 4) to become fairly widespread at present. Approximately 15% to 20% of *H. influenzae* currently isolated from MEFs from our patients in Galveston are ampicillin-resistant.

Branhamella catarrhalis

The role of *Branhamella catarrhalis* (formerly known as *Neisseria catarrhalis*) in the pathogenesis of OM has been controversial because the organism is a normal inhabitant of the nasopharynx and, in MEF cultures, the organism is often mixed with other pathogens. Some early reports on bacteriologic findings in MEFs obtained by needle aspiration listed *B. catarrhalis* as a nonpathogen (30,43,45,91), whereas others considered the organism in pathogen (22,23,36). The significance of *B. catarrhalis* as a pathogen causing systemic disease, including OM, has been recognized since 1981 (27,67).

Reports that *B. catarrhalis* is universally sensitive to ampicillin (52) have recently been challenged (64,65,96). As many as 77% of *B. catarrhalis* strains causing OM have been found to produce β-lactamase, which makes the organism ampicillin-resistant (96). Current studies on the bacteriology of OM ranked *B. catarrhalis* as the third most common causative organism, following only *S. pneumoniae* and *H. influenzae* in incidence. It accounts for 17% to 20% of cases of OM in the studies performed after 1980 (66,96,97). Acute OM caused by *B. catarrhalis* is less common in spring and summer, and the disease is milder than that associated with other bacteria.

Other Middle Ear Pathogens

Group A β-hemolytic streptococcus, *Streptococcus pyogenes,* is the cause of less than 5% of OM cases in the United States (Table 1), but in Europe and Australia it is a more frequent cause of OM, especially in older children with a preceding pharyngitis (10,28,36).

Staphylococcus aureus is an organism whose role as a middle ear pathogen is controversial. Although some investigators consider the organism a nonpathogen (40,45,109), others believe the organism can cause OM (17,32,91,94,96). Since *S. aureus* is a normal inhabitant of nasopharynx and the skin of the external audi-

TABLE 4. *Ampicillin resistance of middle ear isolates of* H. influenzae *obtained in Huntsville, Alabama 1970–1977*[a]

Year	Number of isolates	Resistant strains	Percentage of ampicillin-resistant strains
1970–1972	290	0	0
1973	162	1	0.6
1974	200	2	1.0
1975	209	3	1.4
1976	214	6	2.8
1977	66[b]	9	13.6

[a]Compiled from refs. 105 and 106.
[b]To April 30.

tory canal, it can be considered a significant contributor to OM only if it is recovered from middle ear aspirates, but not from culture of the external canal.

Although most investigators believe that coagulase-negative staphylococcus, *Staphylococcus epidermidis,* is nonpathogenic, it may under certain conditions cause OM. Feigin et al. (29) were able to isolate *S. epidermidis* in pure culture from purulent MEF in 10 of 130 children with acute OM. The organism was not isolated from a concomitant ear canal culture in 5 of the 10 children. All patients were febrile and showed clinical signs and symptoms of middle ear infection. In addition to pure culture, the Gram smear and stain of the purulent fluids revealed Gram-positive cocci within the polymorphonuclear leukocytes. *S. epidermidis* should be considered a pathogen when the organism is isolated in pure culture of MEF, not isolated from external ear canal culture, and when Gram staining of the MEF demonstrates Gram-positive cocci within polymorphonuclear leukocytes.

Gram-negative bacilli are an infrequent cause of acute OM. It is generally believed that the organisms are more common in acute OM in neonates and young infants. Schwartz and Brook (90) reported 11 of 1,143 children with acute OM caused by Gram-negative bacilli; all were more than 14 months old. Gram-negative OM fails to respond to initial empirical antimicrobial therapy designed for *S. pneumoniae* and *H. influenzae*.

The role of anaerobic bacteria in the pathogenesis of acute OM is uncertain. Brook and co-workers (16,17) reported that anaerobic bacteria were isolated from 27% to 41% of MEFs from children with acute OM and almost half of these fluids yielded only anaerobic bacteria. Among the organisms found were *Peptococci, Peptostreptococci, Propionibacterium acnes,* and *Clostridium sp*. These organisms are inhabitants of the skin and nasopharynx, and the reported studies did not include sterilization of the tympanic membranes prior to tympanocentesis or comparison of organisms isolated from middle ear and external ear canal. Therefore, the isolation might represent only contamination from external ear flora. However, Moloy (76) recently argued for the pathogenicity of some anaerobic bacteria. He reported two cases of acute suppurative OM and mastoiditis caused by *Fusobacterium virium* in one case and *Bacteriodes fragilis, B. melanogenicus,* and *Peptococci* in another. Both patients had prolonged and complicated courses of illness.

Sterile Effusions

Nearly one-third of cultures performed on middle ear aspirates from patients with acute OM appear to be bacteria-free (''sterile'') or contain nonpathogens. These cases are clinically and otoscopically indistinguishable from the culture-positive cases. The data suggest nonbacterial causes such as viruses, chlamydia, and mycoplasma. Earlier studies searching for viruses and mycoplasma by tissue culture techniques have yielded little information (60). Recent studies using rapid viral antigen detection, however, support the etiologic role of viruses in the pathogenesis of acute OM (59,86). The study by Chonmaitree et al. (21), using current tissue culture methods for viral isolation, revealed that 20% of MEFs from children with acute OM contain viruses, and that viruses alone can cause acute OM. The role of *Chlamydia trachomatis* in the pathogenesis of acute OM was suggested when chlamydia was isolated from the middle ear of infants with pneumonia (110). Subsequently, chlamydiae were cultured from MEFs in a small number of children with either acute or chronic OM (20,58). With the more effective diagnostic techniques currently available, it is likely that increasing numbers of pathogens causing acute OM will be identified.

Antibody Activity in Acute Otitis Media

Children with acute OM are capable of inducing both local and systemic synthesis of antibodies specific for the causative organism (44,99,100,103). Older children are more capable of producing antibodies than are younger children (63,100). Specific IgG, IgM, IgA, and IgE antibodies have been found in acute and convalescent sera as well as MEFs. IgG was most often found in sera. IgA, if present, was more likely to occur in the MEFs (14,63,99–101). Higher concentrations of antibodies in MEFs are correlated with more rapid clearing of middle ear effusion (102).

The association between the presence of specific antibody and protection against OM caused by the specified organism requires further investigation to determine if antibodies found in acute sera existed before the onset of the infection, or were produced by an immune response to that infection. Only in the latter case could the antibody be interpreted to act against OM. Shurin et al. (95) found that children who had acute OM caused by a nontypable *H. influenzae* strain did not have antibody against this organism in their acute sera, but they developed an antibody response following the infection. These authors suggested that the absence of antibody might be associated with susceptibility to the infection.

RELATIONSHIP BETWEEN BACTERIOLOGIC FINDINGS IN THE MIDDLE EAR FLUIDS AND NASOPHARYNX

Bacteriologic studies of middle ear fluids have provided the only reliable source of information on the bacterial etiology of acute OM. Since the causative bacteria have been thought to ascend from the nasopharynx (NP) through the eustachian tube into the middle ear, attempts to culture bacteria from the NP seem logical. Early studies in the 1950s to 1960s evaluating the accuracy of NP culture in predicting the etiology of acute OM have demonstrated marginally useful (48–60%) correlations (10,30,77,79). Results from NP culture are difficult to interpret because the same bacteria are cultured from the NP of both healthy and sick children, and the nasopharyngeal flora are polymicrobial in nature. However, data from recent studies using both nonquantitative and semiquantitative culture techniques are more encouraging (Table 5). Approximately 75% of cases of acute OM have the same bacterial pathogens isolated from both NP and MEF. Another 20% have mixed pathogens, including the pathogens found in MEF isolated from NP.

The correlation between nasopharyngeal colonization of *S. pneumoniae* and *H. influenzae* and development of OM is still unclear. One study from Finland suggested that children who were in day-care centers that colonized *S. pneumoniae* and *H. influenzae* in NP were not at increased risk for the development of acute OM (82). Another study from Sweden suggested that otitis-prone children who were colonized with *H. influenzae* in NP were at higher risk of developing otitis media compared to those who were colonized with *S. pneumoniae* (31).

DISPARATE CULTURES OF MIDDLE EAR FLUIDS

Disparate results of bacterial cultures of MEFs obtained from children with bilateral OM have been reported by several investigators. In the majority of cases, culture of the MEF is bacteriologically sterile in one ear, whereas pathogenic bacteria are cultured from the other. In some instances, bacterial pathogens isolated from each ear are different. In a series of 122 children with bilateral acute OM, Pelton et al. (81) reported disparate results in one-fourth of the cases. These data suggest that bacteriologic study of acute OM must include aspiration from both ears.

RECURRENT OTITIS MEDIA

Recurrent episodes of acute OM are rather common. Data from bacteriologic studies of recurrent acute OM are similar to those obtained from unselected episodes, except that a slight predominance of *H. influenzae* over other organisms has been reported in the recurrent disease (46,57,70). Recurrences of OM within 1 month have a significant chance of being caused by the same organism, whereas

TABLE 5. *Correlation of nasopharynx and middle ear cultures*[a]

Author, year (reference)	Number of cases	MEF path.[b]	Same NP path.[c]	Percentage having complete correlation	NP Path. +[d]	Percentage having partial correlation	MEF path. not NP[e]	Percentage having no correlation
Howie et al., 1971 (41)	288	182[f]	135	74	179	98	3	1.6
Kamme et al., 1971 (54)	75	60[g]	28	47	59	98	1	1.7
Branefors-Helander et al., 1975 (15)	36	16	NA[i]	NA[i]	15	94	1	6.3
Schwartz et al., 1979 (88)	225	153[h]	124	81	133	87	17	11.1
Totals	624	411	287	73[j]	386	94[j]	22	5.4[j]

[a]MEF, middle ear fluid; NP, nasopharynx; path., pathogens.
[b]Number of cases with pathogens in MEF.
[c]Number of cases with the same pathogens in MEF and NP.
[d]Same pathogen was isolated from both middle ear and nasopharynx, and an additional pathogen was isolated from nasopharynx but not middle ear.
[e]Number of cases with pathogens in MEF, but not in NP.
[f]Path.: *S. pneumoniae, H. influenzae,* group A streptococcus.
[g]Path.: *S. pneumoniae, H. influenzae,* + *Neisseria* sp.
[h]Path.: bacteria mentioned above + *S. aureus*.
[i]NA, not available.
[j]Mean.

later recurrences are usually caused by a different organism (22,39,42,70,78). In studies for which serotyping of *S. pneumoniae* was performed (3,66), all recurrences within 14 days represented infection with organisms of the same serotype. Similarly, the majority of children who experienced *H. influenzae* OM within 1 month were also infected with the same biotype, but late recurrences were usually the result of infection with a new organism (5). However, small numbers of children had late recurrences with the original strains, a result which suggests that strain-specific protective immunity might not develop uniformly during recovery from *H. influenzae* otitis.

CHRONIC OTITIS MEDIA WITH EFFUSION

Otitis media that is persistent for more than 8 weeks is termed *chronic OM*. Chronic middle ear effusions are generally classified into three categories: serous, mucous, and purulent (75). The results of recent studies of bacteriology of chronic OM with effusion suggest that the MEF of asymptomatic children with persistent effusion harbor bacterial pathogens (Table 6). Bacteria were isolated from approximately half of the specimens, and half of them demonstrated common pathogens causing acute OM. In addition, bacteria were seen in 15% to 17% of the Gram-stained smears of the sterile effusions (34,72). Bacterial endotoxin has also been discovered in a number of chronic middle ear effusions (9,25). Common pathogenic bacteria include *H. influenzae* (~25%), *S. pneumoniae* (9%), and *S. aureus* (1%). Other bacteria that account for the smaller number of cases are *B. catarrhalis, S. pyogenes,* and Gram-negative bacilli including *Pseudomonas* (69,71,72,83). Certain biotypes (II and III) account for the majority of the cases of nontypable *H. influenzae* (26). The role of anaerobic bacteria in chronic OM is still debatable. In earlier studies, anaerobic bacteria were isolated from 33% to 58% of the persistent effusions and in 15% of these effusions, the organisms were found in pure culture (18,33,49,56). Unfortunately, these studies did not include methods to sterilize the tympanic membrane prior to tympanocentesis. Therefore

TABLE 6. *Types of effusions and bacterial findings in chronic otitis media*[a]

Type of effusion	Number of specimens	Number that tested positive for bacteria	Percentage
Mucous	207	81	39
Serous	114	63	55
Purulent	75	48	64
Total	396	192	48[b]

[a]Data compiled from refs. 71, 72, and 83. All children received no antibiotic within a month prior to tympanocentesis. Anaerobic cultures were not performed in these studies.
[b]Mean.

some of the isolates might represent contamination from the external ear canal or the tympanic membrane. Teele et al. (107) used sterilization of the external ear canal and the tympanic membrane prior to tympanocentesis and did not recover anaerobic bacteria from any of the 30 samples of persistent effusion tested. However, Brook (19), using a similar method, found pure anaerobic bacteria in 13% and mixed anaerobic with aerobic bacteria in another 38% of MEFs from 68 children with chronic OM. The majority of anaerobic organisms, including *Peptococci, Peptostreptococci, Bacteroides,* and anaerobic Gram-positive bacilli, were isolated from MEF but not from external ear canals.

It is clear that persistent ear effusions may harbor potentially pathogenic bacteria even when there is no sign of inflammation (98). These organisms appear to be capable of stimulating local and systemic immune responses. Lewis et al. (68) reported that 80% of middle ear effusions and 86% of sera from patients with chronic OM contained specific antibody to the bacteria isolated. The antibodies were of IgG, IgM, and IgA classes. IgG was the antibody most commonly found in sera, whereas IgA was most often found in the effusions. The significance of these immune responses in the pathogenesis of chronic OM is yet to be determined.

The role of coagulase-negative staphylococci in middle ear infection has drawn relatively little attention, even though these organisms may be the most frequent isolates from long-standing middle ear effusions. Bernstein et al. (8) have demonstrated these organisms to be the most common single isolate for middle ear effusions in chronic otitis media with effusion, particularly in patients who have been on antibiotics for a long period of time. However, when a multiple biochemical profile system and antibiotic resistance patterns are used, the results suggest that these organisms represent a heterogeneous group of bacteria. Using two classifications for coagulase-negative staphylococci, one can identify at least three or possibly four different subtypes of cocci. In general, these organisms are not contaminants; however, it is not presently possible to differentiate between their causing indolent colonization or representing true pathogens. It is suggested that further work in this area be performed to determine whether certain subtypes of coagulase-negative staphylococci are more frequently found in OM with effusion.

UNCOMMON BACTERIA CAUSING OTITIS MEDIA

A small number of cases of acute, recurrent, or chronic OM appear to be caused by uncommon or uncharacteristic bacteria. Noncholera vibrios were isolated in pure culture of MEFs from children with and without a history of exposure to seawater (4,80). *Pseudomonas putrefaciens* and *Pseudomonas multophilia* were recovered from patients with acute OM and acute OM with mastoiditis, respectively (37,38). Other Gram-negative bacteria that were isolated in pure culture from patients with OM include *Acinetobacter sp.* and *Achromobacter xylosoxidans sp.* (24,111). *Mycobacterium fortuitum* and *Mycobacterium tuberculosis* have also been found to cause OM (2,50,85). The infrequency of these isolations make them interesting but relatively unimportant clinically.

CONCLUSION

Streptococcus pneumoniae and *Haemophilus influenzae* continue to be the most frequently isolated bacteria from acute OM, with β-lactamase-producing *H. influenzae* becoming more common in some population groups. *Branhamella catarrhalis* and *Staphylococcus aureus* have generally been accepted as middle ear pathogens alone and in combination with other organisms. *Staphylococcus epidermidis* and anaerobic bacteria may also have some role in the etiology of OM. The role of viruses in middle ear disease has become more evident, with more sensitive methods of detection and the study of acute cases earlier in the course of the disease. In recurrent OM, the usual pathogens are present in somewhat different percentages as compared with those causing the acute form of OM. Persistent OM has been demonstrated not to be bacteriologically sterile in approximately 50% of MEFs cultured.

REFERENCES

1. American Academy of Pediatrics, Committee on Infectious Diseases (1985): Recommendations for using pneumonoccal vaccine in children. *Pediatrics,* 75:1153–1158.
2. Austin, W.K., and Lockey, M.W. (1976): *Mycobacterium fortuitum* mastoiditis. *Arch. Otolaryngol.,* 102:558–560.
3. Austrian, R., Howie, V.M., and Ploussard, J.H. (1977): The bacteriology of pneumococcal otitis media. *Johns Hopkins Med. J.,* 141:104–111.
4. Back, E., Ljunggren, A., and Smith, H., Jr. (1974): Non-cholera vibrios in Sweden. *Lancet,* I:723–724.
5. Barenkamp, S.J., Shurin, P.A., Marchant, C.D., Karasic, R.B., Pelton, S.I., Howie, V.M., and Granoff, D.M. (1984): Do children with recurrent *Haemophilus influenzae* otitis media become infected with a new organism or reacquire the original strain? *J. Pediatr.,* 105:553–537.
6. Berman, S.A., Balkany, T.J., and Simons, M.A. (1978): Otitis media in the neonatal intensive care unit. *Pediatrics,* 62:198–201.
7. Berman, S.A., Balkany, T.J., and Simons, M.A. (1978): Otitis media in infants less than 12 weeks of age: differing bacteriology among in-patients and out-patients: *J. Pediatr.,* 93:453–454.
8. Bernstein, J.M., Dryja, D., and Neter, E. (1982): The role of coagulase-negative staphylococci in chronic otitis media with effusion. *Otolaryngol. Head Neck Surg.,* 90:837–843.
9. Bernstein, J.M., Praino, M.D, and Neter, E. (1980): Detection of endotoxin in ear specimens from patients with chronic otitis media by means of the limulus amebocyte lysate test. *Can. J. Microbiol.,* 26:546–548.
10. Bjuggren, G., and Tunevall, G. (1952): Otitis in childhood: a clinical and serobacteriological study with special reference to the significance of *Haemophilus influenzae* in relapses. *Acta Otolaryngol.,* 17:311–328.
11. Bland, R.D. (1972): Otitis media in the first six weeks of life: diagnosis, bacteriology, and management. *Pediatrics,* 49:187–197.
12. Bodor, F.F. (1982): Conjunctivitis-otitis syndrome. *Pediatrics,* 69:695–698.
13. Bodor, F.F., Marchant, C.D., Shurin, P.A., and Barenkamp, S.J. (1985): Bacterial etiology of conjunctivitis-otitis media syndrome. *Pediatrics,* 76:26–28.
14. Branefors, P., Dahlberg, T., and Nylen, O. (1980): Study of antibody levels in children with purulent otitis media. *Ann. Otol. Rhinol. Laryngol.,* 89 (3 Suppl. 68, part 2): 117–120.

15. Branefors-Helander, P., Dahlberg, T., and Nylen, O. (1975): Acute otitis media: a clinical, bacteriological and serological study of children with frequent episodes of acute otitis media. *Acta Otolaryngol.,* 80:399–409.
16. Brook, I., Anthony, B.F., and Finegold, S.M. (1978): Aerobic and anaerobic bacteriology of acute otitis media in children. *J. Pediatr.,* 92:13–15.
17. Brook, I. (1979): Otitis media in children: a prospective study of aerobic and anaerobic bacteriology. *Larynogoscope,* 89:992–997.
18. Brook, I. (1979): Bacteriology and treatment of chronic otitis media. *Laryngoscope,* 89:1129–1134.
19. Brook, I. (1980): Chronic otitis media in children: Microbiological studies. *Am. J. Dis. Child.,* 134:564–566.
20. Chang, M.J., Rodriquez, W.J., and Mohla, C. (1982): *Chlamydia trachomatis* in otitis media in children. *Pediatr. Infect. Dis.,* 1:95–97.
21. Chonmaitree, T., Howie, V.M., and Truant, A.L. (1986): Presence of respiratory viruses in middle ear fluids and nasal wash specimens from children with acute otitis media. *Pediatrics,* 77:698–702.
22. Coffey, J.D. (1966): Otitis media in the practice of pediatrics: bacteriological and clinical observations. *Pediatrics,* 38:25–32.
23. Coffey, J.D., Martin, A.D., Booth, H.N., and Miss, N. (1967): *Neisseria catarrhalis* in exudate otitis media. *Arch. Otolaryngol.,* 86:403–406.
24. Dadswell, J.V. (1976): *Acinetobacter* and similar organisms in ear infections. *J. Med. Microbiol.,* 9:345–353.
25. DeMaria, T.F., Prior, R.B., Briggs, B.R., Lim, D.J., and Birck, H.G. (1984): Endotoxin in middle-ear effusions from patients with chronic otitis media with effusion. *J. Clin. Microbiol.,* 20:15–17.
26. DeMaria, T.F., Lim, D.J., Barnishan, J., Ayers, L.W., and Birck H.G. (1984): Biotypes of serologically nontypable *Haemophilus influenza* isolated from the middle ears and nasopharynges of patients with otitis media with effusion. *J. Clin. Microbiol.,* 20:1102–1104.
27. Doern, G.V., Miller, M.J., and Winn, R.E. (1981): *Branhamella (Neisseria) catarrhalis* systemic disease in humans: Case reports and review of the literature. *Arch. Intern. Med.,* 141:1690–1692.
28. Douglas, R.M., Miles, H., Hansman, D., Moore, B., and English, D.T. (1980): Microbiology of acute otitis media: with particular reference to the feasibility of pneumonococcal immunization. *Med. J. Aust.,* 1:263–266.
29. Feigin, R.D., Shackelford, P.G., Campbell, J., Lyles, T.O., Schecter, M., and Lins, R.D. (1973): Assessment of the role of *staphylococcus epidermidis* as a cause of otitis media. *Pediatrics,* 52:569–576.
30. Feingold, M., Klein, J.O., Haslam, G.E., Tilles, J.G., Finland, M., and Gellis, S.S. (1966): Acute otitis media in children: bacteriological findings in middle ear fluid obtained by needle aspiration. *Am. J. Dis. Child.,* 111:361–365.
31. Freijd, A., Bygdeman, S. and Rynnel-Dagoo, B. (1984): The nasopharyngeal microflora of otitis-prone children, with emphasis on *H. influenzae*. *Acta Otolaryngol.,* 97:117–126.
32. Fujita, K., Iseki, K., Yoshioka, H., Sasaki, T., Ando, T., and Nakamuar, M. (1983): Bacteriology of acute otitis media in Japanese children. *Am. J. Dis. Child.,* 137:152–154.
33. Fulghum, R.S., Daniel, H.J. III, and Yarborough, J.G. (1977): Anaerobic bacteria in otitis media. *Ann. Otol.,* 86:196–203.
34. Geibink, G.S., Juhn, S.K., Weber, M.L., and Le, C.T. (1982): The bacteriology and cytology of chronic otitis media with effusion. *Pediatr. Infect. Dis.,* 1:98–103.
35. Gray, B.M., Converse, G.M., III, and Dillon, H.C. (1979): Serotypes of *Streptococcus pneumoniae* causing disease. *J. Infect. Dis.,* 140:979–983.
36. Gronroos, J.A., Kortekangas, A.E., Ojala, L., and Vuori, M. (1964): The aetiology of acute middle ear infection. *Acta Otolaryngol.,* 58:149–158.
37. Harlowe, H.D. (1971): Acute mastoiditis following *Pseudomonal maltophilia* infection: case report. *Laryngoscope,* 82:882–883.
38. Holmes, B., Lapage, S.P., and Malnick H. (1974): Strains of *Pseudomonas putrefaciens* from clinical material. *J. Clin. Pathol.,* 28:149–155.
39. Howard, J.E., Nelson, J.D., Clahsen, J., and Jackson, L.H. (1976). Otitis media of infancy and early childhood: a double-blind study of four treatment regimens. *Am. J. Dis. Child.,* 130:965–970.

40. Howie, V.M., Ploussard, J.H., and Lester, R.L., Jr. (1970): Otitis media: a clinical and bacteriological correlation. *Pediatrics,* 45:29–35.
41. Howie, V.M., and Ploussard, J.H. (1971): Simultaneous nasopharyngeal and middle ear exudate cultures in otitis media. *Pediatr. Digest,* 13:31–35.
42. Howie, V.M., and Ploussard, J.H. (1971): Bacterial etiology and antimicrobial treatment of exudative otitis media: relation of antibiotic therapy to relapses. *South. Med. J.,* 64:233–239.
43. Howie, V.M., and Ploussard, J.H. (1972): Efficacy of fixed combination antibiotics versus separate components in otitis media: effectiveness of erythromycin estolate, triple sulfonamide, ampicillin, erythromycin estolate-triple sulfonamide, and placebo in 280 patients with acute otitis media under two and one-half years of age. *Clin. Pediatr.,* 11:205–214.
44. Howie, V.M., Ploussard, J.H., Sloyer, J.L., and Johnston, R.B., Jr. (1973): Immunoglobulins of the middle ear fluid in acute otitis media: relationship to serum immunoglobulin concentrations and bacterial cultures. *Infect. Immun.,* 7:589–593.
45. Howie, V.M., Ploussard, J.H., and Sloyer, J. (1974): Comparison of ampicillin and amoxicillin in the treatment of otitis media in children. *J. Infect. Dis.,* 129 (Suppl.):S181–S184.
46. Howie, V.M., Ploussard, J.H., Sloyer, J. (1975): The "otitis-prone" condition. *Am. J. Dis. Child.,* 129:676–678.
47. Howie, V.M., Ploussard, J.H., and Sloyer, J.L. (1976): Immunizations against recurrent otitis media. *Ann. Otol. Rhinol. Laryngol.,* 85(2 Suppl. 25, part 2):254–258.
48. Howie, V.M., Ploussard, J., Sloyer, J.L., and Hill, J.C. (1984): Use of pneumococcal polysaccharide vaccine in preventing otitis media in infants: different results between racial groups. *Pediatrics,* 73:79–81.
49. Jagtap, P., and Hardas, U. (1981): Anaerobes in chronic suppurative otitis media. *Indian J. Pathol. Microbiol.,* 24:107–111.
50. Jeang, L.K., and Fletcher, E.C. (1983): Tuberculous otitis media. *JAMA,* 249:2231–2232.
51. Jokippi, A.M.M., and Jokippi, L. (1977): *Haemophilus influenzae* in otitis media and sinusitis: serotypes and susceptibility to ampicillin and amoxycillin *in vitro. Infection,* 5:140–143.
52. Kamme, C. (1970): Evaluation of the *in vitro* sensitivity of *Neisseria catarrhalis* to antibiotics with respect to acute otitis media. *Scand. J. Infect. Dis.,* 2:117–120.
53. Kamme, C., Ageberg, M., and Lundgren, K. (1970): Distribution of *Diplococcus pneumoniae* types in acute otitis media in children and influence of the types on the clinical course in penicillin V therapy. *Scand. Infect. Dis.,* 2:183–190.
54. Kamme, C., Lundgren, K., and Mardh, P. (1971): The aetiology of acute otitis media in children. *Scand. J. Infect. Dis.,* 3:217–223.
55. Kamme, C., and Lundgren, K. (1971): Frequency of typable and non-typable *Haemophilus influenzae* strains in children with acute otitis media and results of penicillin V treatment. *Scand. J. Infect. Dis.,* 3:225–228.
56. Karma, P., Jokippi, L., Ojala, K., and Jokippi, A.M.M. (1978): Bacteriology of the chronically discharging middle ear. *Acta Otolaryngol.,* 86:110–114.
57. Karma, P., Luotonen, J., Pukander, J., Sipila, M., Herva, E., and Gronroos, P. (1983): *Haemophilus influenzae* in acute otitis media. *Acta Otolaryngol.,* 95:105–110.
58. Khurana, C.M. (1980): Importance of myringotomy in treatment failure of otitis media. *Pediatr. Res.,* 14 (part 2):560.
59. Klein, B.S., Dollette, F.R., and Yolken, R.H. (1982): The role of respiratory syncytial virus and other viral pathogens in acute otitis media. *J. Pediatr.,* 101:16–20.
60. Klein, J.O., and Teele, D.W. (1976): Isolation of viruses and mycoplasmas from middle ear effusions: a review. *Ann. Otol. Rhinol. Laryngol.,* 85:140–144.
61. Klein, J.O. (1980): Microbiology of otitis media. *Ann. Otol. Rhinol. Laryngol.,* 89 (3 Suppl. 68, part 2):98–101.
62. Klein, J.O. (1981): Microbiology and antimicrobial treatment of otitis media. *Ann. Otol. Rhinol. Laryngol.* 90 (3 Suppl. 84, part 3):30–36.
63. Koskela, M., Leinonen, M.M., and Luotonen, J. (1982): Serum antibody response to pneumococcal otitis media. *Pediatr. Infect. Dis.,* 1:245–252.
64. Kovatch, A.L., Wald, E.R., and Michaels, R.H (1983): Beta-Lactamase-producing *Branhamella catarrhalis* causing otitis media in children. *J. Pediatr.,* 102:261–264.
65. Lee, W., Fordham, T., and Alban, J. (1981): Otitis media caused by beta-lactamase-producing *Branhamella (Neisseria) catarrhalis. J. Clin. Microbiol.,* 13:222–223.
66. Leinonen, M.K. (1980): Detection of pneumococcal capsular polysaccharide antigens by latex agglutination, counterimmunoelectrophoresis and radioimmunoassay in middle ear exudates in

acute otitis media. *J. Clin. Microbiol.*, 11:135–140.

67. Leinonen, M., Luotonen, J., Herva, E., Valkonen, K., and Makela, P.H. (1981): Preliminary serologic evidence for a pathogenic role of *Branhamella catarrhalis*. *J. Infect. Dis.*, 144:570–574.
68. Lewis, D.M., Schram, J.L., Birck, H.G., and Lim, D.J. (1979): Antibody activity in otitis media with effusion. *Am. Otol.*, 88:392–396.
69. Lim, D.J., and DeMaria, T.F. (1982): Pathogenesis of otitis media: bacteriology and immunology. *Laryngoscope*, 92:278–286.
70. Liston, T.E., Foshee, W.S., and McCleskey, F.K. (1984): The bacteriology of recurrent otitis media and the effect of sulfisoxazole chemoprophylaxis. *Pediatr. Infect. Dis.*, 3:20–24.
71. Liu, Y.S., Lang, R., Lim, D.J., and Birck, H.G. (1976): Microorganisms in chronic otitis media with effusion. *Ann. Otol. Rhinol. Laryngol.*, 85 (2 Suppl. 25, part 2):245–249.
72. Liu, Y.S., Lim, D.J., Lang, R.W., and Birck, H.G. (1975): Chronic middle ear effusions. *Arch. Otolaryngol.*, 101:278–286.
73. Luotonen, J., Herva, E., Karma, P., Timonen, M., Leinonen, M., and Makela, P.H. (1981): The bacteriology of acute otitis media in children with special reference to *Streptococcus pneumoniae* as studied by bacteriological and antigen detection methods. *Scand. J. Infect. Dis.*, 13:177–183.
74. Marchant, C.D., Shurin, P.A., Turcyzk, V.A., Feinstein, J.C., Johnson, C.E., Wasikowski, D.E., Knapp, L.J., and Tutihasi, M.A. (1984): A randomized controlled trial of cefaclor compared with trimethoprim-sulfamethoxazole for treatment of otitis media. *J. Pediatr.*, 105:633–638.
75. Modified report of the Ad Hoc Committee on Definition and Classification of Otitis Media (1980): *Ann. Otol. Rhinol. Laryngol.*, 89 (Suppl. 69):6–8.
76. Moloy, P.J. (1982): Anaerobic mastoiditis: a report of two cases with complications. *Laryngoscope*, 92:1311–1315.
77. Mortimer, E.A., Jr., and Watterson, R.L., Jr. (1956): A bacteriologic investigation of otitis media in infancy. *Pediatrics*, 17:359–366.
78. Nelson, J.D., Ginsburg, C.M., Clahsen, J.C., and Jackson, L.H. (1978): Treatment of acute otitis media of infancy with cefaclor. *Am. J. Dis. Child.;* 132:992–996.
79. Nilson', B.W., Poland, R.L., Thompson, R.S., Morehead, D., Baghdassarian, A., and Carver, D.H. (1969): Acute otitis media: treatment results in relation to bacterial etiology. *Pediatrics*, 43:351–358.
80. Olsen, H. (1978): *Vibrio Parahaemolyticus* isolated from discharge from the ear in two patients exposed to sea water. *Acta. Path. Microbiol. Scand.*, 86:247–248.
81. Pelton, S.I., Teele, D.W., Shurin, P.A., and Klein, J.O. (1980): Disparate cultures of middle ear fluids: results from children with bacterial otitis media. *Am. J. Dis. Child.*, 134:951–953.
82. Prellner, K., Christensen, P., Hovelius, B., and Rosen, C. (1984): Nasopharyngeal carriage of bacteria in otitis-prone and non-otitis-prone children in day-care centers. *Acta Otolaryngol. (Stockh).*, 98:343–350.
83. Riding, K.H., Bluestone, C.D., Michaels, R.H., Cantekin, E.I., Doyle, W.J., and Poziviak, C.S. (1978): Microbiology of recurrent and chronic otitis media with effusion. *J. Pediatr.*, 93:739–743.
84. Rosen, C., Christensen, P., Henrichsen, J., Hovelius, B., and Prellner, K. (1984): Beneficial effect of pneumococcal vaccination on otitis media in children over two years old. *Int. J. Pediatr. Otorhinolaryngol.*, 7:239–246.
85. Ross, P.W., Farquharson, I.M., and Wallace, A.T. (1973): Isolation of *Mycobacterium tuberculosis* from chronic suppurative otitis media. *Practitioner*, 210:401–402.
86. Sarkkinen, H., Ruuskanen, O., Meurman, O., Puhakka, H., Virolainen, E, and Eskola, J. (1985): Identification of respiratory virus antigens in middle ear fluids of children with acute otitis media. *J. Infect. Dis.*, 151:444–448.
87. Schwartz, R., Rodriquez, W.J., Khan, W.N., and Ross, S. (1977): Acute purulent otitis media in children older than 5 years: incidence of *Haemophilus* as a causative organism. *JAMA*, 238:1032–1033.
88. Schwartz, R., Rodriquez, W.J., Mann, R., Khan, W., and Ross, S. (1979): The nasopharyngeal culture in acute otitis media: a reappraisal of its usefulness. *JAMA*. 241:2170–2173.
89. Schwartz, R.H., and Rodriquez, W.J. (1981): Acute otitis media in children eight years old and older: a reappraisal of the role of *Haemophilus influenzae*. *Am. J. Otolaryngol.*, 2:19–21.

90. Schwartz, R.H., and Brook, I. (1981): Gram-negative rod bacteria as a cause of acute otitis media in children. *Ear Nose Throat J.*, 60:9–15.
91. Schwartz, R.H. (1981): Bacteriology of otitis media: a review. *Otolaryngol. Head Neck Surg.*, 89:444–450.
92. Sell, S.H., Wilson, D.A., Stamm, J.M., and Chazen, E.M. (1978): Treatment of otitis media caused by *Haemophilus influenzae:* evaluation of three antimicrobial regimens. *South. Med. J.*, 71:1493–1497.
93. Shurin, P.A., Howie, V.M., Pelton, S.I., Ploussard, J.H., and Klein, J.O. (1978): Bacterial etiology of otitis media during the first six weeks of life. *J. Pediatr.*, 92:893–896.
94. Shurin, P.A., Pelton, S.I., Donner, A., Finkelstein, J., and Klein, J.O. (1980): Trimethoprim-sulfamethoxazole compared with ampicillin in the treatment of acute otitis media. *J. Pediatr.*, 96:1081–1087.
95. Shurin, P.A., Pelton, S.I., Tager, I.B., and Kasper, D.L. (1980): Bactericidal antibody and susceptibility to otitis media caused by nontypable strains of *Haemophilus influenzae. J Pediatr.*, 97:364–369.
96. Shurin, P.A., Marchant, C.D., Kim, C.H., Van Hare, G.F., Johnson, C.E., Tutihasi, M.A., and Knapp, L.J. (1983): Emergence of beta-lactamase-producing strains of *Branhamella catarrhalis* as important agents of acute otitis media. *Pediatr. Infect. Dis.*, 2:34–38.
97. Shurin, P.A., Marchant, C.D., Van Hare, G., Cartelli, N., Johnson, C.E., Fulton, D., and Kim, C.H. (1985): Biology and therapy of acute otitis media caused by *Branhamella catarrhalis. Pediatr. Res.*, 19:304A.
98. Sipila, P., Jokipii, A.M.M., Jokipii, L., and Karma, P. (1981): Bacteria in the middle ear and ear canal of patients with secretory otitis media and with non-inflamed ears. *Acta Otolaryngol.*, 92:123–130.
99. Sloyer, J.L., Jr., Howie, V.M., Ploussard, J.H., Amman, A.J., Austrian, R., and Johnston, R.B., Jr. (1974): Immune response to acute otitis media in children. I. Serotypes isolated and serum and middle ear fluid antibody in pneumococcal otitis media. *Infect. Immun.*, 9:1028–1032.
100. Sloyer, J.L., Cate, C.C., Howie, V.M., Ploussard, J.H. and Johnston, R.B., Jr. (1975): The immune response to acute otitis media in children. II. Serum and middle ear fluid antibody in otitis media due to *Haemophilus influenzae. J. Infect. Dis.*, 132:685–688.
101. Sloyer, J.L., Jr., Ploussard, J.H., and Howie, V.M. (1976): Immunology and microbiology in acute otitis media. *Ann. Otol. Rhinol. Laryngol.*, 85 (2 Suppl. 25, part 2):100–134.
102. Sloyer, J.L., Jr., Howie, V.M., Ploussard, J.H., Schiffman, G., and Johnston, R.B., Jr. (1976): Immune response to acute otitis media: association between middle ear fluid antibody and the clearing of clinical infection. *J. Clin. Microbiol.*, 4:306–308.
103. Sloyer, J.L., Jr., Ploussard, J.H., and Karr, L.J. (1980): Otitis media in young infant: an IgE-mediated disease? *Ann. Otol. Rhinol. Laryngol.* 89 (3 Suppl. 68, part 2):351–356.
104. Sloyer, J.L., Jr., Ploussard, J.H., and Howie, V.M. (1981): Efficacy of pneumococcal polysaccharide vaccine in preventing acute otitis media in infants in Huntsville, Alabama. *Rev. Infect. Dis.* (Suppl.), 3:S119–S123.
105. Syriopoulou, V., Scheifele, D., Howie, V., Ploussard, J., Sloyer, J., and Smith, A.L. (1976): Incidence of ampicillin-resistant *Haemophilus influenzae* in otitis media. *J. Pediatr.*, 89:839–841.
106. Syriopoulou, V., Scheifele, D., Smith, A.L., Perry, P.M., and Howie, V. (1978): Increasing incidence of ampicillin resistance in *Haemophilus influenzae. J. Pediatr.*, 92:889–892.
107. Teele, D.W., Healy, G.B., and Tally, F.P. (1980): Persistent effusions of the middle ear cultures for anaerobic bacteria. *Ann. Ontol. Rhinol. Laryngol.* 89: (3 Suppl. 68, part 2):102–103.
108. Teele, D.W., Pelton, S.I., and Klein, J.O. (1981): Bacteriology of acute otitis media unresponsive to initial antimicrobial therapy. *J. Pediatr.*, 98:537–539.
109. Tetzlaff, T.R., Ashworth, C., and Nelson, J.D. (1977): Otitis media in children less than 12 weeks of age. *Pediatrics.*, 59:827–832.
110. Tipple, M.A., Beem, M.O., and Saxon, E.M. (1979): Clinical characteristics of the afebrile pneumonia associated with *Chlamydia trachomatis* infection in infants less than 6 months of age. *Pediatrics* 63:192–197.
111. Yabuuchi, E., and Ohyama, A. (1971): *Archromobacter xylosoxidans* n. sp. from human ear discharge. *Jpn. J. Microbiol.*, 15:477–481.

Immunology of the Ear, edited by J. Bernstein
and P. Ogra. Raven Press, New York © 1987.

Virologic Aspects of Middle Ear Disease

Peter F. Wright

Departments of Pediatrics, Microbiology, and Pediatric Infectious Disease, Vanderbilt University, Nashville, Tennessee 37232

Acute otitis media (AOM) is most commonly regarded as a disease of bacterial origin. As discussed in the chapter by Chonmaitree and Howie *(this volume),* bacteria are recovered in pure culture from approximately 70% of tympanocentesis cultures done at the onset of AOM. Furthermore, the regular institution of antibiotic therapy in AOM has clearly reduced the long-term morbidity and mortality previously associated with complications of otitis media such as mastoiditis and meningitis. However, several observations have prompted a continued search for a relationship between viral respiratory illness and AOM. These observations fall into three categories:

1. A substantial percentage of AOM is without a provable bacterial etiology.
2. Epidemiologic data link viral illness with AOM.
3. Limited animal and human data suggest mechanisms by which viruses may alter local and systemic defense mechanisms, thus predisposing to secondary bacterial infection.

NONBACTERIAL MICROBIOLOGY OF MIDDLE EAR FLUID

Investigation of a direct role for viruses and other nonbacterial pathogens (chlamydia or mycoplasma) in AOM focused initially on direct recovery of organisms from the middle ear space. A summary of the available literature (16) suggests the relative difficulty in recovering viruses from middle ear fluid (Table 1). Although individual studies may be criticized in terms of technical detail, the great weight of data suggests that viruses are rarely present in middle ear fluid at the time of presentation with clinical otitis media. It should be noted that respiratory syncytial (RS) virus may be an exception to this. In two studies that have been done during RS epidemics, 22 of 71 specimens have yielded this virus (4,9).

More recent research efforts have attempted to demonstrate viral antigen in middle ear fluid by techniques such as enzyme-linked immunosorbent assay (ELISA), which allows detection of small amounts of viral protein. ELISA techniques are not dependent on viral replication and may detect protein from virus that replicated during the initiation of an otitis but is no longer viable at the time the child presents with clinical otitis.

TABLE 1. *Isolation of viruses from middle ear fluid in acute otitis media*

Study	Cases tested	Viruses isolated	Number of positive cases	Reference
A	10	Influenza A	4	Yoshie (30)
B	326	None	0	Gronroos et al. (9)
C	16	None	0	Laxdal et al. (18)
D	60	Respiratory syncytial	16	Berglund et al. (3,4)
E	90	Coxsackie B-4 Adenovirus 3	2	Tilles et al. (24)
F	106	Parainfluenza type 2	1	Halstead et al. (11)
G	11	Respiratory syncytial	6	Gronroos et al. (10)
H	63	Adenovirus type 2	1	Vanderbilt University (*unpublished data*)
	682		30 (4.4% positive)	

Respiratory syncytial virus	22
Influenza A virus	4
Adenovirus	2
Coxsackie virus	2
Parainfluenza virus	1

Several studies in which ELISA techniques have been used on middle ear fluid at the time of presentation with AOM are summarized in Table 2. An overall tabulation of the data demonstrates again the ability of RS to invade the middle ear space. Of interest is the observation in the studies of Serkkinen et al. (22,23) that the clinical picture was similar in those from whom only viruses were recovered and those with bacterial pathogens. Furthermore, the frequency or type of bacterial isolate from the middle ear was not influenced by the presence of a viral pathogen.

Relatively less information is provided by attempts to demonstrate viral antibody in middle ear fluid. A recent study found IgA antibody to purified viral antigens (adenovirus, RS, and parainfluenza type 2) in 31 of 128 ears with chronic effusions (29). An antisecretory component reagent was used to demonstrate that the antibody was of mucosal origin rather than a serum transudate. However, the response detected in middle ear fluid could have been part of a broader respiratory IgA response, and we do not know anything about the temporal relationship of the development of antibody with the onset of middle ear pathology. Alpha interferon has been detected in middle ear fluid and it is suggested that it is of viral origin in that it correlated with the presence of RS antigen in middle ear fluid (21). However, in an earlier study virus could not be isolated from ears with interferon (14).

Finally and most indirectly, you can look for a serum antibody rise to viral pathogens during an episode of AOM. The results of such studies were summarized in 1976 and 1980 by Klein and Teele (15,16). Seventy-two of 249 children (29%) had a serologic response to a virus during the study. Again RS virus would appear to be the leading pathogen from this type of uncontrolled analysis.

In considering how a virus might initiate otitis media without direct penetration

TABLE 2. *Detection of viral antigens in middle ear fluid*

Study	Viruses tested	Number tested	Antigen detected	Percent positive	Reference
A	Adenovirus Influenza A Respiratory syncytial Rotavirus	53	Respiratory syncytial, 10 Influenza, 2 Rotavirus, 1	25	Klein et al. (17)
B	Adenovirus Influenza A and B Parainfluenza 1, 2, 3 Respiratory syncytial	84	Respiratory syncytial, 3 Influenza, 3 Parainfluenza type 3, 2	83	Serkkinen et al. (22)
C	Adenovirus Influenza A and B Parainfluenza 1, 2, 3 Respiratory syncytial	137	Respiratory syncytial, 20 Adenovirus, 4	18	Serkkinen et al. (23)
	Total	274	45	15	
			Respiratory syncytial 33 Influenza A 5 Adenovirus 4 Parainfluenza 3 2 Rotavirus 1		

of the middle ear cavity, it is logical to focus on upper respiratory illness, which is a virtually constant component of otitis. One may therefore look at viruses found in upper respiratory infections and ask if any one virus is more likely to have an associated otitis media with its initiation of infection. In a setting where nasopharyngeal viral cultures were routinely performed on all children less than 2 years of age with respiratory illness, no such virus emerged in that the frequency of viral isolation was the same in those with uncomplicated respiratory infections and those with otitis (Table 3). This would imply that any virus that initiates an upper respiratory infection may predispose to otitis. The presumed sequence of events is depicted at the top of Table 4; other theoretical events for which some evidence may be generated are shown in the lower part of the table and are discussed further in relationship to measles and otitis later on in the chapter.

EPIDEMIOLOGY

In a broad epidemiologic sense it is recognized that the incidence of otitis media is two- to threefold higher in winter months, the traditional respiratory viral season, than in summer months. Likewise, the age-related incidence of otitis, with its peak in the first 2 years of life, parallels the ability to isolate respiratory viruses.

The most detailed epidemiologic study of otitis and viral infections was per-

TABLE 3. *Viruses isolated from the nasopharynx in children with otitis and uncomplicated upper respiratory illness*

	Clinical diagnosis	
	Acute otitis	Coryza
Total cultures	244	159
Positive for virus	67 (28%)	45 (28%)
Adenovirus	26 (11%)	14 (9%)
Parainfluenza	8 (3%)	8 (5%)
Respiratory syncytial	12 (5%)	9 (6%)
Rhinovirus/enterovirus (other than polio)	9 (4%)	3 (2%)
Influenza A	7 (3%)	4 (3%)
Influenza B	—	4
Herpes simplex	2	2
CMV	2	—

TABLE 4. *Viruses in the pathogenesis of acute otitis media*

"Established" sequence of events following viral infection

1. Viral infection of epithelial cells

↓

Epithelial cell damage

Submucosal lymphoid Proliferation avd in specific lymphoid organs—adenoids/tonsils	Edema	Ciliary dysfunction	Goblet cell proliferation Increased mucous production	Cellular exfoliation

2. Eustachian tube blockage and dysfunction

↓

Negative middle ear pressure

3. Middle ear space changes

Fluid accumulation ↘ Bacterial invasion and proliferation ↓

Clinical signs and symptoms of acute otitis media

"Theoretical" events that may occur during viral interference

1. Induction of neutrophil dysfunction. Studies suggest this may occur with influenza (1).
2. Viral/bacterial infections, e.g., viral-destroyed cells may provide a better substrate for bacterial proliferation.
3. Viruses may stimulate protease/antiprotease systems that may damage mucosal surfaces (5).
4. Thermoregulation may be altered by the viral infection to create more optimal bacterial replication.
5. Damage to cilia or virally induced changes in cell surface may alter bacterial adherence.
6. Lysozymes, lactoferrin, and other nonspecific defense proteins may be altered by viral infection.
7. Immune response may be altered.

formed by Henderson et al. (13) in the setting of a day-care center, in which over a period of 14 years careful records of child health have been kept combined with viral, bacterial, and mycoplasmal cultures of every respiratory illness. Additionally, for 3 years of the study, surveillance cultures were obtained every 2 weeks on all participants, whether or not they were ill.

The association of AOM with recovery of either viruses, pathogenic bacteria, or both in the 2 weeks preceding the episodes was examined and compared with the risk of AOM when neither viruses nor pathogenic bacteria were present. Viruses were recovered from the nasopharynx in 26% of AOM (a figure very similar to that shown for Vanderbilt University data in Table 3). The relative risk of otitis was 3.23-fold higher in the period surrounding a virus isolation. Highly significant correlations were seen with RS, adenoviruses, and influenza. These represent the most commonly isolated viruses from the nasopharynx of young children and suggest a universality in the ability of respiratory viruses to trigger otitis media. The only major viral group for which an association with otitis was not evident were rhinoviruses. The temporal association of bacterial colonization with AOM was statistically significant, with a relative risk 1.35-fold higher with pneumococcal colonization and 1.96-fold higher with haemophilus colonization than when neither bacteria was present. Attempts to demonstrate an additive role for viruses plus bacteria were most successful for the group of viruses (parainfluenza, mumps, rhinovirus, enterovirus, and herpes simplex) that did not have as strong a direct association with otitis as did the three major viruses mentioned above.

Sequential influenza epidemics at Vanderbilt University in 1978 suggested that initiation of symptomatic respiratory illness was necessary to induce otitis (28). An initial epidemic was with H3N2 influenza A, which caused a 1.7-fold excess respiratory disease in those who were infected with this influenza strain as compared to uninfected children. In this H3N2 epidemic, 30 episodes of AOM were seen in the 73 children who had evidence of H3N2 influenza as compared to only 19 of 122 children without virus isolation or serologic evidence of influenza (Table 5). This is a 2.7-fold increase in otitis in the influenza group compared to the uninfected group. The H3N2 influenza A epidemic was followed by H1N1 epidemic in which 58 children were infected; however, neither excess respiratory illness nor otitis was seen.

Reports linking chlamydia and mycoplasma to otitis media offer little encouragement that these agents are critical in the pathogenesis of anything but a small minority of cases of otitis media. Reports of attempted chlamydial isolation from the middle ear are few in number. In one report 0 of 68 children had chlamydia in middle ear fluid (12). It is a pathogen that largely occurs in a defined time frame after perinatal acquisition. This timing, 2 weeks to 3 months post-partum, is when there is a low incidence of AOM, which suggests the relative lack of importance of chlamydia in the total problem.

Repeated references are made in the literature to an association of otitis media, particularly bullous otitis media with mycoplasmal pneumonia. This literature was reviewed by Roberts (20), with the finding of only one positive isolate of mycoplasma from middle ear fluid in 771 patients. The original association was based

TABLE 5. *Varying effect of influenza infection of the incidence of otitis during sequential epidemics of influenza*

		Influenza A H3N2		Influenza A H1N1	
Illness	Influenza infection[a]	No. of cases[b]/ No. at risk	Increase	No. of cases[b]/ No. at risk	Increase
Acute otitis media	Yes	30/73	2.7-fold	6/58	0.5-fold
	No	19/122		26/127	
Total illness	Yes	73/73	1.8-fold	27/58	0.9-fold
	No	69/122		68/127	

[a]Seroconversion or isolation of influenza.
[b]cases = No. of clinic visits/No. of children.

on an experimental trial in which, following experimental administration of *Mycoplasma pneumoniae,* 13 of 52 men developed myringitis and 2 had bullae (19). Culture of the bullae in one volunteer did not yield mycoplasma.

In virtually all of the current American literature on AOM and viruses, there is no mention of a viral agent that clearly causes AOM, namely, measles virus. In the older literature, or indeed from clinical experience in developing cultures in which measles virus is not controlled, three major complications of measles are recognized: otitis media, pneumonia, and progressive diarrhea accompanied by weight loss or the appearance of kwashiorkor. In isolated epidemics, the incidence of otitis following measles is 5% to 10% (2).

Otitis following measles is often an acute suppurative process accompanied by perforation of the drum. Series in which bacterial cultures of the ear have been done are difficult to find, but presumably pneumococcus, haemophilus, and group A β-hemolytic streptococci might be found because they are in the acute bacterial pneumonias following measles. No reports of attempts to isolate measles virus directly from the middle ear space are available, although it is recognized that erythema of the drum occurs during the prodromal and exanthematus phase of the disease. Although the pathogenesis of AOM in measles is not established in humans or animals, it provides the best model for discussion of the possible interactions of viruses and bacteria in the pathogenesis of this disease.

As indicated in the schematic flowchart given in Table 6, measles, particularly in the child with underlying defects in cell-mediated immunity, is an extraordinarily aggressive virus in terms of mucosal damage at the entry site for infection—the upper respiratory tract. It can cause inflammatory changes in the ears, severe pharyngitis coryza, and a primary giant cell pneumonia. It is likely that efforts to recover virus from the middle ear in the pre-exanthematous stage of the illness would be successful.

Measles also will initiate acute bacterial invasion of the middle ear space. Most likely, this is through eustachian tube obstruction with fluid stasis and creation of

TABLE 6. *Acute otitis media in measles*

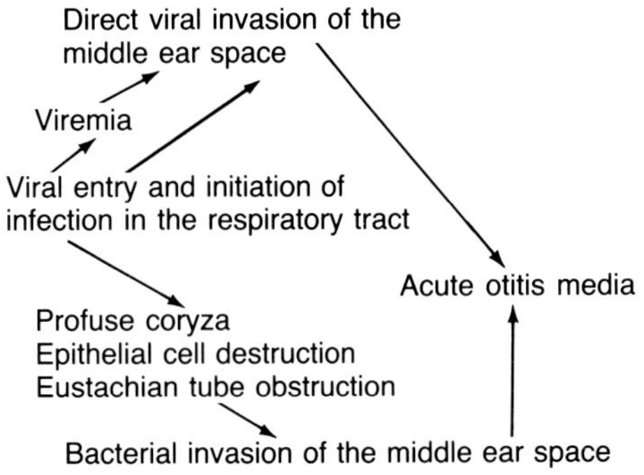

Amplifiers

a. Immunologic changes
   1. Leukopenia, neutropenia (6)
   2. Direct invasion of T lymphocytes (27)
   3. Destruction of thymic tissue (26)
   4. Depressed cell-mediated immunity (25)
   5. Decreased total IgA and IgG (25)

b. Malnutrition
   1. Enhanced viral replication
   2. Further impairment of immune response

an ideal environment in which resident nasopharyngeal bacteria can grow. However, bacterial pneumonia and oral mucosal destruction, noma, suggest that it is more than a passive obstruction and that bacterial growth and invasion are enhanced after measles.

Measles exemplifies the multiple effects that a viral infection can have on the host immune system which may enhance secondary bacterial invasion. Cell-mediated immunity is depressed with direct invasion of the thymus and depletion of lymphocyte subsets. Neutropenia occurs with the additional possibility of neutrophil dysfunction, as demonstrated experimentally for influenza A (1). Hypogammaglobulinemia is present. Finally, overall nutritional status may be impaired, further amplifying the immune incompetence.

Although measles is the prime example of such complex interactions, it is recognized that influenza and perhaps other respiratory viruses have similar effects on immune function.

In summary, viruses may well be a key initiating factor in AOM. Their primary action is most probably in initiating a nasopharyngitis. The degree to which this happens is most marked in measles, RS virus, and influenza. These are the viruses most clearly implicated in the disease. The influence of viruses on systemic or local immunologic factors must not be discounted. Resolution of the importance of such factors may come from animal models of otitis (see the chapter by Giebink, *this volume*).

In one such model, the chinchilla, a synergistic effect of viral (influenza) and bacterial (pneumococcal) infection can readily be demonstrated (8).

It can only be hoped that prevention of effective treatment of additional viral infections will decrease the incidence of otitis as dramatically as has occurred with measles vaccine. Only in the setting of effective prevention of either viral or bacterial disease will we get a true picture of the relative importance of each component in pathogenesis.

REFERENCES

1. Abramson, J.S., Giebink, G.S., Mills, E.L., and Quic, P.G. (1982): Influenza A virus induced polymorphonuclear leukocyte dysfunction in the pathogenesis of experimental pneumococcal otitis media. *Infect. Immun.*, 36:289–296.
2. Bech, V. (1962): Measles epidemic in Greenland (1951–1959). *Am. J. Dis. Child.*, 103:252–253.
3. Berglund, B., Salmivalli, A., and Toivanen, P. (1966): Isolation of respiratory syncytial virus from middle ear exudates of infants. *Acta Otolaryngol.*, 61:475–487.
4. Berglund, B., Salmivalli, A., Groonroos, J.A. (1967): The role of respiratory syncytial virus in otitis media in children. *Acta Otolaryngol.*, 63:445–454.
5. Carlsson, B., and Ohlsson, V. (1983): Localization of antileukoprotease in middle ear mucosa. *Acta Otolaryngol.*, 95:111–116.
6. Debre', R., and Celers, J. (1970): *Measles: Pathogenesis and Epidemiology in Clinical Virology. The Evaluation and Management of Human Viral Infections,* edited by Debre' and Celers, pp. 336–349. W. B. Saunders, Philadelphia.
7. Dossetor, J., Whittle, M.C. and Greenwood, B.M. (1977): Persistent measles infection in malnourished children. *Br. Med. J.*, 1:1633–1635.
8. Giebink, G.S. and Wright, P.F. (1983): Different virulence of influenza A virus strains and susceptibility to pneumococcal otitis media in chinchillas. *Infect. Immun.*, 41:913–920.
9. Gronroos, J.A., Kurterkanges, A.E., Ojala, L., and Vuori, M. (1964): The aetiology of acute middle ear infection. *Acta Otolaryngol.*, 58:149–158.
10. Gronroos, J.A., Vihma, L., Salmivalli, A., and Berglund, B. (1968): Coexisting viral (respiratory syncytial) and bacterial (pneumococcus) otitis media in children. *Acta Otolaryngol.*, 65:505–517.
11. Halsted, C., Lepow, M.L., and Balassarian, N. (1968): Otitis media. Clinical observation, microbiology and evaluation of therapy. *Am. J. Dis. Child.*, 115:542–551.
12. Hammerschlag, M.R., Hammerschlag, P.E., and Alexander, E.R. (1980): The role of chlamydia trachomatis in middle ear effusions in children. *Pediatrics,* 66:615–617.
13. Henderson, F.W., Collier, A.M., Saryal, M.A., Watkins, J.M., Fairclough, D.C., Clude, W.A., and Denny, F.W. (1982): A longitudinal study of respiratory viruses and bacteria in the etiology of acute otitis media with effusion. *N. Engl. J. Med.*, 306:1377–1383.
14. Howie, W., Pollard, R.B., Kleyn, K., Lawrence, B., Peskwic, T., Paucker, K., and Baron, S. (1982): Presence of interferon during bacterial otitis media. *J. Infect. Dis.*, 145:811–814.
15. Klein, J.O. (1980): Microbiology of otitis media. *Ann. Otol. Rhinol. Laryngol.*, 89 (Suppl. 68):98–101.
16. Klein, J.O., and Teale, D.W. (1976): Isolation of viruses and mycoplasma from middle ear effusions: a review. *Ann. Otol. Rhinol. Laryngol.* (2 Suppı. 25, part 2), 85:140–144.
17. Klein, B.S., Dullette, F.R., and Yolken, R.H. (1982): The role of respiratory syncytial virus and other viral pathogens in acute otitis media. *J. Pediatr.*, 101:16–20.
18. Laxdal, O.E., Blake, R.M., Cartmill, T. (1966): Etiology of acute otitis media in infants and children. *Am. Med. Assoc.*, 94:159–163.
19. Rifkind, D., Chanock, R., Kravetz, H. (1962): Ear involvement (myringitis) and primary atypical pneumonia following innoculations of volunteers with Eaton agent. *Am. Rev. Respir. Dis.*, 88:479–485.
20. Roberts, D.B. (1980): The etiology of bullous myringitis and the role of mycoplasms in ear disease: a review. *Pediatrics,* 65:761–766.
21. Saloman, T., Sarkkinen, H.K., and Ruuskanen (1984): Presence of interferon in middle-ear fluid during acute otitis media. *J. Infect. Dis.*, 149:480.
22. Sarkkinen, H.K., Mewman, Q., Salmi, T., Pujakka, H., and Virolainen, E. (1983): Demonstration of viral antigens in middle ear secretions of children with acute otitis media. *Acta Pediatr. Scand.*, 72:137–138.
23. Sarkkinen, H.K., Ruuskanen, O., Mewman, O., Puhakka, M., Virolainen, E., and Eskola, J. (1985): Identification of respiratory viral antigens in middle ear fluid of children with acute otitis media. *J. Infect. Dis.*, 151:444–448.
24. Tilles, J.A., Klein, J.O., Jao, R.L., Haslam, J.E., Feingold, M., Gellis, S.S., and Finland, M. (1967): Acute otitis media in children: serologic studies and attempts to isolate viruses and mycoplasmas from aspirated middle ear fluids. *N. Engl. J. Med.*, 277:613–618.

25. Wesley, A., Coovadis, H.M., and Henderson, L. (1978): Immunologic recovery after measles. *Clin. Exp. Immunol.,* 32:540–544.
26. White, R.O., and Boyd, J.F. (1973): The effect of measles on the thymus and other lymphoid tissues. *Clin. Exp. Immunol.,* 13:343–357.
27. Whittle, M.C., Dossetor, J., Oduloju, A., Bryceson, M., and Greenwood, B.M. (1978): Cell-mediated immunity during natural measles infection. *J. Clin. Invest.,* 62:678–684.
28. Wright, P.F., Thompson, J., and Gerson, D. (1980): Differing virulence of H1N1 and H3N2 influenza strains. *Am. J. Epidemiol.,* 112:814–819.
29. Yamaguchi, T., Urasawa, T., and Kataura, A. (1984): Secretory immunoglobulin A antibodies to respiratory virus in middle ear effusion of chronic otitis media with effusion. *Ann. Otol. Rhinol. Laryngol.,* 93:73–75.
30. Yoshie, C. (1955): On the isolation of influenza virus from middle ear discharge of influenza otitis media. *Jpn. Soc. Med. Biol.,* 8:373–378.

Immunology of the Ear, edited by J. Bernstein and P. Ogra. Raven Press, New York © 1987.

Secretory Immunoglobulin in the Nasopharynx: Implications in Otitis Media

Chr. Hjort Sørensen

E. N. T. Department, Gentofte University Hospital, DK-2900 Hellerup, Denmark

The mucosal membrane of the upper respiratory tract in humans is constantly exposed to a great variety of microorganisms and potential allergens. Especially in small children, high numbers of bacterial colonies can often be cultured from the nasopharynx; increased rates have been found in children with recurrent acute otitis media (47,49,50,71). A well-functioning humoral immunity in the secretions and the mucosa of the nasopharynx is of utmost importance for preventing or combating infections and atopic diseases. In addition, other mechanisms, such as ciliary function and the involvement of nonspecific antimicrobial factors such as mucin, lysozyme, and lactoferrin may also be of major importance in maintaining the subtle balance between invasive and noninvasive inflammatory conditions of the nasopharyngeal membrane (9,30,57,88,89). During childhood, acute otitis media is one of the most common diseases and it starts in the nasopharynx. Although the mechanisms are only partly understood, transient dysfunction of the nasopharyngeal resistance results in growth of microorganisms already present in the secretions, which then spread to the middle ear cavity. Studies of animal models of otitis media, especially in chinchillas, have extended our knowledge of some of the underlying mechanisms involved in the pathogenesis of acute otitis media, i.e., premorbid virus infection in the nasopharynx and negative pressure of the middle ear cavity (see Giebink's chapter, *this volume*).

In this chapter the quantitative and functional aspects of the nasopharyngeal secretory immune system are discussed, and special attention has been focused on children with recurrent attacks of acute otitis media. The involvement of allergic reactions, including the levels of IgE (IgE stands for immunoglobulin E) antibodies, is described in chapter by Welliver (*this volume*).

NASOPHARYNGEAL MUCOSAL IMMUNE SYSTEM

The general aspects of the mucosal immune system have previously been reviewed (4,5). The basic structure and proposed functions of (a) the palatine and nasopharyngeal tonsils and (b) the effector cells of general and local immunity are treated in the chapters by Brandtzaeg, Scicchitano et al., and Cumella *(this vol-*

ume). Therefore, only some of the main principles of the mucosal immune system will be outlined. During the past decade the justification of a classic division of the mucosal immune system into two separate systems, namely the bronchus- and the gut-associated lymphoid tissues (BALT versus GALT, respectively) and system immunity, has been questioned. Evidence of a common mucosal system (MALT) has gained more and more ground (1,14,31). The Peyer's patches of the gut have been shown to be the principal lymphoepithelial tissue, giving rise to primarily IgA precursor cells. Subsequently, these primed lymphocytes recirculate to all mucosal sites and in some cases they "home" near glandular and submucosal tissue to mature into IgA-producing plasma cells (Fig. 1). Several hypotheses concerning the underlying homing mechanism of these lymphoplasts and the stimulus for the final maturation of the cells have been proposed, but exact evidence is lacking (8,12). The observed differences in the distribution of plasma cells and the Ig content in the secretions between BALT and GALT indicate a significant influence of the local mucosal microflora (12,70,82). Moreover, it has been indirectly suggested that priming of precursor cells by lymphoepithelial tissue takes place in crypts of the palatine and nasopharyngeal tonsils (9). However, quantitatively the mass of the lymphoid tissue in the gut far exceeds that of the upper respiratory tract, but during early childhood the almost physiological hyperplasia of the lymphoid tissue of Waldeyer's ring probably upsets the balance between BALT and GALT. In this context, also the qualitative role of the palatine and nasopharyngeal

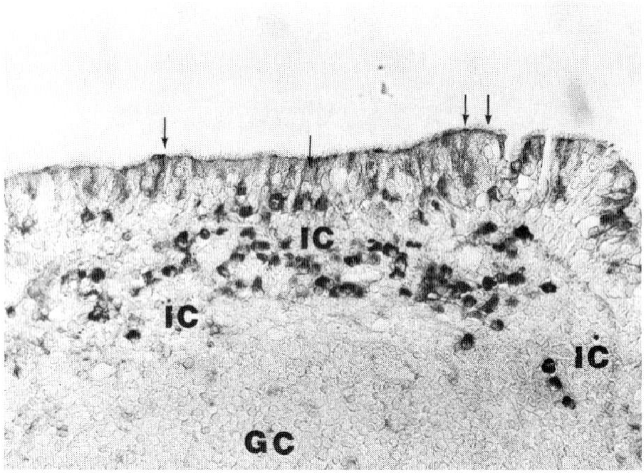

FIG. 1. Immunohistochemical localization of secretory component, secretory IgA, and IgA immunocytes in nasopharyngeal tonsil from a child. The tissue specimen was fixed directly in cold 96% ethanol and finally embedded in paraffin. Thin sections were incubated with a rabbit antiserum (IgG fraction) specific for human secretory component and α-chains of secretory IgA (Dakopatts, Copenhagen), using an indirect enzyme immunohistochemical technique. Numerous IgA-producing immunocytes (IC) are located below the surface epithelium, characterized as the ciliated, pseudostratified columnar type. Arrows indicate the presence of secretory IgA in the epithelial cells, resulting from coupling of dimeric IgA with secretory component. No intracellular IgA immunocytes are seen in the germinal center of the lymphoid follicle (GC). ×144.

tonsils as active immunological organs should be taken into consideration before operative intervention eventually takes place. The long-lasting reduced or absent IgA antibody activity against poliovirus in the nasopharynx of children after adenotonsillectomy clearly demonstrates the importance of these matters (61).

Several models for transport of secretory immunoglobulins through glandular and submucosal tissue have previously been summarized by Brandtzaeg (8). Today, it is generally accepted that incorporation of a joining chain (J chain) into the Ig to be secreted is decisive for the combination with the secretory component (SC) of the epithelial cell. The principles of IgA translocation across the mucosa into the nasopharyngeal secretions as secretory IgA (SIgA) are illustrated in Fig. 1. In addition to this submucosal secretion, the SIgA molecules reach the secretions via glandular transport (8,9). In the nasopharyngeal submucosa, several tubuloalveolar glands are present, mostly of the mucous type (89). The contribution of SIgA to the secretion by means of these glands is not fully elucidated, but quantitatively this contribution must be questioned as the translocation of IgA appears to be limited almost exclusively to serous types of glands (9). Further immunohistochemical studies of the glands in the nasopharynx are needed to clarify these matters.

Stability of Secretory Immunoglobulins

Human SIgA is a stable molecule, which in a broad sense resists proteolysis from both digestive and microbial enzymes normally occurring in external secretions (45,80). Although the basic reason for this resistance is not fully understood, it is likely to be owing, in part, to SC, which for the most part is disulfide-linked to the dimeric IgA (45). The structure of the molecule is further stabilized by several noncovalent interactions, as demonstrated by *in vitro* experiments (30). However, some bacterial species frequently cultured from the nasopharynx of children are able to cleave SIgA by means of extracellular enzymes, the so-called IgA proteases. These matters will be discussed in more detail later on in this chapter.

The SC also associates with 19S IgM during its transfer across epithelial cells (8), but in contrast to SIgA, only minor fractions of the binding complexes are covalently stabilized (7,46). Although the noncovalent binding forces between SC and 19S IgM are stronger than those between SC and 11S IgA, purification of SIgM results in a significant loss of SC from the molecule (7). Therefore, continuing binding of SC with 19S IgM needs excess of free SC in the secretions.

QUANTITATION OF SECRETORY IMMUNOGLOBULIN

Collection of Secretions

Before going into detail about the various methodological obstacles when quantitating SIgA and SIgM in secretions, it is important to state that, basically, the results from Ig measurements are influenced by numerous conditions already inherent in the secretions at the time of collection. First of all, one must be aware of the origin of the secretions obtained. For instance—as will be discussed later on in this chapter—there are marked differences in the SIgA content of salivary and nasopharyngeal secretions. Secondly, the methods of collection of secretions vary greatly in previous studies, mostly dependent on the purpose of the investigation. Nasal and/or nasopharyngeal washes have been used throughout the years in many studies concentrating on the local secretory immune response (15,17,26,33,55,61,65,75,87,94). By use of these methods, it is possible to obtain consecutive secretion samples from the same person. However, in uncooperative children the contamination with tears will be unpredictable and the Ig concentrations cannot be given in absolute values. In this respect the filter-paper and the porous-disk methods, as described by Mygind (57) and Kristiansen (43), respectively, are much easier to handle when investigating the nasal cavity, but the amount of secretion obtained is small (about 50 μliters) and the method is unsuitable for children. Also, the degree of stimulation of secretory activity by the presence of such a piece of paper is difficult to monitor (11). In theory, when quantitating secretory immunoglobulins in nasopharyngeal secretions from children, it is important to obtain undiluted, crude secretions from a well-defined anatomical location and to keep the stimulation of the secretory activity at a fixed minimum.

To fulfill these requirements it is necessary to put the child under general anesthesia. An ethical dilemma may arise because, obviously, children cannot be anesthetized just for the purpose of research only (48). Using a Boyle-Davis gag, it is possible under visual guidance to lift the soft palate and to suck up the secretion puddle (100–500 μliters) located just inferior or lateral to the nasopharyngeal tonsils without touching the mucosal membrane with the suction device. There are two important disadvantages of this collection method: one is the difficulty of obtaining consecutive secretion samples and the other is the time-consuming job of gathering secretion samples from otologically healthy children. This direct method of collection of nasopharyngeal secretions has been used in only a few studies (53,80). Diurnal variations in the content of IgA, IgG, and albumin have been reported in nasal secretions (32,59). Variations in the secretory activity seem responsible for this. However, the ratio of SIgA to IgA remains stable, and for practical reasons we therefore collect the secretion samples between 8 and 9 a.m. (32).

Laboratory Handling of the Secretions

Because of the presence of various microbial, digestive, and other enzymes capable of cleaving the immunoglobulins into small fragments, it is important to freeze immediately the secretions obtained. Previous estimations of the stability of proteins during storage have shown that it is advisable to keep respiratory tract secretions at −80°C (−112°F) (72). The presence of mucoid substance in nasopharyngeal secretions often makes it very difficult to measure the exact volume of the secretion sample; thus, the weight method, with the secretion sample still deep-frozen, is to be preferred (80). After thawing, the diluted samples (weight-to-weight) can be shaken with glass beads to obtain a homogeneous suspension. Subsequent high-speed centrifugation will separate the secretions into well-defined sol and gel fractions. Using chemical agents to break down the gel network is not recommended because most of the agents commercially available also break down the molecular structure of the immunoglobulins, thereby influencing the results of the Ig measurements *(unpublished observations).*

Measuring SIgA and SIgM

Human exocrine secretions contain a mixture of locally produced immunoglobulins as well as plasma immunoglobulins passively diffused to the secretions because of "mucosal leakage" (11,30). Normally, plasma IgA (7S IgA) constitutes only a minor fraction (10–20%) of the total IgA in secretions. However, in the nasopharynx of small children the mucosal membranes are thin and constantly exposed to a variety of microorganisms causing recurrent infections. Therefore, increased amounts of plasma IgA would be expected in the secretions; methodologically, this constitutes a major obstacle when specific quantitation of SIgA is required (30). Moreover, the secretions contain variable concentrations of 10S IgA (SIgA minus SC), heavier aggregates (15S–18S), free SC, and SIgM (11). All in all, the results obtained by quantitation of SIgA using antisera specific for either the heavy chain of IgA or SC will differ according to the ratios of the IgA- and/or SC-associated molecules found in the individual secretions. In this respect, it is worth emphasizing the importance of the specificity of the antisera used. In principle, there are two ways of producing antisera against SC. Employing purified SIgA as the antigen, antibodies against both dimeric IgA and bound SC appear. Subsequently, absorbance with plasma IgA in order to render the antiserum specific for SC (92) does not eliminate antibodies reacting with "polymer" determinants of dimeric IgA (11). In addition to proving the specificity of the various antisera by means of crossed immunoelectrophoresis with intermediate gel technique (2), we also use immunohistochemical analysis of normal intestinal or respiratory mucosa in order to disclose such unwanted specificities (80). Using free SC as the antigen, the above-mentioned obstacles are eliminated. However, most antigenic determinants of SC are hidden when the molecule is associated with dimeric IgA (11), and therefore the validity of such antisera against bound SC is limited. Nevertheless, such antisera have shown excellent precipitating properties with SIgA and SIgM in gel-immunoelectrophoretic techniques, and they are well-suited also for enzyme-linked immunosorbent acid (ELISA) (29,35,80,82).

When quantitating the secretory immunoglobulins it is important to use standards that in most ways resemble the secretion to be quantitated (11,30). Especially in gel-immunoprecipitating techniques, variations in the ratios of the IgA subpopulations influence the results significantly (22). In previous reports, using a serum standard for quantitation of SIgA in secretions, different correction factors have been used in order to convert from monomer to polymer forms of IgA (13,22,28,58,68,90). In this respect, colostrum preparations have shown excellent properties as SIgA standards (21,29,35,80,87,92,96). For other reasons, it is also worth warning against the use of gel-immunoprecipitation techniques, especially radial immunodiffusion. First, the formation of nonimmune precipitates, probably resulting from the reactions of glycoproteins with agarose (72), may lead to misinterpretations for secretions with low levels of SIgA and/or SIgM (Fig. 2A and B). Second, the passive diffusion of these large molecules takes such a long time that the influence during the assay run of proteolytic degradation of immunoglobulins must be taken into consideration (91). Therefore, to overcome the technical obstacles and fulfill the standard requirements just mentioned, new and more specific assays have recently been published (21,29,35,68,80,87,96). In most assays the two different antigenic determinants, the heavy chain of IgA and SC, are utilized in a sandwich technique. The standard used in our assay has been prepared from a pool of human colostrum, and the SIgA content was calculated by immunonephelometry using a World Health Organization (WHO) immunoglobulin preparation for reference (80). It is generally assumed that results from the immunonephelometry method are not affected by the size heterogeneity exhibited by IgA (24,90). The principle of our ELISA for quantitation of nasopharyngeal SIgA is shown in Fig. 3. Interference studies on the influence of coexisting plasma IgA revealed that up to 170% of the original SIgA concentration could be added as plasma IgA without it interfering with the SIgA measurements. In view of this, the contribution of plasma IgA to the nasopharyngeal secretions is negligible, as will be discussed in the following section. However, quantitatively, the monomer form of IgA in middle ear effusions and plasma samples exceeds by far the secretory form of IgA, and for the quantitative measurements of SIgA in these fluids a reverse sandwich model of the one presented in Fig. 3 has proved to be applicable (82).

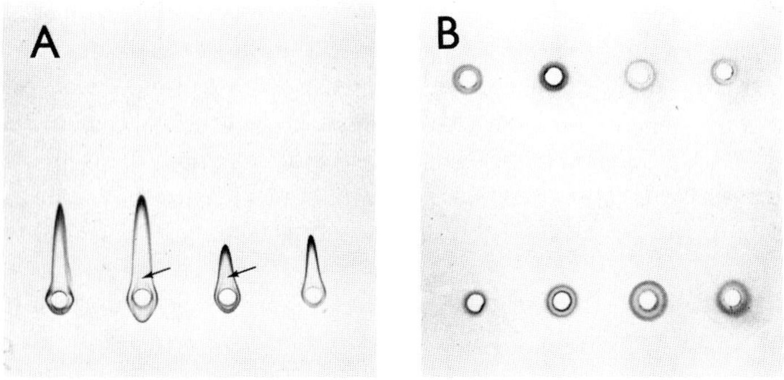

FIG. 2. Formation of nonimmune precipitates in gel-immunoprecipitation techniques. **A:** Rocket immunoelectrophoretic analysis (2) of IgA in four nasopharyngeal secretions. The agarose-gel contained rabbit antiserum (IgG fraction), specific for α-chains of IgA (Dakopatts, Copenhagen). The "extra" rockets inside the true IgA rockets *(arrows)* proved to be nonimmune to reaction because they were restored on control plates without specific antiserum added to the gel. **B:** Radial immunodiffusion of eight middle ear effusions from children with secretory otitis media. Despite no antiserum in the agarose-gel, spontaneous precipitation rings of varying diameter were formed.

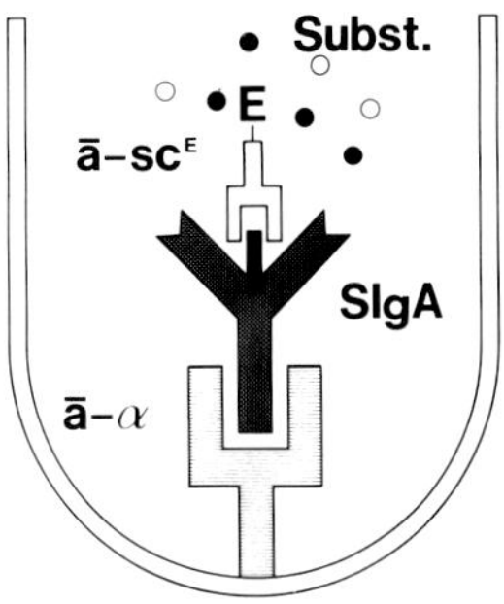

FIG. 3. Principle of enzyme-linked immunosorbent assay (ELISA) for quantitation of SIgA in nasopharyngeal secretion (80). Gamma-irradiated polystyrene microtest plates (Nunc, Copenhagen) are coated overnight with rabbit IgG specific for α-chains of human IgA (ā-α). In the next step, secretion samples and colostrum SIgA standards are added to the wells (SIgA). In the third step, wells are incubated with rabbit IgG specific for SC and conjugated with horseradish peroxidase (ā-SC^E). Finally, chromogenic substrate solution is added to the wells for color development (Subst.) After discontinuing enzyme reaction with sulfuric acid, the absorbance of the colored end-products are read at 492 nm. A washing procedure is carried out between the different steps.

Previously, only a few studies reported on levels of IgM in nasopharyngeal secretions. One reason is that normally this immunoglobulin occurs in small quantities in secretions and is therefore undetectable by use of ordinary gel-immunoelectrophoretic techniques. Another point is the difficulty of making a working standard applicable for the quantitative measurements in exocrine secretions. Normally, IgM appears as a pentamer both in plasma and in secretions, but also monomer forms of IgM occur. In contrast to SIgA, a well-functioning working standard for the measurements of SIgM is difficult to prepare. In theory, purification of SIgM could be done from stimulated parotid secretions or colostrum from a person with selective IgA deficiency, but only 60% to 70% of the molecules retain SC after Sephadex G-200 chromatography (7). For lack of a better one, we have used a nasopharyngeal secretion pool as a working standard, although the content of SIgM could only be calculated arbitrarily (82).

In most reports concerning quantitative measurements by means of ELISA, approximations by a linear function are often done in order to express the relationship between absorbance and SIgA quantity (29,35,96). However, because of saturation of the IgA-binding capacity at high SIgA levels in the first layer of the assay (Fig. 3), and an increasing influence of the background absorbance at low SIgA levels, the analytical range of the standard curve in such an approximation is limited (80). We therefore proposed a model for computation of the standard curve by means of which the analytical range of the standard curve is significantly increased (80). For several reasons, this model has proved to be extremely useful in a variety of ELISAs (82,85).

Levels of Secretory Immunoglobulin

Because of all the methodological obstacles and reservations mentioned in the above section, considerable variations in the results of the Ig measurements are to be expected. Table 1 summarizes the range of mean/median levels of the secretory immunoglobulins in saliva, nasopharyngeal secretions, and serum/plasma from relevant, previous publications. At birth, there are no secretory immunoglobulins in

TABLE 1. *Range of mean/median levels of secretory immunoglobulins in saliva, nasopharyngeal secretions, and serum/plasma from infants, children, and adults*[a]

Substance	SIgA (mg/liter)	IgA (mg/liter)	SIgM (units/liter)	IgM (mg/liter)	Reference
Saliva					
Infants	0–25	0–60			31,33
Children	40–77	30–130		0–7	13,31,33,68,80,95
Adults	15–130	48–210		1–5	11,13,20,35,44,96
Nasopharyngeal secretions					
Infants		117–464			17,33
Children	290–1,200	550–1,800	79	80–92	60,68,75,81,83,85
Adults	900–2,263	750–3,020		7–8	11,29,32,58
Serum/plasma					
Infants	10	(0–750)	ND	(160–2,000)	34,92
Children	(3–18)	(130–2,250)	ND	(400–2,200)	34,35,68,85,92
Adults	(6–40)	(800–3,200)	ND	(300–3,000)	11,20,21,35,92

[a]The 95% confidence limits are indicated in parentheses. ND, not detectable.

exocrine secretions in humans, but already within the first month of life, detectable levels of IgA have been found in secretions from the upper respiratory tract (31,33,73). A significant difference in the IgA but also in the SIgA content between saliva and nasopharyngeal secretions can obviously be seen at all ages. In 4-year-old children, we have calculated the SIgA content of nasopharyngeal secretions to be about 20 times higher than that in unstimulated, whole saliva (80). Although the flow rate of saliva is higher than that of nasopharyngeal secretions, this cannot explain the marked differences observed between the two secretions. Whether or not the same holds true for SIgM is still unknown, but at least in children it seems to be so with regard to the differences in the total IgM content (Table 1). A very high content of IgA was found in nasopharyngeal secretions, in some cases even higher than in serum/plasma. The majority of these immunoglobulins seem to be of local origin as SIgA antibodies, but substantial variations in the individual secretions have been observed (Table 2). Probably, a varying degree of mucosal inflammation more than variations in secretory activity in general is responsible for this (32). The SIgM/IgM ratios are expressed arbitrarily, but nevertheless the interquartile ranges, as listed in Table 2, indicate even greater variations within this secretory system than in the SIgA/IgA system. Such variations have also been described in middle ear effusions, although in addition a pronounced transudation of plasma IgA and plasma IgM occurs (81–83). This means that quantitation of SIgA and/or SIgM instead of total IgA and/or total IgM must be done when examining the local immune response in the nasopharynx and middle ear cavity. Under normal conditions, the contribution of secretory immunoglobulins from plasma to the secretions is negligible (21,92; Table 1).

TABLE 2. *Ratios of SIgA to IgA and SIgM to IgM in nasopharyngeal secretions from children*[a]

Immunoglobulin	Median	IQR[b]
SIgA (mg/liter)	1,180	620–1,970
IgA (mg/liter)	1,720	900–3,540
SIgA/IgA (%)	69	50–85
SIgM (units/liter)	79	46–138
IgM (mg/liter)	92	55–171
SIgM/IgM (units/mg)	0.83	0.47–1.35

[a]Data, in part, from ref. 85.
[b]IQR, Interquartile range.

Levels of Nonsecretory Immunoglobulin

Evidence of an active glandular or mucosal transport of IgG and IgD across epithelial cells has never been furnished (11,30,82). *In vitro* analyses have failed to show any affinity of IgG or IgD for SC (30,82). Although high percentages of J-chain-positive IgG and IgD immunocytes have been found near secretory epithelium, no attachment between the J chain and the intracellular immunoglobulin has been proved. This probably explains the above-mentioned lack of affinity of SC because incorporation of J chain into the immunoglobulin to be secreted is decisive for the combination with the secretory receptor of the epithelial cells. Therefore, the contribution of IgG and IgD to the secretions depends on local, submucosal passive synthesis from plasma cells combined with passive diffusion through epithelial interstices, the so-called mucosal leakage. In newborns, most of the IgG found in serum and secretions are of maternal origin, but at the age of 6 months most of these antibodies disappear. This probably accounts for the high levels of IgG found in nasopharyngeal secretions of infants compared with the levels found in children (86; Table 3). Reliable estimates of the extent of mucosal leakage of plasma proteins to the secretions can be made by calculating the transudation ratio of albumin from plasma to the secretions. In nasopharyngeal secretions from children, the range of this index was found to be 1:7 to 1:12 (85). Therefore, as can be calculated from the data in Table 3, the IgG concentrations in nasopharyngeal secretions of children correspond to those in plasma, when taking into account the transudation index of albumin. However, IgG immunocytes have been demonstrated in the nasopharyngeal submucosa (10,19; see also Brandtzaeg's chapter, *this volume*), indicating a local but passive synthesis of IgG to the secretion, but the cell density is low and therefore the contribution in quantitative terms of IgG locally produced must be regarded as insignificant (15). Recently, the interest in the role of IgD in serum and secretions has increased (18,64,82). During B-lymphocyte differentiation, IgD alone or in combination with IgM is located on the

TABLE 3. *Range of mean/median levels of IgG and IgD in saliva, nasopharyngeal secretions, and serum/plasma from infants, children, and adults*[a]

Substance	IgG (mg/liter)	IgD (mg/liter)	Reference
Saliva			
Infants		ND	70
Children	9.6	0.14	68,95
Adults	14–17	0.14	11,44,69
Nasopharyngeal secretions			
Infants	425–557		17
Children	130–710	1.5–12	60,68,75,83,85
Adults	220–5,000	1.5	29,58,69
Serum/plasma			
Infants	(1,000–9,000)		34
Children	(3,500–13,000)	(1.2–35)	12,34,68,83,85
Adults	(7,200–17,000)	(14–30)	11,12,27,69

[a]The 95% confidence limits are indicated in parentheses. ND, not detectable.

surface of the majority of these cells (18), but very few of these mature into IgD-secreting plasma cells. Therefore, normally only trace amounts of this immunoglobulin are found in serum (12,27,68,70,74). However, increased numbers of IgD immunocytes have been observed in nasopharyngeal tonsils, lacrimal and parotid glands, and lactating mammary glands, as compared with spleen, lymph nodes, and glandular tissue of the gastrointestinal canal (12,30,70; see also Brandtzaeg's chapter, *this volume*). These and other observations (12) indicate that IgD may play an important role in mucosal immunity of the upper respiratory tract. This assumption is supported by the observation of a substantial local synthesis of IgD both to the nasopharynx (83) and to the middle ear cavity (82). Actually, in 18% of the middle ear effusions examined, a content of more than 600 mg/liter of IgD could be calculated.

SPECIFICITY OF THE NASOPHARYNGEAL HUMORAL IMMUNITY AND IMPLICATIONS IN OTITIS MEDIA

It is generally agreed that a continuing stimulation at mucosal sites by means of microorganisms and other antigens is necessary in order to maintain a secretory immune response (30). After oral vaccination with live poliovirus, Ogra (61) was able to demonstrate significant levels of specific nasopharyngeal IgA antibodies even 3 years after the original vaccination, indicating persistence of virus replication in the mucosa. Next to colostrum, nasopharyngeal secretions are the exocrine fluid of humans most enriched with secretory immunoglobulins. Naturally, from a clinical standpoint, it is interesting to study the specificities of all these antibodies found in the secretions. A variety of virus-specific IgA antibodies from adenovirus

(53), respiratory syncytial virus (52,53), parainfluenza virus (53), poliovirus (61,62), influenza A virus (94), coxsackie A virus (15), and rhinovirus (15,26) infections have previously been reported. Also, the role of immunoglobulins other than IgA in the mucosal immunity to virus infection has been described in nasal and nasopharyngeal secretions (15,52,61) and reviewed by Ogra and Karzon (63). Also in middle ear effusions, specific IgA antibodies against a variety of viral antigens have been reported during acute otitis media (79).

Strangely enough, the specificity of the nasopharyngeal secretory immunoglobulins against bacteria has been investigated in only a few articles (55,65). By means of an indirect immunofluorescent technique, Mouton et al. (55) found high titers both of group- and type-specific antipneumococcal antibodies of the IgA isotype in colostrum. However, only occasionally such IgA antibodies could be detected in saliva, nasal secretions, or serum. The existence of a relationship between antibody titer and IgA level as well as the competition from specific IgG antibodies, the so-called masking phenomenon, probably explains the low or absent levels of specific IgA in the secretions. By use of ELISA, we have repeated some of these investigations and, although preliminary, the results seem comparable. In nasopharyngeal secretions of children, the majority of the specific antibodies against the capsule and the cell wall of pneumococci are of the IgG class *(unpublished results)*. In this context, it is important to clarify whether these IgG antibodies are present in the secretions just because of mucosal leakage or whether there is a significant contribution also from local synthesis, but these matters are as yet unsolved. Parenteral vaccination of children with *Hemophilus influenzae* type-b capsular polysaccharides results in a significant increase of specific mucosal as well as serum IgA antibodies (65). In contrast, immunization with an oral-polyvalent-killed bacterial vaccine gave rise to increased levels of specific antibodies of the IgA class against *H. influenzae* in saliva from children but not in serum (16). Evidence of an IgA memory in the upper respiratory tract conducted by bacterial polysaccharides as the only antigen has never been procured. However, recently it has been shown that an inactivated influenza A virus vaccine administered intranasally in children induced a local IgA memory in the nasal cavity with boosting effects (94). Therefore, in theory, oral immunization with bacterial polysaccharides coupled with proteins is advisable to use as an appropriate antigen for the induction of T-cell-dependent immune response. The immune response in the middle ear cavity has been investigated during acute otitis media caused by pneumococci and *H. influenzae* (76,77). Specific IgA, IgG, and IgM antibodies could be detected in middle ear effusions, but the IgA and IgG isotypes dominated. The clearing of the acute infection was significantly associated with the level of the specific Ig at the time of diagnosis (78). However, the origin of these specific antibodies was not investigated. Probably, the majority of the antibodies were of systemic origin because of the high transudation index of plasma proteins to the middle ear cavity, as previously reported (81,82; see also Mogi and Bernstein's chapter, *this volume*).

Within dysfunctions of the B-cell system, selective IgA deficiency is the most common type, found in about one of 500 patients (20). Recurrent infections of the respiratory tract are found in some of these patients, whereas others are quite healthy. A compensatory increase of IgM in the secretions has been reported in some of these patients but not in others (11,30). Thus, the ability to resist infections in IgA-deficient persons is only partially understood (31); however, low levels of IgA have been found in nasal washings from children with protein-calorie malnutrition (75), and high frequencies of mucosal infections in these children are well known. The rate of infections decreased during dietary treatment and the IgA content was normalized (75).

Transient disturbances in the function of the secretory immune system in the nasopharynx of children might serve as a simple and logical explanation of recurrent attacks of acute otitis media (RAOM). Although this has been only partly investigated, the results from several reports do not support these assumptions. No increase in the frequency of immune deficiency syndromes has been found in RAOM patients (3), and no differences in the levels of nasal IgA, IgG, and IgM could be detected between breast-fed and bottle-fed babies despite a reduced morbidity of respiratory diseases in breast-fed infants (87). Mygind and Wihl (60) investigated the protein concentrations in nasal secretions of 14 children during recurrent infections in the upper airways. The Ig concentrations were comparable to the levels found in normal healthy children. Also, we could not demonstrate any significant differences in the SIgA and SIgM levels in 45 children with or without a medical history of RAOM (83). In adults with chronic sinusitis, Hamaguchi et al. (29) reported up to 4 g/liter of SIgA in nasal secretions. Therefore, from a quantitative point of view, it seems that children with RAOM are generally well supplied with secretory immunoglobulins in their nasopharynx, but the qualitative role of these antibodies in the secretory immunity, especially their role in immune exclusion, is still an enigma.

BACTERIUM-INDUCED CLEAVAGE OF SIgA

IgA Proteases

Normally, and especially in small children, a broad spectrum of microorganisms is found in cultures from the upper respiratory tract. It is generally accepted that among several mechanisms, a well-functioning specific secretory immune system, primarily mediated by SIgA antibodies, is crucial in order to maintain the integrity of the mucosal barrier. Under conditions that are only partly understood this subtle balance may shift, resulting in mucosal and/or systemic infections. However, very few microorganisms seem capable of such an invasion, and therefore it was most interesting when it was discovered that the majority of these microorganisms were capable of cleaving IgA into Fab and Fc fragments. This IgA cleavage was caused by enzymes excreted from the bacteria. Studies have demonstrated such enzymatic activity in *Hemophilus influenzae, Streptococcus pneumoniae, Neisseria gonorrhoeae, N. meningitidis,* some strains of *S. sanguis,* and *S. mitior* (36,38,51,66,67). Furthermore, some bacteroides and capnocytophaga species, which are suspected as being principal etiological agents in destructive periodontal diseases, also excrete these so-called IgA proteases (36). Detailed information from comprehensive surveys of bacteria, mycoplasma, fungi, and viruses capable and not capable of cleaving IgA has been published (40,42).

Characteristics of IgA Proteases

Most proteases yet examined belong to the metallo class of endopeptidases and appear extracellularly. Inhibition of enzyme activity by ethylenediaminetetraacetic acid has been found to vary between different bacterial species (39). Probably one of the most interesting features of these IgA proteases is the fact that they selectively cleave IgA subclass 1, but not subclass 2. In humans IgA1 is the predominant subclass in serum (up to 95% of total IgA), but in secretions subclass 2 is significantly increased compared to serum (up to 40%) (25). The principal molecular difference between the two subclasses is the deletion in IgA2 of a 13-amino-acid sequence found in the hinge region of IgA1. All known IgA proteases cleave within this sequence of the hinge region (39,42) and leave IgG, IgM, IgD, and IgE isotypes of human immunoglobulins and porcine and bovine SIgA uncleaved (38). In these reports immunoelectrophoresis has been used to identify IgA degradation products, i.e., Fab and Fc fragments. However, using a thin-layer enzyme plate assay, it has recently been suggested that the majority of 102 strains of *S. pneumoniae* were capable of degrading not only human SIgA but also IgG and IgM (93).

Previous studies have indicated that purified colostrum SIgA is only partially cleaved by IgA proteases (38,39). Although, in general, coupling of SC with dimer IgA makes the SIgA molecule resistant to proteolysis, immunochemical analyses have shown that the cleavage products of SIgA after treatment with IgA proteases can be described as $(Fc_\alpha)_2 \cdot SC$ and Fab_α, respectively (39,41). Therefore, SC by itself does not protect against attacks by IgA proteases. An important point is that approximately one-third of colostrum SIgA belongs to the IgA2 subclass (25), which is resistant to cleavage. Another point is that colostrum antibodies have shown neutralizing properties of IgA1 protease activity (39). Whether these antibodies belong to the IgA1 or IgA2 subclass is unknown. In this respect, it is worth noting that degradation of SIgA by nonspecific proteases does not result in intact Fc_α fragments (6).

In Vivo Activity of IgA Proteases

Obviously, the discovery that the three principal causes of bacterial meningitides in humans, *H. influenzae, N. meningitidis,* and *S. pneumoniae,* all produce IgA proteases and that nonpathogenic species of the genera *Neisseria* and *Hemophilus* lack the property (38,56) indicates that these enzymes may be important virulent factors on mucosal surfaces. However, very few papers have focused on the evidence for such an *in vivo* activity. Intact Fc_α fragments have been described in vaginal secretions of women with gonococcal infections and in cerebrospinal fluid from patients with *H. influenzae* meningitis (6,40). Recently, we examined nasopharyngeal secretions from small children and reported the presence of IgA cleavage products in 18 of 97 children (84). Immunochemical analysis of the cleavage products included rocket immunoelectrophoresis (Fig. 4) and further characterization by high-pressure liquid chromatography followed by analysis in two different ELISA systems (41). The molecular structure of these *in-vivo*-produced Fc fragments of SIgA could be described as $(Fc_\alpha)_2 \cdot SC$. Therefore, it is most likely that the observed cleavage of SIgA is caused by bacterial IgA proteases. Of particular interest is the significant correlation between the presence of IgA cleavage products in the secretions and a history of atopic disease (Table 4). Previously, circulating antibodies to food proteins have been demonstrated in sera from IgA-deficient subjects, and also it has been suggested that the atopic condition in children was associated with a transitorily reduced production of IgA (86). We provided evidence that despite a normal content of IgA (Table 4), the defect in the IgA system may be of local nature induced by IgA-protease-producing bacteria. Whether this degradation is primary or secondary in the development of the atopic condition is at present unknown. Furthermore, cleavage products were found more frequently in the youngest children. There are several reports indicating that significantly increased numbers of *H. influenzae, S. pneumoniae,* and *S. mitior* are found in cultures from the nasopharynx of children suffering from recurrent acute otitis media and secretory otitis media (47,49,50,71; see also Chonmaitree and Howie's chapter, *this volume*). However, the prevalence of Fc fragments was evenly distributed in the nasopharyngeal secretions examined (Table 4), and no correlation could be demonstrated between IgA cleavage and a history of recurrent acute otitis media.

During the prephase of acute otitis media in small children caused by either *S. pneumoniae* or *H. influenzae,* pure cultures of the causative agent can often be obtained from the nasopharynx (see Chonmaitree and Howie's chapter, *this volume*). Undoubtedly, the bacterium-induced impairment of the immune barrier of

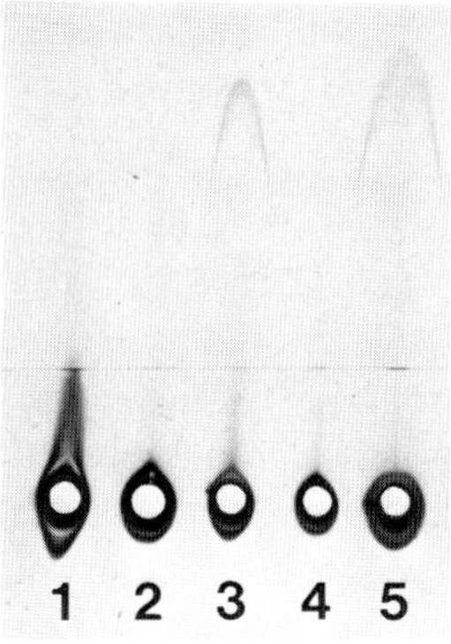

FIG. 4. Rocket immunoelectrophoretic analysis of nasopharyngeal secretions used to detect IgA cleavage. Lower gel contained antiserum against lambda- and kappa-type light chains (Dakopatts, Copenhagen). Top gel contained antiserum specific for heavy chains of IgA (Dakopatts, Copenhagen). The intermediate gel was free of antiserum. **1–3:** Samples of nasopharyngeal secretions from three different subjects. Fc_α (complement-binding fraction of alpha heavy chain) fragments are demonstrated in sample 3. **4** and **5:** Nasopharyngeal secretions incubated for 2 hr at 37°C with buffer and *H. influenzae,* respectively. (From ref. 84.)

TABLE 4. *Prevalence of IgA cleavage products in nasopharyngeal secretions of 97 children related to age, level of IgA, history of atopic disease, and recurrent acute otitis media*[b]

Parameter	IgA cleavage products present ($N = 18$)	IgA intact ($N = 79$)	Confidence level[a]
Age			
Median	3.5 years	4.8 years	
Range	2.6–5.1	4.1–5.7	$p < 0.03$
IgA			
Median	1,500 mg/liter	1,700 mg/liter	
Range	900–2,400	900–3,700	NS
Atopic disease			
Present (13)	61.5%	38.5%	
Absent (84)	11.9%	88.1%	$p < 0.001$
Recurrent acute otitis media			
Present (54)	18.5%	81.5%	
Absent (43)	18.6%	81.4%	NS

[a]NS, nonsignificant.
[b]Data, in part, from ref. 84.

the nasopharyngeal mucosa might thereby indirectly influence the invasion of the bacteria through the mucosa and to the middle ear cavity. However, no data are available to support such speculations. The significance, in a biological sense, of the IgA cleavage products, Fc_α and Fab_α is not fully understood. Recently, Manza and Kilian (51a) have shown that *in vitro* cleavage of different IgA1 myeloma proteins into Fab and Fc fragments by IgA proteases did not influence the antigen-binding capacity of the Fab portion. Therefore, it seems reasonable to assume that in secretions with a high prevalence of IgA-protease-producing bacteria, a significant part of the microorganisms and other antigens will be covered by specific Fab's rather than intact SIgA. In addition to being the predominant Ig in nasopharyngeal secretions, IgA constitutes the first isotype of antibody that antigens meet during penetration of the mucosal barrier (Fig. 1). However, if microorganisms are ''protected'' by means of the Fab fragments, the immune elimination most likely occurs deeper in the lamina propria, primarily by means of IgG, complement, and IgE antibodies. Presumably, also activated T cells are involved in these reactions, but very little is known about the role of cell-mediated immunity in the nasopharyngeal submucosa. Nevertheless, enhancement of both humoral and cellular immune reactions tend toward a state of chronic mucosal inflammation, the so-called second line of defense (9,30). In the clinics, we often treat small children with chronic inflammation of the nasopharynx and with enlarged nasopharyngeal tonsils. It is putative to think that this pathotopic potentiation of the local immunity in some way or another is associated with an increased prevalence of the IgA-protease-producing microflora in the nasopharyngeal secretions.

Speculations concerning the possible prevention of severe bacterial infection and/or atopic diseases, in which IgA proteases may play a significant role, led to studies on the ability of such proteases to induce neutralizing antibodies. In rabbits, highly specific inhibitory antibodies against IgA1 proteases could be raised from a variety of *H. influenzae* (37,40). However, these investigations have disclosed such a complexity in the specificities on the IgA proteases, not only with regard to the cleaving site at the hinge region but also in the pattern of inhibition by rabbit neutralizing antibodies, that it is at present impossible to point out the appropriate composition of a protease vaccine.

The local immune system at the level of the nasopharynx is critical in the prevention of acute suppurative otitis media. This chapter has reviewed the humoral immune mechanisms that may play a role in the eradication of pathological microflora in the nasopharyngeal tonsil area. The important interaction of the microflora, the production of IgA proteases, and secretory immunoglobulins will need to be thoroughly evaluated before one can make any conclusions as to the exact roles played by each participant in this immunobiological scenario. Also, the role of intranasal vaccination and possibly the potential role of bacteriophage against specific bacteria may be exciting new areas to investigate in the prevention and/or eradication of otitis media, particularly in the otitis-prone child.

ACKNOWLEDGMENTS

Financial support was received from "C.L. Davids Legat for Slaegt og Venner" and "Danmarks Astma- og Allergiforbund." I thank Mrs. Birgitte Jepsen and Mrs. Elisabeth Simonsen for their skillful technical assistance.

REFERENCES

1. Arnold, R.R., Mestecky, J., and McGhee, J.R. (1976): Naturally occurring secretory immunoglobulin A antibodies to *Streptococcus mutans* in human colostrum and saliva. *Infect. Immun.*, 14:355–362.
2. Axelsen, N.H., Krøll, J., and Weeke, B. (1973): A manual of quantitative immunoelectrophoresis. *Scand. J. Immunol.*, 2 (Suppl. 1):15–83.
3. Berdal, P., Brandtzaeg, P., Frøland, S.S., Henriksen, S.D., and Skrede, S. (1976): Immunodeficiency syndromes with otorhinolaryngological manifestations. *Acta Otolaryngol.*, 82:185–192.
4. Bernstein, J.M., and Ogra, P.L. (1980): Mucosal immune system: implications in otitis media with effusion. *Ann. Otol. Rhinol. Laryngol.*, 89 (Suppl. 68):326–332.
5. Bienenstock, J., and Befus, A.D. (1980): Mucosal immunology. *Immunology,* 41:249–270.
6. Blake, M., Holmes, K.K., and Swanson, J. (1979): Studies of gonococcus infection. XVII. IgA_1-cleaving protease in vaginal washings from women with gonorrhea. *J. Infect. Dis.*, 139:89–92.
7. Brandtzaeg, P. (1975): Human secretory immunoglobulin M. An immunochemical and immunohistochemical study. *Immunology,* 29:559–570.
8. Brandtzaeg, P. (1981): Transport models for secretory IgA and secretory IgM. *Clin. Exp. Immunol.*, 44:221–232.
9. Brandtzaeg, P. (1984): Immune functions of human nasal mucosa and tonsils in health and disease. In: *Immunology of the Lung and Upper Respiratory Tract,* edited by J. Bienenstock, pp. 28–95. McGraw-Hill, New York.

10. Brandtzaeg, P., Fjellanger, I., and Gjeruldsen, S.T. (1967): Localization of immunoglobulins in human nasal mucosa. *Immunochemistry,* 4:57–60.
11. Brandtzaeg, P., Fjellanger, I., and Gjeruldsen, S.T. (1970): Human secretory immunoglobulins. I. Salivary secretions from individuals with normal or low levels of serum immunoglobulins. *Scand. J. Haematol.* (Suppl.), 12:1–83.
12. Brandtzaeg, P., Gjeruldsen, S.T., Korsrud, F., Baklien, K., Berdal, P., and Ek, J. (1979): The human secretory immune system shows striking heterogeneity with regard to involvement of J chain-positive IgD immunocytes. *J. Immunol.,* 122:503–510.
13. Bratthall, D., and Ellen, R.P. (1982): Determination of immunoglobulin A in saliva by immunobead enzyme-linked immunosorbent assay: comparison with single radial immunodiffusion. *J. Clin. Microbiol.,* 16:766–769.
14. Burns, C.A., Ebersole, J.L., and Allansmith, M.R. (1982): Immunoglobulin A antibody levels in human tears, saliva, and serum. *Infect. Immun.,* 36:1019–1022.
15. Butler, W.T., Waldmann, T.A., Rossen, R.D., Douglas, R.G., Jr., and Couch, R.B. (1970): Changes in IgA and IgG concentrations in nasal secretions prior to the appearance of antibody during viral respiratory infection in man. *J. Immunol.,* 105:584–591.
16. Clancy, R.L., Cripps, A.W., Husband, A.J., and Buckley, D. (1983): Specific immune response in the respiratory tract after administration of an oral polyvalent bacterial vaccine. *Infect. Immun.,* 39:491–496.
17. Cohen, A.B., Goldberg, S., and London, R.L. (1970): Immunoglobulins in nasal secretions of infants. *Clin. Exp. Immunol.,* 6:753–760.
18. Cooper, M.D., Kuritani, T., Chen, C., Lehmeyer, J.E., and Gathings, W.E. (1982): Expression of IgD as a function of B-cell differentiation. *Ann. NY Acad. Sci.,* 399:146–154.
19. Crabbe, P.A., and Heremans, J.F. (1967): Distribution in human nasopharyngeal tonsils of plasma cells containing different types of immunoglobulin polypeptide chains. *Lab. Invest.,* 16:112–123.
20. D'Amelio, R., Palmisano, L., Le Moli, S., Seminara, R., and Aiuti, F. (1982): Serum and salivary IgA levels in normal subjects: comparison between tonsillectomized and non-tonsillectomized subjects. *Int. Arch. Allergy Appl. Immun.,* 68:256–259.
21. Delacroix, D.L., and Vaerman, J.P. (1981): A solid phase, direct competition, radioimmunoassay for quantitation of secretory IgA in human serum. *J. Immunol. Methods,* 40:345–358.
22. Delacroix, D.L., Meykens, R., and Vaerman, J.P. (1982): Influence of molecular size of IgA on its immunoassay by various techniques. I. Direct and reversed single radial immunodiffusion. *Mol. Immunol.,* 19:297–305.
23. Delacroix, D.L., Dehennin, J.P., and Vaerman, J.P. (1982): Influence of molecular size of IgA on its immunoassay by various techniques. II. Solid-phase radioimmunoassays. *J. Immunol. Methods,* 48:327–337.
24. Delacroix, D.L., and Vaerman, J.P. (1982): Influence of molecular size of IgA on its immunoassay by various techniques. III. Immunonephelometry. *J. Immunol. Methods,* 51:49–55.
25. Delacroix, D.L., Dive, C., Rambaud, J.C., and Vaerman, J.P. (1982): IgA subclasses in various secretions and in serum. *Immunology,* 47:383–385.
26. Douglas, R.G., Jr., Rossen, R.D., Butler, W.T., and Couch, R.B. (1967): Rhinovirus neutralizing antibody in tears, parotid saliva, nasal secretions and serum. *J. Immunol.,* 99:297–303.
27. Dunnette, S.L., Gleich, G.J., Miller, R.D., and Kyle, R.A. (1977): Measurement of IgD by a double antibody radioimmunoassay: demonstration of an apparent trimodal distribution of IgD levels in normal human sera. *J. Immunol.,* 119:1727–1731.
28. Greenberg, S.B., Rossen, R.D., Six, H.R., Baxter, B.D., and Couch, R.B. (1978): Determination of immunoglobulin A concentrations in human nasal secretions with a serum immunoglobulin A standard. *J. Clin. Microbiol.,* 8:465–467.
29. Hamaguchi, Y., Ohi, M., Sakakura, Y., and Mukojima, T. (1982): Quantitation of nasal secretory IgA by enzyme-linked immunosorbent assay. *Int. Arch. Allergy. Appl. Immunol.,* 69:1–6.
30. Hanson, L.A., and Brandtzaeg, P. (1980): The mucosal defense system. In: *Immunological Disorders in Infants and Children,* edited by E.R. Stiehm and V.A. Fulginiti, pp. 137–164. Saunders, London.
31. Hanson, L.A., Ahlstedt, S., Andersson, B., Carlsson, B., Cole, M.F., Cruz, J.R., Dahlgren, U., Ericsson, T.H., Jalil, F., and Khan, S.R. (1983): Mucosal immunity. *Ann. NY Acad. Sci.,* 409:1–21.
32. Harada, T., Hamaguchi, Y., Sakakura, Y., and Miyoshi, Y. (1984): Circadian variation of secretory IgA in nasal secretions from normal subjects. *Acta Otolaryngol. (Stockh),* 97:359–362.

33. Haworth, J.C., and Dilling, L. (1966): Concentration of A-globulin in serum, saliva, and nasopharyngeal secretions of infants and children. *Lab. Clin. Med.*, 67:922–933.
34. Isaacs, D., Altman, D.G., Tidmarsh, C.E., Valman, H.B., and Webster, A.D.B. (1983): Serum immunoglobulin concentrations in preschool children measured by laser nephelometry: reference ranges for IgG, IgA, IgM. *J. Clin. Pathol.*, 36:1193–1196.
35. Ishiguro, Y., Kato, K., Ito, T.., Nagaya, M., and Tsuda, M. (1983): Specific quantitation of secretory immunoglobulin A with enzyme immunoassay using activated thiol-sepharose for separation method. *J. Immunol. Methods,* 56:109–116.
36. Kilian, M., and Holmgren, K. (1981): Ecology and nature of immunoglobulin A1 protease-producing streptococci in the human oral cavity and pharynx. *Infect. Immun.*, 31:868–873.
37. Kilian, M., and Thomsen, B. (1983): Antigenic heterogeniety of immunoglobulin A1 proteases from encapsulated and non-encapsulated *Haemophilus influenzae*. *Infect. Immun.*, 42:126–132.
38. Kilian, M., Mestecky, J., and Schrohenloher, R.E. (1979): Pathogenic species of the genus *Haemophilus* and *Streptococcus pneumoniae* produce immunoglobulin A1 protease. *Infect. Immun.*, 26:143–149.
39. Kilian, M., Mestecky, J., Kulhavy, R., Tomana, M., and Butler, W.T. (1980): IgA1 proteases from *Haemophilus influenzae, Streptococcus pneumoniae, Neisseria meningitidis, and Streptococcus sanguis:* comparative immunochemical studies. *J. Immunol.*, 124:2596–2600.
40. Kilian, M., Thomsen, B., Petersen, T.E., and Bleeg, H.S. (1983): Occurrence and nature of bacterial IgA proteases. *Ann. NY Acad. Sci.*, 409:612–623.
41. Kilian, M., Reinholdt, J., Mortensen, S.B., and Sørensen, C.H. (1983): Perturbation of mucosal immune defence mechanisms by bacterial IgA proteases. *Clin. Respir. Physiol.*, 19:99–104.
42. Kornfeld, S.J., and Plaut, A.G. (1981): Secretory immunity and the bacterial IgA proteases. *Rev. Infect. Dis.*, 3:521–534.
43. Kristiansen, B.-E. (1984): Collection of mucosal secretion by synthetic discs for quantitation of secretory IgA and bacteria. *J. Immunol. Methods,* 73:251–257.
44. Lems-Van Kan, P., Verspaget, H.W., and Pena, A.S. (1983): ELISA assay for quantitative measurement of human immunoglobulins IgA, IgG, and IgM in nanograms. *J. Immunol. Methods,* 57:51–57.
45. Lindh, E. (1975): Increased resistance of immunoglobulin A dimers to proteolytic degradation after binding of secretory component. *J. Immunol.*, 114:284–286.
46. Lindh, E., and Bjork, I. (1976): Binding of secretory component to human immunoglobulin M. *Eur. J. Biochem.*, 62:271–278.
47. Long, S.S., Henretig, F.M., Teter, M.J., and McGowan, K.L. (1983): Nasopharyngeal flora and acute otitis media. *Infect. Immun.*, 41:987–991.
48. Lowe, C.U., Alexander, D., and Mishkin, B. (1974): Nontherapeutic research on children: an ethical dilemma. *J. Pediatr.*, 84:468–472.
49. Lundberg, C. Lonnroth, J., and Nord, C.E. (1982): Identification of attached bacteria in the nasopharynx of the child. *Infection,* 10:58–62.
50. Lundberg, C., Lonnroth, J., and Nord, C.A. (1982): Adherence in the colonization of *Streptococcus pneumoniae* in the nasopharynx in children. *Infection,* 10:63–66.
51. Male, C.J. (1979): Immunoglobulin A1 protease production by *Haemophilus influenzae* and *Streptococcus pneumoniae*. *Infect. Immun.*, 26:254–261.
51a. Manza, and Killian, M. (1986). *Infect. Immun.*, 52:171–174.
52. McIntosh, K., McQuillin, J., and Gardner, P.S. (1979): Cell-free and cell-bound antibody in nasal secretions from infants with respiratory syncytial virus infection. *Infect. Immun.* 23:276–281.
53. Meurman, O.H., Sarkkinen, H.K., Puhakka, H.J., Virolainen, E.S., and Meurman, O.H. (1980): Local IgA-class antibodies against respiratory viruses in middle ear and nasopharyngeal secretions of children with secretory otitis media. *Laryngoscope,* 90:304–311.
54. Mogi, G. (1975): Secretory immunoglobulin A in oral and respiratory passages in man. *Ann. Otol. Rhinol. Laryngol.*, 84:3–23.
55. Mouton, R.P., Stoop, J.W., Ballieux, R.E., and Mul, N.A.J. (1970): Pneumococcal antibodies in IgA of serum and external secretions. *Clin. Exp. Immunol.*, 7:201–210.
56. Mulks, M.H., and Plaut, A.G. (1978): IgA protease production as a characteristic distinguishing pathogenic from harmless *Neisseriaceae*. *N. Engl. J. Med.*, 299:973–976.
57. Mygind, N. (1978): *Nasal Allergy*. Blackwell Scientific Publishers, London.
58. Mygind, N., Weeke, B., and Ullman, S. (1975): Quantitative determination of immunoglobulins in nasal secretion. *Int. Arch. Allergy Appl. Immun.*, 49:99–107.

59. Mygind, N., and Thomsen, J. (1976): Diurnal variation of nasal protein concentration. *Acta Otolaryngol.*, 82:219–221.
60. Mygind, N., and Wihl, J.-A. (1976): Concentration of immunoglobulins in nasal secretion from children with recurrent infections in the upper airways. *Acta Otolaryngol.*, 82:216–218.
61. Ogra, P.L. (1971): Effect of tonsillectomy and adenoidectomy on nasopharyngeal antibody response to poliovirus. *N. Engl. J. Med.*, 284:59–64.
62. Ogra, P.L., and Karzon, D.T. (1969): Distribution of poliovirus antibody in serum, nasopharynx and alimentary tract following segmental immunization of lower alimentary tract with poliovaccine. *J. Immunol.*, 102:1423–1430.
63. Ogra, P.L., and Karzon, D.T. (1970): The role of immunoglobulins in the mechanism of mucosal immunity to virus infection. *Ped. Clin. N. Am.*, 17:385–400.
64. Olson, J.C., and Leslie, G.A. (1982): IgD: a component of the secretory immune system? *Ann NY Acad. Sci.*, 399:97–104.
65. Pichichero, M.E., and Insel, R.A. (1983): Mucosal antibody response to parenteral vaccination with *Haemophilus influenzae* type b capsule. *J. Allergy Clin. Immunol.*, 72:481–486.
66. Plaut, A.G., Genco, R.J., and Tomasi, T. (1974): Isolation of an enzyme from *Streptococcus sanguis* which specifically cleaves IgA. *J. Immunol.*, 113:289–291.
67. Plaut, A.G., Gilbert, J.V., Artenstein, M.S., and Capra, J.D. (1975): *Neisseria gonorrhoeae* and *Neisseria meningitidis:* extracellular enzyme cleaves human immunoglobulin A. *Science,* 190:1103–1105.
68. Plebani, A., Mira, E., Mevio, E., Monafo, V., Notarangelo, L.D., Avanzini, A., and Ugazio, A.G. (1983): IgM and IgD concentrations in the serum and secretions of children with selective IgA deficiency. *Clin. Exp. Immunol.*, 53:689–696.
69. Plebani, A., Avanzini, M.A., Massa, M., and Ugazio, A.G. (1984): An avidin-biotin ELISA for the measurement of serum and secretory IgD. *J. Immunol. Methods,* 71:133–140.
70. Rowe, D.S., Crabbe, P.A., and Turner, M.W. (1968): Immunoglobulin D in serum, body fluids and lymphoid tissues. *Clin. Exp. Immunol.*, 3:477–490.
71. Ruokonen, J., Sandelin, K., and Makinen, J. (1979): Adenoids and otitis media with effusion. *Ann. Otol. Rhinol. Laryngol.*, 88:166–171.
72. Schiøtz, P.O., Clemmensen, I., and Høiby, N. (1980): Immunoglobulins and albumin in sputum from patients with cystic fibrosis. *Acta Pathol. Microbiol. Scand. (C),* 88:275–280.
73. Selner, J.C., Merrill, D.A., and Claman, H.N. (1968): Salivary immunoglobulin and albumin: development during the newborn period. *J. Pediatr.*, 72:685–689.
74. Sewell, H.F., Matthews, J.B., Flack, V., and Jefferis, R. (1979): Human immunoglobulin D in colostrum, saliva and amniotic fluid. *Clin. Exp. Immunol.*, 36:183–188.
75. Sirisinha, S., Suskind, R., Edelman, R., Asvapaka, C., and Olson, R.E. (1975): Secretory and serum IgA in children with protein-calorie malnutrition. *Pediatrics,* 55:166–170.
76. Sloyer, J.L., Jr., Howie, V.M., Ploussard, J.H., Amman, A.J., Austrian, R., and Johnston, R.B., Jr. (1974): Immune response to acute otitis media in children. I. Serotypes isolated and serum and middle ear fluid antibody in pneumococcal otitis media. *Infect. Immun.*, 9:1028–1032.
77. Sloyer, J.L., Jr., Cate, C.C., Howie, V.M., Ploussard, J.H., and Johnston, R.B., Jr. (1975): The immune response to acute otitis media in children. II. Serum and middle ear fluid antibody in otitis media due to *Haemophilus influenzae*. *J. Infect. Dis.*, 132:685–688.
78. Sloyer, J.L., Jr., Howie, V.M., Ploussard, J.H., Schiffman, G., and Johnston, R.B., Jr. (1976): Immune response to acute otitis media: association between middle ear fluid antibody and the clearing of clinical infection. *J. Clin. Microbiol.*, 4:306–308.
79. Sloyer, J.L., Jr., Howie, V.M., Ploussard, J.H., Bradac, J., Habercorn, M., and Ogra, P.L. (1977): Immune response to acute otitis media in children. III. Implications of viral antibody in middle ear fluid. *J. Immunol.*, 118:248–250.
80. Sørensen, C.H. (1982): Secretory IgA enzyme immunoassay. Application of a model for computation of the standard curve. *Scand. J. Clin. Lab. Invest.*, 42:577–583.
81. Sørensen, C.H. (1982): The ratio of secretory IgA to IgA in middle ear effusions and nasopharyngeal secretions. *Acta Otolaryngol, (Suppl.),* 386:91–93.
82. Sørensen, C.H. (1983): Quantitative aspects of IgD and secretory immunoglobulins in middle ear effusions. *Int. J. Pediatr. Otorhinolaryngol.*, 6:247–253.
83. Sørensen, C.H. (1984): IgD and secretory immunoglobulins in secretions from the upper respiratory tract of children with secretory otitis media. In: *Recent Advances in Otitis Media with Effusion,* edited by D.J. Lim, pp. 150–152. B.C. Decker, Toronto.

84. Sørensen, C.H., and Kilian, M. (1984): Bacterium-induced cleavage of IgA in nasopharyngeal secretions from atopic children. *Acta Pathol. Microbiol. Scand. (C)*, 92:85–87.
85. Sørensen, C.H., and Larsen, P. (1985): Humoral immunity in the nasopharynx of children. In: *Immunobiology, Autoimmunity and Transplantation in Otorhinolaryngology*, edited by J.E. Veldman, pp. 247–250. Kugler Publications, Amsterdam.
86. Taylor, B., Norman, A.P., Orgel, H.A., Stokes, C.R., Turner, M.W., and Soothill, J.F. (1973): Transient IgA deficiency and pathogenesis of infantile atopy. *Lancet*, ii:111–113.
87. Taylor, C.E., and Toms, G.L. (1984): Immunoglobulin concentrations in nasopharyngeal secretions. *Arch. Dis. Chlid.*, 59:48–53.
88. Tos, M. (1975): Goblet cells in the developing rhinopharynx and pharynx. *Arch. Otorhinolaryngol.*, 209:315–324.
89. Tos, M. (1977): Mucous glands in the developing human rhinopharynx. *Laryngoscope*, 87:987–995.
90. Virella, G., and Fudenberg, H.H. (1977): Comparison of immunoglobulin determinations in pathological sera by radial immunodiffusion and laser nephelometry. *Clin. Chem.*, 23:1925–1928.
91. Virella, G., Goudswaard, J., and Boackle, R.J. (1978): Preparation of saliva samples for immunochemical determinations of immunoglobulins and for assay of lysozyme. *Clin. Chem.*, 24:1421–1422.
92. Waldman, R.H., Mach, J.P., Stella, M.M., and Rowe, D.S. (1970): Secretory IgA in human serum. *J. Immunol.*, 105:43–47.
93. Wikstrom, M.B., Dahlen, G., Kaijser, B., and Nygren, H. (1984): Degradation of human immunoglobulins by proteases from *Streptococcus pneumoniae* obtained from various human sources. *Infect. Immun.*, 44:33–37.
94. Wright, P.F., Murphy, B.R., Kervina, M., Lawrence, E.M., Phelan, M.A., and Karzon, D.T. (1983): Secretory immunological response after intranasal inactivated influenza A virus vaccinations: evidence for immunoglobulin A memory. *Infect. Immun.*, 40:1092–1095.
95. Østergaard, P.A., and Blom, M. (1977): Whole salivary immunoglobulin levels in 60 healthy children: determined by a sensitive electroimmunotechnique after prior carbamylation. *J. Clin. Chem. Clin. Biochem.*, 15:393–396.
96. Akerlund, A.S., Hanson, L.A., Ahlstedt, S., and Carlsson, B. (1977): A sensitive method for specific quantitation of secretory IgA. *Scand. J. Immunol.*, 6:1275–1282.

Immunology of the Ear, edited by J. Bernstein
and P. Ogra. Raven Press, New York © 1987.

Immune Mechanisms in Otitis Media with Effusion

*Goro Mogi and **Joel M. Bernstein

**Department of Otolaryngology, Medical College of Oita, Oita 879-56, Japan; and **Departments of Otolaryngology and Pediatrics, State University of New York at Buffalo, Buffalo, New York 14214, and Division of Infectious Diseases, Children's Hospital of Buffalo, Buffalo, New York 14222*

Otitis media with effusion (OME) in humans is an inflammatory disease that is acquired through the mucosal portals of the nasopharynx, the eustachian tube, and the middle ear. It appears that the outcome of this infection may be determined to a large extent by the nature of the initial cell-virus or cell-bacterial interaction at the mucosal site. The characteristics of the induced immunological reactivity may result in immunological protection or may give rise to immunopathological changes in the middle ear mucosa. The purpose of this chapter is to review the various immunological mechanisms that are known to be present in the middle ear cleft and to discuss their contribution to either immune protection or to the immunopathology that may result when this immunological activity is present for a long period of time associated with continued eustachian tube dysfunction.

IMMUNOGLOBULINS

In an effort to clarify the origin and nature of middle ear effusions (MEEs), investigators (1,3,10,31,57) have analyzed the protein components of MEE and, in general, have demonstrated little qualitative difference between the protein component of serum and those of MEE. Mogi and Honjo (31), however, have suggested that the alpha-2 fraction in MEE is lower than it is in sera. Based on these results, and the results of disk electrophoretic analysis, it has been postulated that the decrease in alpha-2 fraction in MEE is because of the absence or presence of only very small quantities of haptoglobin and alpha-2 macroglobulin in MEE. Thus, except for immunoglobulins and perhaps secretory component (SC), the major protein components that appear in the middle ear represent transudation of serum proteins. There is abundant evidence that the increased concentration of immunoglobulin in MEE is the result of local synthesis of these proteins by plasma cells in the lamina propria of the middle ear mucosa (3,20,25,36). Quantitative analysis of IgG, IgA, and IgM using radioimmunodiffusion reveals that the mean levels of IgG and IgA in MEE are significantly greater than that in the serum of the same patients (3,26,32,59). In general, IgM has been found to be at least the same or slightly greater in the MEE than in the sera. Thus, there is evidence of local production of the major classes of immunoglobulins by almost all investigators.

IgD is a minor, but very important, immunoglobulin in human sera. The function of IgD in the immune response and its biological properties in humoral immunity are not entirely known. This immunoglobulin is usually present on the surface of human B cells together with IgM, and very few of these B lymphocytes mature into IgD-producing plasma cells. Nevertheless, it has been reported that an increased number of IgD-producing plasma cells was observed in lymphoid tissue from the upper respiratory tract compared with other lymphoid tissues such as the spleen and lymph nodes. IgD measurement in MEE has been undertaken by several investigators and it has been shown that IgD, like other immunoglobulins, appears to be greater in the MEE than in the corresponding serum in some effusion samples, although substantial variations have been noted (51,59). Sørensen (51) has recently reported increased mean levels of IgD in MEE and nasopharyngeal samples compared to the mean level in the corresponding sera. From the results of his investigation, Sørensen postulated that IgD and secretory IgM in MEE are produced locally in the tympanic cavity and that IgD-producing plasma cells in the middle ear mucosa probably originate from precursor B cells in the palatine and nasopharyngeal tonsils. (see Sørensen's chapter, *this volume*).

The role of IgE-mediated hypersensitivity in MEE is reviewed in a chapter by Welliver *(this volume)*. Briefly, however, allergy has been considered to play an etiologic role in MEE for over 30 years and some authors have reported a high incidence of OME in allergic patients (14,28,46). However, since the discovery of specific assays for IgE (21), which is now known to be the reaginic antibody, the role of atopic disease or specifically IgE-mediated allergy in the upper respiratory tract has been considerably clarified. In general, the studies that have been published generally suggest that IgE-producing plasma cells are very sparse in the middle ear mucosa and that local production of IgE in middle ear fluids is low (3,4,24,34), similar to human milk (58). Thus, IgE in the middle ear fluid is derived from the sera. Figure 1 shows the relationship of IgE concentration between MEE and sera.

Specific IgE antibody against a number of allergens has also been detected in MEE, but again the concentrations of these antibodies is rarely higher in the MEE fluid than in the corresponding sera. The role of IgE-mediated hypersensitivity in MEE has not yet been completely understood. However, recent evidence suggests that allergen reacting with mucosal mast cells in the nose, nasopharynx, or eustachian tube may result in eustachian tube dysfunction and subsequent otitis media (OM) (13,15,17). The middle ear may also be a target organ in probably less than 10% of cases (4,38). Viral infection in the nasopharynx may also lead to an IgE-mediated response in the nasopharynx with subsequent mast cell degranulation and eustachain tube inflammation (17,45,61). Finally, it should be emphasized that al-

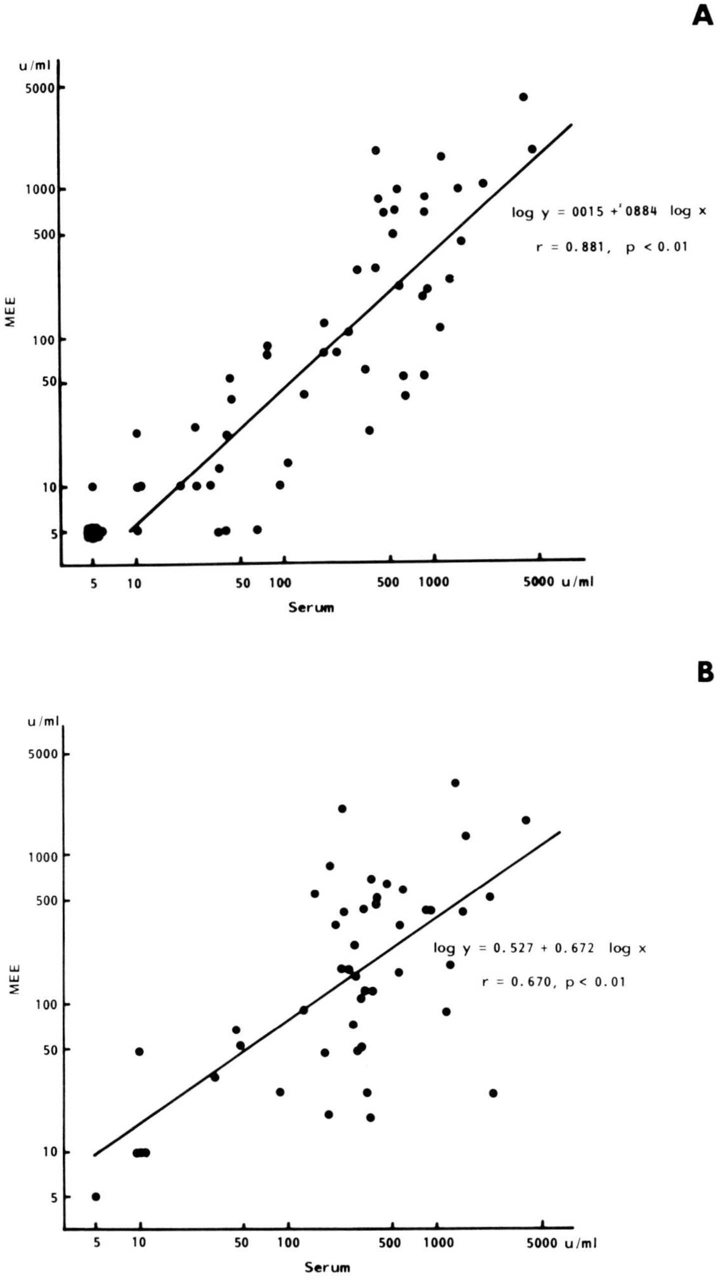

FIG. 1. Relationship of IgE concentrations between MEEs and sera. **A:** Serous effusions. **B:** Mucoid effusions.

lergy, or more specifically IgE-mediated hypersensitivity, may be responsible for recurrent OM in about one-third of children with chronic OME.

MUCOSAL IMMUNITY OF THE MIDDLE EAR

In OME the subepithelial mucosal sites are characterized by the presence of T and B cells (Palva et al., *this volume*). Furthermore, the T cells are primarily of a helper inducer variety (Palva et al., *this volume*). The source of these cells is not known, but one would speculate that they derive their origin from gut-associated lymphoid tissue (GALT), bronchus-associated lymphoid tissue (BALT), or from the tonsils and adenoids.

It has been demonstrated by numerous investigators that the major immunoglobulin synthesized by the plasma cells of the middle ear mucosa is IgA and that at least one-third to one-half of this is the 10S dimer (3,23,25,26,32,33,35,50). During its transport across the mucosal epithelium, this dimer acquires the SC by a complex sequence of events on the luminal surface as a complete secretory IgA (sIgA) molecule [dimeric IgA and joining (J) chain + SC].

Available evidence suggests that the development of a humoral immune response and a cell-mediated immune respone in the middle ear is determined, among other factors, by the availability of sufficient antigenic mass to the mucosal immunocompetent tissue and the nature of the available bacterial or viral antigens (39,40,43,49). The remainder of this chapter will address humoral and cell-mediated immune responses that have been demonstrated in the middle ear mucosa and in MEE.

Information on the mucosa of the normal middle ear has suggested that the middle ear mucosa shares a number of features in common with the mucosal system in the intestinal and respiratory tract (31,40,41,42,56). The anterior/inferior portion of the middle ear mucosa possesses a ciliated epithelium with goblet cells and therefore also possesses the potential for a mucociliary system (55). The presence of sIgA in the middle ear, as well as the significant difference in the IgG/IgA ratio and the local *in vitro* synthesis of IgA and SC in the middle ear mucosa, strongly suggests that middle ear mucosa in OME has characteristics of a common immune mucosal system (3,20,33,35,36,39,41,56). In the normal middle ear without inflammation, the remainder of the middle ear posterior to the above-mentioned areas possesses mainly basal cells, nonciliated cells with very few goblet cells, and very few inflammatory cells. In general, the normal middle ear cavity contains a paucity of mucous glands, a low density of goblet cells, and a characteristic absence of organized lymphoid follicles and very sparse presence of plasma cells or lymphocytes. However, in OME the middle ear mucosa bears a striking resemblance to the immunological features observed in the peripheral mucosal sites of the common mucosal system.

The results of immunological studies performed on middle ear secretions and middle ear tissues strongly indicate that the effusion in OME is caused by a local reaction. The effusion SC is a protein unique to external secretions and found in serum in only small amounts, usually below the level detectable by the techniques of routine immunochemistry. In studies performed in various laboratories, SC has been identified in over 80% of MEEs (3,33,43,51). It appears to be antigenically identical to SC found in other external secretions, such as colostrum and nasal fluid (3,39,40,43). The SC in the middle ear appears in bound form with 10S IgA as evidenced by its position on sucrose density gradient ultracentrifugation (3,43). Recent studies have suggested that the ratio of sIgA to monomeric IgA is different in nasal secretions and the nasopharynx than in the MEE (36,51) (see Fig. 2 and also Sørensen's chapter, *this volume*).

Further evidence for the local secretory basis of fluid is based on analysis of immunoglobulin content of the fluid. These findings suggest that the IgA/IgG ratios are significantly lower in MEE than in serum. This is the result of an increase in local synthesis of IgA in the middle ear mucosa. Lactoferin and lysozyme are two other proteins found in MEE and rarely found in the sera (22). An observation of particular importance is viral-specific IgA antibody activity in MEE (3,30,62). These observations provide evidence for the existence of a distinct system of local immunity functioning in the middle ear of patients with OME.

The mechanism underlying the production of sIgA antibody in middle ear mucosa appears to be the local availability of immunologically active antigen to immunocompetent cells in the middle ear mucosa or to immunocompetent tissue in the nasopharynx (49). Although IgG and IgA classes of viral specific antibody were detected in the middle ear, the proportion of viral-specific antibody of the IgA class was 2 to 6 times higher than those of the IgG class antibody (3,30,62). In view of these observations, it has been suggested that the middle ear mucosa is capable of mounting a specific local antibody response after appropriate antigen stimulus. Recent evidence also suggests local antibody response in MEEs against a variety of bacterial agents, including the M protein of *Streptococcus pyogenes*

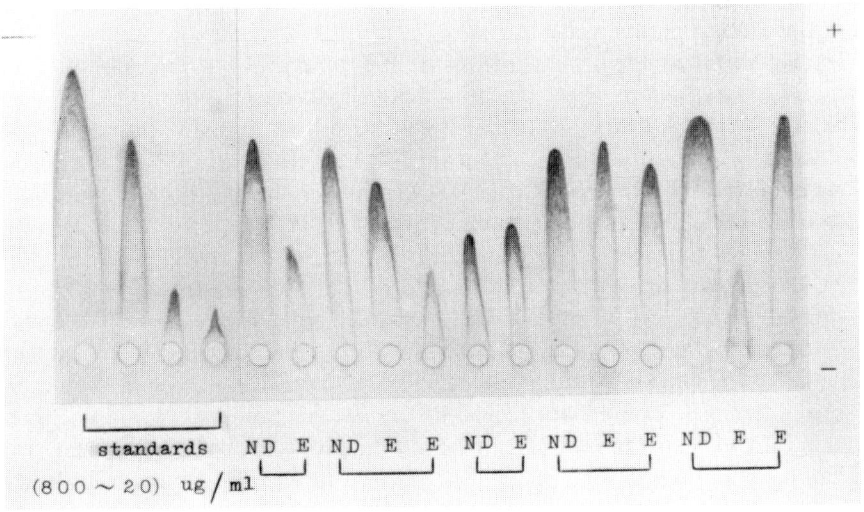

FIG. 2. Electroimmunodiffusion patterns of sIgA in MEEs (E) and nasal discharges (ND).

(37,52,60). This specific antibody directed against the M protein may prevent adherence of the bacteria to the middle ear mucosa and prevent suppurative OM.

The source of B-cell precursors that give rise later to IgA in the middle ear is not entirely known. A complete description of this has been reviewed in several chapters (Scicchitano et al. and Cumella, *this volume*) and will only be considered here very briefly. IgA-bearing B lymphocytes are abundant in GALT and/or BALT (9). It is also possible that the tonsils and adenoids could be sites for precursor B cells that will infiltrate the middle ear mucosa following OME (52). After sensitization with antigen in the GALT or BALT or adenoids or tonsils, precursors of IgA-producing cells will enter the general circulation from the thoracic duct and eventually settle in mucosal tissue of the antigen-stimulated organ, as well as in distant secretory sites, such as the genital tract, the salivary glands, the lacrimal gland, and the middle ear cleft (9,12). The presence of IgA-producing cells in distant mucosal tissues is considered evidence of a common mucosal immune system, as discussed in several preceding chapters (Scicchitano et al. and Cumella, *this volume*).

Mucosal surfaces are in constant contact with a myriad of substances, and the mucosal immune system has a powerful regulatory mechanism that allows it to react selectively to many, or most, substances found in the mucosal environment. These regulatory mechanisms result because the regular administration of oral antigen induces the formation of mucosa-derived suppressor T cells that may act on IgG and IgM lymphocytes, but apparently not on IgA B lymphocytes (53). In contrast, the IgA response may be enhanced because of the induction of antigen-specific helper T cells for IgA response upon mucosal antigen administration (48). Recently, Strober (53) was successful in cloning Peyer's patch T cells, which act as "switch" cells that induce IgM B lymphocytes to differentiate directly into IgA B lymphocytes. The switch T cells operate only on IgM B lymphocytes, not on IgA B lymphocytes, and do not mediate the differentiation of IgA B lymphocytes to IgA-producing plasma cells.

The sIgA in the middle ear fluids, as mentioned above, has been identified in many MEEs, particularly of the mucoid variety. The concentration of IgA_2 appears to be higher in sIgA than in 7S or serum IgA (33,50). Apparently IgA_2 molecules are less susceptible to digestion by bacterial IgA protease, which is produced by *Hemophilus influenzae* and *Streptococcus pneumoniae,* the two most common bacterial organisms found in acute suppurative OM (19). Therefore, sIgA is relatively less susceptible to bacterial enzymatic digestion than serum or 7S IgA.

Although Bernstein et al. (3) and Mogi et al. (33,36) consider SC in MEEs to be primarily bound to IgA, other investigators have reported that the SC/sIgA ratio is much greater in MEEs from patients with OME than in patients with recurrent acute OM (51). Obviously more studies in this regard need to be done in order to resolve differences of opinion. Recent studies also suggest that the sIgA/7S IgA ratio in MEEs is approximately 1:1 in the mucoid effusions, but approximately 1:6 in the serous effusions (40). This is demonstrated in Table 1. On the other hand, nasopharyngeal secretions reveal a much higher sIgA/IgA serum ratio as noted in Table 1. These findings suggest MEE is a mixture of exudation of middle ear se-

TABLE 1. *Mean levels of sIgG and serum-type IgA in MEE, NS, and sera*[a]

	Mucoid group			Serous group		
	MEE ($N = 87$)	NS ($N = 28$)	Serum ($N = 65$)	MEE ($N = 54$)	NS ($N = 27$)	Serum ($N = 49$)
sIgA	2 712.6 (A) ± 2 267.4	3 672.8 (B) ± 2 747.4	— (C)	854.6 (D) ± 1 060.8	3 096.5 (E) ± 2 713.0	— (F)
Serum-type IgA	2 919.3 (a) ± 2 308.9	576.9 (b) ± 458.5	2 342.9 (c) ± 1 872.1	4 862.4 (d) ± 3 387.4	452.7 (e) ± 2 843.4	2 998.0 (f) ± 2 195.8

[a]sIgA, secretory IgA; MEE, middle ear effusion; NS, nasal secretion.

Note: All figures represent mean ± SD,μg/ml. Significant differences: A > D, $p < 0.001$; a < d, $p < 0.001$; a > b, $p < 0.001$; B > b, $p < 0.001$; D < E, $p < 0.001$; d > e, $p < 0.001$; d > f, $p < 0.005$; d > D, $p < 0.005$; E > e, $p < 0.001$. Significant correlation between: A and a, $p < 0.05$, $r = 0.309$; A and B, $p < 0.05$, $r = 0.439$; B and b, $p < 0.01$; $r = 0.562$; d and f, $p < 0.05$, $r = 0.336$.

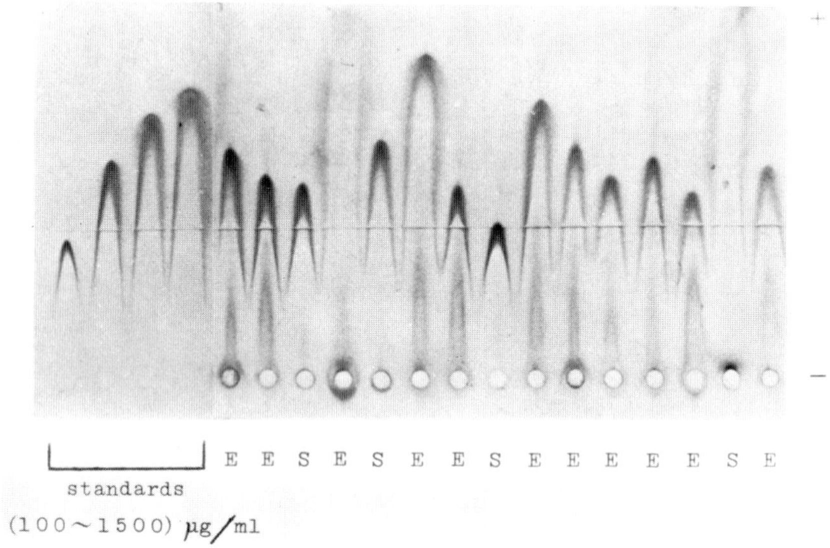

FIG. 3. Electroimmunodiffusion patterns of serum-type IgA in MEEs (E) and sera (S). Two equal-sized gel layers are made on a glass plate. The gel on the cathodal side has an antisecretory component antibodies, whereas the gel on the anodal side has anti-IgA antibodies. Rocket-shaped immunoprecipitations on the cathodal gel layer are sIgA and free SC, whereas those on the anodal gel layer are serum-type IgA.

cretions from the middle ear mucosa, as well as transudation from the serum (see Fig. 3). It also appears likely that some of the middle ear secretions may be related to retrograde reflux of mucus from the eustachian tube because there are abundant glands secreting both 10S IgA and SC in the lamina propria and epithelium of the eustachian tube, respectively (39).

As mentioned above, sIgA plays an important role in protection against bacterial and viral diseases. In MEE and in nasopharyngeal secretions, the presence of specific antibody activity of the IgA class to respiratory viruses, even if these viral infections do not appear to be causative for OME, could be explained by the common mucosal immune system. After sensitization of precursor of IgA B lymphocytes in the special lymphoid tissue of the mucosal-associated lymphoid tissue (MALT) with such viruses, precursor B cells enter the circulation and apparently migrate to mucosal tissue of the nasopharynx and middle ear, as well as other distant sites. At the present time, the exact source of IgA B-cell precursors and their route to the middle ear mucosa is still not known.

In addition to viruses there is evidence that sIgA may be directed against various bacteria in the middle ear, such as coagulase-negative staphylococci and corynebacterium (6), suggesting that these organisms may not necessarily be contaminants when found in middle ear cultures. Other investigators have identified class-specific antibody to isolated bacteria in MEE and sera by the use of direct immunofluorescent methods. In general, IgA antibodies are detected more frequently in MEE than in sera (19). Antibodies directed against *Streptococcus pneumoniae* and *Hemophilus influenzae* have been obtained from patients with recurrent OM and those with OME (23,52). Furthermore, in animal models, it appears that a primary infection with a specific organism will render the host more resistant to infection by that specific organism than from another bacteria (19,23,37). Locally derived antibodies to bacterial organisms appear to have a beneficial role in elimination of effusions, eradication of the infectious agent, and probably in the protection against reinfection with the same homologous organism. The exact mechanism of sIgA in viral and bacterial infections in the middle ear is not known. The most commonly suggested mechanism is that of immune adherence, in that sIgA is capable of blocking bacterial adherence to mucosal surfaces, preventing the colonization of bacteria (40). On the other hand, it may be possible that sIgA, by surrounding the organism, may also prevent phagocytosis by IgG antibody, which fixes complement, and in this way it is possible that IgA may actually act as a blocking antibody rather than as a protective antibody.

Thus, the presence in MEE of sIgA implies that mucosal immunity occurs in middle ears involved in OME. Furthermore, it should be noted that IgA and lysozyme levels are significantly higher in culture-negative MEE than in the culture-positive effusions (22).

The development of mucosal immunity requires constant adequate antigenic stimuli. From results of the studies mentioned so far in this chapter, it can be suggested that local synthesis of IgA, as well as other classes of immunoglobulins, is latent in the lining membrane of the normal tympanic cavity. This evidence is attributed to the fact that anatomically the middle ear has less frequent opportunity to undergo antigenic stimulation than other areas of the upper respiratory tract and alimentary tracts. Inasmuch as there is no normal bacterial flora in the normal tympanic cavity, there would be no opportunity for antigenic stimulation of the normal middle ear mucosa (16). Figure 4 represents immunofluorescent observation of the middle ear mucosa from a patient with chronic OME, demonstrating numerous IgA-synthesizing plasma cells. Undoubtedly, therefore, once antigenic stimulation from bacteria or virus takes place in the middle ear mucosa, a transformation of the middle ear mucosa occurs. Chemotaxis for inflammatory cells into the middle ear mucosa would then follow from the bloodstream, and presumably precursor B cells from GALT, BALT, adenoids, or tonsils would then be stimulated by local antigen present in the middle ear to produce sIgA. In this way, the middle ear mucosa can develop an immune response. The induction of experimental OM in developing guinea pigs by inoculation of killed type III *Streptococcus pneumoniae* or bovine albumin will result in marked accumulation of IgA-forming cells in the middle ear mucosa of these animals (Fig. 5), even though the presence of IgA-forming cells is very rare in the uninjected animals. Thus, the middle ear mucosa is a potential site of immunological reactivity, and a developing middle ear possesses all of the requirements for immunological responsiveness. Because younger children possess a more immature immune system, it is more likely that in this

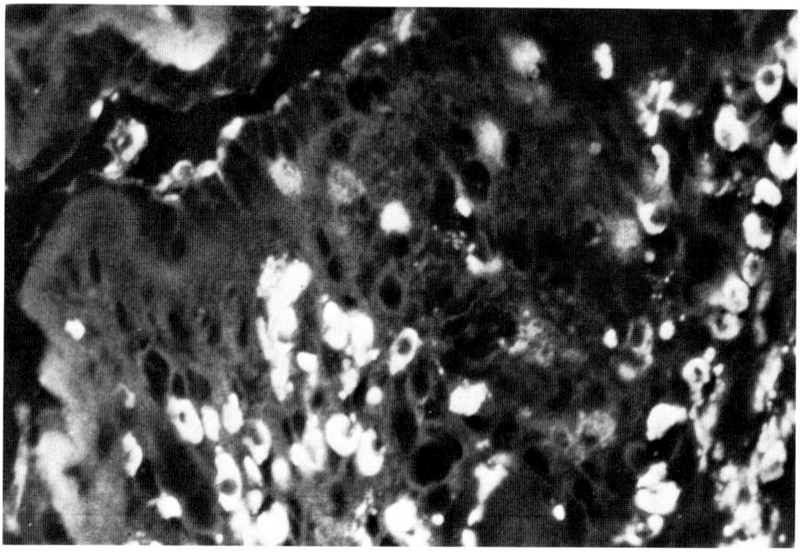

FIG. 4. Immunofluorescent pattern of the middle ear mucosa obtained from a patient with chronic OME, showing numerous IgA-forming cells.

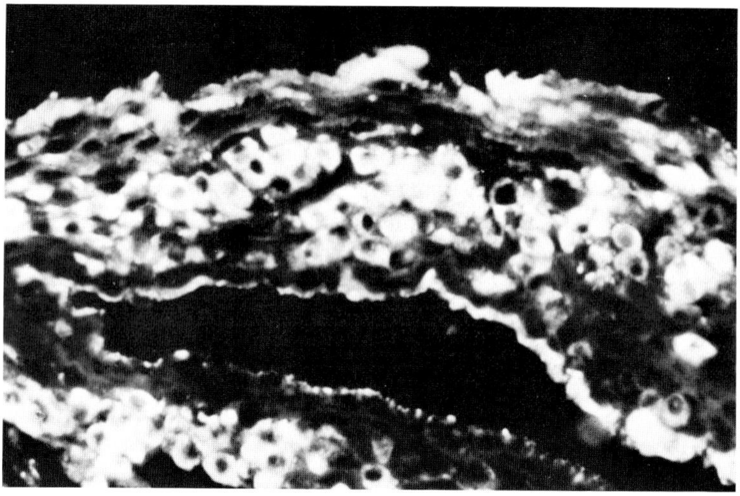

FIG. 5. Immunofluorescent photograph. Heavy infiltration of IgA-forming cells is seen in the mucous membrane of tympanic bulla of a developing guinea pig with experimental OME.

age group, poor development of middle ear mucosal immune response may be one of the factors leading to infection proneness of the middle ear that leads to recurrent suppurative OM and to OME (see Dagöö's chapter, *this volume*).

IMMUNOLOGICAL MECHANISMS AND INFLAMMATORY REACTIONS IN OTITIS MEDIA

In addition to the above-mentioned humoral immune mechanisms that may play a role in the eradication and perhaps prevention of OM, the same immune mechanisms may be responsible for the prolongation and chronicity of OM if eustachian tube function remains abnormal. Therefore, IgE-mediated hypersensitivity (this subject is covered completely in Welliver's chapter, *this volume*), immune complexes, delayed hypersensitivity, activated complements, bacterial toxins, lysosomal enzymes, prostaglandins, rheumatoid factors, and other mediators may be harmful to the middle ear and may be related to the chronicity and prolongation of the inflammatory response in the middle ear mucosa (see van Cauwenberger and Bernstein, *this volume*).

The presence of soluble immune complexes in middle ear fluids has been reported and therefore it has been suggested that immune complex may be responsible for immunopathology in the middle ear (27,42,44,49,54). Some investigators not only strongly support this opinion, but consider it to be a common cause of OME (27). At the recent Symposium on Acute Otitis Media and Secretory Otitis Media in Jerusalem in 1985, the panel on immunology suggested that immune complexes are present in the middle ear fluid, but probably represent a process of immunoelimination rather than a process leading to immunopathology. There has not been any demonstration by any investigation that, in human OM, immune complexes are deposited in the basement membrane of the epithelium or in the basement membrane of the blood vessels of the middle ear mucosa or mastoid mucosa (7). Furthermore, soluble immune complexes do not represent necessarily a pathological situation, but rather represent only the possibility that bacteria and antibody have complexed and perhaps fixed complement in the fluid phase. This is found in normal inflammatory situations without immune complex immunopathology.

Even if immune complexes do not deposit in the middle ear mucosa, there is adequate evidence that the complement system is activated via both the classic pathway and the alternative pathway (5,18,29). The role of complement in OM is thoroughly discussed in Prellner's chapter *(this volume)*. Furthermore, pneumococcal polysaccharide capsular antigens and endotoxin of *Hemophilus influenzae* may also activate the complement system nonspecifically via the alternate pathway. Thus, breakdown products of complement components of C2, C4, C3, and C5 have all been found in the middle ear and may give rise to inflammatory products, which may cause activation of mast cells, chemotaxis for neutrophils, and, in general, maintain the inflammatory situation in the middle ear (11,18,29). As shown in Figs. 6 and 7, the mean concentrations of C3a and C5a in MEE are significantly

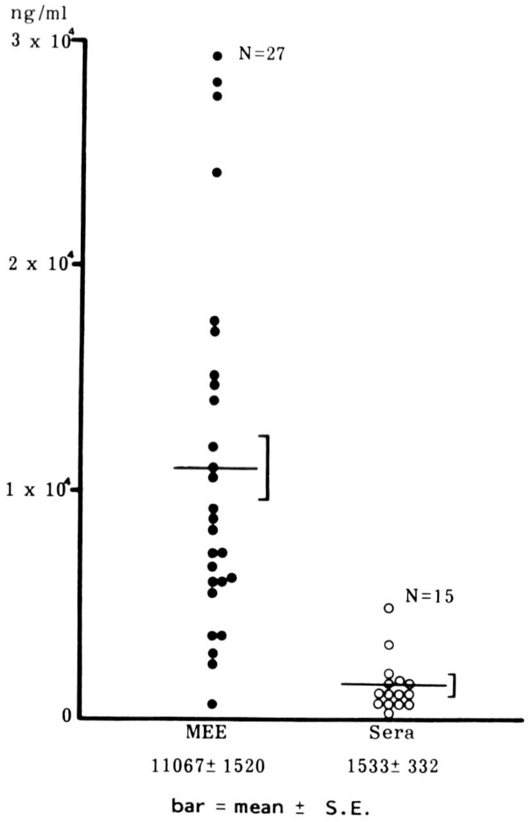

FIG. 6. C3a levels in MEEs and sera.

greater than those in the corresponding sera. In addition, the mean histamine level in MEE exceeds significantly that in sera (Fig. 8). All of these findings strongly suggest that there is an active inflammatory process in OM similar to that of other inflammatory conditions in other sites in the body. Furthermore, lysosomal enzymes are released as a result of neutrophil activation following ingestion of immune complexes in the middle ear (2,11). Granulocyte proteases that are released may also activate the alternative pathway of the complement system (2,5,27). The activity of granulocyte protease is quite high in MEE, and this has been noted in a chapter by Jhun, et al., *(this volume)*. As shown in the schematic drawing in Fig. 9, immune complexes and other substances in the MEE may activate complement components, leading to the production of inflammation-generating fragments that, in turn, may activate mast cells releasing inflammatory mediators producing vasodilation and mucosal edema, as well as neutrophil chemotaxis. These neutrophils would then ingest the immune complexes and, in turn, release the granulocytic proteases and produce tissue injury. Therefore, the vicious cycle between these substances may maintain the inflammatory condition in the middle ear.

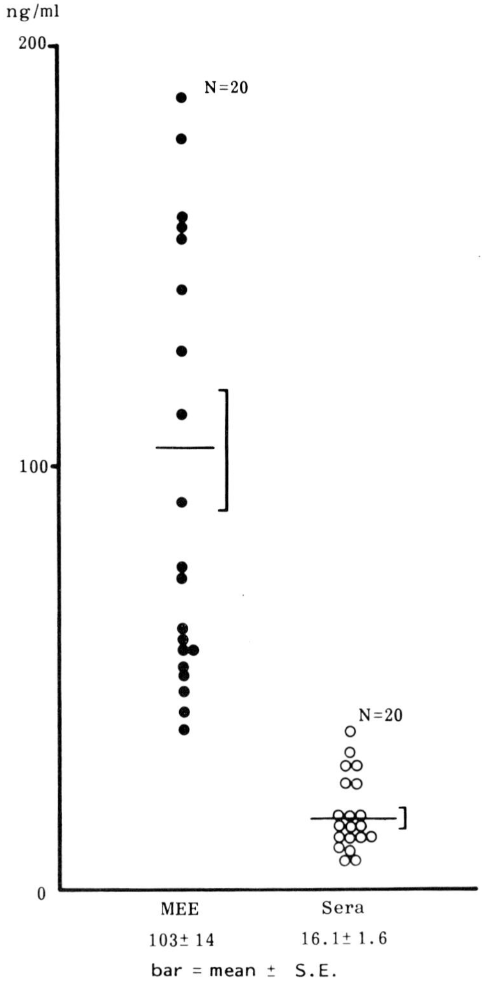

FIG. 7. C5a levels in MEEs and sera.

CELL-MEDIATED MECHANISMS AND MACROPHAGE-LYMPHOCYTE RELATIONS IN THE MIDDLE EAR

Little information is available regarding the role of cellular immune mechanisms in protection or in the pathogenesis of OM. Using cell surface receptors on T and B lymphocytes and macrophages, it is now evident that T cells predominate in all MEEs (see Palva et al.'s chapter, *this volume*). However, there is some evidence that B cells appear to predominate in the mucoid effusions (again, see Palva et al.'s chapter, *this volume*). Furthermore, macrophages represent the most common mononuclear cell in the sediment of all chronic MEEs, except for the purulent form of OM in which neutrophils are the most common cells found (8). Using monoclonal antibodies directed against specific determinants on the surface of T

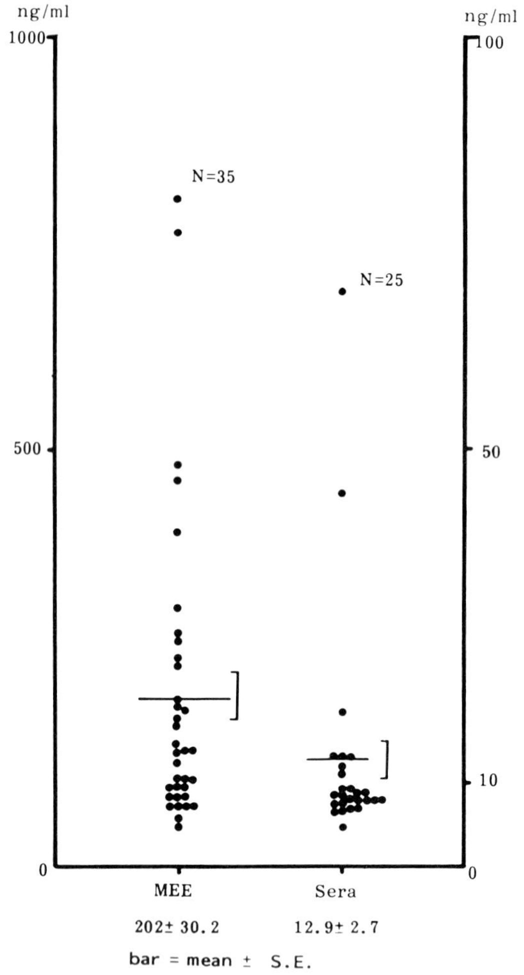

FIG. 8. Histamine levels in MEEs and sera.

cells, T helper-inducer cells, and T suppressor-cytotoxic cells, there is now abundant information regarding T-cell subsets and B cells in different MEEs. This is thoroughly discussed in Palva et al.'s chapter *(this volume)*.

Recent studies have suggested that macrophages may play a critical role in the modulation of T- and B-cell activity in the middle ear (8). The characteristics of cellular elements in MEEs, peripheral blood, and adenoidal tissue, as well as the effects of middle ear macrophage on the functional activity of lymphocytes, have been examined in patients with chronic OME. The proliferative responses induced by phytohemagglutinin (PHA) or pokeweed mitogen (PWM) of middle ear lymphocytes are generally low compared with the responses observed in peripheral blood and adenoidal lymphocytes. Co-cultures of middle ear macrophages with adenoidal lymphocytes result in a significant depression of proliferative response in

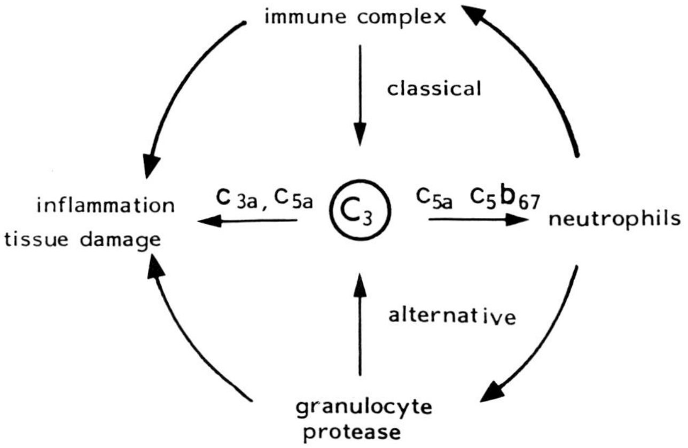

FIG. 9. Schematic drawing of a vicious cycle that maintains inflammatory change in the middle ear affected by OME.

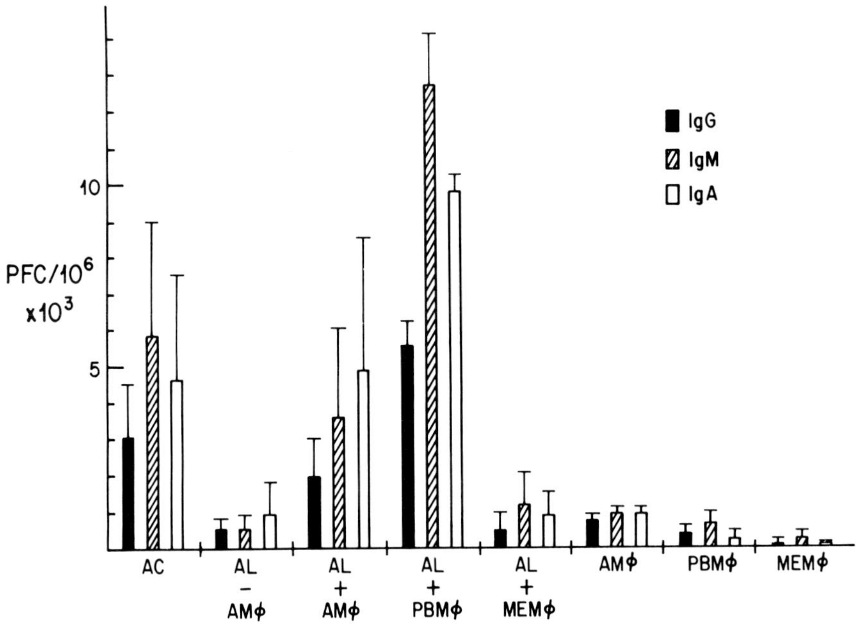

FIG. 10. The effect of co-cultivation of adenoidal macrophages (AM), peripheral blood monocytes (PBM), and middle ear macrophages (MEM) in patients with chronic OME on the synthesis of polyclonal IgG, IgM, and IgA antibodies by adenoidal lymphocytes (AL) after *in vitro* stimulation by pokeweed mitogen. Data are mean plaque-forming counts (PFC)/10^3. The bars represent standard deviation. (AC) Adenoidal cells (unfractionated).

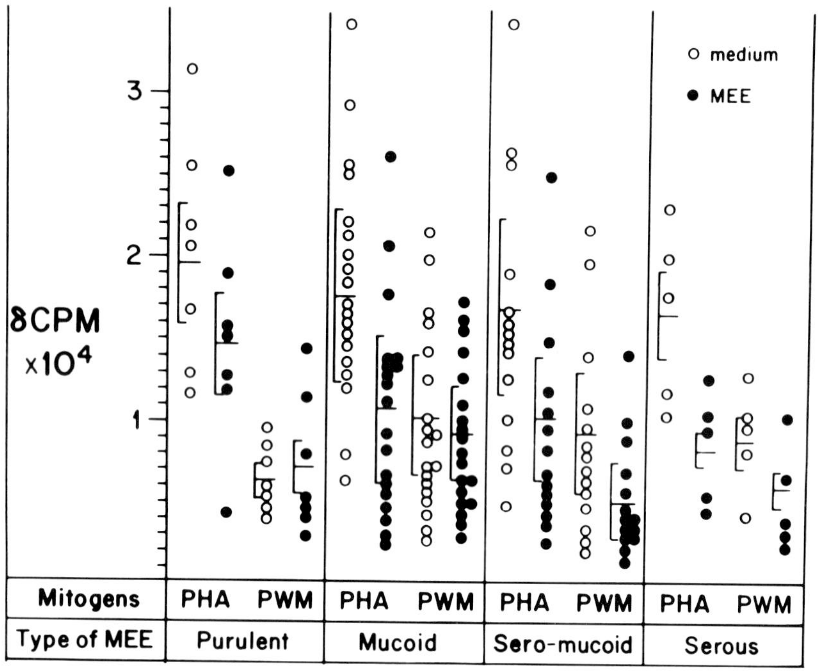

FIG. 11. Effect of different types of MEEs on proliferative response to PHA or PWM in adenoidal lymphocytes.

both immunoglobulin synthesis and lymphocyte transformation, as demonstrated in Figs. 10 and 11. These observations suggest that macrophages in the middle ear may have a profound influence on the regulation of the immune response in OME patients. The hyporesponsiveness of middle ear cells to PWM and PHA may be a reflection of the relatively large proportion of macrophages observed in the MEEs. These observations, taken together, suggest that the adherent cell population, which most likely consists of macrophages, is functionally distinct from the peripheral blood monocytes and exerts a profound suppressive effect on the proliferative response of MEE lymphocytes to PWM, as well as on the *in vitro* synthesis of major immunoglobulins. Further studies on the immunological aspects of OME revealed the nature of the cell-mediated immunoresponsive activity in middle ear fluid by fractionating pooled middle ear fluid. The effects of these different pools on lymphocyte transformation and polyclonal immunoglobulin synthesis have been studied. The immunosuppressive activity appears to be limited to a soluble factor with molecular weight of approximately 50,000, as demonstrated in Fig. 12. The degree of immunosuppression appears to be most marked with serous or seromucinous forms of MEE. Further studies are needed to determine whether the material that was used in the middle ear fractionation was the result of macrophage secretion or lymphocyte secretion. On the basis of these observations, it is proposed that in certain chronic forms of OME, there is a relative preponderance of macro-

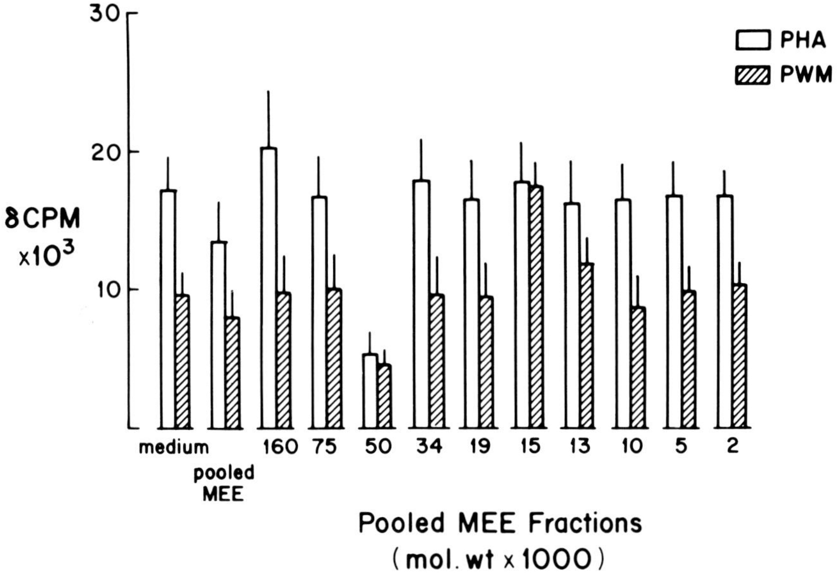

FIG. 12. Effects of different column fractions of pooled MEEs on proliferative response to adenoidal lymphocytes, PHA, and PWM. Unfractionated MEE and tissue cultures medium were included as controls.

phages that are actively immunosuppressive for the proliferative response to mitogen and specific antigens as well as suppressive to the synthesis of specific immunoglobulin. Such immunological hyporesponsiveness may be related to the pathogenesis of chronic OME.

NATURAL KILLER CELL ACTIVITY IN MIDDLE EAR SUPERNATANTS

The role of cytotoxic T cells, antibody-dependent cytotoxicity, and natural killer (NK) cell activity has only recently been investigated in MEEs. Initial studies suggest that the numbers of lymphocytes in the MEEs are too small to evaluate the presence of NK cells. However, when using peripheral blood cytotoxic T cells against effector cells, which are known to respond specifically to NK cells, one can observe the role of middle ear fluids on the modulation of NK cells in peripheral blood. This effect is shown in Fig. 13. It appears that middle ear fluid supernatant may have an effect on the percentage of NK activity in the peripheral blood. In general, there may be either augmentation of NK cell activity or there may be actual depression of NK cell activity in some middle ear fluids. Prostaglandin E2 (PGE2) has been measured in these fluids and there is some evidence that PGE2 may be found in higher concentrations in those middle ear fluids that depress NK cell activity.

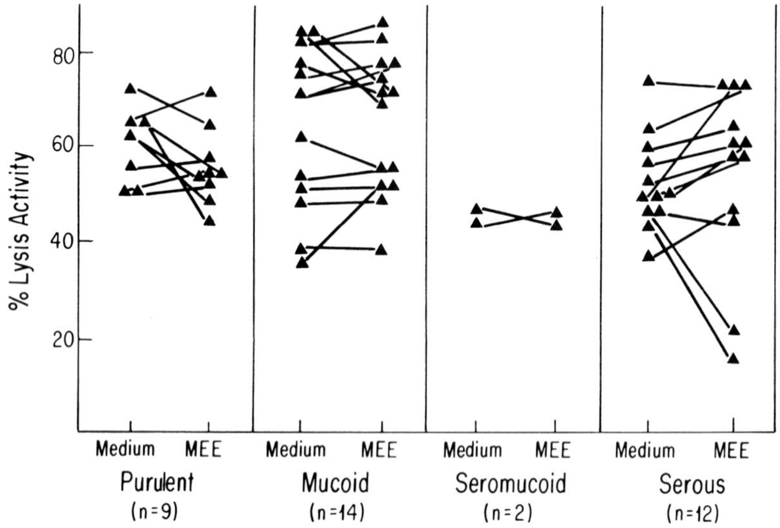

FIG. 13. The effect of middle ear supernatants of different MEEs on NK cell activity from peripheral blood lymphocytes. There is a relationship between the decrease in NK cell activity by peripheral blood lymphocytes and the concentration of PGE2 in the middle ear fluids. Augmentation of NK activity was also seen in some middle ear fluids. However, there was no detection of interferon in any of these middle ear supernatants.

CONCLUSIONS

The secretory immune system is a composite of T cells and T-cell subsets, antibodies, macrophages, and other cellular effectors, which function in a unique and somewhat compartmentalized manner. Available evidence to date suggests that B cells and antibody production and function, as well as T-cell-mediated reactivity, in the mucosal surfaces of gastrointestinal tract, respiratory tract, genital tract, mammary glands, nasopharynx and salivary glands, and upper respiratory airway mucosa share a common function. The bulk of the sIgA reactivity observed in these mucosal sites appears to be a reflection of initial antigenic exposure and lymphoid activation in the GALT and BALT. The mucosa of the middle ear during inflammatory states has now been shown to function in a manner similar to other secretory sites listed above and appears to respond to antigenic stimuli in a similar manner.

The role of immunologic reactivity in middle ear pathology, however, remains to be defined. The source of immunocompetent cells in the middle ear particularly needs to be elucidated to aid further development of efficient vaccines against middle ear infection. The role of antibiotics in modulating or depressing an effective immune response in the middle ear needs to be studied. The duration of the humoral and cellular immune response should be investigated, particularly with regard to specific T and B cells. This may have a bearing on reinfection in otitis-prone children. Finally, further studies on IgG subclasses and bacterial adherence in the nasopharynx need to be evaluated in children with recurrent OME.

REFERENCES

1. Aro, M.J.T., and Kouvalainnen, K. (1967): Proteins of middle ear secretion in serous otitis. An electrophoretic and immunoelectrophoretic study. *Acta Otolaryngol.*, 244(Suppl.):385–389.
2. Berger, G., Hawke, M., Propps, D.W., Ranadive, N.S., and Wong, D. (1984): Granulocyte protease in middle ear effusions. *Ann. Otol. Rhinol. Laryngol.*, 91:76–81.
3. Bernstein, J.M., Tomasi, T.B., and Ogra, P.L. (1974): The immunochemistry of middle ear effusions. *Arch Otolaryngol.*, 99:320–326.
4. Bernstein, J.M., and Reisman, R. (1974): The role of acute hypersensitivity in secretory otitis media. *Trans. Am. Acad. Ophthal. Otolaryngol.*, 78:120–127.
5. Bernstein, J.M., Shenkheim, H.A., Genco, R.J., and Bartholomew, W.R. (1978): Complement activity in middle ear effusions. *Clin. Exp. Immunol.*, 33:340–346.
6. Bernstein, J.M., Myers, D., Losinski, D., Nisengard, R., and Wicher, K. (1980): Antibody coated bacteria in otitis media with effusion. *Ann. Otol. Rhinol. Laryngol.*, 89(Suppl. 68, No. 3, part 2):104–109.
7. Bernstein, J.M., Brentjens, J., and Vladutiu, A. (1982): Immune complexes determination in otitis media with effusion. *Am. J. Otolaryngol.*, 3:20–25.
8. Bernstein, J.M., Yamanaka, T., Cumella, J., and Ogra, P.L. (1984): Characterisitcs of lymphocyte and macrophage reactivity in otitis media with effusion. *Acta Otolaryngol.*, 414(Suppl.):131–137.
9. Bienenstock, J., Johnston, N., and Perey, D.Y.E. (1973): Bronchial lymphoid tissue. II. Functional characteristics. *Lab. Invest.*, 28:693–698.
10. Carlson, L.A., and Lokk, T. (1955): Protein studies of transdates of the middle ear. *Scand. J. Clin. Lab. Invest.*, 7:43–48.
11. Carlsson, B., Lundberg, C., and Ohlsson, K. (1982): Granulocyte protease in middle ear effusions. *Ann. Otol. Rhinol. Laryngol.*, 91:76–81.
12. Craig, S.W., and Cebra, J.J. (1971): Peyer's patches. An enriched source of precursors for IgA producing immunocytes in the rabbit. *J. Exp. Med.*, 134:188–200.
13. Doyle, W.J., Takahara, T., and Fireman, P. (1985): The role of allergy in the pathogenesis of otitis media with effusion. *Arch. Otolaryngol.*, 111:502–506.
14. Draper, W.L. (1967): Secretory otitis media in children: a study of 540 children. *Laryngoscope*, 77:636–653.
15. Friedman, R.A., Doyle, W.J., and Cassellbrant, M.L. (1983): Immunologic-mediated eustachian tube obstruction: a double-blind crossover study. *J. Allergy Clin. Immunol.*, 71:442–447.
16. Goycoolea, M.V., Valenzuela, E.M., Nartinez, G.C., and Maldonado, A.B. (1984): Is there a normal microflora in the middle ear cavity? In: *Recent Advances in Otitis Media with Effusion*, edited by D.J. Lim, C.D. Bluestone, J.O. Klein, and J.D. Nelson, pp. 139–141. B.C. Decker, Philadelphia/Toronto.
17. Hambling, M.H. (1964): A survey of antibodies to respiratory syncytial virus in the population. *Br. Med. J.*, 1:1223–1225.
18. Harada, T., Ogino, S., Suzawa, Y., Matsunaga, T., Hong, K., and Inoue, K. (1984): Complement anaphylotoxins activity in middle ear effusion. *Auris Nasus Larynx*, 12(Suppl. 1):188–190.
19. Howie, V.M., Ploussard, J.H., Sloyer, J.L., and Johnston, R.B., Jr. (1973): Immunoglobulins of the middle ear fluid in acute otitis media: relationship to serum immunoglobulin concentrations and bacterial cultures. *Infect. Immun.*, 7:589–593.
20. Hussl, B., and Lim, D.J. (1974): Experimental middle ear effusion: an immunofluorescent study. *Ann. Otol. Rhinol. Laryngol.*, 83:332–342.
21. Ishizaka, K., Ishizaka, T., and Hornbrook, M.M. (1966): Physicochemical properties of human reaginic antibodies. IV. Presence of a unique immunoglobulin as a carrier of reaginic activity. *J. Immunol.*, 97:75–85.
22. Lang, R.W., Liu, Y.S., Lim, D.J., and Birck, H.G. (1976): Antimicrobial factors and bacterial correlation in chronic otitis media with effusion. *Ann. Otol. Rhinol. Laryngol.*, 85(Suppl. 25, No. 2):145–151.
23. Lewis, D.M., Schram, J.L., Birck, H.G., and Lim, D.J. (1979): Antibody activity in otitis media with effusion. *Ann. Otol. Rhinol. Laryngol.*, 88:392–396.
24. Lewis, D.M., Schram, J.L., Lim, D.J., Birck, H.G., and Gleick, G. (1978): Immunoglobulin E in chronic middle ear effusions. Comparison of RIST, PRIST and RIA techniques. *Ann. Otol. Rhinol. Laryngol.*, 87:197–201.

25. Lewis, D.M., Schram, J.L., Meadema, S.J., and Lim, D.J. (1980): Experimental otitis media in chinchillas. *Ann. Otol. Rhinol. Laryngol.*, 89(Suppl. 89, No. 3):344–350.
26. Liu, Y.S., Lim, D.J., Lang, R.W., and Birck, H.G. (1975): Chronic middle ear effusions. Immunological and bacteriological investigations. *Arch. Otolaryngol.*, 101:278–286.
27. Maxim, P.E., Vetri, R.W., and Sprinkle, P.M. (1979): Chronic serous otitis media: an immune complex disease. *Trans. Am. Acad. Ophthal. Otolaryngol., ORL*, 84:234–238.
28. McGovern, J.P., Haywood, T.J., and Fernandez, A.A. (1967): Allergy and secretory otitis media. An analysis of 512 cases. *JAMA*, 200:134–138.
29. Meri, S., Lehtinen, T., and Palva, T. (1984): Complement in chronic secretory otitis media. C breakdown and C splitting activity. *Arch. Otolaryngol.*, 110:774–778.
30. Meurman, O.H., Sarkkinen, H.K., Puhakka, H.J., Virolainen, E.S., and Meurman, O.H. (1980): Local IgA-class antibodies against respiratory viruses in middle ear and nasopharyngeal secretions of children with secretory otitis media. *Laryngoscope*, 90:304–311.
31. Mogi, G., and Honjo, S. (1972): Middle ear effusion. Analysis of protein components. *Ann. Otol. Rhinol. Laryngol.*, 81:99–105.
32. Mogi, G., Yoshida, T., Honjo, S., and Maeda, S. (1973): Middle ear effusions. Quantitative analysis of immunoglobulins. *Ann. Otol. Rhinol. Laryngol.*, 82:196–202.
33. Mogi, G., Honjo, S. Maeda, S., and Yoshida, T. (1973): Secretory immunoglobulin A (SIgA) in middle ear effusions. Observation of 160 specimens. *Ann. Otol. Rhinol. Laryngol.*, 82:302–310.
34. Mogi, G., Honjo, S., Maeda, S., Yoshida, T., and Watanabe, N. (1974): Immunoglobulin E (IgE) in middle ear effusions. *Ann. Otol. Rhinol. Laryngol.*, 83:393–398.
35. Mogi, G., Honjo, S., Maeda, S., Yoshida, T., and Watanabe, N. (1974): Secretory immunoglobulin A (SIgA) in middle ear effusions. A further report. *Ann. Otol. Rhinol. Laryngol.*, 82:92–101.
36. Mogi, G., Honjo, S., Maeda, S., Yoshida, T., and Watanabe, N. (1974): Quantitative determination of secretory immunoglobulin A (SIgA) in middle ear effusions. *Ann. Otol. Rhinol. Laryngol.*, 83:239–246.
37. Mogi, G., Maeda, S., Yoshida, T., and Watanabe, N. (1976): Otitis media with effusion: specific antibody activities against exotoxins in middle ear effusion. *Laryngoscope*, 86:1043–1055.
38. Mogi, G., Maeda, S., Yoshida, T., and Watanabe, N. (1979): Role of atopic allergy in otitis media with effusion. *J. C. E. O. R. L. and Allergy*, 41:43–45.
39. Mogi, G., Maeda, S., and Watanabe, N. (1980): The development of mucosal immunity in guinea pig middle ears. *Int. J. Pediatr. Otorhinolaryngol.*, 1:331–349.
40. Mogi, G., Maeda, S., Umehara, T., Fujiyoshi, T., and Kurono, Y. (1984): Secretory IgA, serum Iga and secretory component in middle ear effusion. In: *Recent Advances in Otitis Media with Effusion*, edited by D.J. Lim, C.D. Bluestone, J.O. Klein, and J.D. Nelson, pp. 147–149. B.C. Decker, Philadelphia/Toronto.
41. Mogi, G. (1985): Biochemical and immunological characteristics of middle ear effusion. In: *New Dimension in Otorhinolaryngology—Head and Neck Surgery*, vol. 1, edited by E. N. Myers, pp. 271–274. Excepta Medica.
42. Mravec, J., Lewis, D.M., and Lim, D.J. (1978): Experimental otitis media with effusion: an immune-complex-mediated response. *Trans. Am. Acad. Ophthal. Otolaryngol. ORL*, 86:258–268.
43. Ogra, P.L., Bernstein, J.M., Yurchak, A.M., Copolla, P.R., and Tomasi, T.B., Jr. (1974): Characteristics of secretory immune system in human middle ear: implications in otitis media. *J. Immunol.*, 112:488–495.
44. Palva, T., Lehtinen, T., and Rinne, J. (1983): Immune complexes in middle ear fluid in chronic secretory otitis media. *Ann. Otol. Rhinol. Laryngol.*, 92:42–44.
45. Parrott, R.H., Kim, H.W., Bell, J.A., and Chanock, R.M. (1962): Respiratory diseases of viral etiology. III. Myxoviruses: parainfluenza. *Am. J. Public Health*, 52:907–917.
46. Phillips, M.J., Knight, N.J., Manning, H., Abbott, A.L., and Tripp, W.G. (1974): IgE and secretory otitis media. *Lancet*, 2:1176–1178.
47. Potter, C.W., and Shedden, W.I.H. (1963): The distribution of adenovirus antibodies in normal children. *J. Hyg. (Lond.)*, 61:155–160.
48. Richman, L.K., Graeff, A.S., Yarchoan, R., and Strober, W. (1981): Simultaneous induction of antigen specific IgA helper T cells and IgG suppressor T cells in the murine Peyer's patch after protein feeding. *J. Immunol.*, 126:2079–2083.

49. Ryan, A.F., Cleveland, P.H., Hartman, M.T., and Catanzaro, A. (1982): Humoral and cell-mediated immunity in peripheral blood following introduction of antigen into the middle ear. *Ann. Otol. Rhinol. Laryngol.,* 91:70–75.
50. Sipila, P., Koskela, M., Karjalainen, H., and Luotenen, J. (1985): Secretory IgA, secretory component and specific antibodies in the middle ear effusion during an attack of acute and respiratory otitis media. *Auris Nasus Larynx,* 12(Suppl. 1):180–182..
51. Sørensen, C.H. (1982): The ratio of secretory IgA to IgA in middle ear effusions and nasopharyngeal secretions. *Acta Otolaryngol.,* 396(Suppl.):91–93.
52. Sørensen, C.H. (1984): IgD and secretory immunoglobulins in secretions from the upper respiratory tract of children with secretory otitis media. In: *Recent Advances in Otitis Media with Effusion,* edited by D.J. Lim, C.D. Bluestone, J.O. Klein, and J.D. Nelson, pp. 150–152. B.C. Decker, Philadelphia/Toronto.
53. Strober, W. (1982): The regulation of mucosal immune system. *J. Allergy Clin. Immunol.,* 70:225–230.
54. Tachibana, M., Morioka, H., Tanimura, F., Tanaka, T., Machino, M., Amagi, T., Imanishi, J., and Mizukoshi, O. (1985): Experimental immune complex otitis media: localization of IgG by protein A-gold technique. *Auris Nasus Larynx,* 12(Suppl. 1): 86–88.
55. Takasaka, T., and Kawamoto, K. (1985): Mucocilliary dysfunction in experimental otitis media with effusion. *Am. J. Otolaryngol.,* 6:232–236.
56. Tomasi, T.B., Jr., Tan, E.M., Solomon, A., and Prendergast, R.A. (1965): Characteristics of an immune system common to certain external secretions. *J. Exp. Med.,* 121:101–124.
57. Tonder, O., and Gunderson, T. (1971): Nature of the fluid in serous otitis media. *Arch. Otolaryngol.,* 93:473–478.
58. Underdown, R.J., Knight, A., and Papsin, F.R. (1976): The relative paucity of IgE in human milk. *J. Immunol.,* 116:1435–1438.
59. Veltri, R.W., and Sprinkle, P.M. (1973): Serous otitis media. Immunoglobulin and lysozyme levels in middle ear fluids and serum. *Ann. Otol. Rhinol. Laryngol.,* 82:297–301.
60. Watanabe, N., DeMaria, T.F., Lewis, D.M., Mogi, G., and Lim, D.J. (1982): Experimental otitis media in chinchillas. II. Comparison of the middle ear immune response to *S. pneumoniae* types 3 and 23. *Ann. Otol. Rhinol. Laryngol.,* 91(Suppl. 93, No. 3, part 3):9–16.
61. Welliver, R.C., Wong, D.T., Sun, M., Middleton, E., Jr., Vaughan, R.S., and Ogra, P.L. (1981): The development of respiratory syncytial virus-specific IgE and the release of histamine in nasopharyngeal secretions after infection. *N. Eng. J. Med.,* 305:841–846.
62. Yamaguchi, T., Urasawa, T., and Kataura, A. (1984): Secretory immunoglobulin A antibodies to respiratory viruses in middle ear effusion of chronic otitis media with effusion. *Ann. Otol. Rhinol. Laryngol.,* 93:73–75.

Immunology of the Ear, edited by J. Bernstein and P. Ogra. Raven Press, New York © 1987.

Inflammatory Cell Subpopulations in Secretory Otitis Media

*Tauno Palva, **Eero Taskinen, **Pekka Hayry, and ***Joel M. Bernstein

**ENT Department and **Transplantation Laboratory, University of Helsinki, Helsinki, Finland; and ***Departments of Otolaryngology and Pediatrics, State University of New York at Buffalo, Buffalo, New York 14214, and Division of Infectious Diseases, Children's Hospital of Buffalo, Buffalo, New York 14222*

It has been well established that all types of inflammatory cells are present in both acute and chronic otitis media with effusion (OME). Thus, polymorphonuclear leukocytes (PMN), various types of lymphocytes, and other mononuclear cells, as well as eosinophils, basophils, natural killer (NK) cells, and probably interepithelial lymphocytes are all present in this inflammatory disorder (3–5,12,17,18,24). The integrity of these cells, however, is sometimes related to the chronicity of the disease, and in long-standing chronic effusions there is occasionally marked degeneration of polymorphonuclear leukocytes.

Over 30 years ago, Bryan (4) published a study correlating the cellular characteristics of middle ear effusions (MEEs) and the chronicity of chronic middle ear and mastoid disease. Using a conventional stain (Wright's method of supravital staining), PMN leukocytes were present in highest proportion and they exhibited active mobility associated with protoplasmic streaming and evidence of phagocytosis. Lymphocytes of various sizes and nuclear detail were present and varied from blast form to mature lymphocytes (5). Bryan's thesis was that large phagocytes in the secretion indicated a severe infection with prolonged recovery and mastoid involvement. Conversely, the absence of large phagocytes was regarded as an indication of a relatively mild disease of short duration. Further studies of the cellular pattern of prolonged OME studied suggested that in the first few days of acute OME, PMN predominated (17,18). After the third to fourth day, macrophages of various sizes were seen. After five days or more, macrophages were the most predominant finding in the secretion. It is interesting to note that in more recent work by other investigators, macrophages and lymphocytes appear to predominate in the chronic effusions (3,17,18). In general, both studies of MEE aspirates and serially sectioned temporal bones possess predominantly cells of the mononuclear type. Recent advances in surface receptors and the development of monoclonal antibodies have led to a more specific identification of cells that are present in middle ear mucosal tissue as well as in middle ear fluid. These studies will be thoroughly discussed in this chapter.

BASIC CYTOLOGY OF MIDDLE EAR ASPIRATES IN OME

The study of middle ear fluids received new impetus when the incidence of OME was noted to be an extremely common problem and truly a widespread disease. The first classification of chronic OME was made by Senturia et al. (24) almost 30 years ago. They distinguished between (a) serous effusions which contained few inflammatory cells; (b) purulent effusions that possessed abundant acute inflammatory cells, particularly PMN cells; (c) mucopurulent effusions that contained a moderate number of inflammatory cells, cellular remnants, and mucus; and finally (d) mucoid effusions that contained a moderate number of chronic inflammatory cells and many mucoid strands. In general, the cause of these effusions was considered to be an inflammatory disorder caused by infection. In experimental animals, cautery of the naospharyngeal orifice of the eustachian tube resulted in effusions in all middle ears (21,23). Sequential study of MEEs in these experimental animals (mongrel dogs) revealed that PMN leukocytes were the predominant cells in the early stage of the disease. Lymphocytes also appeared in all ears, but represented less than 10% of all cells. Monocytes were seen in later stages, accounting for only about 1% of inflammatory cells, and eosinophils were never observed. Bacteria were cultured from 22 of 24 effusions, and it was concluded that trauma to the nasopharyngeal orifice of the eustachian tube produces an inflammatory reaction in the middle ear cleft.

Senturia and his group continued their studies of the cytology of OME in the 1960s. In a series of 223 specimens, eosinophils occurred in only 11; allergy was not felt to be an important etiological factor in most cases (24). Of the serous specimens, 35% had positive bacteriological cultures.

In studies done in the laboratory of Palva, inflammatory cells consisted mainly of PMN leukocytes and lymphocytes, whereas macrophage appeared in smaller numbers than the lymphocytes and neutrophils and giant phagocytes were infrequent (13,15,17,18). Eosinophils and basophils were rare and in no case did either of these cells appear in moderate numbers. Mucous strands and various numbers of red blood cells were also common findings. An example of the general appearance of the inflammatory cells is seen in Fig. 1. In general, these studies suggest that all inflammatory cells are present and that PMN leukocytes predominate in the early stages of the inflammation, but appear to be present in effusions in moderate numbers no matter how long the inflammation has persisted (3). However, lymphocytes and other mononuclear cells appear to predominate in the later stages of the effusion. Because of the predominance of mononuclear cells in the late stages, some investigators have suggested that the cellular infiltrate in long-standing OME suggests the possibility of delayed hypersensitivity (3). This mechanism of immunological reactivity appears to be plausible inasmuch as various putative mediators of delayed hypersensitivity such as macrophage inhibition activity, interferon, and chemotactic activity for both neutrophils and macrophage have all been found in MEE (2).

Thus, prior to the availability of specific antisera to identify subpopulations of

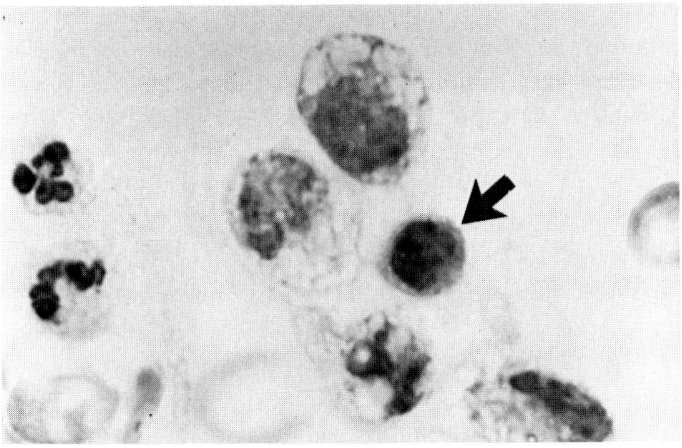

FIG. 1. General morphology of cells as seen in MEF with May-Grünwald-Giemsa stain. Two polymorphonuclear leukocytes are shown *(left)* and one small lymphocyte is in the center *(arrow)*, encircled by four phagocytes. Also shown are some cell rests *(left)*, and an erythrocyte *(right)*. ×800.

various inflammatory cells in MEE, most investigators had suggested that MEE and middle ear tissue have a predominance of cells that would be consistent with chronic inflammation and possibly delayed hypersensitivity or cell-mediated immunological reactivity.

SUBPOPULATIONS OF WHITE BLOOD CELLS

Lymphocyte subpopulations were first classified by two principal methods: the sheep red blood cells (SRBC) rosetting technique and the acetyl-naphthyly-lacetate esterase (ANAE) staining. Bernstein et al. (3) used the SRBC technique on serous, seromucinous, and mucoid MEEs. The average cell count varied from 4×10^5 cells/ml in the serous variety to 1×10^6 cells/ml in the seromucinous type. Macrophages and lymphocytes were most prevalent, although PMN leukocytes comprised anywhere from 50% to 80% of all cells in a few specimens.

In studies using specific erythrocyte-antibody (EA) and erythrocyte-antibody-complement (EAC) rosetting, which utilize both IgG and IgM rabbit antibody directed against ox red blood cells and guinea pig complement, T cells were found primarily in serous and seromucinous types of effusions, whereas they appeared to be in lower concentrations in the mucoid fluids. B cells appeared to predominate in the mucoid fluids, whereas they were in lower percentages in the serous and seromucinous varieties of MEEs. However, more recent data by Bernstein using monoclonal antibodies (this chapter) suggest that the original study reported by his laboratory is no longer acceptable because monoclonal antibodies directed against specific determinants on T cells as well as T helper (Th) and T suppressor (Ts) cells strongly suggest now that T cells predominate in all MEE, including the mucoid variety. However, B cells continue to predominate in mucoid effusions.

Other approaches to the determination of subpopulations of T cells and B cells in MEE have utilized the ANAE staining reaction as markers of T cells (18–20). Using this technique, Palva's laboratory has demonstrated that the PMN leukocyte was the predominant cell in 67% of 54 serous fluids and the ANAE-positive T cells comprised more than 50% of the lymphocytes in 68% of these samples (14,15,17,18). The granulocytic predominance was slightly less marked (56%) in the mucoid than in the serous fluids. Also, in the mucoid fluid the proportion of ANAE-positive lymphocytes was over 50% in almost half of the specimens. More than 50% of the lymphocytes were ANAE positive in 63% of the fluids in which lymphocytes and macrophages made up the bulk of the cells (Figs. 2 and 3). Thus,

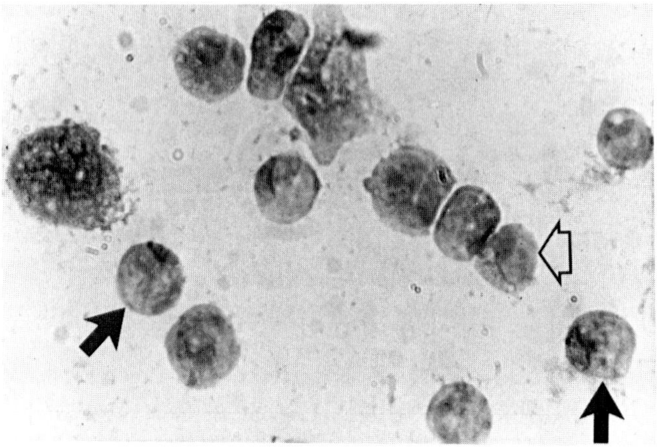

FIG. 2. Mononuclear cells in middle ear fluids, stained with the ANAE technique. One ANAE-positive phagocyte is seen *(left).* Most of the lymphocytes are ANAE-positive T cells *(filled arrows),* showing a reddish-brown reactive dot in their cytoplasma. An ANAE-negative lymphocyte (B cells) is also shown *(unfilled arrow).* ×800.

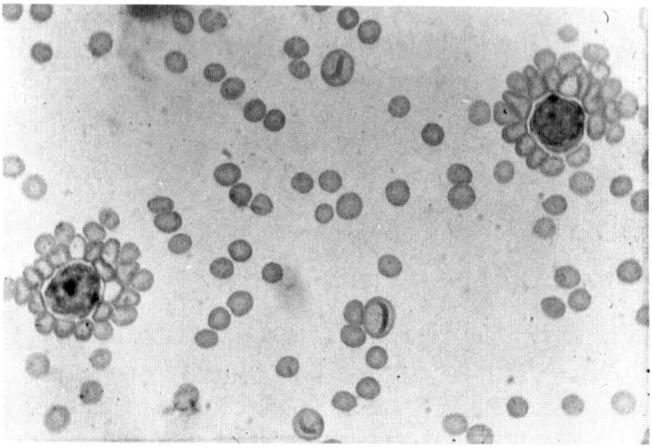

FIG. 3. Combination of ANAE-staining and E-rosetting technique. Two ANAE-positive lymphocytes form distinct rosettes with sheep erythrocytes. ×800.

both Bernstein and Palva now would agree that the predominant lymphocyte cell in the MEE is the T cell. The subpopulations of T cells will be discussed later in this chapter. In subsequent studies, Palva examined the ANAE-positive cells in middle ear mucosal biopsies. Representative biopsies from eight ears demonstrated that PMN leukocytes were mostly absent from the subepithelial tissue and that the inflammatory cells consisted mainly of lymphocytes, macrophages, and plasma cells (Fig. 4). The occurrence of T and B cells and plasma cells suggests a normal cellular and humoral immune response occurring in the middle ear mucosa in OME.

MONOCLONAL ANTISERA IN THE CELLULAR ANALYSIS OF MIDDLE EAR MUCOSA IN OME AND IN MIDDLE EAR FLUIDS

Utilizing specific monoclonal antibodies (26) directed against antigenic determinants on Th and Ts cells, biopsy specimens of middle ear mucosa from patients with OME, or with chronic otitis media (OM) with or without cholesteatoma, have been performed.

Using the OKT series of monoclonal antibodies, tissue samples were obtained from six ears with OME. The mononuclear cell infiltrates in the subepithelial tissue consisted mainly of OKT-3-positive cells, which represent the PAN T cells (70–80%). OKT-4-positive cells, which represent the marker for T helper-inducer cells, seem to concentrate in aggregates whereas the OKT-8-positive cells, which represent the T suppressor cytotoxic cells, appear to be evenly distributed throughout the whole subepithelial area, but comprised only 20% to 30% of the lymphocytes whereas the T helper cells comprised approximately 50% to 60% of the total

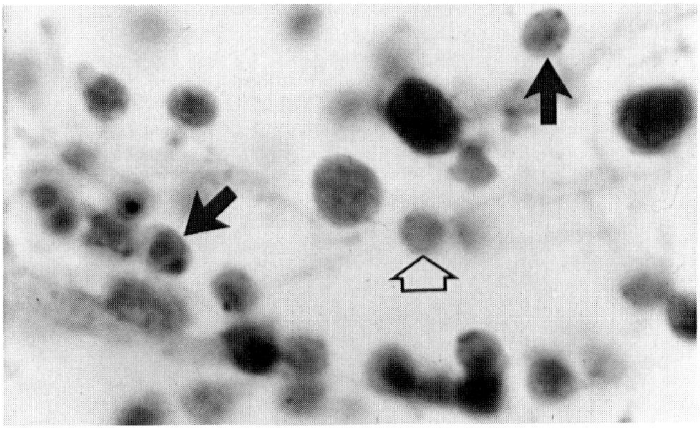

FIG. 4. ANAE staining of immunocompetent cells in middle ear submucosa. There are several T lymphocytes displaying the dot-like ANAE-positive reaction product *(filled arrows)* and some ANAE-negative B lymphocytes *(unfilled arrow).* Two larger phagocytes show a diffuse ANAE-positive staining of their cytoplasm. The plasma cell in the center remains ANAE-negative. ×1,000.

lymphocytes. The Ts cells were also seen in areas adjacent to the basement membrane and seemed to penetrate through the epithelium into the middle ear lumen. All together 80% to 90% of the cells were Ia-positive, suggesting that these cells were in an active state immunologically. The presence of Ia antigen on the surface of the T lymphocytes suggests that they have been activated by antigen.

Further studies on the distribution of T-cell subpopulations using monoclonal antibodies were performed in mucoid MEEs. OKT-11 was used as a marker for all T cells, OKT-4 for helper cells, OKT-8 for suppressor cells, B1 for B lymphocytes, and HNK-1 for NK cells. In addition, small biopsy specimens were also taken and were compared with the results in the MEE. The analysis of the lymphocyte subgroups in the MEE as well as in the biopsies was performed with the immunoperoxidase technique and with monoclonal antibodies. In the specimens and effusions the positive reactions were visualized by aminoethylcarbazoledimethylformamide staining. The background was stained with hemalum, both in cytologic and histologic specimens.

BIOPSIES

At the present time an analysis of 25 biopsies will be reported. The interpretation of the findings, however, is hampered by the fact that the biopsy specimens are necessarily small and often the total cell count is less than 100 cells and sometimes is based on the number of positive cells in five consecutive oil immersion visual fields. Nevertheless, the overall evaluation of the data of the whole material is probably indicative of the character of the reactive process. Representative fields of one tissue section stained for reactions with OKT-11, OKT-4, OKT-8, B1, and HNK-1 antisera are seen in Fig. 5a to d. This specimen revealed a follicular type of lymphocyte aggregation in the subepithelial tissue as well as diffusely scattered lymphocytes at the periphery.

In two of 17 representative specimens the Th/Ts ratio was less than 1, in one it was 1.0, and in all others it was greater than 1.

The percentage of B cells varied from 0 to 30 in all biopsy preparations. As a rule, they were far less than the number of OKT-11-positive cells, but in one case the figure for OKT-11- and B1-positive cells was identical. Usually, NK cells occurred in the same frequency as B1 cells.

MUCOID EFFUSION FLUID

The total number of inflammatory cells varied considerably. Of 38 centrifuged[22] specimens, eight (21%) contained so few cells that no reliable counting was possible. This finding did not depend on the size of the sample. In 14 (37%) samples, the total number was approximately 10^4 cells; in 10 (26%) samples, counts of 10^5 cells were made. Only six samples (16%) had more than 10^6 cells. The detailed analysis of lymphocyte cell subpopulations is based mainly on the 16 samples in which more than 10^5 cells were present. In the remaining 22 samples, the total number of cells was too small to allow reliable estimates of the distribution of individual cells.

Polymorphonuclear-Mononuclear Cell Relationships

In the analysis of the total number of white cells, degenerated cells (22) were counted separately and their percentages were recorded (Fig. 6). There were three samples in which all white cells were degenerated. Among the rest of the 35 samples there were five (14%) in which the PMNs were in the minority, comprising less than 50% of all leukocytes. In 30 (86%) samples the PMNs comprised 50% or more of the white cell population, and in 26 specimens (74%) more than 70% of all inflammatory cells were PMN leukocytes. The percentage of PMN leukocytes was as low as 6 and 3 in two cases, and in these samples 95% and 81% of the respective white cell populations were degenerated. In six samples, more than 70% of the white cells showed degeneration. Three of them exhibited a pronounced mononuclear cell predominance, whereas three showed a PMN predominance similar to that of the samples with lower percentages of degenerated cells. In the specimens with degeneration percentages below 70, lymphocytes and monocytes were equally frequent, the average figures being around 5% to 15% for both cells (Fig. 7). Stimulated lymphocytes accounted for 1% to 5% of the cells in 19 samples (54% of all specimens) whereas lymphoblasts were seen in four samples (11%), comprising 1% of the cells.

Red blood cells were seen in varying numbers in nearly all samples, despite the fact that the tympanic membrane surface had been pretreated with saturated phenol. The blood presented contamination from the paracentesis margins, but it could also have leaked from the middle ear capillaries as a result of suction. These blood cells are artifactual because siderophages, which would be indicative of old bleeding, were not present. In specimens with large numbers of inflammatory cells, the presence of blood apparently has very little effect on the cellular picture.

Subgroups of Lymphocytes

The percentage for all T cells (OKT-11) varied from 44 to 73 (average 57%) in the samples with 10^5 cells or more. In 13 of these samples, the percentage of Th cells ranged from 21 to 60 (average 47%) and that of Ts cells ranged from 28 to 47 (average 36%). The Th/Ts ratio was above 1 in ten samples and below 1 in three. In two children with bilateral disease, one ear showed a ratio below 1 and the other ear showed a ratio above 1. The percentage for B cells varied from 2 to 43 (average 20%), and in all secretions their number was smaller than the number of OKT-11-positive cells. For NK cells, percentages varied from 1 to 29 (average 10%) and, as a rule, they were clearly less frequent than B cells. Representative microscopic fields of various lymphocyte subgroups are shown in Fig. 8a to f.

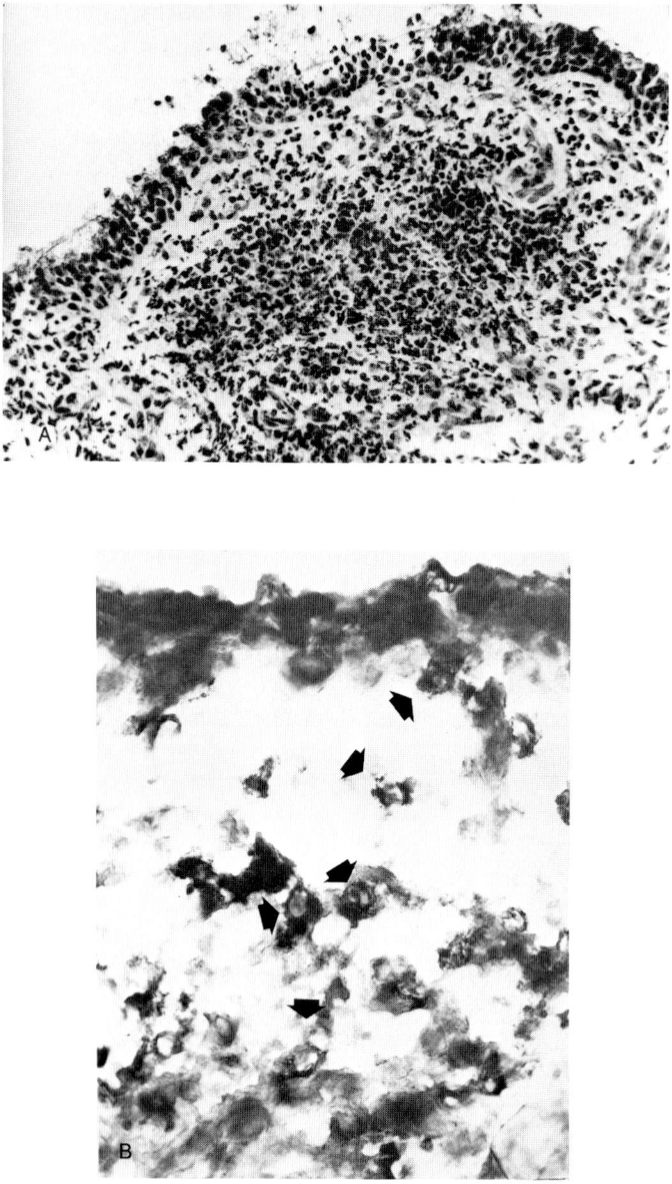

FIG. 5. (a) Subepithelial follicular lymphoid infiltration of the middle ear mucosa. The patient was a 14-month-old boy with bilateral serous OM. Deep-frozen tissue section and toluidine blue staining. ×480. Analysis of the lymphoid subsets was performed by using monoclonal antibodies and an immunoperoxidase technique. The tissue infiltrate contained 27% T cells, 37% Th cells, and 26% Ts cells; 5% of the infiltrate were B cells and 5% were NK cells. The following series of photomicrographs demonstrates the appearance of these T-cell subsets in the middle ear mucosa. Positive cells are indicated *(arrows)*. **(b)** OKT-11-positive T cells. ×1,200. **(c)** OKT-4-positive Th cells. ×480. **(d)** OKT-8-positive Ts cells. ×1,200.

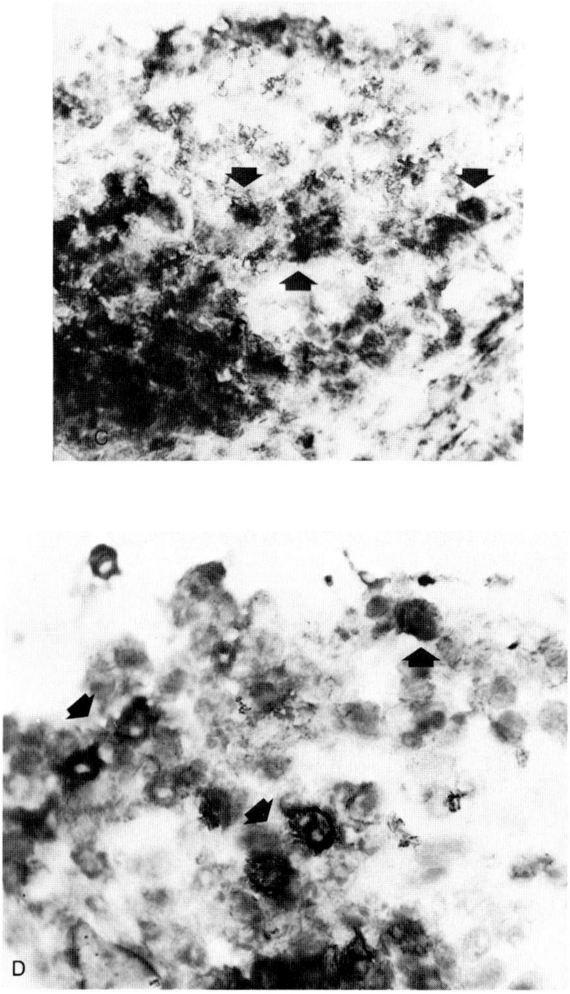

Fig. 5. *(See legend on facing page.)*

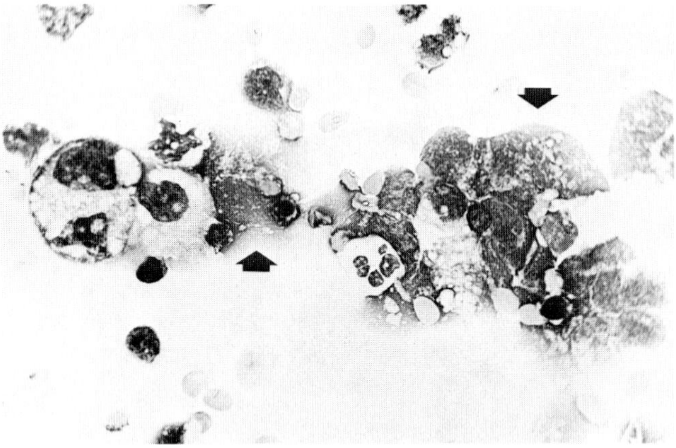

FIG. 6. Degenerated cellular debris *(arrows)* among well-preserved inflammatory cells in mucous middle ear fluid. The proportion of degenerated cells was 68% of the total cell number counted. The patient was a 6-year-old boy with bilateral serous OM. The cytologic specimen contained 35% lymphoid cells. Enzyme-dispersed cytocentrifuge specimen, May-Grünwald-Giemsa staining. ×1,200.

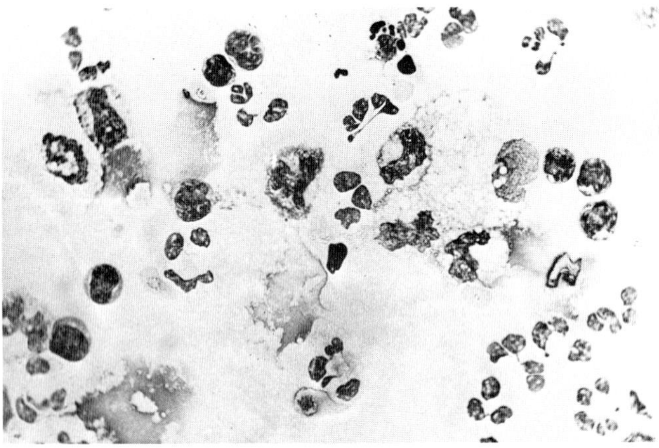

FIG. 7. Lymphocytosis (16% of all inflammatory cells) in the mucous middle ear fluid from a 53-month-old girl with bilateral serous OM. Enzyme-dispersed cytocentrifuge specimen, May-Grünwald-Giemsa staining. ×1,200.

Other Observations

Mast cells, although few in number, were identified in practically all specimens. Their proportion was difficult to assess but it was definitely less than 1%. Some slides showed granules that might have been derived from mast cells after cellular rupture. Phagocytic cells with ingested material (Fig. 9) were mainly represented by erythrophages and not by siderophages. The phagocytes were occasionally found to have engulfed PMN leukocytes or homogeneous mucoid material, but in view of the long-standing fluid retention the event was relatively infrequent. Similar studies from the laboratory of Bernstein suggest that the T-cell subpopulation in different MEEs may be significantly different. Table 1 summarizes the data for lymphocyte subpopulations in different MEEs using monoclonal antibodies. Several important findings appear to be present. There is a significantly greater number of B cells in the mucoid and purulent effusions than in the serous effusions. A significantly greater number of Ts cells also occurs in the mucoid fluid as compared to the Ts cells in the serous fluid. The Th/Ts ratios are significantly less in the mucoid effusions than in the serous effusions. The number of B cells in the purulent effusions is greater than in the serous effusions.

Natural killer cells were found in some of the MEEs, but they represented an extremely small number, averaging less than 2%. They were found in all fluids, including the serous, mucoid, and purulent effusions.

COMMENTS

Chronic OME is not characterized by a systemic reaction on the part of the host. In general, the sedimentation rate and the number and differential white count is usually normal, and the C-reactive protein is not elevated in most patients with OME. Therefore, the disease can be considered a local inflammatory response. It may be assumed that the findings in the fluid and in the mucosal tissue represent a local inflammatory reaction at the level of the middle ear mucosa and that it is not significantly altered by systemic changes in inflammatory cells. Although there are signs of distinct white cell degeneration in many of the middle ear fluids, a general distinction between T and B cells may be accurately performed. The results of studies from the laboratories of Palva and Bernstein strongly suggest that T cells predominate in all effusions, although the percentage of B cells may be significantly greater in the mucoid variety of MEEs. Furthermore, PMN leukocytes appear to predominate also in all effusions that are well preserved. The degeneration of the PMNs may be related to the toxic nature of the middle ear fluids in which, for example, complement activation has been well documented (10). Leukocytic breakdown and liberation of lysosomal enzymes is also a factor that may contribute to the constant irritation of the middle ear mucosa (1,6,8). From a clinical point of view, these data emphasize the need for MEE evacuation either by tympanostomy and/or the use of a ventilation tube. The mononuclear cell infiltrates in the middle ear mucosa reveal the predominance of Th cells. They appear

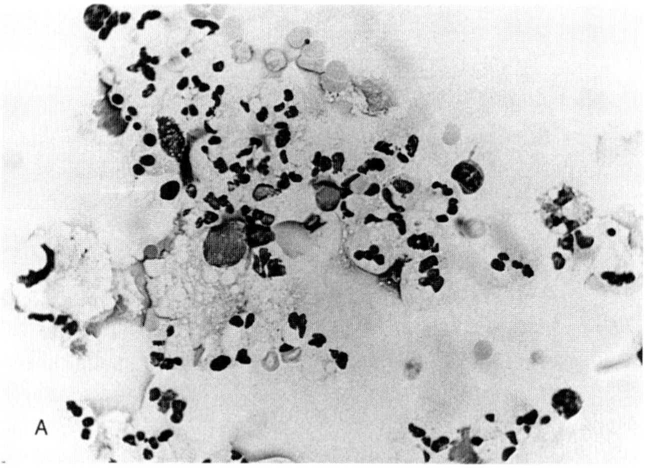

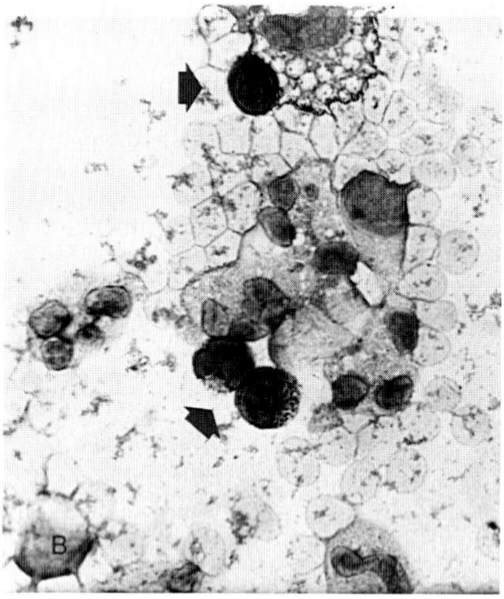

FIG. 8. (a) A typical cytologic finding in a cytocentrifuge specimen prepared from enzyme-dispersed mucous middle ear fluid, May-Grünwald-Giemsa staining. ×1,200. This 1½-year-old girl had bilateral serous OM, and this left-sided mucous secretion contained 81% neutrophils and 5% lymphocytes. Surface markers of the lymphoid population were analyzed by using monoclonal antibodies and an immunoperoxidase technique. Distribution of the various subtypes were as follows: T cells 73%, Th 55%, Ts 38%, B cells 18%, and NK cells 5%. The Th/Ts ratio was 1.45. The following series of photomicrographs demonstrates the appearance of the subsets in this same specimen. ×1,200. Positive cells are indicated *(arrows)*. **(b)** OKT-11-positive T cells. **(c)** OKT-4-positive Th cells. **(d)** OKT-8-positive Ts cells. **(e)** B1-positive B cells. **(f)** Leu-7-positive HNK-1 cells.

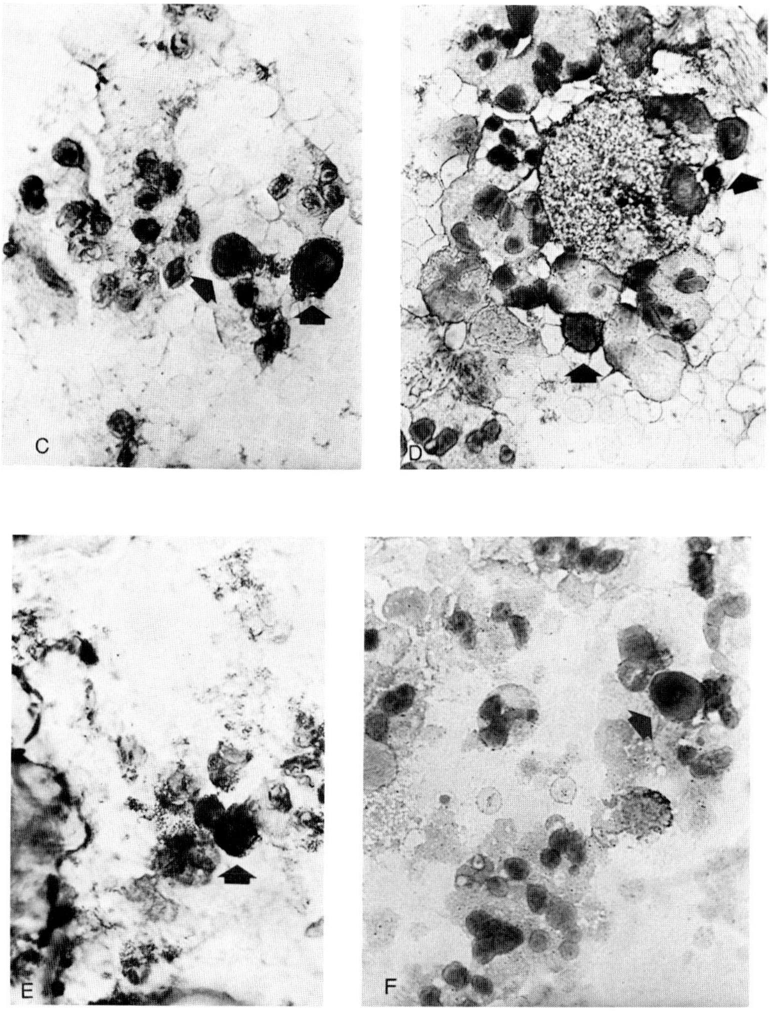

Fig. 8. *(See legend on facing page.)*

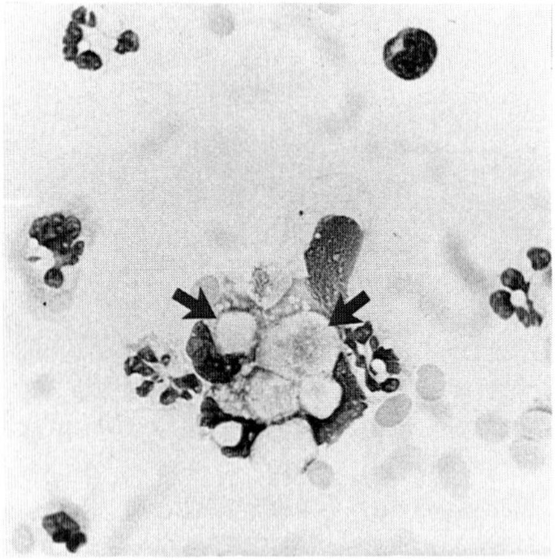

FIG. 9. Two macrophages *(arrows)*, containing phagocytosed erythrocytes and mucous fluid, in the mucous middle ear fluid from a 14-month-old boy with bilateral serous OM. Enzyme-dispersed cytocentrifuge specimen, May-Grün-wald-Giemsa staining. ×1200.

TABLE 1. *Summary of the T-cell subpopulations and B cells in different MEEs*

	Serous n=14	Mucoid n=13	Purulent n=4
T	*485±204	705±344	441±119
B	188±69	423±196	416±277
	p<.01		
T_H	450±202	481±197	353±16
T_S	170±48	309±204	156±23
	p<.01		
T_H/T_S	2.64	1.5	2.26
	p<.01		

* = cells/ul of MEE

to be twice as frequent as Ts cells. Furthermore, Th cells appear to be in an aggregated form, whereas Ts cells appear to be spread more uniformly throughout the submucosa. Also, Th cells appear to be more frequent than Ts cells in the majority of MEEs, that is, the cells in the fluid reflect the pattern seen in tissues. However, 15% of ears with chronic OME reveal both tissue and fluid specimens where the Th/Ts ratio is less than 1, suggesting a predominance of Ts cells in that particular sample. This also may be true more for the mucoid effusions than for the serous effusions, suggesting that as the disease progresses Ts cells may increase in the MEE. This might have interesting ramifications in that as the effusion becomes more chronic there may be a down regulation of the immune response. This has also been suggested by other investigators, who believe that a down regulation of the immune response may occur because of the presence of an increased number of macrophages, which may down regulate the lymphocyte function in the MEE (see Mogi and Bernsteins's chapter, *this volume*). Nevertheless, despite the potential increase of Ts cells, it is quite obvious that Th cells predominate in the great majority of effusions and are present in sufficient numbers to activate antigen-specific B cells. This is because there certainly is no deficiency in OM in the production of immunoglobulins, and the levels of IgG, IgA, and IgD are clearly higher than in the serum. Although B cells are present in all effusions, they do seem to be statistically greater in the mucoid effusions. One possible reason for this may be that microbial antigen present in purulent and mucoid effusions may directly stimulate B cells to proliferate and differentiate. It is well known, for example, that lipopolysaccharide (LPS), found in the cell walls of most gram-negative bacilli, including nontypable *Hemophilus influenzae,* may be a potent B-cell mitogen. Furthermore, pneumococcal capsular polysaccharides may also directly cause B-cell differentiation without the help of T cells. Macrophages appear to be present in all specimens in adequate or increased numbers; thus all the cells required for a normal immune response are present.

Natural killer cells are seen in small numbers both in the mucosa and in the MEEs. Recent studies (see Wright's chapter, *this volume*) provide more evidence that viruses attack the upper respiratory tract and the middle ear and may represent the trigger in the activation of bacteria in the nasopharynx for suppurative OM. In the youngest age group, respiratory syncytial virus and, to some extent, parainfluenza viruses and adenoviruses may be the main agents responsible for this triggering affect (11). Natural killer cells might play a role as a first line of defense against these viruses.

Finally, it should be mentioned that the findings reported in the above-mentioned studies have relevance to the cellular interaction of the immune response in OME. We can now demonstrate important surface determinants on MEE lymphocytes. The key interaction of the immune response involves the cooperation of macrophage with Th cells. This essentially involves four components: First, antigenic determinants on the surface of the macrophage following processing of complex antigen must be recognized by other cells to produce an antigen-specific response. Second, a factor that must be present on the macrophage is the class II HLA antigenic determinant, the so-called Ia determinant. Third, a component that must be present is the receptor on the Th cell that recognizes antigen. Fourth and finally, there must be a receptor on both the Th cell and the Ts cell that recognizes the class II and class I HLA antigenic determinants coded for by the HLA A, B, C, and D region of the human histocompatability locus on chromosome 6, respectively. It is now evident that all of these elements are present on the cells in MEE and in middle ear mucosa. Not only are the T markers that have been presented in these studies important in the identification of the types of lymphocyte subpopulations that occur in MEEs, but it has now been established that these markers also play an important role in the T-cell receptors that are responsible for antigen recognition. The T-4 antigen is considered to be important in binding the D-locus surface determinant of the macrophage and plays a role in facilitating the subsequent recognition by a complex that includes T3 and another antigenic determinant and which constitutes the recognition site for the specific antigen in this model. Thus, the surface markers T3, T4, and T8, which are used to subtype lymphocytes, also participate in a functional way in recognizing the A, B, C, and D loci antigens and the specific antigen that is presented by the macrophage. Thus, this recognition includes (a) the T4 on the helper cell (which recognizes the D locus) and (b) the T3 (which is present on all T cells), which supplies a structural framework for the specific recognition on the T lymphocyte, presumably an immunoglobulin-like molecule that recognizes specific antigen.

CONCLUSION

It has been established that T cells, B cells, Th cells, Ts cells, and NK cells are all found in MEEs. These cells may not only be responsible for antibody production and, with complement, may eliminate bacteria, virus, or injured tissue, but, in a closed space, if these products are not removed, they may lead to tissue injury as the result of immune complex disease (2,16) or delayed hypersensitivity. Furthermore, a second mechanism is that of cell-mediated immunity. The Th cells may give rise to delayed hypersensitivity with the release of lymphokines which will result in the increase and activation of macrophages. These macrophages may produce factors that are capable of tissue breakdown or they may be responsible for the elimination of viruses and other foreign cells (25). Finally, NK cells that are present in the middle ear may also be protective but may also cause injury to target cells on which antigenic determinants have been changed as a result of chronic inflammation. An understanding of these extremely sophisticated and complex cellular interactions of the immune response may be important in understanding the pathogenesis of OME and hopefully may lead to specific and selective medical treatment of this problem.

REFERENCES

1. Barrett, A.J. (1977): *Proteinases in Mammalian Cells and Tissues: A Review. Vol. 2.* North-Holland Publishing Co., New York.
2. Bernstein, J.M., Brentjens, J., and Vladutiu, A. (1982): Are immune complexes a factor in the pathogenesis of otitis media with effusion? *Am. J. Otolaryngol.*, 3:20–25.
3. Bernstein, J.M., Szymanski, C., Albini, B., Sun, M., and Ogra, P.L. (1978): Lymphocyte subpopulations in otitis media with effusion. *Pediatr. Res.*, 12:786–788.
4. Bryan, W.T.K. (1953): The identification and clinical significance of large phagocytes in the exudates of acute otitis media and mastoiditis. *Laryngoscope*, 63:559–580.
5. Bryan, M.P., and Bryan, W.T.K. (1976): Cytologic and immunologic response revealed in middle ear effusions. *Ann. Otol. Rhinol. Laryngol.*, 85(Suppl.):238–244.
6. Horwitz, A.L., Hance, A.J., and Crystal, R.G. (1977): Granulocyte collagenase: selective digestion of type I relative to type III collagen. *Proc. Natl. Acad. Sci. USA*, 74:897–901.
7. Kähönen, K., Palva, T., Bergroth, V., Konttinen, Y.T., and Reitamo, S. (1984): Immunohistochemical identification of inflammatory cells in secretory and chronic otitis media and cholesteatoma using monoclonal antibodies. *Acta Otolaryngol. (Stockh.)*, 97:431–436.

8. Kuhn, C., and Senior, R.M. (1978): The role of elastases in the development of emphysema. *Lung,* 155:185–198.
9. Liu, Y.S., Lim, D.J., Lang, R.W., and Birck, H.G. (1975): Chronic middle ear effusions, immunochemical and bacteriological investigations. *Arch. Otolaryngol.,* 101:278–286.
10. Meri, S., Lehtinen, T., and Palva, T. (1984): Complement in chronic secretory otitis media. C3 breakdown and C3 splitting activity. *Arch. Otolaryngol.,* 110:774–778.
11. Meurman, O.H., Sarkkinen, H.K., and Puhakka, H.J. (1980): Local IgA-class antibodies against respiratory viruses in middle ear and nasopharyngeal secretion of children with secretory otitis media. *Laryngoscope,* 90:304–311.
12. Ojala, L., and Palva, T. (1955): Macrophages in aural secretions and their clinical significance. *Laryngoscope,* 65:670–692.
13. Palva, T., Holopainen, E., and Karma P. (1976): Protein and cellular pattern of glue ear secretions. *Ann. Otol. Rhinol. Laryngol.,* 85(Suppl. 25):103–109.
14. Palva, T., Häyry, P., and Ylikoski, J. (1978): Lymphocyte morphology in mucoid middle ear effusions. *Ann. Otol. Rhinol. Laryngol.,* 87:421–425.
15. Palva, T. Häyry, P., and Ylikoski, J. (1980): Lymphocyte morphology in middle ear effusions. *Ann. Otol. Rhinol. Laryngol.,* 89 (Suppl. 68):143–146.
16. Palva, T., Lehtinen, T., and Virtanen, H. (1983): Immune complexes in the middle ear fluid and adenoid tissue in chronic secretory otitis media. *Acta Otolaryngol. (Stockh.),* 95:539–543.
17. Palva, T., Reitamo, S., Konttinen, Y.T., Häyry, P., and Rinne, J. (1981): Inflammatory cell subpopulations in the middle ear mucosa of ears with effusion. *Int. J. Pediatr. Otorhinolaryngol.,* 3:71–78.
18. Palva, T., Taskinen, E., and Häyry, P. (1985): T lymphocytes in secretory otitis media. In: *Immunology, Autoimmunity and Transplantation in Otorhinolaryngology, Proceedings of the 1st International Conference, Utrecht, The Netherlands, April 11–12,* pp. 45–50. Kugler Publications, Amsterdam.
19. Ranki, A. (1978): Nonspecific esterase activity in human lymphocytes. Histochemical characterization and distribution among major lymphocyte subclasses. *Clin. Immunol. Immunopathol.,* 10:47–58.
20. Ranki, A., Tötterman, T.H., and Häyry, P.P. (1976): Identification of resting human T and B lymphocytes by acid alpha-naphthyl acetate esterase staining combined with rosette formation with Staphylococcus aureus strain Cowan 1. *Scand. J. Immunol.,* 5:1129–1138.
21. Sadé, J., Carr, C.D., and Senturia, B.H. (1959): Middle ear effusions produced experimentally in dogs. I. Microscopic and bacteriologic findings. *Ann. Otol. Rhinol. Laryngol.,* 68:1017–1027.
22. Scelsi, R., Bassi, P., and Poloni, M. (1976): Cytomorphologic changes in the cerebrospinal fluid sediment; a comparative study by cytocentrifugation and cytosedimentation techniques. *Boll. Soc. Ital. Biol. Sper.,* 52:1229–1233.
23. Senturia, B.H., Gessert, C.F., Carr, C.D., and Baumann, E.S. (1958): Studies concerned with tubotympanitis. *Ann. Otol. Rhinol. Laryngol.,* 67:440–467.
24. Senturia, B.H., Gessert, C.F., Carr, C.D., and Baumann, E.S. (1960): Middle ear effusions: causes and treatment. *Trans. Am. Acad. Ophthalmol. Otolaryngol.,* 64:60–75.
25. Sissons, J.G.P., and Oldstone, M.B.A. (1980): Killing of virus-infected cells by cytotoxic lymphocytes. *J. Infect. Dis.,* 142:114–119.
26. Stites, D.P., Stobo, J.D., Fudenberg, H.H., and Wells, J.V. (editors) (1984): *Basic and Clinical Immunology,* 5th ed. Lange Medical Publications, Los Altos, Cal.

Immunology of the Ear, edited by J. Bernstein
and P. Ogra. Raven Press, New York © 1987.

Biochemistry of Middle Ear Effusion

*Steven K. Juhn, *Yukiyoshi Hamaguchi,
and **Timothy T. K. Jung

**Department of Otolaryngology, University of Minnesota Medical School, Minneapolis, Minnesota 55455; and **Division of Otolaryngology, Loma Linda University School of Medicine, Loma Linda, California 92354*

The availability of middle ear effusions (MEEs) for laboratory analyses provides the possibility of identifying several biochemical markers that may characterize the types and stage of inflammation in the middle ear cavity. Epithelial and subepithelial cells of the middle ear mucosa, microorganisms, inflammatory cells, and plasma are known to contribute to the composition of MEE. The effects of treatment on the composition of middle ear fluid have also been reported. An overview of the biochemical and immunochemical parameters studied in the past is shown in Table 1. Although many parameters have been studied, correlative studies between the disciplines (biochemistry versus bacteriology or cytology or clinical features) are still lacking. It is clear that complex inflammatory reactions including immunological defense mechanisms take place in the middle ear cavity. Future endeavors should focus on the identification of several key factors responsible for chronicity of otitis media (OM) and should determine methods of eliminating those factors. This will result in better management and prevention of chronicity and recurrence of OM (Fig. 1).

PROTEIN COMPOSITION

Middle ear effusions contain both plasma proteins and secretions derived from the middle ear mucosa (MEM), as well as cellular elements composed of both inflammatory and epithelial cells (45,55,60). Protein analyses of various types of MEE (serous, mucoid, and purulent) demonstrate that serous MEE, among other types of effusions, consists mainly of plasma components that, in turn, usually depend on the selective vascular permeability in the middle ear mucosa (25,32,52). Mucoid MEE contains a higher concentration of high-molecular-weight glycoprotein than it does of plasma (32,60).

The concentration ratio of each plasma protein to albumin has been used as the parameter reflecting the degree of plasma leakage. A lower ratio of the concentration of α_2-macroglobulin to albumin in comparison to that in plasma indicates that the vascular permeability does not completely appear to be damaged during the course of otitis media with effusion (OME) (6,24).

TABLE 1. *Biochemical and immunochemical composition of middle ear effusion*

	Author	Date	Reference number
Protein and enzyme analysis			
General analysis	Sade	1979	60
General analysis	Palva et al.	1976	54
General analysis and enzymes (CPK, GOT, etc.)	Lupovich and Harkins	1972	45
General analysis and electrolytes	Juhn and Huff	1976	32
General analysis and cytology	Paparella et al.	1970	52
LDH and isoenzyme	Juhn et al.	1973	31
Hexosamine	Juhn et al.	1977	33
Glycoproteins	Palva et al.	1975	55
Glycoproteins	Kobayashi et al.	1984	40
Lactoferrin and secretory IgA	Mogi et al.	1980	48
Immunological analysis			
Secretory IgA	Mogi et al.	1974	47
Mucosal immunity in guinea pig	Mogi et al.	1980	50
Immunoglobulins	Watanabe et al.	1982	64
Specific antibody of IgG, IgA, IgM	Watanabe et al.	1982	65
Secretory IgA and secretory component	Sipila et al.	1985	61
Cellular immunity	Drucker et al.	1979	15
T cell and B cell	Bernstein and Park	1985	4
Immune complex	Palva et al.	1983	56
Immune complex (animal model)	Takasaka et al.	1983	62
Immune complex	Yamanaka et al.	1984	67
Rheumatoid factor	DeMaria et al.	1984	12
Endotoxin	DeMaria et al.	1983	11
Endotoxin	Iino et al.	1985	28
Endotoxin (animal model)	Okazaki et al.	1984	51
C_3, C_5a, chemotaxin, and lactoferrin	Giebink et al.	1985	17
$C_{1q,r,s}$	Prellner	1985	59
Complement	Prellner and Nillson	1982	58
Immune complex	Bernstein et al.	1982	3
Immune complex (animal model)	Kyogoku and Hozawa	1984	41
IgE	Mogi et al.	1976	49
Immunoglobulin and bacteriology	Liu et al.	1975	44
Proteases			
Prekallikrein-kallikrein	Hamaguchi et al.	1985	25
Elastase and collagenase	Carlsson et al.	1982	7
Collagenase	Juhn	1985	36
Collagenase	Paparella et al.	1985	53
Collagenase	Granstrom et al.	1985	18
Lysosomal hydrolases	Diven et al.	1981	13
Cathepsin B and cathepsin H	Hamaguchi et al.	1985	25
Cathepsin B	Hamaguchi et al.	1986	23
Cathepsin B (cholesteatoma)	Iwanaga et al.	1985	30
Lysosomal hydrolases	Hara et al.	1984	26
Neuraminidase	LaMarco et al.	1984	42
Lysosomal hydrolases	Diven et al.	1985	14
Lysozyme	Juhn	1982	34
Lysozyme	Juhn et al.	1984	35

TABLE 1. *Biochemical and immunochemical composition of middle ear effusion*

	Author	Date	Reference number
	Protease inhibitors		
α_1-Antitrypsin and α_2-macroglobulin, etc.	Carlsson et al.	1981	6
α_1-Antitrypsin and α_1-antichymotrypsin, etc.	Hamaguchi et al.	1986	24
Proteases and inhibitors	Hochstrasser et al.	1981	27
Antileukoprotease	Carlsson and Ohlsson	1983	8
Antileukoprotease	Carlsson et al.	1983	9
Antiplasmin	Hamaguchi et al.	1985	19
Plasminogen and α_2-plasmin inhibitor	Hamaguchi and Sakakura	1985	20
	Other mediators		
Histamine	Berger et al.	1984	1
Kallikrein-kinin	Bernstein et al.	1978	2
Kallikrein-kinin	Hamaguchi et al.	1986	21
Prostaglandin E	Willis	1970	66
Prostaglandins	Jung et al.	1983	38
Prostaglandins	Jung et al.	1982	37
	Cytology		
Cytology and microbiology	Lim et al.	1976	43
Macrophage induction in ME	McGhee et al.	1983	46
Cytology	Ishii et al.	1980	29

Variable amounts of enzymes [lactic acid dehydrogenase (LDH), creatine phosphokinase (CPK)] (31,54) and glycoproteins are observed in different types of MEE, suggesting that locally produced proteins contribute significantly to the composition of MEE. The levels of amino sugars [*N*-acetylglucosamine (Glu-Nac) and *N*-acetylgalactosamine (Gal-Nac)] (33) and sialic acid containing acid glucosaminoglycans have been measured by many investigators (40,55,60). Locally produced high-molecular-weight acid glycoproteins containing hexosamine and sialic acid contribute to the viscoelasticity of mucoid MEE in chronic OME. In general, secretory glycoproteins have many tight disulfide (S-S) linkages to maintain their structures. This S-S linkage is the most important factor in mucoid effusions.

Dithiothreitol (DTT), a mild S-S linkage splitting agent (10), is usually used for liquefying middle ear samples in the biochemical analyses of mucoid MEE. It would be desirable to find S-S splitting agents to liquefy mucoid MEE for future clinical applications.

IMMUNOLOGICAL ASPECTS

The immunological factors in OME are addressed in a chapter by Mogi and Bernstein (*this volume*). However, immunological reactivity as it relates to bio-

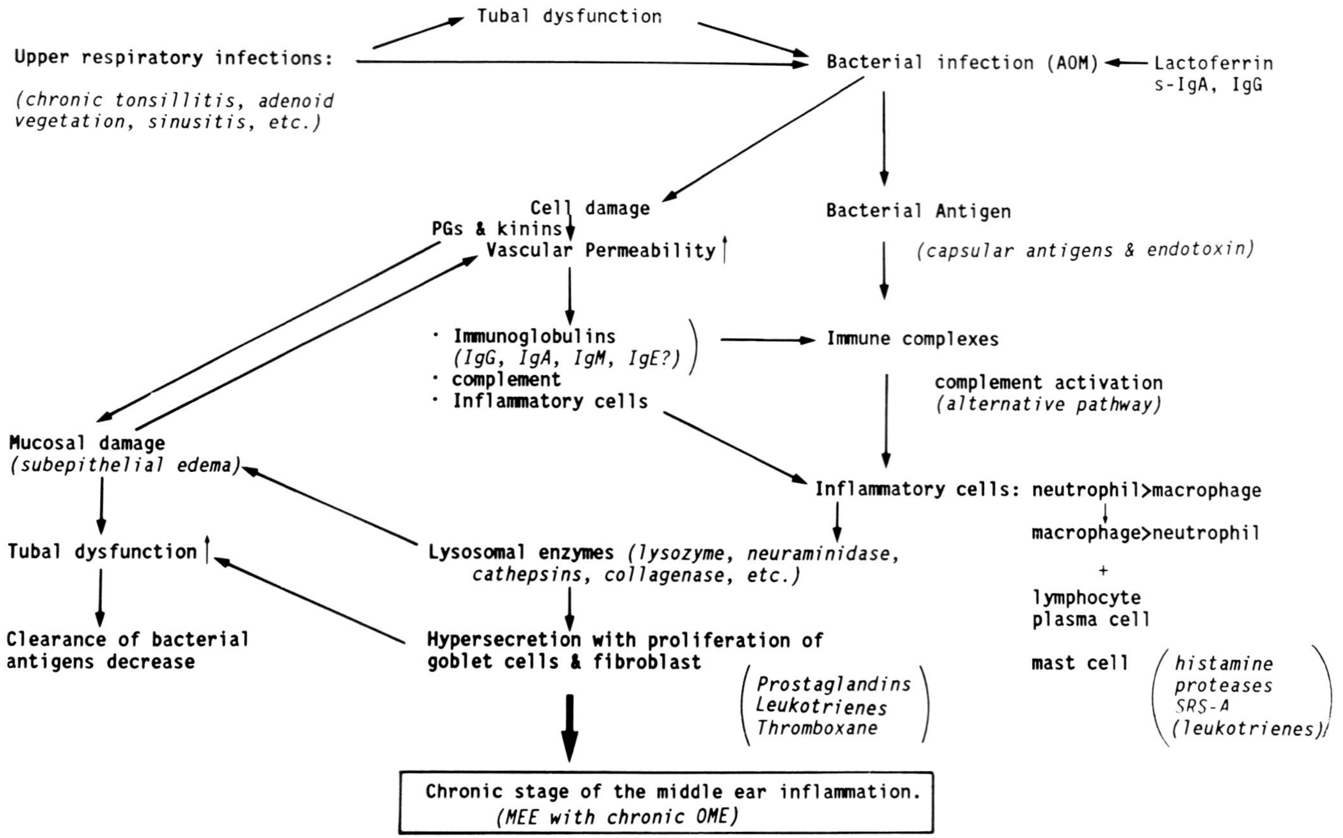

FIG 1. Pathogenesis of chronic OM.

chemical entities will be briefly considered. Secretory IgA is the major immunoglobulin in the MEM and middle ear fluids and plays a key role as a first-line defense against both bacteria and viruses (63). The presence of specific IgA antibody in MEE after pneumococcal infection suggests that once immunocompetent cells are stimulated by specific antigen, the IgG- and IgA-mediated defense system can develop in the MEM (65). Many investigators have now measured specific secretory IgA antibody against *Streptococcus pneumoniae* and *Hemophilus influenzae* in human MEE by enzyme-linked immunosorbent assay method (ELISA) (61). Both serum- and secretory-type antibodies to the infectious agents indicate that the local production of antigen-specific antibodies occurs in MEM. The local immune system comprises not only mucosal immunoglobulins, but also cell-mediated immunity existing in the middle ear (4). The kinetics of the cellular immune system in pediatric patients with OME has been performed by analysis of T- and B-cell subpopulations and interleukin-2 (IL-2) production in both patient plasma and MEE samples (4). Imbalance of T-cell subsets as well as decrease in B-cell function along with decreased production of IL-2 may indicate the presence of defective immunoregulatory function in some pediatric patients with OME (4).

Immune complexes have been identified by many investigators (55,62,67). However, the exact role of immune complexes in OME is still controversial. Although most investigators would agree with regard to the presence of immune complexes in the middle ear fluid in the fluid phase, further investigation is necessary to determine whether this immune mechanism is responsible for the pathogenesis of OME. Rheumatoid factor has also been identified in many middle ear samples and may also contribute to the role of the inflammatory process in OME (12). Endotoxin and lipopolysaccharide (LPS), which are cell-wall components of gram-negative bacteria, have been examined by the Limulus assay in MEE (11). A higher percentage of endotoxin-positive MEE was observed in children with recurrent OME than in adult patients, indicating that endotoxin levels may be an important factor in delayed recovery from OME in children (28). Since nontypable *H. influenzae* do not contain the polyribophosphate capsule that partially masks endotoxin on the surface of bacteria, more endotoxin may be in direct contact with middle ear epithelial surface in acute OM caused by *H. influenzae* (51). More recently, the relationship between chemotaxin and complement components has been studied (17). Inasmuch as neutrophil chemotaxin content correlated poorly with the C3a and C5a content of the MEE, it was suggested that the chemotaxin probably is derived mainly from bacterial peptides and not from the complement system in OM.

The levels of C1q, C1r, C1s, and C1q complexes have been measured (58). Lower levels of C1q have been found in children with recurrent OM as compared to normal children. Furthermore, a high level of C1r-C1s complexes have been found in the MEE of patients with OME (59). These investigators concluded that (a) children with recurrent OME have an inability to synthesize antibody and (b) there exists an aberration within the complement system that is characterized by generalized immunological incompetence in children who are otitis-prone (58). In contrast, Bernstein et al. (3) isolated immune complexes in only four of 63 MEEs and could not demonstrate immune complex deposition in the MEM, indicating that immune complexes probably do not contribute to the pathogenesis of OME. Therefore, it has not yet been established whether or not immune complexes play any role whatsoever in the pathogenesis of human OME.

PROTEASES AND INHIBITORS

Inflammatory cells, particularly neutrophils and macrophages, are observed in various types of MEE. Their role in inflammation in general is thoroughly discussed in Tillinghast et al.'s chapter (*this volume*). It has been established that these cells are present in large numbers in acute as well as chronic OME. These cells are capable of releasing lysosomal enzymes into the middle ear fluid. Such enzymes as glucosidase, collagenase, and cathepsins have all been identified in MEE (7–9). Granuloproteases, such as elastase and collagenase, may play a key role in proteolytic damage to MEM, and these enzymes can also activate other precursor proteins such as the complement system, plasminogen, and kininogen, which may reach the MEM or MEE by transudation from inflamed mucosa. Collagenolytic activity in MEE has been demonstrated in the chinchilla model. The collagenase activity in MEE from the purulent otitis media (POM) model was significantly higher than in the serous otitis media (SOM) model, indicating that infiltrating neutrophils and macrophages can contribute to collagenolytic activity (36). A significant difference in lysosomal hydrolases has been reported in culture-positive as compared to culture-negative cases in OM (13). The activity of lysosomal thiol proteases, mainly cathepsin B, has also been reported in MEE (22). These thiol proteases appear to be derived mainly from macrophages and they each function as a major proteolytic enzyme that may induce mucosal injury. Mucosal destruction may be a result of strong collagenolytic activity and insufficient amounts of available thiol protease inhibitors (22,23).

The activity of collagenolytic cathepsin B in tissue extracts from cholesteatoma has also been reported (30). A significant increase of cathepsin B activity in the subepithelial granulation has been shown to be very important in the degradation of collagen fibers in granulation tissue.

Activity of lysosomal enzymes, such as cathepsin D, acid phosphatase, etc., has been examined in both extra- and intracellular portions of MEE. The high activity of these enzymes observed in the extracellular portion may contribute to direct tissue damage of MEM (26). Moreover, bacterial enzymes released into the middle ear may also play a significant role in inducing inflammation. Human MEEs yield positive cultures for *S. pneumoniae*, and MEEs from infected chinchillas contain high concentrations of neuraminidase (42). As mentioned above, neuraminidase was present in higher concentrations in culture-positive cases as compared to those MEEs that were culture-negative (14). Thus, it may be that neuraminidase from *S. pneumoniae* may play a key role in the infectious disease process in OME.

Lysozyme is one of the major lysosomal enzymes found in inflammatory cells.

It is active against peptidoglycans of bacterial cell walls and can act synergistically with complement and specific antibodies to destroy a variety of bacteria. Lysozyme concentration has been found to be higher in mucoid effusions than in serous effusions and was much higher in MEE from the POM chinchilla model than from the SOM model (35). The concentration of lysozyme decreased significantly with penicillin treatment, suggesting that the level of this enzyme may be a good indicator of inflammation in OM (33). Proteolytic enzyme activity in MEE can only be considered in relation to the inhibitor levels. The presence of protease-inhibitor complexes, unsaturated free proteases, and free inhibitors [α-protease inhibitors and low-molecular-weight (LMW) inhibitors] will determine whether or not tissue injury may occur. It has been determined that LMW trypsin inhibitors have the most important and specific inhibitory function against granuloproteases, such as elastase and cathepsin G, in chronic OME (8). In MEE from acute OME, free LMW inhibitors are completely saturated with granuloproteases, and most of α_1-antitrypsin found in MEE was not active (9). In the fibrinolytic system, antitrypsin, antiplasmin, and plasminogen have been examined in both serous and mucoid forms of MEE in human OME (19). The bulk of α_1-antitrypsin was not bound to proteases and, therefore, antitrypsin activity was preserved in serous MEE. Since the specific inhibitor for plasmin (α_1-plasmin inhibitor) was in higher concentrations than plasmin and the conversion of plasminogen to plasmin was reduced, large amounts of plasminogen have been observed in serous forms of MEE. On the other hand, in mucoid MEE, the level of free α_1-antitrypsin was low because of the large amounts of lysosomal proteases that are present. Most plasminogen in mucoid MEE is activated to plasmin by the various proteases (20). Thus, in mucoid effusions, an active inflammatory state exists in which fragments of serum proteins are present and may contribute to tissue injury.

CHEMICAL MEDIATORS OF INFLAMMATION

Despite the fact that the levels of IgE are generally low in most MEE (49), a significant amount of histamine has been measured in middle ear fluid sample (1). However, the levels of histamine in MEE are significantly lower than that found in the nasal secretions in allergic rhinitis. Recently it has been suggested that tubal dysfunction may occur often in allergic patients and that the incidence of OME in allergic patients may be higher than in patients without allergy (5). It is possible that histamine released by mast cells in the nasopharynx can induce an inflammatory response of the tubal mucosa following specific allergic provocation. This, in turn, can trigger OME.

Kinins, such as bradykinin and kallidin, are vasoactive mediators similar to histamine and have been demonstrated in MEE by a number of investigators (2,21). The kallikrein-kinin system appears to be relatively active in serous effusions; however, the activity of this system in mucoid effusions appears to be less. Prekallikrein, which is activated into kallikrein, can be used as one of the sensitive parameters reflecting the level of plasma leakage of this mediator (25). The kallikrein-kinin system may be an important factor in the pathogenesis of acute OME, but not in chronic OM of the mucoid variety.

Prostaglandins (PGs) are polyunsaturated fatty acids arising from arachidonic acid following cell membrane perturbation.

It has been established that PGs have potent bioactive functions, including vasodilation, and enhance vascular permeability and release of lysosomal enzymes. In general, PGs are always present in all acute inflammatory fluids (66). Higher levels of PGE_2 and 6-keto-$PGF_{2\alpha}$ are present in human mucoid MEEs compared to serous effusions (38). In the animal model, both levels of PGE_2 and $PGF_{2\alpha}$ were higher in MEE from the POM model than from the mucoid otitis media (MOM) model. Cyclo-oxygenase, the enzyme that synthesizes various types of PGs, was localized in MEM of human and animal models (37). Furthermore, MEE from the SOM model demonstrated a predominance of 6-keto-$PGF_{1\alpha}$ whereas MEE from the MOM model had higher concentrations of PGE_2 (38). Other metabolites catalyzed by the enzyme lipoxygenase, such as the leukotrienes (LT), have been identified in MEE, and LTD_4 has an apparent cooperative function with PGs (57). It is interesting to note that LTB_4 has a remarkable activity on neutrophil chemotaxis, which is about 100 times more potent than hydroxyeicosatetraenoic acid (HETEs) (16). Therefore, PGs and LTs may play important roles in the initiation and/or the maintenance of the inflammatory state in OME.

SUMMARY

When viral and bacterial antigens injure MEM through immunological and/or nonimmunological mechanisms, many bioactive substances derived from inflammatory cells are produced. These products include enzymes; fatty acids; and plasma proteins, such as kallikrein-kinin, plasmin, complement components, and immunoglobulins. These substances may sustain middle ear inflammation. It is unclear, however, which factors are more important in the development of chronicity. If one can identify the specific factors responsible for the chronicity, one may be able to inhibit those specific factors and prevent chronic inflammation from occurring in middle ear inflammation. It is, therefore, important to identify the source of these specific factors. The correlation between the biochemical or immunochemical components of MEE and cytological as well as bacteriological findings is essential in the identification of the specific factors. Animal models have provided valuable information and will further add to our fundamental understanding of the mechanisms of sequential inflammatory changes in the middle ear cavity. The information obtained from animal studies will help establish a list of biochemical or immunochemical parameters that may lead to irreversible tissue injury. The incorporation of laboratory data on MEE with the clinical features of OM is critical in our understanding of the immunopathology of human MEM in OME. Since the collection of human samples is restricted to the time of tympanostomy, the follow-up studies recording the initial MEE data are important in identifying the factors related to chronicity. The effect of various therapeutic managements of the biochemical or immunological parameters in MEE should be studied extensively to establish the guidelines for better treatment. Multidisciplinary approaches in MEE analyses are desirable, and accumulation of available data on (a) MEE bacteriology and cytology and (b) biochemical and immunochemical parameters, together with the history and clinical findings, will be necessary to evaluate the inflammatory stages in OME.

REFERENCES

1. Berger, G., Hawke, M., Proops, D.W., and Ranadive, N.S. (1984): Histamine levels in middle ear effusions. *Acta Otolaryngol. (Stockh.)*, 98:385–390.
2. Bernstein, J.M., Steger, R., and Back, N. (1978): The kallikrein-kinin system in otitis media with effusion. *ORL J. Otorhinolaryngol. Relat. Spec.*, 86:249–255.
3. Bernstein, J.M., Brentjens, J., and Vladutia, A. (1982): Are immune complexes a factor in the pathogenesis of otitis media with effusion? *Am. J. Otolaryngol.*, 3:20–25.
4. Bernstein, J.M., and Park, B.H. (1985): Defective immunoregulation in children with chronic otitis media with effusion. Presented at the International Symposium on Recent Advances in Otitis Media with Effusion in Kyoto, January, 1985.
5. Bluestone, C.D. (1983): Eustachian tube function: physiology, pathophysiology, and role of allergy in pathogenesis of otitis media. *J. Allergy Clin. Immunol.*, 72:242–251.
6. Carlsson, B., Lundberg, C., and Ohlsson, K. (1981): Protease inhibitors in middle ear effusions. *Ann. Otol. Rhinol. Laryngol.*, 90:38–41.
7. Carlsson, B., Lundberg, C., and Ohlsson, K. (1982): Granuloproteases in middle ear effusions. *Ann. Otol. Rhinol. Laryngol.*, 91:76–81.
8. Carlsson, B., and Ohlsson, K. (1983): Localization of antileukoprotease in middle ear mucosa. *Acta Otolaryngol. (Stockh.)*, 95:111–116.
9. Carlsson, B., Lundberg, C., and Ohlsson, K. (1983): Granulocyte protease inhibition in acute and chronic middle ear effusion. *Acta Otolaryngol. (Stockh.)*, 95:341–349.
10. Clelland, W.W. (1964): Dithiothreitol: a new productive agent for SH-groups. *Biochemistry*, 3:480–482.
11. DeMaria, T.F., Priop, R.B., Briggs, B., Lim, D.J., and Birck, H.G. (1983): Endotoxin in middle ear effusions from patients with chronic otitis media with effusion. In: *Recent Advances in Otitis Media with Effusion*, edited by D.J. Lim, C.D. Bluestone, et al., pp. 123–124. B.C. Decker, Philadelphia.
12. DeMaria, T.F., McGee, R.B., Jr., and Lim, D.J. (1984): Rheumatoid factor in otitis media with effusion. *Arch. Otolaryngol.*, 110:279–280.
13. Diven, W.F., Glew, R.H., and Bluestone, C.D. (1981): Lysosomal hydrolases in middle ear effusions. *Ann. Otol. Rhinol. Laryngol.*, 90:148–153.
14. Diven, W.F., Glew, R.H., and LaMarco, K.L. (1985): Hydrolase activity in acute otitis media with effusion. *Ann. Otol. Rhinol. Laryngol.*, 94:415–518.
15. Drucker, M., Drucker, J., Neter, E., Bernstein, J.M., and Ogra, P.L. (1970): Cell mediated immune responses to bacterial antigens on human mucosal surfaces. In: *Secretory Immunity and Infection*, edited by J.R. McGhee, J. Mestecky, and J.L. Babb, pp. 479–488. Plenum Press, New York.
16. Ford-Hutchinson, A.W., Bray, M.A., Doig, M.V., Shipley, M.E., and Smith, M.J.H. (1980): Leukotriene B, a potent chemokinetic and aggregating substance released from polymorphonuclear leukocytes. *Nature*, 285:264–265.
17. Giebink, G.S., Carlsson, B.A., Hetherington, S.V., Hostetter, M.K., and Le, C.T. (1985): Bacterial polymorphonuclear contribution to middle ear inflammation in chronic otitis media with effusion. *Ann. Otol. Rhinol. Laryngol.*, 94:398–402.
18. Granstrom, G.,Holmquist, J., Jarlstedt, J., and Renvall, V. (1985): Collagenase activity in middle ear effusions. *Acta Otolaryngol. (Stockh.)*, 100:405–413.
19. Hamaguchi, Y., Ohi, M., Sakakura, Y., and Miyoshi, Y. (1985): Activities of antiplasmin and antiplasminogen activator in serous middle ear effusions. *Ann. Otol. Rhinol. Laryngol.*, 94:293–296.

20. Hamaguchi, Y., and Sakakura, Y. (1985): Protein and enzymes in middle ear effusion. In: *The Latest Medical Book: Otitis Media With Effusion*, edited by K. Kawamoto, pp. 117–126. Igaku-kyoikusha, Tokyo.
21. Hamaguchi, Y., Majima, Y., Ukai, K., Sakakura, Y., and Miyoshi, Y. (1986): Significance of kallikrein-kinin system in otitis media with effusion. *Ann. Otol. Rhinol. Laryngol.*, 95 (Suppl. 124): 5–8.
22. Hamaguchi, Y., Sakakura, K., Majima, Y., and Sakakura, Y. (1986): Lysosomal thiolproteases in middle ear effusions. *Ann. Otol. Rhinol. Laryngol.*, 95 (Suppl. 124): 9–12.
23. Hamaguchi, Y., Sakakura, K., Majima, Y., and Sakakura, Y. (1986): Lysosomal thiolproteases (cathepsin B-like proteases) in serous middle ear effusions from adult patients. *Acta Otolaryngol. (Stockh.)*, 101:257–262.
24. Hamaguchi, Y., Majima, Y., Ikai, K., Sakakura, Y., and Miyoshi, Y. (1985): The significance of protease inhibitors in the pathogenesis of otitis media with effusion. *Auris Nasus Larynx*, 12 (Suppl. I): 145–147.
25. Hamaguchi, Y., Sakakura, Y., Majima, Y., Ukai, K., and Miyoshi, Y. (1985): Plasma component of middle ear effusion evaluated by prekallikrein level. *ORL J. Otorhinolaryngol. Relat. Spec.*, 47:145–150.
26. Hara, H., Takasaka, T., and Kawamoto, K. (1984): Lysosomal enzyme activity in middle ear effusions. *Jpn. J. Otorhinolaryngol.*, 87:594–602.
27. Hochstrasser, K.,Arnold, W., and Naumann, R. (1981): Proteinase and proteinase inhibitors in middle ear effusions. In: *Recent Advances in Otitis Media with Effusion*, edited by D.J. Lim, C.D. Bluestone, et al., pp. 184–189. B.C. Decker, Philadelphia.
28. Iino, Y., Kaneko, Y., and Takasaka, T. (1985): Endotoxin in middle ear effusions tested with Limulus Assay. *Acta Otolaryngol. (Stockh.)*, 100:42–50.
29. Ishii, Y., Totiyama, M., and Suzuki, J. (1980): Histopathological study of otitis media with effusion. *Ann. Otol. Rhinol. Laryngol.* (Suppl. 68), 89:83–86.
30. Iwanaga, M., Yamamota, E., and Fukumoto, M. (1985): Cathepsin activity in cholesteatoma. *Ann. Otol. Rhinol. Laryngol.*, 94:309–312.
31. Juhn, S.K., Huff, J.S., and Paparella, M.M. (1973): Lactate dehydrogenase activity and isozyme patterns in serous middle ear effusions. *Ann. Otol. Rhinol. Laryngol.*, 82:192–195.
32. Juhn, S.K., and Huff, J.S. (1976): Biochemical characteristics of middle ear effusions. *Ann. Otol. Rhinol. Laryngol.*, 85:110–115.
33. Juhn, S.K., Paparella, M.M., and Kim, C.S. (1977): Pathogenesis of otitis media. *Ann. Otol. Rhinol. Laryngol.*, 86:481–492.
34. Juhn, S.K. (1982): Pathogenesis of otitis media. Studies on middle ear effusions. *Laryngoscope*, 92:287–291.
35. Juhn, S.K., Sipila, P., Jung, T.T.K., and Edlin, J. (1984): Biochemical pathology of otitis media with effusion. *Acta Otolaryngol. (Stockh.)*, 414:45–51.
36. Juhn, S.K. (1985): Inflammatory changes reflected in middle ear effusions in otitis media. *Auris Nasus Larynx*, 12 (Suppl. I): 63–66.
37. Jung, T.T.K., Juhn, S.K., and Jonathan, M.G. (1982): Identification of prostaglandins and other arachidonic acid metabolites in experimental otitis media. *Prostaglandins Leukotrienes Med.*, 8:249–261.
38. Jung, T.T.K., Huang, E., and Juhn, S.K. (1983): Prostaglandins in middle ear fluids, cholesteatoma and granulation tissue (Abstr.). In: *The Third International Symposium on Recent Advances in Otitis Media with Effusion*, edited by D.J. Lim, and C.D. Bluestone, p. 53.
39. Jung, T.T.K., and Juhn, S.K. (1985): Prostaglandins and other arachidonic acid metabolites in the middle ear fluids. *Auris Nasus Larynx,* 12 (Suppl. I): 148–150.
40. Kobayashi, K., Somekawa, Y., Yamanaka, N., and Kataura, A. (1984): Composition of sugar of glycoprotein fractions in the human middle ear effusions. *Ear Res. J.*, 14:27–29.
41. Kyogoku, M., and Hozawa, K. (1984): Studies of pathogenesis of chronic inflammation. In case of rheumatoid arthritis and otitis media with effusion. *J. Jpn. Bronchoesophageal Soc.*, 35:66–75.
42. LaMarco, K.L., Diven, W.F., Glew, R.H., Doyle, W.J., and Cantekin, E.I. (1984): Neuraminidase activity in middle ear effusions. *Ann. Otol. Rhinol. Laryngol.*, 93:76–84.
43. Lim, D.J., Lewis, D.M., Schram, J.L., and Birck, H.G. (1976): Otitis media with effusion. Cytological and microbiological correlates. *Arch. Otolaryngol.*, 105:404–412.
44. Liu, Y.S., Lim, D.J., Lang, R.W., and Birck, H.G. (1975): Chronic middle ear effusions. Immunological and bacteriological investigations. *Arch. Otolaryngol.*, 101:278–286.

45. Lupovich, P., and Harkins, M. (1972): Symposium on prophylaxis and treatment of middle ear effusions. IV. The pathophysiology of effusion in otitis media. *Laryngoscope*, 82:1647–1653.
46. McGhee, R.B., Jr., DeMaria, T.A., Okazaki, N., and Lim, D.J. (1983): Selective induction of macrophages in the middle ear. *Ann. Otol. Rhinol. Laryngol.*, 92:510–517.
47. Mogi, G., Honjo, S., Maeda, S., Yoshida, T., and Watanabe, N. (1974): Secretory immunoglobulin A (s-IgA) in middle ear effusions, a further report. *Ann. Otol. Rhinol. Laryngol.*, 83:92–101.
48. Mogi, G., Honjo, S., Maeda, S., and Yoshida, T. (1973):Secretory immunoglobulin A(SI_gA) in middle ear effusions. Observations of 160 specimens. *Ann. Otol. Rhinol. Laryngol.*, 82:302–310. The development of mucosal immunity in guinea pig middle ear. *Int. J. Pediatr. Otolaryngol.*, 1:331–349.
49. Mogi, G., Maeda, S., Yoshida, T., and Watanabe, N. (1976): Radioimmunoassay of IgE in middle ear effusions. *Acta Otolaryngol. (Stockh.)*, 86:26–30.
50. Mogi, G., Maeda, S., Watanabe, N. (1980): The development of mucosal immunity in guinea pig middle ears. *Int. J. Pediatr. Otolaryngol.*, 1:331–349.
51. Okazaki, N., DeMaria, T.A., Briggs, B.R., and Lim, D.J. (1984): Experimental otitis media with effusion induced by nonviable *Haemophilus influenzae*. *Am. J. Otolaryngol.*, 5:80–92.
52. Paparella, M.M., Hiraide, F., Juhn, S.K., and Kaneko, Y. (1970): Cellular events involved in middle ear fluid production. *Ann. Otol. Rhinol. Laryngol.*, 79:1–15.
53. Paparella, M.M., Sipila, P., Juhn, S.K., and Jung, T.T.K. (1985): Subepithelial spaces in otitis media. *Laryngoscope*, 95:414–420.
54. Palva, T., Holopainen, E., and Karma, P. (1976): Protein and cellular pattern of glue ear secretion. *Ann. Otol. Rhinol. Laryngol.*, 85(Suppl. 25): 103–109.
55. Palva, T., Raunio, V., Nousiainen, R. (1975): Middle ear specific proteins in glue ears. *Acta Otolaryngol. (Stockh.),* 79:160–165.
56. Palva, T., Lehtinen, T., and Rinne, J. (1983): Immune complexes in the middle ear fluid in chronic secretory otitis media. *Ann. Otol. Rhinol. Laryngol.*, 92:42–44.
57. Peck, M.M., Piper, P.J., and Williams, T.J. (1981): The effect of leukotrienes C and D on the microvasculature of guinea pig skin. *Prostaglandins*, 21:315–321.
58. Prellner, K., and Nillson, N.I. (1982): Complement aberration in serum from children with otitis media due to *S. pneumoniae* or *H. influenzae*. *Acta Otolaryngol. (Stockh.)*, 94:275–282.
59. Prellner, K.: Antigens, specific antibodies and complement in otitis media. *(Submitted for publication.)*
60. Sade, J. (1970): The nature of middle ear effusion. The biochemical aspect. In: *Secretory Otitis Media with Effusion and Its Sequelae*, edited by J. Sade, pp. 144–153. Churchill Livingstone, New York.
61. Sipila, P., Koskela, M., Karjalainen, H., and Luotonen, J. (1985): Secretory IgA, secretory component and pathogen specific antibodies in the middle ear effusion during an attack of acute and secretory otitis media. *Auris Nasus Larynx,* 12 (Suppl. I): 180–182.
62. Takasaka, T., Kaku, Y., Shibahara, Y., Hozawa, K., Takeyama, M., Kaneko, Y., and Kawamoto, K. (1983): Experimental otitis media with effusion: an immunoelectron microscopic study. In: *Recent Advances in Otitis Media With Effusion*, edited by D.J. Lim, C.D. Bluestone, et al., pp. 88–91. B.C. Decker, Philadelphia.
63. Tomasi, T.B., Jr. (1972): Secretory immunoglobulins. *N. Engl. J. Med.*, 287:500–506.
64. Watanabe, N., Briggs, B.R., and Lim, D.J. (1982): Experimental otitis media in chinchillas. I. Baseline immunological investigations. *Ann. Otol. Rhinol. Laryngol.*, 83:92–101.
65. Watanabe, N., DeMaria, T.F., Lewis, D.M., Mogi, G., and Lim, D.J. (1982): Comparison of middle ear responses to *S. pneumoniae* types 3 and 23. *Ann. Otol. Rhinol. Laryngol.* (Suppl. 93), 91:9–16.
66. Willis, A.L. (1970): Identification of prostaglandin E in rat inflammatory exudate. *Pharmacol. Res. Comm.*, 2:297–304.
67. Yamanaka, N., Somekawa, H., and Kataura, A. (1984): Pathogenesis of chronic otitis media with effusion in children. Immune complex levels in middle ear effusions. Ear Res. J., 14:24–26.

Immunology of the Ear, edited by J. Bernstein
and P. Ogra. Raven Press, New York © 1987.

Inflammatory Mediators in Middle Ear Disease

*Paul B. van Cauwenberge and **Joel M. Bernstein

**Department of Otolaryngology, State University Hospital, B-9000 Ghent, Belgium; and **Departments of Otolaryngology and Pediatrics, State University of New York at Buffalo, Buffalo, New York 14214, and Division of Infectious Diseases, Children's Hospital of Buffalo, Buffalo, New York 14222*

The resolution of otitis media (OM) requires the eradication of bacteria or virus from the middle ear space and a return of normal ventilation to the tympanum. The latter requires normal eustachian tube function and the former requires nonimmunological and immunological mechanisms that lead to the phagocytosis and subsequent killing of pathological microorganisms.

However, when eustachian tube dysfunction continues and middle ear effusion (MEE) persists, the immunological activity in these effusions is maintained by the persistence of antibody and/or mediators of cell-mediated immune mechanisms. The persistence of these mediators of inflammation may then lead to tissue injury to the soft tissue as well as to the bony structures in the middle ear cleft. This section has already addressed (a) some of the immunological mechanisms that are present in MEEs, (b) the inflammatory cells present in the effusions, and (c) the biochemistry of the effusions.

This chapter will specifically review those mediators of inflammation that may have an effect on (a) the blood flow to the mucosa, (b) the glandular secretion of the mucosa, and (c) bone resorption in the middle ear cleft.

Inflammatory mediators in the middle ear cleft may arise from at least three different sources: (a) Serum proteins may enter the middle ear as a result of transudation and may be broken down nonspecifically by enzymes released either from epithelial cells of the middle ear cleft or from inflammatory cells in the middle ear space. Proteins such as fibrinogen, the complement cascade, the clotting factors, and plasminogen may all be broken down to active inflammatory products. (b) The release of mediators from inflammatory cells may infiltrate into the middle ear space and tissue following an inflammatory process. Neutrophils, eosinophils, and mast cells may be involved. These cells can release lysosomal enzymes that are capable of breaking down tissue protein, thus leading to tissue necrosis in the middle ear space. (c) The breakdown and necrosis of the tissue in the middle ear itself may lead to collagenolysis, and the products of collagenolysis may be chemotactic even in nanogram amounts and are capable of (a) attracting neutrophils, (b) aggregating platelets, and (c) clumping erythrocytes. Inflammatory reactions in the middle ear space can be looked upon in terms of two key elements that characterize the inflammatory reaction: (a) vasopermeability changes and (b) the arrival of leukocytes from the circulation. The increased vascular permeability is a result of the transient opening in the endothelial junctions permitting egress of soluble substances such as plasma proteins, electrolytes, and water. The mechanism by which these mediators are currently presumed to work is through their ability to induce contraction of the active contractile elements in endothelial cells. This causes them to become shrunken, leaving gaps in the junctional zone between the endothelial cells (27).

MEDIATORS OF INFLAMMATION IN THE MIDDLE EAR

The following mediators of inflammation have been identified in the middle ear cleft and are thought to be associated with the inflammatory state in OM.

Histamine

Histamine is a potent pharmacological mediator of inflammation which influences smooth muscles, thus resulting in increased permeability of blood vessels. It has been shown experimentally that histamine causes vasodilation and increases the permeability of the middle ear mucosa (11). There are a few reports on the histamine content of MEEs. Jackson (quoted in ref. 11), with a biological assay technique, found that histamine was either absent or present in small amounts. Furthermore, using a modification of the fluorometric assay of Shore et al. (32), Berger et al. (3) found high levels of histamine in MEEs. The concentration varied greatly, ranging from 0 to 3,650 ng/ml, with a mean value of 449 ng/ml. In the same study, the mean histamine blood count concentration was only 49 ng/ml. There was also a significant difference between the mucoid and serous varieties of MEEs. The mucoid type had significantly higher histamine concentration than the serous type. No significant difference was found between the purulent and mucoid or between the serous and the purulent types. Finally, there was no difference between the middle ear fluids in patients with allergy and those who were nonatopic.

Skoner et al. (33) used a modified single isotopic-enzymatic assay with sensitivities in the picogram range and a high degree of specificity for histamine. They reported lower levels than in the Berger et al. study (3). This is likely a result of the higher specificity of the radioenzymatic assay for histamine. In the latter study, 22 human MEEs were studied and the range of histamine concentration was 1.3 to 112 ng, with a median value of 21 ng/ml. The mean plasma level was only 0.7 ng/ml. Finally, in preliminary studies of experimentally induced effusions in chinchillas, marked histamine elevations were found after middle ear infection with various organisms (D. P. Skoner et al., *unpublished results*). The highest amounts were found after *Pseudomonas aeruginosa* was artifically placed in the middle ear.

The conclusion from these studies is that although the absolute values of histamine show marked variations between studies, it is obvious that histamine concentrations are significantly and markedly elevated in MEEs compared to the serum levels. Furthermore, the presence of elevated levels of histamine in most of the MEEs supports the hypothesis that this substance might be involved in the production and maintenance of an inflammatory response in otitis media with effusion (OME). Histamine may originate from the serum, but more likely it is locally produced by release from both mucosal mast cells and connective tissue mast cells that are known to occur in middle ear mucosa. Although type-1 hypersensitivity may be responsible for activation of the mast cells in OME, it is more likely that the mast cells are nonspecifically activated by C_3 and perhaps by immune complexes that are known to be present in middle ear fluids. Finally, neurotransmitters such as substance P and vasoactive intestinal polypetide (VIP) may also play a role. They are potent histamine releasers from mast cells and/or basophils and they are involved in every type of inflammatory reaction so far described. Thus, it is likely that histamine is the initial inflammatory mediator causing increased vascular permeability in the middle ear mucosa in OME.

Leukotactic Factors

Once histamine, and perhaps other vasoactive substances, enhance vascular permeability in the middle ear, inflammatory cells such as polymorphonuclear (PMN) leukocytes and monocytes may then migrate to the middle ear space. It is likely that this migration is the result of active chemotaxis from chemotaxins that are present in the middle ear. Such chemotaxins may be bacterial products that are known to be present in the middle ear. Chemotaxins may also result from activated complement components that have been repeatedly demonstrated in MEEs and have been critically analyzed in several chapters in this volume. Finally, breakdown products of tissue collagen may be chemotactic for PMN leukocytes, and it is possible that polypeptides released by activated lymphocytes, the so-called lymphokines, may be chemotactic for a number of inflammatory cells. Thus, the important features of this early increased vascular permeability are (a) the arrival into the middle ear space of serum proteins that can be broken down into activated inflammatory mediators and (b) the migration of inflammatory cells from the tissue spaces as well as from the circulating blood.

Bradykinins

In addition to histamine, a group of small polypeptides formed by enzymatic mechanisms have potent pharmacological actions that dilate blood vessels and may also enhance white blood cell migration. The kallikrein-kinin system is activated by the proteolytic activity of a variety of enzymes, including plasmin and trypsin, and by activation of Hageman factor and by acidification and dilution (1) (Fig. 1). Kallikrein is a highly specific kinin-forming enzyme that acts by converting kinin-

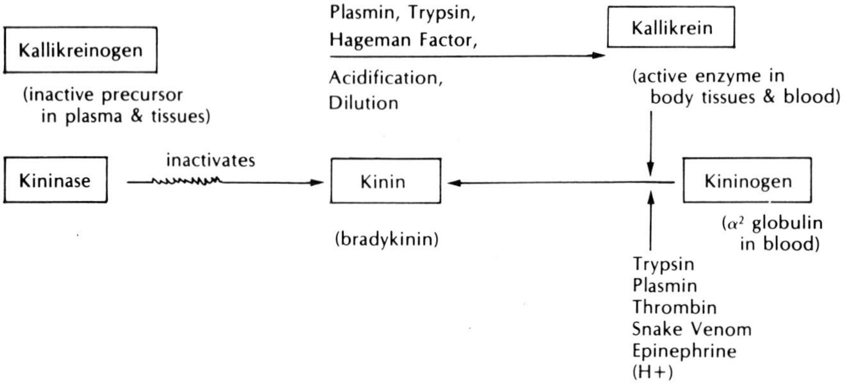

FIG. 1. The kallikrein-kinin system. (Reproduced with permission of the *American Journal of Otolaryngology*, Vol. 1, 1979, p. 31.)

ogen into kinin. The conversion of kininogen to kinin can also occur through nonspecific enzymatic degradation by trypsin, plasmin, thrombin, and lysosomal hydrolases. The kallikrein-kinin system appears to be present in human MEEs, and although considerable variability in kinin activity was observed in different middle ear fluids, the concentrations of kinin and kininogen appear to be greatest in the serous and seromucinous effusions and lowest in the mucoid effusions (5). This finding may be of some importance in determining the duration of the disease because it has been shown that kinins appear in the early phase of acute inflammation. This might suggest that, in general, serous and seromucinous effusions may precede the mucoid type of MEE.

Kallikrein has not been found in middle ear fluids as yet. This is probably because of the elevated levels of α-1 antitrypsin, which is known to be present in middle ear fluid and which actively inhibits proteases (9,28). The conversion of kininogen to kinin in the effusion is, consequently, a result of nonspecific enzymatic degradation, possibly by lysosomal hydrolases. These may originate from neutrophils or macrophages present in most MEEs or from mast cells. Another possibility is that the conversion of kininogen to kinin results from a kallikrein-like substance demonstrated in neutrophils.

With regard to the possible role of the kinin system in OME, it has been shown that injection of bradykinin produces (a) gaps in the venular side of the vascular bed in vessels with a diameter of greater than 60 nm and (b) an accumulation of high-molecular-weight plasma proteins in the interstitium, followed by tissue edema (27). Finally, Dennis et al. (11) has demonstrated that bradykinin induces an increased vascular permeability and vasodilation leading to edema of the middle ear and eustachian tube mucosa for about 10 min.

Plasminogen-Plasmin System

Factor XII (Hageman factor), not only induces the breakdown of prekallikrein to kallikrein and the subsequent release of bradykinin from kininogen, but may also be involved in activation of plasminogen to plasmin. This fibrinolytic system is also present in MEE, which can cause fibrinolytic dissolution of human fibrin clots. The highest levels of fibrinolytic activity appear to be present in the serous effusions (6). Mucoid effusions possess lower levels of fibrinolytic activity, which is a logical finding in view of the nature of these effusions. The role of this activity in OME is unknown; however, plasmin is present in MEEs and is probably responsible for this lytic activity. Plasmin, an active protease of the fibrinolysin system, is capable of activating a number of proteolytic systems, including the intrinsic coagulation system, the vasoactive peptide system, and the complement system. The relation of these systems to inflammation in the middle ear may have a profound influence on the possible conversion of a simple MEE into a chronic OM. It is also interesting to note that the lack of fibrinolytic activity promotes the development of a fibrin mesh. This could contribute to connective tissue synthesis and a progressive fibrosis, with eventual development of adhesive OM (6) (Figs. 2 and 3).

Prostaglandins

If histamine is the earliest mediator of inflammation in the middle ear following the initial insult of the mucous membrane from bacterial invasion, and the kininogen-kinin and plasminogen-plasmin system follows, the later stage of acute in-

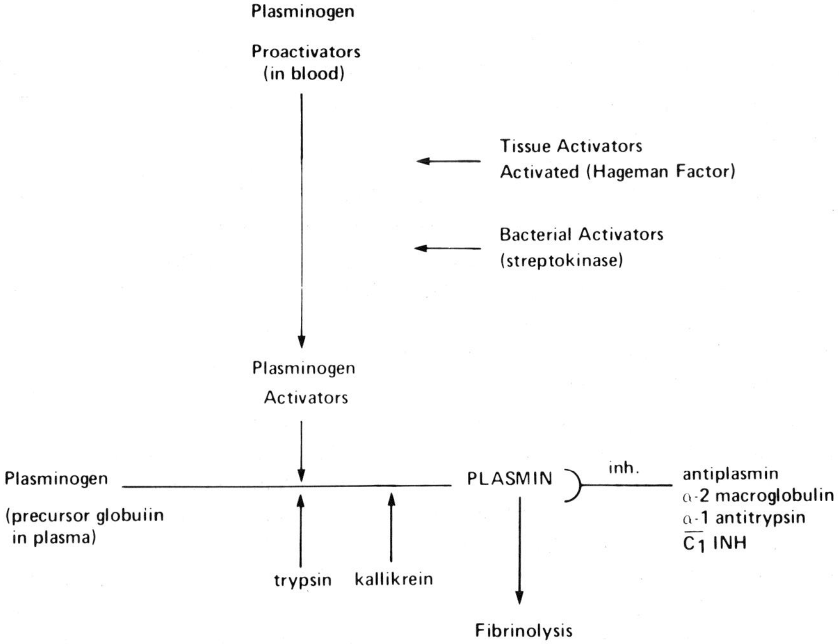

FIG. 2. Fibrinolysin system. (Reproduced with permission of the *American Journal of Otolaryngology*, Vol. 1, 1979, p. 31.)

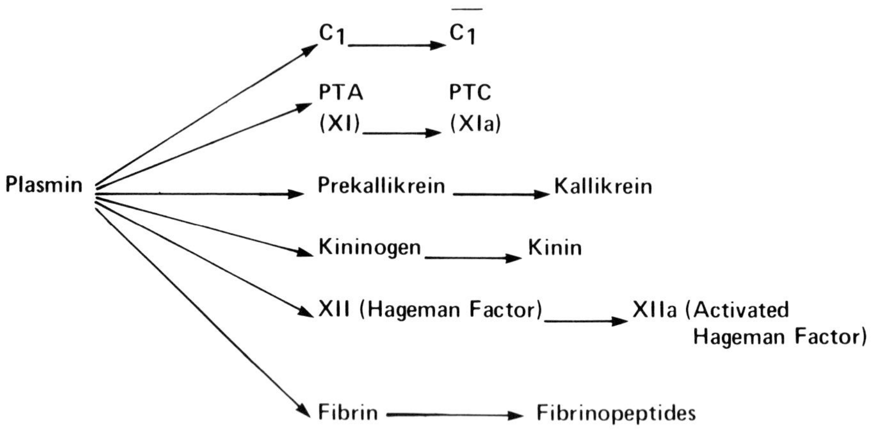

FIG. 3. The potential pathways for plasmin in the inflammatory response. (Reproduced with permission of the *American Journal of Otolaryngology*, Vol. 1, 1979, p. 31.)

flammation is most likely related to the release of prostaglandins (PGs) into the middle ear. Details of the chemistry and function of the PG system have been reviewed in a chapter by Tillinghast and Metcalfe (*this volume*). The possible role that may be played by PGs in the middle ear, however, will be briefly reviewed in this chapter.

Prostaglandins are naturally occurring cyclic unsaturated fatty acids that mediate or modulate a wide variety of potent biological activities, including inflammation, contraction of smooth muscles, increase in intraocular pressure, and stimulation of bone resorption. They are ubiquitous in their distribution and synthesized by virtually every tissue in the body.

Davis et al. (10) has demonstrated that topical application of 50 ng of PGE_1 can cause a reduction in the patency of the eustachian tube. The same dose given via the carotid artery has the same effect. Dennis et al. (11) showed that PGs of the E series can induce vasodilation, increased vascular permeability, and edema in the middle ear and eustachian tube mucosa. It has been shown that PGF_2 and PGE_2 are present in high concentrations in both the serous and mucoid effusions (4,21,22). It is possible that PGs may play a role in causing increased capillary permeability in MEEs which could lead to tissue edema in OME. Furthermore, PGE-like material in granulation tissue has been found in chronic OM (22). High concentrations of PGE_2 are present in purulent OM and may be present in higher concentrations in acute suppurative disease than in chronic secretory OM.

In experimental animals it has been found that the injection of PGE_2 may result in a significant elevation of lactic acid dehydrogenase (LDH), acid phosphatase, and calcium and protein concentrations in the middle ear (20). This suggests an important role for PGs in middle ear mucosal inflammation. Indeed, the elevated protein level may be a result of local vasodilation and increased permeability of the blood-aqueous barrier of the middle ear. Lactic acid dehydrogenase has also been used as an indicator of inflammation, so elevation of the LDH level after administration of PGE_2 may suggest an inflammatory reaction (21). Finally, elevation of acid phosphatases and calcium may signify an initiation of bone resorption activity, and the alkaline phosphatase may participate in new bone formation often seen in OME.

All of these studies strongly indicate that PGs of the E and F series may be synthesized locally in the middle ear cavity and that they probably play an important role in the pathophysiology of all kinds of middle ear inflammation.

Leukotrienes

Whereas cyclooxygenase converts arachidonic acid (AA) into the PG series, lipoxygenase enzymes convert AA into substances that also have a profound effect on smooth muscles. These substances, which were originally collectively labeled "slow-reacting substance of anaphylaxis" (SRS-A), are now known as the leukotrienes. At least two potent leukotrienes (LTs) have been identified in the middle ear fluids: LTB4 and LTC4 (Table 1). The exact function of leukotrienes in the

TABLE 1. *Concentration of LTB_4 in 18 MEEs*

Patient	LTB_4[a]	LTC_4
	Serous	
L.C.	0.001	0.001
M.C.	0.003	0.002
C.R.	0.005	0.002
	Seromucinous	
G.L.	0.002	0.001
J.M.	0.0	0.002
J.P.	0.006	0.001
A.F.	0.004	0.002
V.H.	0.013	0.018
C.L.	0.0	0.001
	Mucoid	
M.H.	0.004	0.003
K.G.	0.003	0.001
C.J.	0.020	0.007
J.L.	0.027	0.005
K.C.	0.001	0.001
	Purulent	
K.F.	0.009	0.002
M.S.	0.006	0.002
L.D.	0.007	0.006
B.M.	0.052	0.006

[a]Nanograms of LTB_4 per milligram of albumin; double-antibody radioimmunoassay.

middle ear space and middle ear mucosa is not known. It is most likely that these substances, derived by the action of membrane-associated phospholipases, act on the smooth muscle of the blood vessels of the middle ear mucosa and represent one more pathway that leads to increased capillary permeability and inflammatory cell migration. In this regard, it should be emphasized that LTB4 is an extremely potent chemotactic agent for neutrophils and could be responsible for the influx of PMN leukocytes into the middle ear space.

Platelet-Activating Factor

In addition to the AA metabolites mentioned above, platelet-activating factor (PAF) has been shown to be present in the middle ear fluids. (J. M. Bernstein, *unpublished results*). The presence of PAF is reviewed in Table 2. The active component of PAF has been found to be an acetylglycerylether phosphoryl choline. Aside from inducing aggregation and degranulation of platelets, PAF produces contraction of smooth muscle and stimulates aggregation, chemotaxis, and granular secretion of PMN neutrophils and monocytes. Furthermore, PAF is, on a molar basis, 10^3 to 10^4 times more potent than histamine in increasing vascular permeability. Finally, PAF has a strong hypotensive action. It has been demonstrated that PAF may be released not only from basophils, but also after appropriate stimulation from cells of the monocyte/macrophage series and from PMNs, platelets, and endothelial cells. It is likely that in the middle ear fluid, PAF is derived from all of the above-mentioned cells. Although the precise role of PAF has not been defined, it has been suggested that this substance has an important function in the entangled web of humoral and cellular effectors of inflammation (8). In this regard, mast cells may release PAF following association of specific IgE with antigen or by stimulation by activated complement, and in this way C5a may stimulate the neutrophil or basophil to release PAF. Finally, it is possible that thymus-derived lymphocytes (T cells) may release PAF. Inasmuch as all of these cells and immunological mechanisms are known to exist in the middle ear, it is not surprising that this inflammatory mediator has been found, sometimes in significant

TABLE 2. *Concentration of PAF*[a] in MEE

Patient[b]	PAF[c]
M.G.	7.4
A.G.	3.5
K.C.	4.3
A.L.	4.2
L.J.	2.2

[a]Measured by platelet aggregation in an aggregometer.
[b]Five of 15 patients demonstrated measurable levels of PAF in the MEE.
[c]Nanograms of PAF per milliliter of MEE.

amounts. Like histamine and bradykinins, PAF has been shown to act on the endothelial walls of blood vessels. Furthermore, PAF appears to also be active in local recruitment and activation of inflammatory cells. Thus, PAF is a potent inflammatory mediator that not only can produce increased capillary permeability, but also has the effect of recruiting inflammatory cells into the middle ear space.

Lysosomal Enzymes

The mediators mentioned so far have two basic common denominators. One is increased vascular permeability and the other is recruitment of inflammatory cells. Once these inflammatory cells are present, interaction with various mediators of inflammation may activate the surface of these cells and result in the release of more inflammatory mediators. Among these will be lysosomal enzymes. These lysosomal enzymes may, in turn, break down serum proteins into activated inflammatory mediators, such as kinins, plasmins, and fibrins. In this way, the inflammatory response is maintained in the middle ear space. The concept that lysosomal enzymes may mediate tissue injury in OME by directly injuring middle ear tissues has not been thoroughly explored, although it has been suggested that tympanosclerosis and nonotosclerotic fixation of the stapediovestibular joint may result from the action of lysosomal hydrolases (7). It has been demonstrated that lysosomal enzymes produce inflammation by increasing capillary permeability, stimulating chemotaxis, and activating plasminogen and complement, causing depolymerization of basement membrane and even mediating cell lysis. Thus, the presence of lysosomal enzymes in MEEs may lead to a cascade of biologic mechanisms, including the complement system, the kinogen-kinin vasoactive peptide system, and the plasminogen-plasmin fibrinolytic system (Fig. 4). These systems may contribute to the effect of chronic inflammation in the middle ear cavity in OME (7,12,15,23,35) (Fig. 5).

1. $C_1 \xrightarrow{L^*} C_1$ (classic complement pathway)
2. $C_3 \xrightarrow{L} C_{3a} + C_{3b}$ (alternate complement pathway)
   Chemotaxis, increased vascular permeability, cell lysis
3. Kininogen $\xrightarrow{L}$ kinin → increased vascular permeability, smooth muscle concentration
4. Plasminogen $\xrightarrow{L}$ plasmin → activation of complement fibrinolysis, activation of kinogen
5. C_{3b} → macrophages → release of lysosomal enzymes that directly effect bone resorption
6. Direct proteolytic, lipolytic, glycolytic effects on cells and tissues

*Lysosomal hydrolases.

FIG. 4. Potential pathways for the effect of lysosomal enzymes in MEEs. (Reproduced with permission of the *American Journal of Otolaryngology*, Vol. 1, 1979, p. 31.)

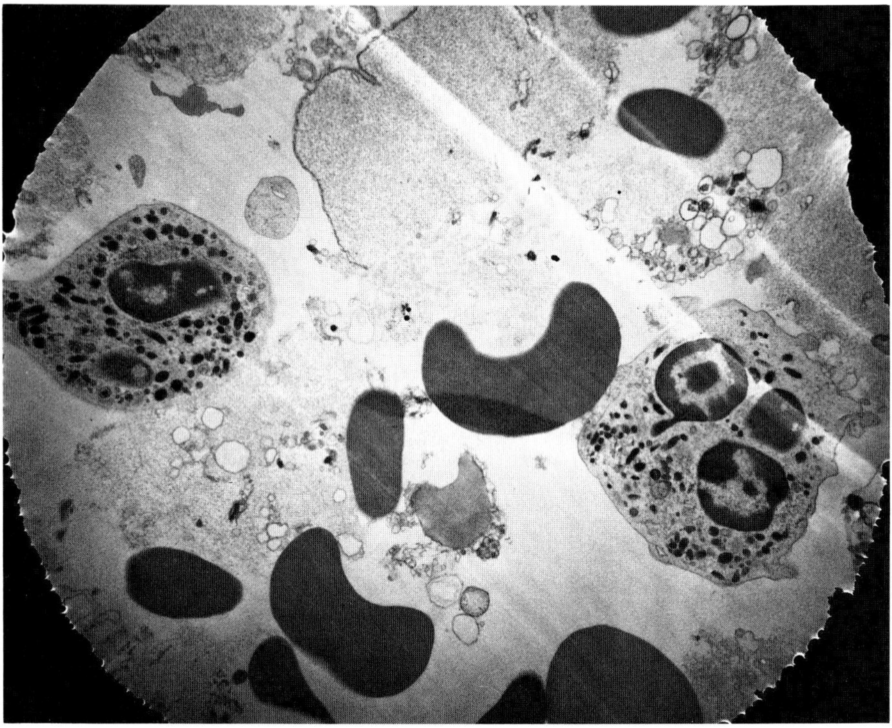

FIG. 5. Electron photomicrograph of sediment of seromucinous MEE showing neutrophils packed with lysosomes.

Lysozymes

Lysozymes are α-1,4 glycan hydrolases (12–14,16). Lysozyme from different animal species, and sometimes from different organs or secretions of the same animal, are chemically different (16). Despite the wealth of information concerning lysozymes, accumulated during the last 50 years, the full range of functions of the diverse lysozyme system is not fully known (26). Its bacterial activities are now well established. However, the action of lysozyme alone is relatively weak against bacteria, but it can act synergistically with the complement system and specific antibodies. In a recent study, heating of the middle ear liquid to 60°C for 30 min to destroy complement also deprived the middle ear liquid of its bacteriostatic effect (25). Lysozyme may play a role in the calcification of cartilage and in the lysis of a seminal clot (24). It has also been reported that rheological properties of mucus in the MEEs are not effected by lysozyme. In patients with OME that are microbiologically sterile, lysozyme levels appear to be elevated. The middle ear/serum ratios may range to almost 200 in paired middle ear fluid and serum

(34). Although lysozyme alone is not very active against pathogenic bacteria, as mentioned above, in combination with other enzymes, such as lipases or proteases, it can synergistically destroy various types of pathogenic bacteria. Immunocytochemical localization of lysozyme demonstrates that lysozyme is localized in the mucigen granules of the secretory cells as well as in the specific granules of PMN leukocytes and macrophage (26). The specimens obtained from patients with mucoid effusions also show numerous secretory cells containing lysozyme; this is in sharp contrast to the serous type, in which only a few secretory cells containing this enzyme can be found. The localization of lysozyme in the secretory granules is confined to the light granules and is not found in the dark cores. These morphological findings are in agreement with the biochemical findings that demonstrate higher lysozyme levels in mucoid effusions than in serous effusions. It has been demonstrated that lysosomal enzymes in middle ear fluids are primarily of cellular origin rather than just the result of transudation from plasma. Using B-D-N-acetyl hexosaminidase as a marker, it has been demonstrated that this enzyme is present in the middle ear fluid as a result of cellular release rather than from transudation. In general, most enzymes found in MEEs appear to be significantly higher in mucoid effusions than in serous effusions. These latter findings again strongly support the idea that the release of lysosomal enzymes into the middle ear fluid occurs mainly as a result of active secretion from inflammatory cells present in the MEE (7).

Other Enzymes

There are many other enzymes that have been found in MEE. These include LDH and its isoenzymes (17,18), malic dehydrogenase (2), alkaline phosphatase (19,30,31), acid phosphatase (19,30,31), leucine aminopeptidase (19,31), nonspecific esterases (29), and transaminases (30). It is likely that these enzymes do not represent true inflammatory mediators, but are most likely the result of the active oxidative metabolism that occurs in the inflammatory cells and possibly in the epithelial cells in middle ear tissue. It is highly unlikely that these glycolytic enzymes are involved in the inflammatory process.

CONCLUSION—A UNIFYING CONCEPT FOR INFLAMMATION IN THE MIDDLE EAR MUCOSA

It is proposed that the earliest change in the inflammatory response in OM is the production of modified tissue proteins in the middle ear mucosa as a result of viral and/or bacterial infection. Eustachian tube dysfunction may also lead to modified tissue proteins just on the basis of altered environmental gases. These proteins can alter complement and lead to the release of histamine, kinins, and PG. In addition, the coagulation system becomes activated, which, in turn, can activate certain complement components and lead to release of vasoactive amines. The complement system also contains characteristic factors that may play a role in the nonimmune inflammatory response. Other mediators, such as LTs and PAF, also are present in MEEs and may play a role in both increased vascular permeability and in the migration of inflammatory cells into the middle ear space. Whether or not this acute inflammation will lead to healing or to chronic inflammation depends on the persistence of chronic inflammatory cells, such as macrophages and lymphocytes, and on the mediators that can be released from these inflammatory cells (36). Perhaps the most important message to leave with the reader is that these inflammatory mediators can cause tissue injury and may lead to permanent damage to the mucous membrane of the middle ear, to the tympanic membrane, and to the ossicular chain. Furthermore, there is some evidence that these inflammatory mediators may penetrate the round window membrane and lead to permanent sensorineural hearing loss. For all these reasons, it is strongly emphasized that these effusions should be evacuated if they persist for longer than 90 days and do not respond to medical management.

REFERENCES

1. Back, N. (1966): Fibrolysin system and vasoactive kinins. *Fed. Proc.*, 25:77.
2. Balough, K., and Cohen, R.B. (1961): Histochemical demonstration of diaphorases and dehydrogenases in normal leukocytes and platelets. *Blood*, 17:491.
3. Berger, G., Hawke, M., Proops, D.W., et al. (1984): Histamine levels in middle ear effusions. In: *Recent Advances in Otitis Media with Effusion*, edited by D.J. Lim, C.D. Bluestone, J.O. Klein, and J.D. Nelson, pp. 195–198. B.C. Decker, Philadelphia.
4. Bernstein, J.M. (1976): Biological mediators of inflammation in middle ear effusions. *Ann. Otol. Rhinol. Laryngol.*, 85(Suppl. 25):90.
5. Bernstein, J.M., Steger, R., and Back, N. (1978): The kallikrein-kinin system in otitis media with effusion. *Trans. Am. Acad. Ophthalmol. Otolaryngol.*, 86:249.
6. Bernstein, J.M., Steger, R., and Back, N. (1979): The fibrinolysin system in otitis media with effusion. *Am. J. Otolaryngol.*, 1:28.
7. Bernstein, J.M., Villari, E.M., and Ratazzi, M.C. (1979): The significance of lysosomal enzymes in middle ear effusions. *Otolaryngol. Head Neck Surg.*, 87:845.
8. Camussi, G., Brentjens, J., Bussolino, F., and Tetta, C. (1986): Role of platelet activating factor in immunopathological reactions. In: *Advances in Inflammation Research, Vol. II*, edited by I. Otterness et al., pp. 97–109. Raven Press, New York.
9. Carlsson, L., and Lokk, G. (1955): Protein studies of transidates of the middle ear. *Scand. J. Clin. Invest.*, 7:43.
10. Davis, L.J., Sheffield, P.A., and Jackson, R.T. (1970): Drug-induced patency changes in the eustachian tube. *Arch. Otolaryngol.*, 92:325.
11. Dennis, R.G., Whitmire, R.N., and Jackson, R.T. (1976): Action of inflammatory mediators on middle ear mucosa. A method for measuring permeability and swelling. *Arch. Otolaryngol.*, 102:420.
12. Diven, W.F., Glew, R.H., and Bluestone, C.D. (1981): Lysosomal hydrolases in middle ear effusions. *Ann. Otol. Rhinol. Laryngol.*, 90:148.
13. Fleming, A. (1929): Arris and Gale lecture on lysozyme. A bacteriolytic ferment found normally in tissues and secretions. *Lancet*, 1:217.
14. Glynn, A.A., Bernier, I., Finch, S.C., and Salton, M.R.J. (1974): Notes on nomenclature. In: *Lysozyme.*, edited by E.F. Osserman, R.F. Canfield, and S. Beychok, p. 27. Academic Press, New York.
15. Hayashi, M. (1967): Comparative histochemical localization of lysosomal enzymes in rat tissues. *J. Histochem. Cytochem.*, 15:83.

16. Jolees, P. (1967): Relationship between chemical structures and biological activity of hen egg-white lysozyme and lysozymes of different species. *Proc. R. Soc. Lond. (Biol.)*, 167:350.
17. Juhn, S.K., Huff, J.S., and Paparella, M.M. (1971): Biochemical analyses of middle ear effusions. Preliminary report. *Ann. Otol. Rhinol. Laryngol.*, 80:347.
18. Juhn, S.K., Huff, J.S., and Paparella, M.M. (1973): Lactate dehydrogenase activity and isoenzyme patterns in serous middle ear effusions. *Ann. Otol. Rhinol. Laryngol.*, 82:192.
19. Juhn, S.K., and Huff, J.S. (1976): Biochemical characteristics of middle ear effusions. *Ann. Otol. Rhinol. Laryngol.*, 85(Suppl. 25):110.
20. Juhn, S.K. (1984): Biochemistry of middle ear effusion: state of the art. In: *Recent Advances in Otitis Media with Effusion.* edited by D.J. Lim, C.D. Bluestone, J.D. Klein, and J.D. Nelson, pp. 181–184. B.C. Decker, Philadelphia.
21. Jung, T.T.K., Smith, D.M., Juhn, S.K., and Gerrard, J.M. (1980): Effect of prostaglandin on the composition of chinchilla middle ear effusion. *Ann. Otol. Rhinol. Laryngol.*, 89(Suppl. 68):153.
22. Jung, T.T.K., Huang, D., and Juhn, S.K. (1983): Prostaglandins in middle ear fluids, cholesteatoma and granulation tissue (abstr.). *Third Int. Symp. Recent Adv. OME,* 53.
23. Kellermeyer, R.W., and Graham, R.C. (1968): Kinins—possible physiologic and pathologic roles in man. *N. Engl. J. Med.*, 279:802.
24. Kottner, K.E., Gunther, H.C., Halper, J., et al. (1968): Lysozyme in preosseous cartilage. *Calcif. Tissue Res.*, 1:298.
25. Lahikainen, E.A. (1953): Clinico-bacteriologic studies on acute otitis media. *Acta. Otolaryngol. (Stockh.)* (Suppl.):107.
26. Lim, D.J., Liu, Y.S., and Birck, H. (1976): Secretory lysozyme of the human middle ear mucosa: Immunocytochemical localization. *Ann. Otol. Rhinol. Laryngol.*, 85(Suppl. 25):50.
27. Majno, G., and Palade, G.E. (1961): Studies on inflammation. I. The effect of histamine and serotonin on vascular permeability: an electron microscopic study. *J. Biophys. Biochem. Cytol.*, 11:571.
28. Ohlsson, K. (1975): Alpha 1-antitrypsin and alpha 2-macroglobulin. Interactions with human neutrophil collagenase and elastase. *Ann. NY Acad. Sci.*, 256:409.
29. Palva, T., and Palva, A. (1975): Mucosal histochemistry in secretory otitis. *Ann. Otol. Rhinol. Laryngol.*, 84:112.
30. Paparella, M.M., and Dito, W.R. (1964): Enzyme studies in serous otitis media. *Arch. Otolaryngol.*, 79:393.
31. Paparella, M.M., Hiraide, F., Juhn, S.K., and Kaneko, Y. (1970): Cellular events involved in middle ear fluid production. *Ann. Otol. Rhinol. Laryngol.*, 79:1–15.
32. Shore, P.A., Burkhalter, A., and Cohn, V.H. (1959): A method for the fluorometric assay of histamine in tissues. *J. Pharm. Exp. Ther.*, 127:182.
33. Skoner, D.P., Doyle, W.J., Tanner, E., and Fireman, P. (1985): Histamine concentration in middle ear effusions (abstr.). *Ann. Allergy*, 54:4.
34. Veltri, R.W., and Sprinkle, P.M. (1973): Serous otitis media. Immunoglobulin and lysozyme levels in middle ear fluids and serum. *Ann. Otol. Rhinol. Laryngol.*, 82:297.
35. Virtanen, S., and Lahikainen, E. (1979): Lysozyme activity and immunoglobulins in middle ear effusion fluid in acute purulent otitis media and in otitis media with effusion. *Scand. J. Infect. Dis.*, 11:63.
36. Willoughby, D.A., and DiRosa, L. (1971): A unifying concept for inflammation: a new appraisal of some old mediators. In: *Immunopathology of Inflammation*, edited by B.K. Forscher and J.C. Hauch, pp. 28–38. Excerpta Medica, Amsterdam.

Immunology of the Ear, edited by J. Bernstein and P. Ogra. Raven Press, New York © 1987.

Complement and Other Amplification Mechanisms in Otitis Media

Karin Prellner

Department of Otorhinolaryngology, University Hospital, 221 85 Lund, Sweden

The main functions of the serum proteins of the complement system are related to their ability to participate in the induction of an acute inflammatory response serving to (a) limit the spread of injurious agents and (b) facilitate their destruction by phagocytosis and/or lysis. Along with its protective role, activation of the complement system also results in the formation of biologically active components capable of contributing to tissue damage.

In acute purulent otitis media (APOM), protective effects mediated by the complement sequence, such as killing of the infecting bacteria and the confinement of infection to the middle ear, are probably the most important. By contrast, it has been suggested that there may be harmful effects in conjunction with complement activation in chronic otitis media with effusion (chronic OME), such as the release of factors said to be responsible for the chronic inflammatory state and for tissue damage to middle ear mucosa.

Thus, in otitis media, factors generated as a result of complement activation may have either a protective or a destructive effect.

This chapter includes a general review of the complement system, the current knowledge of activating substances (such as immune complexes), and the complement factors in otitis media. Some implications of aberrations in, and activation of, the complement system in recurrent APOM and in chronic OME will also be discussed.

COMPLEMENT ACTIVATION

Complement is the principal effector system of humoral immunity. It consists of a group of distinct plasma proteins, some of which are proenzymes. The components of the complement system are capable of sequential activation in processes characterized by the generation of complement component complexes and by the release of biologically active peptides.

Two main pathways of complement activation are distinguished: the classical pathway and the alternative pathway (Fig. 1). The classical complement system comprises nine components, designated C1 through C9. In the alternative path-

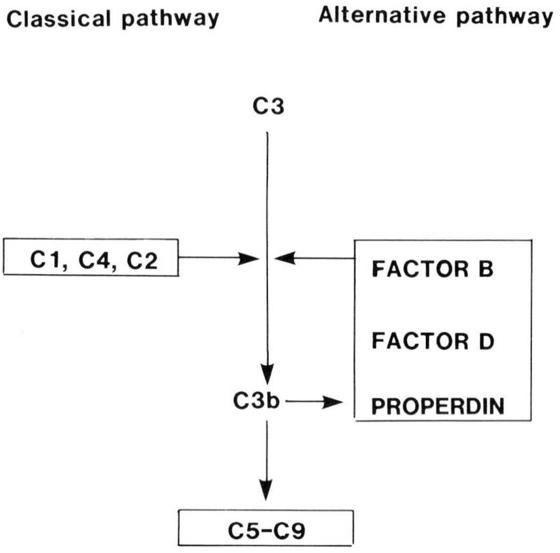

FIG. 1. Complement activation.

way, C1, C2, and C4 are not required, but the activated form of C3 (C3b), factor B, factor D, and properdin (P) are involved. C3 and the terminal sequence C5 to C9 may be activated by either pathway.

Activation is regulated by spontaneous decay of activated complexed components and by inhibitors.

Classical Pathway

The first component of the classical pathway, C1, is a macromolecular complex of three proteins, C1q, C1r, and C1s, held together with Ca^{2+} (Fig. 2).

In serum an equilibrium exists between free and macromolecularly bound C1 subcomponents. This equilibrium is strongly shifted toward the C1 macromolecule.

The most important biological activators of C1 are immune complexes containing IgG or IgM. IgG and IgM have binding sites for C1q in their Fc (complement-combining fragment of immunoglobulin) regions (as illustrated for IgG in Fig. 2). One IgM molecule in complex with antigen is sufficient to activate C1, whereas at least two IgG molecules in close proximity are required. Activation of the early components of complement (C1 to C5) leads to their enzymatic cleavage. The smaller fragments thus generated are freely diffusible and are important soluble mediators of the inflammatory response. The larger fragments become bound to the surface of the activating substance, where they serve as ligands.

The C1q molecule consists of six peripheral globular structures, representing the Fc-binding regions, connected by fibrillary strands to a central portion (Fig. 2) representing the C1r- and C1s-binding sites. On C1 activation after the binding of

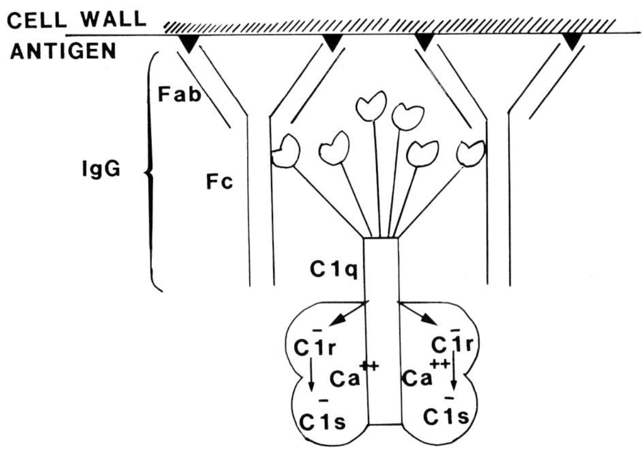

FIG. 2. Subcomponents of C1 and their reactions with cell-surface-associated IgG.

C1q, C1r is converted to the enzyme, $C\overline{1}r$, which acts on C1s, converting it to $C\overline{1}s$. $C\overline{1}s$ splits C4; later in the sequence it splits C2 into two fragments each. A complex of the larger C4 and C2 fragments then splits C3 into C3a and C3b, of which C3b binds to cell walls and immune complexes. C5 is then cleaved into the fragments C5a and C5b. C5b binds to the cell surface and fuses successively with C6 through C9. Insertion of cell membranes by the complex C5b6789 produces an aperture through which water, ions, and other substances can flow. This flow of water and ions results in the osmotic rupture of the cell.

Regulator proteins may block the complement activation at various levels. Thus, C1 inactivator inhibits $C\overline{1}r$ and $C\overline{1}s$.

Alternative Pathway

This pathway was originally described by Pillemer et al. (20) in 1954 as the properdin system; and it is distinct from the classical pathway with which it converges at the C3 level. The alternative pathway does not require antibody for its activation. The alternative pathway is in a constant state of subdued activation, the product of which is C3b. This state is maintained by the regulatory proteins, factors H and I. Additional presence of activating substances results in unrestricted activation of the pathway and, as an effect of factor D, the generation of C3bBb. Although this C3bBb complex is labile, binding of properdin enhances its stability. C3bBb cleaves more C3, leading to the deposition of additional C3b molecules on the cell surface. Cooperation of C3b and the C3bBb complex leads to cleavage of C5. Thus, the alternative pathway converges with the classical pathway for the C5-C9 sequence.

An essential part of the alternative pathway is the C3b-generating feedback mechanism (Fig. 1), called the *amplification loop*, in which, by cleaving C3,

C3bBb recruits more C3b for its own formation. This feedback mechanism may also be initiated by C3b obtained through activation of the classical pathway.

Activating Substances

Immune complexes are well-documented activators of the classical pathway. Immune complexes are formed when antibodies combine with their corresponding antigen. The antigens may be either tissue-fixed or free in serum or other body fluids.

C1 is activated either by immune complexes containing any of the immunoglobulin IgG1, IgG2, IgG3, or IgM, or by these immunoglobulins themselves when physically aggregated.

Anti-immunoglobulins known as *rheumatoid factors* (RF) are another possible source of immune complex formation. IgM-RF and IgG-RF are both capable of inducing classical pathway activation.

In addition to immune complexes, the classical pathway may be activated by any of a number of substances, including polyanions, polyanion-polycation complexes, certain viruses, and C-reactive protein in complex with the common pneumococcal cell-wall polysaccharide (C-polysaccharide).

The alternative pathway is activated by a variety of substances, such as microbial polysaccharides, without their prior sensitization with antibodies, although the presence of IgG antibodies has been shown to enhance activation.

Besides the activating substances described above, certain polyanions and microbial polysaccharides (24) are capable of binding C1q without causing successive activation of C1.

Proteolytic enzymes (e.g., plasmin, trypsin, collagenase, elastase, and other proteases from granulocytes) can activate individual complement components from either the classical pathway or the alternative pathway, and thus produce biologically active fragments.

BIOLOGICAL ACTIVITIES OF COMPLEMENT

Various combinations of different biological activities or mechanisms are responsible for the vital role of complement in host defense against either bacteria, immune complexes, or certain viruses; however, the same mechanisms may also cause the release of important mediators that can result in tissue damage.

Immune adherence is the binding of particles or immune complexes carrying C3b on their surfaces to different cells equipped with specific receptors. The immune adherence to phagocytic cells is the basis of opsonization in the presence of complement and may also trigger the release of lysosomal enzymes. A complement function of possible importance in immune complex diseases is the capacity of complement to modify immune complexes. Thus, classical pathway components inhibit precipitation of immune complexes, whereas an intact alternative pathway is required to solubilize already formed immune complexes (32).

A complement-mediated neutralization of certain viruses has been observed, which is probably dependent on the presence of C4b. C3a and C5a are anaphylatoxins, i.e., their binding to receptors on mast cells and basophils results in the release of vasoactive amines such as histamine and slow-reacting substances, which are important mediators of inflammation. C5a also has a chemotactic effect on polymorphonuclear leukocytes. Deposition of the C5b-9 complex on cell membranes by activation of the classical or alternative pathways leads to cytolysis.

METHODS FOR THE STUDY OF COMPLEMENT AND IMMUNE COMPLEXES

Complement

Complement can be measured by functional assays to determine the overall activity of the classical and alternative pathway. The functional assay most frequently used is the CH50 test, a test yielding information about the integrity of the classical complement system. Although specific functional assays have been developed for all components in both pathways, immunochemical assays are most frequently used in routine work.

In studies of the complement profile, the pattern of the individual complement components in serum or other body fluids may yield information on mechanisms of complement activation during disease. In disease, complement activation may lead to manifest hypocomplementemia. Thus, low levels of C1q, C4, C2, and C3 indicate activation of the classical pathway, whereas alternative pathway activation is characterized by low concentrations of C3, B, and/or P, in conjunction with normal concentrations of C1q, C4, and C2.

It should be kept in mind that certain complement proteins (e.g., C3, C4, C1s, and B) behave like acute-phase reactants in inflammation. Thus, apparently normal serum concentrations of these factors during disease may be the result of consumption due to complement activation being offset by an increase caused by an acute-phase reaction.

Detection of activation products, in the form of fragments or complexes of complement components in clinical specimens, will yield further information. Thus, even in the absence of hypocomplementemia, C1 activation may be detected by measuring $C\bar{1}r$-$C\bar{1}s$-$C\bar{1}$ inactivator complexes. Classical pathway activation may also be assessed by measuring C4d or by analyzing C2 cleavage products; and a technique for measuring certain C3b complexes (i.e., indicating activation of the alternative pathway) has recently been described (17). The measurement of C3 split products provides another tool for demonstrating C3 activation. Assays are also available for measuring the anaphylatoxins, C3a and C5a.

Immune Complexes

Many methods have been reported for detecting immune complexes (ICs) (12). These techniques are based on the physical properties of IC, including their specific recognition by free molecules—such as complement components and RFs—and their interaction with various cell receptors for the Fc part of immunoglobulins or for complement. Commonly used tests, based on specific recognition by complement components, are the C1q-binding assay (C1q BA) and C1q-deviation test (C1q DT), whereas in the Raji cell tests, cells with receptors for split products such as C3b represent the detection principle. The wide variety of methods for detecting IC in biological fluids are based on different principles, each of which imposes its own limitations on the capacity of the test to detect IC. Since, for example, the complement-receptor-dependent tests fail to detect IC that cannot activate and bind complement, complement-dependent tests do not detect IC containing only IgA, IgD, or IgE. The different methods are subject to interference by various substances in addition to IC—for example, monomeric IgG, DNA, bacterial polysaccharides, and antibodies reacting with cell-surface structures. No method is yet available for distinguishing true IC (antigen-antibody complexes) from nonspecifically aggregated immunoglobulins.

COMPLEMENT IN DISEASE OTHER THAN OTITIS MEDIA

Genetic and Inherited Abnormalities

Although genetically determined deficiencies have been described for many complement components, such deficiencies are rare and are inherited as autosomal recessive traits (30). Deficiencies of the classical components C1r, C1s, C2, and C4 are associated mainly with clinical manifestations of chronic immune-complex-associated diseases such as systemic lupus erythematosus. C3 deficiency enhances susceptibility to bacterial infection, as does deficiency of the C3b inactivator. Deficiencies of any of the complement proteins from C5 to C9 are often found in association with disseminated infections of the *Neisseria* genus. Hereditary angioedema is caused by a partial deficiency of the C1 inactivator.

Complement Activation in Disease

Involvement of the complement system has been described in many conditions, including immune complex diseases, infections, and shock. A prominent feature of immune complex diseases, whether inherited or acquired, is the presence of reduced concentrations of classical pathway components in serum as a sign of complement activation. Although many bacterial infections are associated with normal or increased serum concentrations of complement factors, hypocomplementemia is seen in fulminant septic conditions. In bacteriemia caused by gram-negative bacteria, mainly alternative pathway activation is seen, which is attributable to effects of bacterial lipopolysaccharides. In septic shock resulting from gram-positive pneumococci, marked activation of both classical and alternative pathways has been reported. In adults with less severe pneumococcal infections, the complement profile is consistent with a more moderate activation of both pathways (23) (see Table 1).

COMPLEMENT AND OTITIS MEDIA

Those bacteria commonly associated with otitis media are, *in vitro*, susceptible to complement-mediated phagocytosis or destruction, and it is a reasonable assumption that the localization and healing of a bacterial middle ear infection is partly due to the protective effects resulting from complement activation.

The protective effect of the complement system is clearly demonstrated by the striking susceptibility to bacterial infections, including recurrent APOM, of patients who are genetically deficient in certain complement factors (30).

In addition to its protective role, activation of the complement system also results in the formation of components capable of contributing to tissue damage; and unrestricted complement activation—caused by, e.g., immune complexes—has been suggested to be responsible both for the induction of chronic OME and for its prolonged course. The most common varieties of childhood otitis media that cause problems, not only for the patients and their families but also for pediatricians and ENT specialists, are recurrent episodes of APOM and chronic OME, both of which are accompanied not only by activation of the complement system but also by aberrations within it.

As with other diseases, the pathogenic significance of complement activation in disease is not always clearly understood but may be related to the mediation of symptoms and possibly to the derangement of normal protective functions of the complement system.

TABLE 1. *Complement activation, serum concentrations of C1q and C-reactive protein (CRP), and presence of abnormal C1r-C1s complexes, in various pneumococcal infections and in chronic OME*[a]

	Chronic OME in children	APOM in children		APOM in adults, single episode	Meningitis or pneumonia in adults
		Single episode	Recurrent		
Classical pathway activation	+	+	+	N	++
Alternative pathway activation	+	N	+	N	+(+)[b]
C1q	N	N	−−	N	N
C1r-C1s complexes	+	+	++	NP	OIP
CRP	N	+	+	+	+++

[a]N, normal; +, increase; −, decrease; NP, not present; OIP, only infrequently present.
[b]+(+) is more than + but less than ++.

Microbial Antigens Associated with Otitis Media and Their Interaction with the Complement System

A viral infection often precedes APOM. Although it has not been established, complement-mediated virus neutralization might constitute a defense mechanism at this stage of the middle ear infection.

Although it is generally agreed that APOM is caused by bacteria, it is widely disputed whether the bacteria isolated from middle ear effusions in chronic OME are primary causative agents or secondary invaders. However, both in APOM and in chronic OME, pneumococci and *Hemophilus influenzae* are the two bacteria most commonly isolated. For normal phagocytosis or killing of pneumococci and *H. influenzae*, their surfaces need to be coated with antibody and certain complement components.

The pneumococcus is a gram-positive bacterium and, like all gram-positive bacteria, is not susceptible to complement-mediated cell lysis. The virulence of pneumococci is largely dependent on its ability to resist phagocytosis in the host. When the pneumococcus is coated with specific capsular antibodies, the bacterium is ingested by granulocytes and macrophages, but only slowly. The rate of ingestion is markedly enhanced following the binding of C3b to the bacterial surface. C3b is the most important opsonin for invasive pneumococci.

In pneumococcal otitis media, there are several possibilities for the formation of C3b (Fig. 3). The alternative pathway can be activated either by intact pneumococci or by pneumococcal cell constituents (6,21,24,36). Furthermore, together with specific antibodies, these pneumococcal bacterial antigens can form immune complexes, which then activate the classical pathway. Complexes between C-reactive protein and the common pneumococcal cell-wall polysaccharide (C-polysaccharide) constitute another possible complement activator in otitis media (11,24).

Hemophilus influenzae is a gram-negative bacterium and, like most gram-nega-

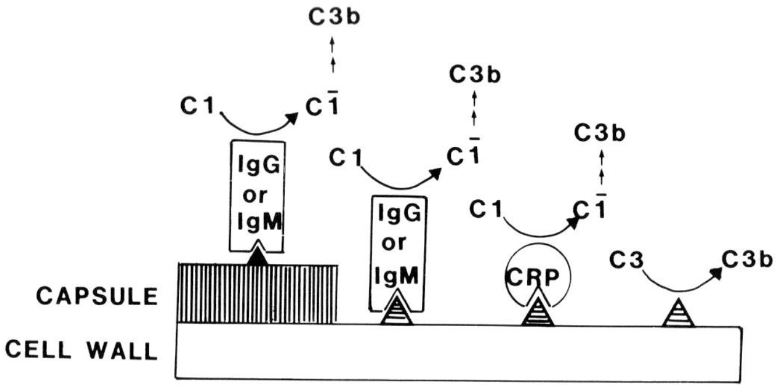

FIG. 3. Schematic presentation of the complement activation and generation of C3b by pneumococcal antigens. (▲) Type-specific capsular polysaccharide. (▲) Teichoic acid of the common pneumococcal cell-wall polysaccharide (C-polysaccharide). (CRP) C-reactive protein.

tive bacteria, is susceptible to complement-mediating killing. The insertion of the C5b-9 complex into the outer bacterial membrane results in membrane disorganization and cellular death. Strains of *H. influenzae* that are nontypable (NT)—inasmuch as they do not belong to the known capsular types—are isolated in 85% of otitis media episodes caused by the *Hemophilus* genus. Although many immunological studies concerning capsulated strains have been performed, few investigations concerning NT strains have been reported. In complex with their specific antibodies, their outer membrane proteins—which vary from one NT strain to another (33,34)—constitute possible activators of the classical pathway of complement in otitis media. Alternative pathway activation could be elicited by the lipopolysaccharide of the cell wall of these bacteria.

Thus in otitis media, complement activation can be elicited by any one of several antigens or their complexes. Furthermore, many enzymes (3,9), e.g., different granulocyte proteases released in the middle ear during inflammation, are potent activators of the complement system. In addition to activating the complement system, certain bacterial constituents can interact with complement components so as to block the activation. Among others, teichoic acid from pneumococci—the main constituent of the C-polysaccharide—can bind C1q without eliciting complement activation (24). Pronounced C1q binding capacity for whole bacteria has also been demonstrated for certain pneumococcal types associated with otitis media, NT *H. influenzae*, and *Branhamella catarrhalis* (22). A striking difference between typable and NT *H. influenzae* has been observed, with the NT strain exhibiting a far more pronounced direct C1q-binding capacity than the typable strain.

Acute Purulent Otitis Media

Complement Profile

In purulent middle ear effusion, it is possible to demonstrate the presence of many substances—e.g., bacteria, bacterial-product, antibodies, and enzymes—capable of interacting with the complement system, although reliable data concerning complement factors in the effusions in APOM is scant.

However, although otitis media is an infection localized to the middle ear, changes in humoral factors are often noticed in specimen blood. In cases of APOM, complement studies have been performed in serum and plasma. During an APOM episode, children, unlike adults, exhibit activation of the complement system together with aberrations within the first complement factor (8,23,26,27) (see Table 1). The complement profile in serum is similar whether the APOM is caused by pneumococci or by *H. influenzae*. In children with recurrent APOM the aberrations in the C1 subcomponents are far more pronounced than in children with single episodes. Both classical and alternative pathway activation—as indicated by increased amounts of $C\bar{1}r$-$C\bar{1}s$-$C\bar{1}$ inactivator complexes and decreased levels of P, respectively—is present to moderate degrees in about one-third of children with recurrent APOM. But, more important, pronounced aberrations within C1 factor, present in almost all children with recurrent APOM, suggest inadequate presence of prerequisite factors for optimal complement activation. In children with recurrent APOM, the C1q concentrations are aberrantly low, whereas those of C1r and C1s are normal or slightly increased. The C1q concentrations do not vary with those of $C\bar{1}r$-$C\bar{1}s$-$C\bar{1}$ inactivator complexes, but together with these low C1q concentrations, children with recurrent APOM exhibit high amounts of circulating, abnormal C1r-C1s complexes (Fig. 4) (Table 1).

This indicated that the low C1q concentrations are not caused by classical pathway activation. The C1r-C1s complexes are probably formed because of the relative excess of C1r and C1s. The aberrations reach a maximum in conjunction with an APOM episode, and persist to some extent in between episodes, but are not present in individuals investigated some years after their APOM episodes have ceased (26–28).

Anti-immunoglobulins (RF) are present in about one-third of sera from children with recurrent APOM (*unpublished observation*). Increased amounts of circulating substances capable of binding C1q are present in many children with recurrent APOM (26). These C1q binding substances might represent either circulating immune complexes or other C1q binding substances such as bacterial constituents, and the amounts are higher in APOM caused by pneumococci than in APOM caused by *H. influenzae* (26).

The concentrations of C-reactive protein is often moderately increased in patients with APOM caused by pneumococci (26).

Implications

Although some C activation does occur during APOM, the low C1q concentrations seen in children with recurrent APOM suggest a dysfunction of complement activation and thus suboptimal complement-mediated opsonization and/or killing of the causative bacteria. Although the C1q deficiency might be of primary nature, it could also be a result of C1q consumption. Whether or not low C1q concentrations pre-exist in children who will become otitis prone is unknown, but prospective studies are in progress. C1q consumption in conjunction with the APOM episodes is perhaps a more probable explanation. C1q-binding substances are available in both sera (26) and in purulent ear effusions (*unpublished observation*). In *in vitro* studies it has been shown that (among other agents) teichoic acid from the pneumococcal C-polysaccharide is capable of binding C1q so as to prevent complement activation (24).

Taken together with the fact that children with recurrent APOM often lack specific antibodies to NT *H. influenzae* (33) and to the pneumococcal types associated with APOM (7,10,27,28), the findings outlined above suggest the following interpretation: In children with recurrent APOM, there may be competition for C1q available in the middle ear effusion between non-complement-activating bacterial

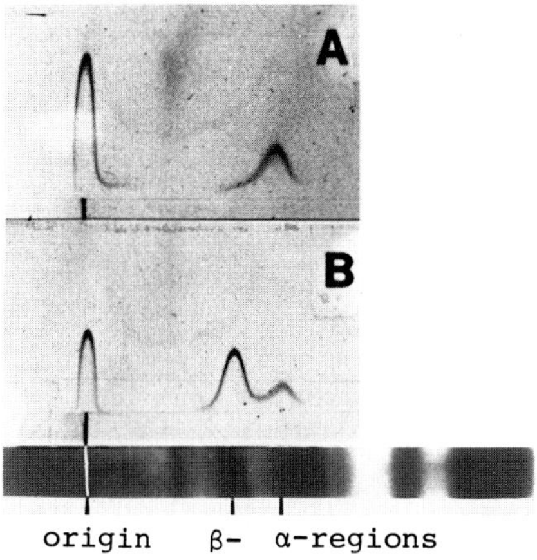

FIG. 4. Crossed immunoelectrophoresis with anti-C1s in the gel. The peak demonstrated in the beta region represents C1r-C1s complexes, and that in the alpha region represents $C\bar{1}r$-$C\bar{1}s$-$C\bar{1}$ inactivator complexes. The peak to the left represents the native C1q-C1r-C1s complex. **A**: Normal serum. **B**: Serum from a patient with recurrent episodes of APOM.

constituents (e.g., teichoic acid in the C-polysaccharide) on the one hand, and, on the other, substances capable of complement activation (e.g., bacterial antigens complexed with specific antibodies, C-polysaccharide complexed with C-reactive protein, complexes of immunoglobulins and anti-immunoglobulins (RF), or proteolytic enzymes); and, in the absence of specific antibodies, for instance, certain bacterial antigens such as pneumococcal C-polysaccharide perhaps interfere with the C1 subcomponents by binding C1q without causing C1 activation (see Fig. 5).

Interestingly, in an adult patient with selective immunoglobulin deficiency—including absence of specific pneumococcal antibodies—and repeated pneumococcal infections, C1 aberrations closely resembling those of children with recurrent APOM were demonstrated (29). This is in contrast to observations in adult patients with pneumococcal infections but without antibody deficiencies, where complement activation but almost no C1 aberrations are seen (23) (Table 1). Further supporting the interpretation outlined above, pneumococcal C-polysaccharide could be demonstrated in the circulation of this adult patient with selective immunoglobulin deficiency state, even during infection-free periods (29).

The same interpretation might also help to explain the C1 aberrations found in children with recurrent APOM. Although the complement aberrations tend to normalize, low concentrations of C1q and presence of C1r-C1s complexes persist in many patients 2 to 4 weeks after APOM episodes (26). It is a reasonable assumption that, whatever the reason for low C1q concentration, bacteria invading the middle ear cavity of a child partially deficient in C1q are less easily phagocytosed or killed, owing to impaired activation of the classical pathway, and thus are more prone to cause infection than in a child with a normal C1q concentration. Theoretically, as a prophylactic measure in cases of recurrent APOM, it might be beneficial to introduce certain substances capable of optimizing complement activation, such as specific antibodies to capsular or cell-wall components, C-reactive protein, or purified C1q.

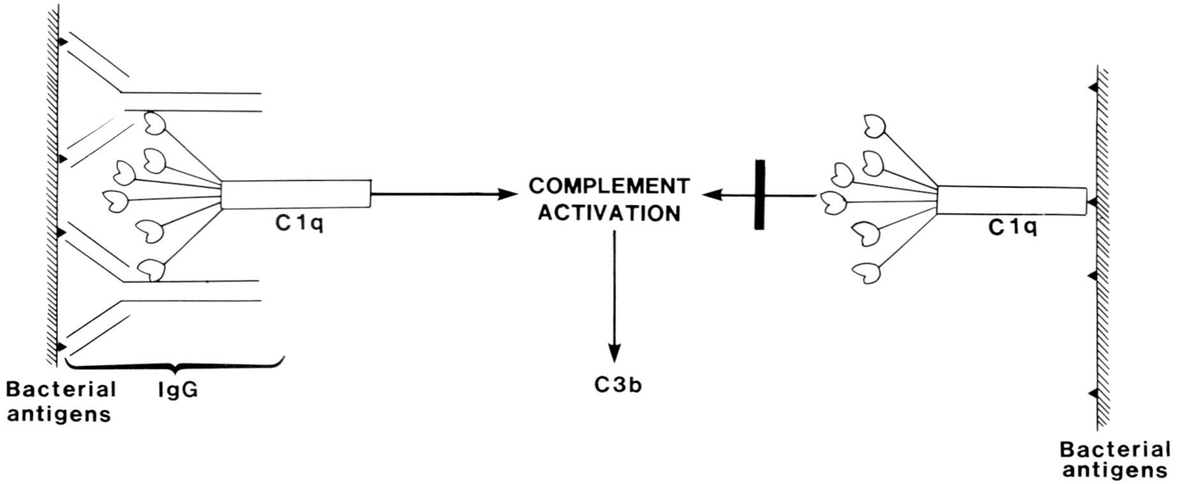

FIG. 5. Schematic representation of the competition for available C1q. In the presence of specific IgG antibodies (*left*), complement activation will occur, whereas absence of antibody may result in the blockage of activation (*right*).

Chronic Otitis Media with Effusion

Complement Profile

In serous or mucoid middle ear effusions from patients with chronic OME, the concentration of separate complement factors—as measured both functionally (C2;C4;C3 and C5) (1) and immunochemically (C4;C3 and B) (3,13,16,35)—is considerably lower than that estimated in the corresponding serum. When the amount of C3 was calculated in relation to the total protein content, however, the concentrations in serum and effusions were quite similar (35). The presence of split products from C3 (C3c and C3d) (1,16) in addition to very low (or even absent) total hemolytic complement activity (CH50) suggest that a local utilization of complement has taken place in the middle ear effusions. This receives strong support from the demonstration of C3 splitting activity in the effusions (1,16,35).

In sera from patients with chronic OME, increased amounts of $C\bar{1}r$-$C\bar{1}s$-$C\bar{1}$ inactivator complexes—present in one of four patients—indicate activation of the classical pathway, whereas moderately decreased P concentrations present in many patients suggest activation of the alternative pathway (14,25).

The low C1q concentrations and the presence of C1r-C1s complexes seen in almost all patients with recurrent APOM are also present in 40% of patients with chronic OME (14,25), although the C1 aberrations are far less pronounced in chronic OME.

Immune Complexes

The concept that chronic OME is mediated by IC was first suggested by Veltri and Sprinkle (35). Although attempts have been made (2), it has not been found possible to demonstrate deposition of IC in the blood vessels or the basement membrane epithelia of the middle ear mucosa.

In the middle ear effusions in chronic OME, it is often possible to demonstrate the presence of the prerequisites for IC formation—i.e., bacteria and/or bacterial products and specific antibodies—but whether actual ICs are present is controversial. The reported frequency with which ICs occur in middle ear effusion varies widely (from 3 to 85%) (Table 2) (2,14–16,18,19,25). These discrepancies are probably partly resulting from differences in the sensitivity and specificity of the assays used (see IC tests). Although the assays used are common tests for IC, it should be kept in mind that the Raji cell test, both that used by Maxim et al. (15) and that used by Bernstein et al. (2), and the C1q BA and C1q DT tests used by Prellner and co-workers (14,25), are only capable of detecting ICs that interact with the complement system. Substances other than ICs (e.g., bacterial polysaccharides) that can interact with the complement system may also interfere with these tests, especially with the C1q DT test.

The results of tests based on RFs, besides detecting only IC-containing IgG or

TABLE 2. *Investigations on ICs in chronic OME*

Investigators	Frequency (%) of ICs in: Middle ear or mastoid (mast) mucosa	Middle ear effusion[a]	Serum	Assay used
Maxim et al., 1977 (ref. 15)		75 (18/24)	0 (0/12)	Raji cell fluorescent assay
Laurell et al., 1980 (ref. 14)		85 (17/20)	28 (16/57)	C1q BA and/or C1q DT
Bernstein et al., 1982 (ref. 2)	0 (0/21) 0 (mast) (0/16)			Immunohistologic C3 detection
		0 (0/22) 13 (c) (2/15)	10 (2/22)	Raji cell RIA[b] using ^{125}I protein A
		8 (2/26) 0 (c) (0/7)	5 (1/22)	Agglutination inhibition using polyclonal RF
Palva et al., 1983 (ref. 19)		26 (30/113)		Detection of pneumococcal antigens by counterimmuno-electrophoresis with antiserum
Meri et al., 1984 (ref. 16)		3 (1/36)		Same as for Palva et al.

[a](c), concentrated.
[b]RIA, radioimmunoassay.

IgA, are highly dependent on the affinity of the RF for the immunoglobulins present in the IC. Presence of RF in the effusions may also interfere with the results. As reported by DeMaria and colleagues (5), 85% of effusions from patients with chronic OME contain RF.

The tests used by Palva and Meri and their colleagues (16,19) are no ordinary IC tests but have been designed to detect specific pneumococcal antigens in IC.

It should also be kept in mind that none of the tests used for IC detection are capable of distinguishing nonspecifically aggregated immunoglobulins from IC. Since ICs are not the only substances that react with C1q in the C1q BA or C1q DT tests, it is perhaps more accurate to refer to substances detected by these IC methods as *C1q-binding substances*. Increased amounts of C1q-binding substances are demonstrated in serum from about one in four patients with chronic OME (14,25), and RF is reported in 8% of sera from patients (5).

In animals, the injection of IC (18), or an antigenic challenge in the middle ear of a sensitized animal (4), results in the production of middle ear inflammation, effusion, or both. The fact that complement is an important mediator in this middle ear inflammation is indicated by the finding that animals depleted of complement generate much less effusion than nondepleted animals after the same challenge (31). But the fact that even complete suppression of serum complement did not totally eliminate immune-mediated production of middle ear effusion suggests that in addition to complement, other mechanisms also contribute to this phenomenon.

Implications

It seems clear that activation of the complement system does take place in the middle ear effusions, and it is also generally agreed that the potent mediators thus elicited are capable of maintaining an inflammatory response in the middle ear mucosa in chronic OME. However, it is disputed whether the complement activation is caused by immune complexes.

The alternative pathway seems to be the major route for complement activation in the effusions (16), but classical pathway activation has also been demonstrated in chronic OME (14,25). Although IC composed of bacterial antigens and their respective antibody, or of immunoglobulins and anti-immunoglobulins (RF)—as well as other substances such as complexes of C-reactive protein and pneumococcal C-polysaccharide—present in the effusions might be responsible for the classical pathway activation, IC is not a main activator of the alternative pathway. Thus it is reasonable to assume that the complement activation seen in middle ear effusions is largely caused by factors (e.g., bacterial polysaccharides and/or proteolytic enzymes) other than IC. Although ICs are probably present in some middle ear effusions, their role in the pathogenesis of chronic OME is still unclear. The suggestion that IC deposited in the middle ear mucosa might induce complement activation and tissue damage (a mechanism proposed in the case of glomerulonephritis) has not found support in the extensive studies performed by Bernstein et al. (2).

Although complement activation—whether induced by IC or by other factors—probably plays an important role in the maintenance of the inflammatory state in the middle ear mucosa, other immune-mediated factors might also be of importance, as indicated by studies of experimental OME (31).

CONCLUDING REMARKS

Complement activation is commonly demonstrated in children with otitis media. In children with recurrent APOM the activation is of a moderate degree, but pronounced aberrations in the complement system is almost inevitably present. In children with chronic OME, pronounced complement activation is present in most effusions.

The role the complement system plays during chronic serous or mucoid otitis media may be different from that during APOM. During APOM, complement activation is probably important for proper phagocytosis and elimination of the invading bacteria, and thus interference with complement activation—as indicated by the complement aberrations in this disease—might predispose for recurrence. In chronic OME, it has been determined that bacteria, bacterial products, ICs, proteolytic enzymes, or other complement-activating substances that, owing to poor tubal ventilation or defective absorption, are trapped in the middle ear cavity, lead to continuous complement activation and generation of potent mediators of inflammation that cause tissue damage.

REFERENCES

1. Bernstein, J.M. (1976): Biological mediators of inflammation in middle ear effusions. *Ann. Otol. Rhinol. Laryngol.*, 85 (Suppl. 25):90–96.
2. Bernstein, J.M., Brentjens, J., and Vladutiu, A. (1982): Are immune complexes a factor in the pathogenesis of otitis media with effusion? *Am. J. Otolaryngol.*, 3:20–25.
3. Carlsson, B., Lundberg, C., and Ohlsson, K. (1982): Granulocyte proteases in middle ear effusions. *Ann. Otol. Rhinol. Laryngol.*, 91:76–81.
4. Catanzaro, A., Ryan, A., Batcher, S., Black, V., Harris, J., and Wasserman, S. (1984): Local antibody in a model of otitis media with effusion. In: *Recent Advances in Otitis Media with Effusion,* edited by D.J. Lim, C.D. Bluestone, J.O. Klein, and J.D. Nelson, pp. 219–220. B. C. Decker, Philadelphia/Toronto.
5. DeMaria, T.F., McGhee, R.B., and Lim, D. (1984): Rheumatoid factor in otitis media with effusion. *Arch. Otolaryngol.*, 110:279–280.
6. Fine, D. (1975): Pneumococcal type-associated variability in alternative complement pathway activation. *Infect. Immun.*, 12:772–778.
7. Freijd, A., Hammarström, L., Persson, M.A.A., and Smith, C.I.E. (1984): Plasma anti-pneumococcal antibody activity of the IgG class and subclasses in otitis prone children. *Clin. Exp. Immunol.*, 56:233–238.
8. Johnson, U., Kamme, C., Laurell, A.-B., and Nilsson, N.I. (1977): C1 subcomponents in acute pneumococcal otitis media in children. *Acta Pathol. Microbiol. Scand. (C),* 85:10–16.
9. Juhn, S.K. (1984): Biochemistry of middle ear effusion: state of the art. In: *Recent Advances in Otitis Media with Effusion,* edited by D.J. Lim, C.D. Bluestone, J.O. Klein, and J.D. Nelson, pp. 181–184. B.C. Decker, Philadelphia/Toronto.
10. Kalm, O., Prellner, K., and Pedersen, F.K. (1984): Pneumococcal antibodies in families with recurrent otitis media. *Int. Arch. Allergy Appl. Immun.*, 75:139–142.
11. Kaplan, M., and Volanakis, J. (1974): Interaction of C-reactive protein complexes with the complement system. I. Consumption of human complement associated with the reaction of CRP with pneumococcal C-polysaccharide and with the cholin phosphatides, lecithin and sphingomyelin. *J. Immunol.*, 112:2135–2139.
12. Lambert, P.H., Dixon, F.J., and Zubler, R.H., et al. (1978): A WHO collaborative study for the evaluation of eighteen methods for detecting immune complexes in serum. *J. Clin. Lab. Immunol.*, 1:1–15.
13. Lang, R.W., Liu, Y.S., Lim, D.J., and Birck, H.G. (1976): Antimicrobial factors and bacterial correlation in chronic otitis media with effusion. *Ann. Otol. Rhinol. Laryngol.*, 85(Suppl. 25):145–151.
14. Laurell, A.-B., Nilsson, N.-I., and Prellner, K. (1980): Immune complexes and complement in serous and mucoid otitis media. *Acta otolaryngol.* 90:290–296.
15. Maxim, P., Veltri, R., and Sprinkle, P. (1977): Chronic serous otitis media: an immune complex disease. *Trans. Am. Acad. Ophthalmol. Otolaryngol.*, 84(2):234–238.
16. Meri, S., Lehtinen, T., and Palva, T. (1984): Complement in chronic secretory otitis media. C3 breakdown and C3 splitting activity. *Arch. Otolaryngol.*, 110:774–778.
17. Milgrom, H., Curd, J.G., Kaplan, M., et al. (1980): Activation of the fourth component of complement (C4): assessment by rocket immuno-electrophoresis in correlation with metabolism of C4. *J. Immunol.*, 124:2780.
18. Mravaec, J., Lewis, D.M., and Lim, D.J. (1978): Experimental otitis media with effusion: an immune-complex-mediated response. *Otolaryngology*, 86:258–268.

19. Palva, T., Lehtinen, T., and Rinne, J. (1983): Immune complexes in middle ear fluid in chronic secrectory otitis media. *Ann. Otol. Rhinol. Laryngol.*, 92:42–44.
20. Pillemer, L., Blum, L., Lepow, I.H., Ross, O.A., Todd, E.W., and Wardlaw, A.C. (1954): The properdin system and immunity. I. Demonstration and isolation of a new serum protein and its role in immune phenomena. *Science*, 120:279.
21. Prellner, K. (1979): Complement activation by pneumococci associated with acute otitis media. *Acta Pathol. Microbiol. Scand. (C)*, 87:213–217.
22. Prellner, K. (1980): Bacteria associated with acute otitis media have high C1q binding capacity. *Acta Pathol. Microbiol. Scand. (C)*, 88:187–190.
23. Prellner, K. (1981): Complement in pneumococcal infections with varying degrees of severity. *Scand. J. Infect. Dis.*, 13:263–268.
24. Prellner, K. (1981): C1q binding and complement activation by capsular and cell wall components of *S. pneumoniae* type XIX. *Acta Pathol. Microbiol. Scand. (C)*, 89:359–364.
25. Prellner, K.J., Nilsson, N.-I., Johnson, U., and Laurell, A.-B. (1980): Complement and C1q binding substances in otitis media. *Ann. Otol. Rhinol. Laryngol.*, 89:129–132.
26. Prellner, K., and Nilsson, N.-I. (1982): Complement aberrations in serum from children with otitis media due to *S. pneumoniae* or *H. influenzae*. *Acta Otolaryngol. (Stockh.)*, 94:275–282.
27. Prellner, K., Kalm, O., and Pedersen, F.K.: (1984): Complement and pneumococcal antibodies during and after recurrent otitis media. In: *Recent Advances in Otitis Media with Effusion*, edited by D.J. Lim, C.D. Bluestone, J.O. Klein, and J.D. Nelson, pp. 162–165. B.C. Decker, Philadelphia/Toronto.
28. Prellner, K., Kalm, O., and Pedersen, F.K. (1984): Pneumococcal antibodies and complement during and after periods of recurrent otitis. *Int. J. Pediatr. Otorhinolaryngol.*, 7:39–49.
29. Prellner, K., Braconier, J.H., and Sjoholm, A.C. (1985): Combined IgG2, IgG4 and IgA deficiency: low C1q concentrations and the presence of excess C1r and C1s in an adult patient with recurrent pneumococcal infections. *Acta Pathol. Microbiol. Scand. (C)*, 93:257–263.
30. Ross, S.C., and Densen, P. (1984): Complement deficiency state neisserial and other infections in an immune deficiency. *Medicine*, 63:243–273.
31. Ryan, A.F., and Vogel, C.-W. (1984): Complement depletion by cobra venom factor: effect on immune mediated middle ear effusion and inflammation. In: *Recent Advances in Otitis Media with Effusion*, edited by D.J. Lim, C.D. Bluestone, J.O. Klein, and J.D. Nelson, pp. 166–168. Decker, Philadelphia/Toronto.
32. Schifferli, J.A., and Peters, D.K. (1983): Complement, the immune-complex lattice, and the pathophysiology of the complement-deficiency syndrome. *Lancet*, 2: 957–959.
33. Shurin, P., Pelton, S., Tager, I., and Kasper, D. (1980): Bactericidal antibody and susceptibility to otitis media caused by non-typable strains of *Hemophilus influenzae*. *J. Pediatr.*, 97:364–367.
34. Shurin, P.A., Marchant, C.D., and Howie, W.M. (1984): Bactericidal antibody to antigenically distinct nontypable strains of *Hemophilus influenzae* isolated from acute otitis media. In: *Recent Advances in Otitis Media with Effusion*, edited by D.J. Lim, C.D. Bluestone, J.O. Klein, and J.D. Nelson, pp. 155–157. B.C. Decker, Philadelphia/Toronto.
35. Veltri, R.W., and Sprinkle, P.M. (1976): Secretory otitis media. An immune complex disease. *Ann. Otol. Rhinol. Laryngol.*, 85 (Suppl. 25):135–139.
36. Winkelstein, J., and Tomasz, A. (1978): Activation of the alternative complement pathway by pneumococcal cell wall teichoic acid. *J. Immunol.*, 120:174–178.

Immunology of the Ear, edited by J. Bernstein
and P. Ogra. Raven Press, New York © 1987.

Immune Deficiency and Otitis Media

Britta Rynnel-Dagöö and Anders Freijd

*Departments of Otorhinolaryngology and Clinical Immunology,
Huddinge University Hospital, and Karolinska Institute, Stockholm, Sweden*

It has long been recognized that some children suffer from more frequent infections than others and that most grow out of their problems. A minority of infection-prone children develop overwhelming infections and, if they survive, are recognized as being severely immunodeficient. There is today evidence of heterogeneity of immune response in humans and in various other species. Variation in immunocompetence within the normal range will probably contribute to proneness to infection (65). Such vulnerability is relative, depending in part on environmental factors that might not harm individuals with better immune function.

In general, infections resulting from defects of nonimmunological systems such as, for instance, malfunction of the eustachian tube, are bacterial and characterized by recurrence in the same location. However, such localized infections can sometimes occur as the initial consequence of an immune disorder. Relapsing episodes of purulent otitis media have earlier not indicated an underlying immunological disorder. There is, however, increasing evidence for minor immunodeficiencies contributing to proneness to infections such as otitis media. It has also been shown that many patients, later recognized as having primary immunodeficiencies, start with recurrent episodes of otitis media before they develop more serious infections like pneumonia and meningitis.

Knowledge of the normal age-dependent maturation and function of the immune system is important for the understanding of immunodeficiency diseases.

IMMUNOCOMPETENCE

Immunocompetence is defined as the humoral and cell mediated immune responses to bacteria and viruses of the upper respiratory tract. In the following sections, we will discuss the various developmental and immunological factors involved.

Differentiation of Normal Human B Lymphocytes

The earliest progenitors of immunoglobulin-synthesizing cells are identified in the liver during fetal development and later in ontogeny among bone marrow cells

(26). Antigen-reactive B (bone marrow-derived) lymphocytes arise without contact with antigen. All normal individuals have the capacity to generate millions of B-cell clones, each of which expresses a unique set of immunoglobulin heavy- and light-chain genes determining antibody specificity. This diversity of the B-cell repertoire is derived from a system of gene rearrangements involving chromosomal segments that code portions of the heavy and light immunoglobulin chains (68). First, the cell synthesizes IgM, which can be detected in the cytoplasm prior to expression of surface immunoglobulin (17). Such cytoplasmic-positive cells, known as pre-B cells, are thought to give rise to immature B lymphocytes, which express intact IgM molecules or IgM and IgD on their cell surfaces. Within each B-cell clone, some members switch from the expression of IgM (and IgD) to the expression of IgG or IgA or IgE (41) (Fig. 1).

Once B cells are surface-membrane immunoglobulin positive they become antigen responsive either directly or together with signals provided by macrophages and T cells. The final result of this process is differentiation to antibody-secreting plasma cells.

Genetic Control of the Immune Response

It has long been known that the immunocompetence is genetically controlled, and a number of specific immune response genes have been described in laboratory animals. Two major gene complexes are known: One is known to be linked

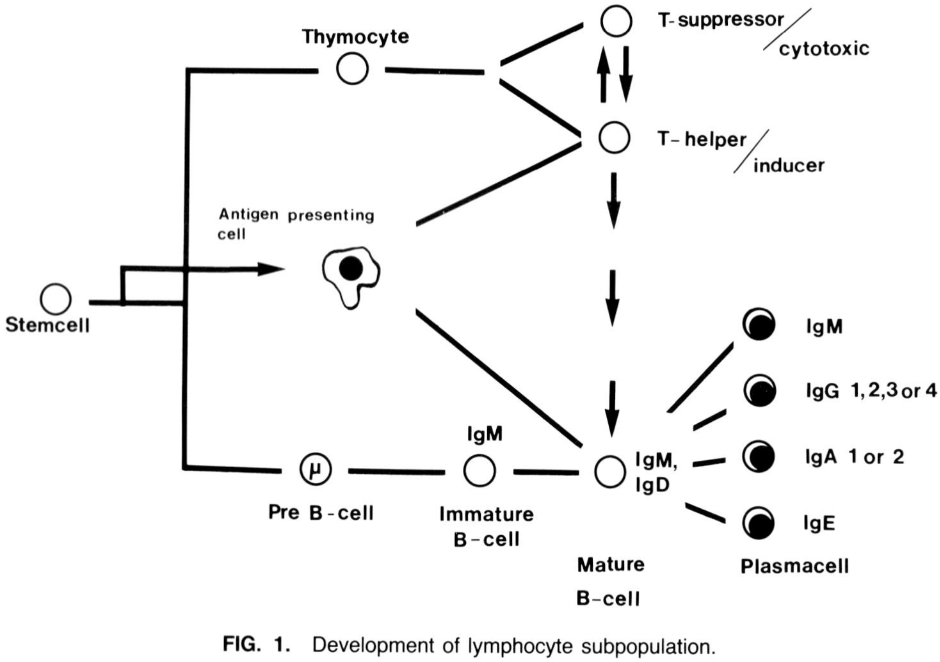

FIG. 1. Development of lymphocyte subpopulation.

to the HLA complex in mice and guinea pigs (64), and the other is linked to the genes that regulate the allogenic determinants of the antibody heavy chains, the so-called allotypes (7). An example of genetic aberration leading to immunodeficiency is the CBA-N mouse strain, which has a mutation on the X chromosome, the so-called X-linked immunodeficiency syndrome, or Xid (3). The hemi- or homozygote form leads to a deficiency of the B-lymphocyte function. This mouse strain was found not to respond to a number of pneumococcal polysaccharide antigens, and this inability was found to be inherited in an X-linked fashion. The defect could be corrected if thymectomized, and irradiated mice received bone marrow transplants from normal donors (39). Mice with this defect have normal total levels of serum immunoglobulin, although the IgM is somewhat reduced (49); however, the main defect concerns the IgG3 subclass, which is heavily reduced (the murine IgG3 subclass corresponds to the human IgG2).

Pandey et al. (47) have described an association between immunoglobulin allotypes and immune response to *Haemophilus influenzae* and a meningococcal polysaccharide. They found a strong correlation between the KM-1 allotype and the strength of the response to these antigens. KM-1 positive children lacked a response, whereas KM-1 negative children did respond to *H. influenzae* polysaccharide. The contrary relation was found for meningococcal type-C polysaccharide. A plausible explanation to these findings could be that the immune response genes on chromosome 6 which regulate the immunoresponse to *H. influenzae* polysaccharides exist in a linkage nonequilibrium with the gene coding for the KM-1 allotype.

Subclasses of IgG

Immunoglobulin G can, in most species, be separated into distinct subclasses on the basis of antigenic and physiochemical characteristics (28,67). Human IgG can be divided into four subclasses, namely, IgG1 to IgG4. The proportions in normal serum from adults are: IgG1, 60% to 70%; IgG2, 14% to 20%; IgG3, 4% to 8%; and IgG4, 2% to 6% (45). These subclasses show different biological features, but their significance remains unclear (66). It has been shown that different antigens give rise to antibody responses within single subclasses (70). In humans, antibodies to diphtheria and tetanus toxins are of IgG1 and IgG4 type, Rh factor is of IgG1 and IgG3 type, coagulation factor is of IgG4 type, and carbohydrate antigens are of IgG2 type. It is conceivable that variable heavy regions may be restricted to particular IgG subclasses and that the immunoregulation of subclass expression occurs at the level of the antibody-forming cell. The subclass restriction by serum antigens is thought to be regulated at the T-cell (thymus-derived lymphocyte) level. In a number of species it has been shown that carbohydrated antigens seem to stimulate the antibody information within a single subclass that quantitatively represents a very small portion of normal serum immunoglobulins. Perlmutter et al. (48) have shown in mice that antibodies directed against group A and C streptococci, pneumococcal polysaccharide, and phosphorylcholine were restricted only to IgG3 subclass although this portion is only 0.1 mg/ml. It has therefore been assumed that IgG3 is especially efficient in creating immunity toward bacteria. IgG3 in mice passes the placenta six times faster than other subclasses. However, an observation speaking against this notion is the report that this subclass is a poor activator of complement (10). Guinea pigs have a very poor reaction toward the group A streptococci and pneumococcal polysaccharide type 3 and are therefore especially sensitive to infection for these bacteria. They seem to lack an IgG3-like subclass.

Results from studies where different haptens have been coupled to polysaccharide conjugates indicate that the subclass selection is mediated by interaction between the antigenic determinant and its binding site on the antibody. Antibodies against different determinants on the same antigen can have different isotype distribution. Another factor that can regulate the isotype pattern is the type of immunization. Antibodies to phospholipase, which is a component of bee venom, have been studied in beekeepers (1). It has been found that chronically exposed beekeepers had antibodies of the IgG4 type, whereas persons who had been stung a few times and also those stung early in the bee season had antibodies of IgG1 type. *In vitro* studies have shown that the type of adjuvant used in inducing an antibody response has influenced the subclass pattern toward different haptens (29).

Different Principles for B-Cell Activation with Respect to Protein and Polysaccharide Antigen

Subcategorization of mature human B cells similar to that done for mice has not yet been accomplished, although studies of newly synthesized monoclonal reagents will likely uncover more diversity, which could explain differences in immune response to antigens of protein or polysaccharide nature.

The structural differences of protein and polysaccharide molecules are reflected in their immunobiological reactivity. Proteins or polypeptides, with a unique secondary and tertiary structure, have a surface consisting of amino acid residues with different electrical charges, randomly distributed. The antigenic determinants of protein molecules consist of four to eight spatially adjacent amino acid residues. The surface of the molecule therefore consists of a large number of different determinants, and identical determinants appear in very low numbers (low epitope density). This is in contrast to polysaccharides, which are built up by repeated subunits of a few different types of oligosaccharide, each functioning as an antigenic determinant, therefore giving rise to a high number of very few different types of (or identical) determinants (high epitope density).

Characteristically high epitope density antigens induce a specific B-cell response without the cooperation of T-helper cells (16). In higher concentrations they can also activate different B-cell clones (subpopulations) and induce a polyclonal antibody response (4). In contrast to proteins, which induce a strong secondary IgG response, polysaccharides mainly induce production of IgM antibodies, and this response is of longer duration compared to the IgG response brought on by proteins. Proteins need the cooperation of other auxiliary cells in inducing an antibody response. The mechanism may be that the antigenic determinants are concentrated on the surface of macrophages and T cells before they are presented to the B cells, the process being facilitated by soluble helper factors. This process is not necessary in the case of polysaccharides, which themselves have a sufficient epitope density to induce the activation process. It is possible to manipulate the antipolysaccharide response. A covalent binding to proteins can induce a strong IgG response. The surface of bacteria can be analogous to a polysaccharide protein complex. It is also known that pneumococci induce an antipolysaccharide response by the IgG and the IgM classes.

Another difference between proteins and polysaccharides is the influence on immunogenicity by molecular size. The immunostimulatory effect by proteins is independent of molecular size, i.e., small protein molecules like tetanus toxoid have good immunogenicity. On the other hand, small polysaccharide molecules lack immunogenicity, which demands a certain minimum molecular size. Also, immunogenicity increases with increasing molecular size.

Owing to a lack of necessary enzymes, polysaccharides are often not degraded in animals (32), in contrast to proteins that have a relatively short half-life *in vivo*. The immunostimulatory effect of polysaccharides is therefore much longer than that brought about by proteins.

Immunity to Pneumococci and *H. influenzae*

The complex structure of bacterial cell-wall antigens makes study of immunity to bacterial antigens difficult. It is, however, facilitated in species with a well-defined cell-wall capsule. The capsule is often a relevant antigen in the study of protective antibodies.

Immunity to pneumococcal infections is closely associated with levels of complement and specific antibodies against the capsular polysaccharide (12). Immunization of certain adult patient groups with purified pneumococcal capsular antigens is now widely used. Among a huge number of different pneumococcal serotypes only a few are clinically important as a cause of otitis media, and they also show different immunobiological characteristics. Type 19 is one of the most common serotypes. Cowan et al. (18) showed that this serotype gave a poor immune response at the same time that it showed one of the highest preimmunization antibody levels. The opposite was observed with serotype 3. Douglas et al. (20) found increasing levels of naturally occurring antibodies to each studied pneumococcal serotype in children up to 5 years of age. The poor efficacy to vaccination in early childhood depends probably not only on the poor response to immunization but also on low preimmune antibody levels (55).

The hapten phosphorylcholine (Pc) is the dominant immunogen in the cell wall of a number of common microorganisms such as pneumococci, streptococci, and certain fungi and helminths. Pc is a part of the C substance of the pneumococcal capsule, and anti-Pc antibodies appear after vaccination with pneumococcal polysaccharide (11).

Anti-Pc antibodies have been shown to protect against pneumococcal infections, and in mice it has been shown experimentally that the T15 idiotype, which dominates the immune response, efficiently protects the mice against intravenous infection with type-3 pneumococci.

Perhaps even more than pneumococci, *H. influenzae* creates problems when we are treating otitis media. Infections caused by *H. influenzae* are described as the most common infectious agents in immunodeficient patients. This organism occurs with or without a cell-wall capsule. The encapsulated forms are much more pathogenic than the other types, but the unencapsulated form is the one most commonly found in association with upper respiratory tract infections. Great interest has been taken in developing a study to define the antigen that is most appropriate in eliciting protective antibody formation. The capsule polysaccharide is considered the most important target antigen for bactericidal and opsonizing antibodies directed against encapsulated *H. influenzae* type B. However, there is evidence that bactericidal and opsonizing antibodies directed at noncapsular cell-wall antigens are present in immune sera from both animals and humans. The target antigen of antibodies against cell-wall components is the proteinaceous part of the outer membrane of the cell wall and the lipopolysaccharide. Hansen et al. (30) has shown that a monoclonal antibody against *H. influenzae* cell-membrane protein protects rats against *H. influenzae* type B disease. Shurin et al. (58) studied the immune response in association with otitis media against unencapsulated *H. influenzae* strains by using a bactericidal antibody assay. They found that a significant number of convalescent children developed a rise in titers against the infecting organism.

Neonatal and Infant Antibody Production

There is a relationship between the maturation of the immune response and the changing pattern of susceptibility to infections in childhood (46). Andersson (5) has studied the human B- and T-cell ontogeny from early infancy. A strong T-cell suppressor function was found in newborns. T cells from cord blood were found to suppress human lymphocytes in co-culture with adult cells but not in co-culture with cells from newborns. After adding gamma-interferon antisera this suppression was abolished, indicating that the mechanism is mediated by gamma-interferon. It has been assumed that this paradoxical fact that newborns have strongly expressed suppression, but not susceptibility to it, could serve the purpose of preventing the survival of potentially harmful maternal immunocompetent cells entering the fetus. This might, however, be harmful to some children during the first months or year of life and increase their susceptibility to infection.

Antibodies synthesized by the human fetus are mainly IgM (25). The newborn infant starts to produce IgM at birth and reaches adult levels by the end of the first year of life. The levels of IgG in the full-term newborn infant are the same as or slightly higher than in the mother as a result of transplacental transference of antibodies during the last month of gestation. Thus premature children can have a serious hypogammaglobulinemia and suffer from severe infections.

As a result of catabolism of maternal IgG the levels decline during the first 6 months of life. Subsequently, IgG levels increase in a distinct pattern of appearance for each subclass (42,44,57). The level of IgG2 declines more proportionally and rises more slowly than IgG1 and does not reach adult levels until adolescence (see Fig. 2). As a result of the delayed onset of IgG production, a period of physiological hypogammaglobulinemia is observed between the ages 4 to 9 months.

PRIMARY IMMUNODEFICIENCY DISORDERS

The first documented association between recurrent infections and immunodeficiency was described by Bruton (13) in 1952. An 8-year-old boy suffered from recurrent pneumococcal sepsis and otitis media and was unable to produce anti-

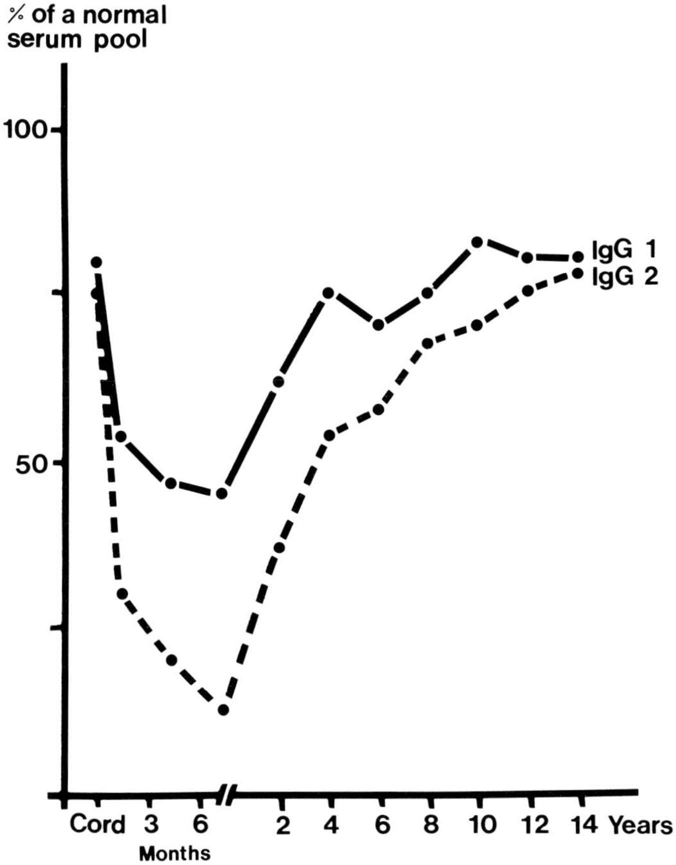

FIG. 2. The concentration of IgG1 and IgG2 relative to a normal adult serum pool. (Data from Oxelius, *personal communication*.)

bodies against pneumococcal polysaccharides. On substitution with human gammaglobulin he became free from infections.

Since this report, a large number of disorders affecting the immune system have been described (52). Lymphocytes of the B- and T-cell lineage pass through a series of stages prior to their development into immunocompetent cells. The signals and processes involved are so complex that inborn or acquired defects interfering with normal antibody production are not improbable. Defects of terminal B-cell differentiation, plasma cell function, and antibody secretion are described and affect the system at various levels, causing a heterogeneous group of diseases (22).

Defects of Cellular Immunity

Defective B- and T-cell function causes combined immunodeficiency, a severe disease with a high mortality rate. Disorders of cell-mediated immunity are caused by a defective function of T lymphocytes. Infections are mainly caused by pathogens such as viruses, protozoa, fungi, and some intracellular bacteria. Since T lymphocytes have an important control over the function of B lymphocytes, the capacity to make antibodies was also invariably affected in cases of T-cell abnormalities. In many B-cell defects, a concomitant T-cell deficiency is found (53).

Incidence of Immune Disorders

Immunodeficiencies are rare diseases. A nationwide survey of symptomatic primary immunodeficiency disorders in children has been performed in Sweden, which has a population of 8.3 million people (21). The study was performed during the period 1974 to 1979 and 201 cases of immunodeficiency disorder were found. Antibody deficiencies were the most frequent (40.0%), followed by phagocytic disorders (22.0%) and combined T-cell and B-cell disorders (20.8%). The prevalence of primary immunodeficiency disorders was 8.4 cases per 100,000 children during the time of the survey. Since these disorders comprise a heterogeneous group and are easily overlooked, the number of cases found in this study must be looked upon as a minimum figure.

Immunodeficiency Diseases Involving B-Cell Dysfunction—Antibody Deficiency Syndromes

The X chromosome appears to play a major role in normal B-cell function, and an immunoregulatory locus has tentatively been assigned to the short arm of X chromosome in humans (22). Several immunodeficiency disorders in humans as well as the major B-cell defect in mice (Xid) are X-linked.

Table 1 shows the major categories of mainly genetically determined human immunodeficiency disorders with associated B-cell dysfunction (22).

TABLE 1. *Human immunodeficiency disorders with B-cell dysfunction*

Deficiencies of humoral immunity
Transient hypogammaglobulinemia of infancy
X-linked agammaglobulinemia
Sporadic agammaglobulinemia
X-linked lymphoproliferative disorder
Selective immunoglobulin deficiencies
High IgM
Low IgA
Low-IgG subclass
Common variable immunodeficiency (heterogeneous)

Clinical Findings

Individuals with antibody-deficiency syndromes usually present with a history of recurrent pyogenic infections of the respiratory tract (40). The infections have increased frequency, increased severity, and prolonged duration. Infants are usually asymptomatic from birth to about 6 months of age because of placentally transferred maternal antibodies. The bacterial infections are mainly caused by capsulated pyogenic bacteria such as *Streptococcus pneumoniae* and *Haemophilus influenzae*. Usually, the upper respiratory tract is affected several years prior to the lower respiratory tract (37). Thus relapsing otitis media and sinusitis is common in children, often prior to the advent of more serious infection such as pneumoniae and meningitis. The number of viral infections is not increased in these patients. Lymphoid tissue such as tonsils and adenoids is reported to be poorly developed.

Immunological Findings

The measurement of serum immunoglobulins is an important screening test for the diagnosis of deficiencies in immunity. Measurement of IgG subclasses has been performed in only a few laboratories because antisera to IgG subclasses have been scarce. With the use of commercially available monoclonal antibodies, the method will probably become more common. Certain individuals may lack specific antibodies despite normal immunoglobulin levels. The determination of antibody activity against various antigens of protein and polysaccharide nature will give information about the ability of an individual to mount a specific immune response. Immunoelectrophoresis not only detects components—monoclonal antibody production in patients with multiple myeloma—but it can also give some information about the IgG2 level in individuals above 2 years of age.

Whereas enumeration of T and B cells is essential in the assessment and monitoring of primary immunodeficiencies, the study of T- and B-cell subsets is mainly useful for research purposes. The same holds true for the determination of lymphocyte response to mitogens (polyclonal T- and/or B-cell activators). For the investigation of cell-mediated immunity, delayed-hypersensitivity skin testing using antigens like PPD or candida is used.

Immunodeficiencies with Agammaglobulinemia

X-linked agammaglobulinemia, also called Bruton's disease, is characterized by the early onset of recurrent, purulent infections. These patients have low serum concentrations of all immunoglobulin classes and have no circulating B cells. There is a maturational block in early B-cell lymphocyte development (69).

Common variable agammaglobulinemia, earlier called "acquired" primary hypogammaglobulinemia, represents a heterogeneous group of disorders (40) with serum immunoglobulin levels not being as severely depressed as in X-linked agammaglobulinemia. The onset is variable in time and both sexes are equally affected. The B-cell differentiation seems to be blocked at various levels in the different groups of patients.

Transient Hypogammaglobulinemia in Infancy

Between 4 and 9 months of age a period of physiological hypogammaglobulinemia occurs. Transient hypogammaglobulinemia is a prolongation of this period, resulting from delay in the onset of production of immunoglobulins in some infants (40). Recurrent otitis media and bronchitis are the most common findings in these patients. Asymptomatic infants with this type of hypogammaglobulinemia have incidentally been found among relatives of individuals with other immunodeficiencies.

Serum IgG levels are usually between 1.5 to 3.0 g/liter, and IgG subclasses are reported to be uniformly depressed. Since the number of circulating B cells is reported to be normal, the defect might involve the terminal differentiation of B cells into antibody-producing plasma cells. However, Siegel et al. (60) found a numerical as well as a functional deficiency of helper T cells which could be responsible for the deficiency in immunoglobulin production. By definition, all patients recover usually in the first or second year of life. The majority of patients do not require gammaglobulin replacement. Watchful expectancy until normal serum levels of IgG are reached is recommended.

Selective IgA Deficiency

Selective IgA deficiency is characterized by a reduced level of serum IgA, namely, 0.05 g/liter (2). This condition is the most common form of immunodeficiency, with an incidence of about 1 in 700 (31). The frequency varies, however, with groups investigated and the methods employed for detection, making comparisons difficult.

IgA antibodies are the dominating antibody in secretions, as has been earlier described. With only a few exceptions the deficiency of serum IgA is accompanied by a deficiency of secretory IgA in secretions. Even if the IgA system is an important defense mechanism for the mucous membranes, a number of individuals with this deficiency are healthy. The majority of such persons have been found by screening blood donors (31). About 50% of patients with IgA deficiency have recurrent infections, mainly of the upper respiratory tract, and about 25% have autoimmune or collagen vascular diseases. Acute otitis media is not very common. Of 35 infection-prone children with complete deficiency of IgA, only 4 suffered from recurrent otitis media (15).

In most cases the infections described are mild to moderately severe. When more severe respiratory tract infections occur in IgA-deficient patients a concomitant deficiency of the IgG2 subclass can be suspected. Oxelius et al. (45) have described the combined IgA and IgG2 deficiency in 7 of 37 IgA-deficient patients.

In the IgA-deficient individual, there are only a few IgA-containing cells in the mucosa (19). Instead, there is a probable compensatory increase of IgM-producing cells (8). Korsrud and Brandzaeg (38) found a striking compensatory increase, not only of IgM but also of IgG- and IgD-producing cells in the parotid gland from IgA-deficient individuals.

So far, no specific treatment for the underlying immune defect has been successful except for immunoglobulin substitution for IgG2 deficiency. The potential risk for immunization against IgA must be considered (6).

Selective IgG Deficiency

Some highly infection-prone individuals with normal or slightly decreased levels of total IgG in serum have been found to have low or nonexistent levels of certain subclasses, especially IgG2 (56). Oxelius (43) has described IgG2 and IgG4 subclass deficiency in two siblings and their mother, all of whom were abnormally susceptible to recurrent infections. The mother suffered for many years from recurrent otitis media, resulting in deafness in one ear. The most common bacteria among these patients are *H. influenzae* and pneumococci, since antibodies against capsular antigens are largely restricted to the IgG2 subclass.

Patients lacking one or several IgG subclasses require the same substitution with gammaglobulin as patients with hypogammaglobulinemia.

IMMUNE RESPONSE IN OTITIS MEDIA

In 1975 Howie et al. (33) coined the term "otitis-prone condition" for children with recurrent episodes of acute otitis media. Recent epidemiologic investigations show clearly that recurrent otitis media is a disease of early childhood. Ingvarsson et al. (34) have shown that the highest number of episodes per 100 children was registered among children 1 to 2 years of age (Fig. 3). Among children having had their first episode before 1 year of age, 14% had six or more attacks during their first 2 years of life.

Local and Humoral Immune Response to Single Episodes of Otitis Media

The antibody response in association with attacks of acute otitis media has been studied in serum as well as in middle ear fluid. Sloyer et al. (61) found that one-third of the attacks of acute otitis media was caused by pneumococci. It was found that 25% of the children had an immune response, as judged by an increased antibody level in convalescent serum, and the percentage of responders increased with age; 12% of the infants less that 12 months of age and 48% of the children over 24 months of age showed a significant response.

The antibody responses to the homologous *H. influenzae* strains in serum and middle ear fluid were also investigated in 40 children less than 2 years of age (62). Bactericidal or indirect antibody fluorescent tests were used. Fourteen patients had significant increases of specific antibody in convalescent sera. In another study (63), the specific antibody content of any class was positively correlated to a swift clearing of the middle ear in 80 patients under 3 years of age.

Immunology of the "Otitis-Prone" Condition

Children with recurrent upper respiratory tract infections have been studied with regard to serum immunoglobulin levels. Buckley et al. (14) found that 44% of 600

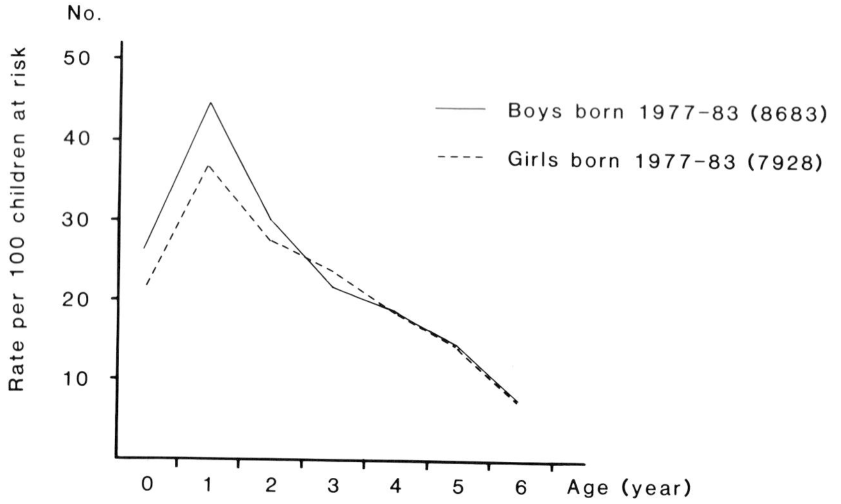

FIG. 3. Incidence rate of acute otitis media in relation to sex. (Data from Ingvarsson, *personal communication.*)

children who were reported to be subject to frequent respiratory tract and cutaneous infections had concentrations of one or more immunoglobulin outside the normal findings for age. This was in contrast to only 7.7% of 181 normal subjects of comparable ages. Isaacs et al. (35), on the other hand, found no correlation between serum immunoglobulin levels and proneness to infection. In other investigations, attempts have been made to correlate the tendency to acquire otitis media with serum levels of immunoglobulins in otitis-prone children. So far, no aberrations in these children have been noticed as compared to healthy children (9,27).

In a recently performed prospective study, 150 children with different degrees of otitis proneness were monitored from the first episode of otitis media up to 3 years of age (24). The first episode always occurred before 1 year of age. Serum samples were obtained at intervals during the observation time and every episode was recorded. The 20 children who were in the otitis-prone group (8–17 episodes of otitis media) were compared with a healthy control group (1–2 otitis media). Serum samples from these two groups of children were analyzed with regard to IgG subclasses and samples of 10 to 12 months and 32 months were analyzed. There was no difference with regard to IgG1, IgG3, and IgG4, but a significant difference concerning IgG2 was found; otitis-prone children had lower levels of IgG2 both at 12 months and 32 months of age (Fig. 4).

The theoretical linkage between IgG2 and antibodies for polysaccharide antigens was discussed earlier in this chapter. Siber et al. (59) showed that the antibody response in connection with immunization against pneumococcal antigen was correlated to the serum-IgG2 level before vaccination. Thus patients with high IgG2 levels did mount a higher antibody response than patients with low levels. This finding, together with the finding of low IgG2 levels in otitis-prone children, could explain the tendency toward recurrent episodes in this group. These findings indicate the importance of the IgG2 subclass since this isotype only constitutes 25% to 30% of the entire IgG pool.

It has long been recognized that boys, to a greater extent than girls, are affected by infections, and this was also true in the study of otitis-prone children. The infection-prone group contained a significantly higher number of boys. In the control group, the sexes were evenly distributed. The connection of antibody response via the X chromosome described in CBA mice is, in this context, interesting.

Prellner et al. (51) found a reduced ability of otitis-prone children to respond with IgG antibodies to pneumococcal types encountered in acute otitis media. Thus fifteen 2-year-old children with recurrent episodes of otitis media had no detectable IgG antibodies against pneumococcal capsular polysaccharide 6A or 19F, in contrast to non-otitis-prone children.

Specific antipneumococcal polysaccharide antibodies, with regard to IgG-subclass distribution, have also been investigated in otitis-prone children, normal children, and adults. For this, a recently developed enzyme-linked immunosorbent assay (ELISA) technique (50) using anti-IgG-subclass monoclonal antibodies was used. An interesting discovery was made concerning specific antibodies of the IgG1 subclass. It was shown that children have significantly higher values than adults and that healthy children have higher levels than otitis-prone children (23).

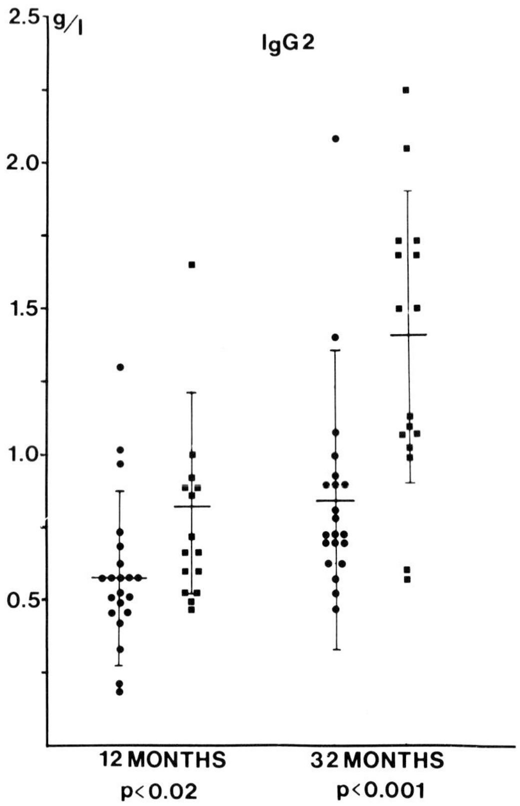

FIG. 4. Plasma IgG2 levels (arithmetic means ± SD) at 12 and 32 months of age in otitis-prone (•) and age-matched controls (■). (From ref. 24.)

On the contrary, as was expected, adults have the highest levels of IgG2 antibodies, followed by healthy children and otitis-prone children. Somewhat different patterns are observed when pneumococcal polysaccharides of the different serotypes are analyzed. Type 6, which is one the most common serotypes in connection with otitis media, gave the greatest differences. Type 3, which is a very pathogenic serotype per se, but not in connection with otitis media, gave no significant difference in any of the groups with regard to IgG1 and gave a significant difference only between adults and healthy children with regard to IgG2.

The mechanisms resulting in different isotype patterns in adults and children is unknown. In later studies it has been found that a switch of isotype pattern occurs at 7 to 10 years of age (54). Different mechanisms with regard to immunization might be responsible. Children are more or less constantly colonized with bacteria and often have bacterial infections, in contrast to adults who are rarely colonized. It is possible that immunization in connection with acute bacterial infections involving cellular mechanisms such as T-helper cells results in significant IgG1 production. Adults have perhaps an endogenous non-antigen-dependent immunization process, owing to nondegraded polysaccharides using a more T-cell-independent immunization process, thus leading to production of IgG2 antibodies.

Conclusion

Recurrent episodes of purulent otitis media occur in otitis-prone children who are defectively immunocompetent. Until appropriate immunoprophylaxis is available it is important that this group of children receive a specialist's care for their infections.

The pattern of recurrent infections in various locations can easily be overlooked, causing a dangerous delay of diagnosis and treatment of immunodeficiency disorders (36). Many of the diseases have only recently been recognized. IgG-subclass defects have not generally been looked for partly because of limited diagnostic resources and partly because of the fact that many of these children have recurrent episodes of acute otitis media and/or respiratory infections, a symptomatology earlier not linked to immunodeficiency. Even if such deficiencies may be more common than previously recognized, they are rare disorders. Thus physicians must keep the possibility of an immunodeficiency in mind much more often than they can expect to diagnose one.

A careful analysis of the patient's history is the most important clue to a diagnosis. General practitioners, pediatricians, and otorhinolaryngologists should have the best opportunity to detect patients with hypogammaglobulinemia. One episode of meningitis, septicemia, osteomyelitis, or pyogenic arthritis with an episode of pneumonia or with recurrent otitis media should raise suspicion of the possibility of an immunodeficiency disorder.

Help in interpreting results and suggestions for further investigation in order to achieve a final diagnosis has to be given by a clinical immunological laboratory.

REFERENCES

1. Aalbeerse, R., van der Gaag, R., and van Leeuwen, J. (1983): Serologic aspects to IgG4 antibodies. Prolonged immunization results in IgG4 restricted response. *J. Immunol.*, 130:722–726.
2. Amman, A.J., and Hong, R. (1980): Disorders of the IgA system. In: *Immunological Disorders in Infants and Children*, edited by R.T. Stiehm and V. Fulginiti, pp. 260–273. W.B. Saunders, Philadelphia.
3. Amsbaugh, D., Hansen, C., Prescott, P., et al. (1972): Genetic control of the antibody response to type III pneumococcal polysaccharide in mice. Evidence that an X-linked gene plays a decisive role in determining responsiveness. *J. Exp. Med.*, 136:931–949.
4. Andersson, J., Sjöberg, O., and Möller, G. (1972): Mitogens as probes for immunocyte and cellular cooperation. *Transplant. Rev.*, 11:131–177.
5. Andersson, U. (1982): Ontogenic development of human lymphocyte functions. Thesis. Department of Immunology, Karolinska Institute and Department of Pediatrics, Danderyd Hospital, Stockholm, Sweden.
6. Björkander, J., Hammarström, L., Smith, C.I.E., Buckley, R.H., Cunningham, Rundbes, C., and Hansson, L.Å. (1986): Immunoglobulin prophylaxis in patients with antibody deficiency syndromes and anti IgA antibodies. *J. Clin. Immunol.* (*in press*).

7. Blomberg, B., Geckaler, W.R., and Wiegert, M. (1972): Genetics of the antibody response to dextran in mice. *Science*, 177:178–180.
8. Brandtzaeg, P., Fjellanger, I., and Gjeruldsen, S.T. (1968): Immunoglobulin M: local synthesis and selective secretion in patients with immunoglobulin A deficiency. *Science*, 160:789–791.
9. Branefors-Helander, P., et al. (1975): Otitis media acuta. A clinical, bacteriological and serological study of children with frequent episodes of acute otitis media. *Acta Otolaryngol. (Stockh.)*, 80:399–406.
10. Briles, D.E., and Davie, J.M. (1975): Detection of isoelectric focused antibody by autoradiography and hemolysis of antigen coated erythrocytes of comparison of methods. *J. Immunol. Methods*, 8:363–369.
11. Briles, D.E., Forman, C., Hudak, S., and Claflin, J.L. (1982): Anti-phosphorylcholine antibodies of the T15 idiotype are optimally protective against *Streptococcus pneumoniae*. *J. Exp. Med.*, 156:1177–1185.
12. Brown, E.J., et al. (1982): A quantitative analysis of the interactions of antipneumococcal antibody and complement in experimental pneumococcal bacteremia. *J. Clin. Invest.*, 69:85–98.
13. Bruton, C.O.C. (1952): Agammaglobulinemia. *Pediatriacs*, 9:722–728.
14. Buckley, R.H., Dees, S.C., and O'Fallon, W.M. (1968): Serum immunoglobulins. II. Levels in children subject to recurrent infection. *Pediatrics*, 42:50–60.
15. Burgio, G.R., Duse, M., Monafo, V., Ascione, A., and Nespoli, L. (1980): Selective IgA deficiency: clinical and immunological evaluation of 50 pediatric patients. *Eur. J. Pediatr.*, 133:101–106.
16. Coutinho, A., and Möller, G. (1975): Thymus independent B-cell induction and paralysis. *Adv. Immunol.*, 21:114–127.
17. Cooper, M.D. (1981): Pre-B cells, normal and abnormal development. *J. Clin. Immunol.*, 1:81–89.
18. Cowan, M.J., Amman, A.J., Wara, D.W., Howie, V.M., Schutz, L., Doyle, N., and Kaplan, M. (1978): Pneumococcal polysaccharide immunization in infants and children. *Pediatrics*, 62:721–727.
19. Crabbé, P.A., and Heremans, J.F. (1966): The distribution of immunoglobulin-containing cells along the human gastrointesinal tract. *Gastroenterology.*, 51:305–316.
20. Douglas, R.M., Paton, J.C., Duncan, S.J., and Hansman, D.J. (1983): Antibody response to pneumococcal vaccination in children younger than five years of age. *J. Infect. Dis.*, 148:131–137.
21. Fast, A. (1982): Primary immunodeficiency disorders in Sweden: cases among children. 1974–1979. *J. Clin. Immunol.*, 2:86–92.
22. Filipovich, A.H., and Kersey, J.H. (1983): B-lymphocyte function in immunodeficiency disease. *Immunology Today*, 4:50–55.
23. Freijd, A., Hammarström, L., Persson, M.A.A., and Smith, C.I.E. (1984): Plasma anti-pneumococcal activity of the IgG class and subclasses in otitis prone children. *Clin. Exp. Immunol.*, 56:233–238.
24. Freijd, A., Oxelius, V.-A., and Rynnel-Dagöö, B. (1985): A prospective study demonstrating an association between plasma IgG2 concentrations and susceptibility to otitis media in children. *Scand. J. Infect. Dis.*, 17:115–120.
25. Fudenberg, H.H., and Fudenberg, B.R. (1964): Antibody to hereditary human gamma-globulin (m) factor resulting from maternal fetal incompatibility. *Science*, 145:170–171.
26. Gathings, W.E., Lawton, A.R., and Cooper, M.D. (1977): Immunofluorescent studies of the development of pre-B cells, B lymphocytes and immunoglobulin isotype diversity in humans. *Eur. J. Immunol.*, 7:804–810.
27. Gebharddt, H. (1981): Tympanotomy tubes in the otitis-media prone child. *Laryngoscope*, 91:849–866.
28. Grey, H., and Kunkel, H. (1964): H chain subgroups of myeloma proteins and normal 7S-globulins. *J. Exp. Med.*, 120:253–266.
29. Hadjipetrou-Korounakis, L., and Möller, E. (1984): Adjuvants influence the immunoglobulin subclass distribution of immune responses *in vivo*. *Scand. J. Immunol.*, 19:219–225.
30. Hansen, E., Robertsson, S., Gulig, P., Frisch, C., and Haanes, E. (1982): Immunoprotection of rats against *Haemophilus influenzae* type 6 disease mediated by monoclonal antibody against a *Haemophilus* outer-membrane protein. *Lancet*, i:366–367.
31. Hansson, L.A., Björkander, J., and Oxelius, V.-A. (1983): Selective IgA deficiency. In: *Pri-*

mary and Secondary Immunodeficiency Disorders, edited by R.K. Chandra, pp. 62–84. Churchill/Livingstone, Edinburgh.

32. Howard, J. (1972): Cellular events in the induction and loss of tolerance to pneumococcal polysaccharides. *Transplant. Rev.*, 8:50–75.
33. Howie, W., Plussard, J., and Sloyer, J. (1975): The "otitis-prone" condition. *Am. J. Dis. Child.*, 129:676–678.
34. Ingvarsson, L., Lundgren, K., Olofsson, B., and Wall, S. (1982): Epidemiology of acute otitis media in children. *Acta Otolaryngol. (Stockh).*, (Suppl.):388.
35. Isaacs, D., Webster, A.D.B., and Valman, H.B. (1984): Immunoglobulin levels and function in pre-school children with recurrent respiratory infections. *Clin. Exp. Immunol.*, 58:335–340.
36. Johnston, R.B. (1984): Recurrent bacterial infections in children. *N. Engl. J. Med.*, 310:1237–1243.
37. Karlsson, G., Petrusson, B., Björkander, J., and Hansson, L.A. (1985): Infections of the nose and paranasal sinuses in adult patients with immunodeficiency. *Arch. Otolaryngol.*, 111:290–293.
38. Korsrud, F.R., and Bradtzaeg, P. (1980): Quantitative immunohistochemistry of immunoglobulin- and J-chain producing cells in human parotid and submandibular salivary glands. *Immunology.*, 39:129–140.
39. Kung, J.T., and Paul, W.E. (1983): B-lymphocyte subpopulations. *Immunology Today*, 4:37–41.
40. Leung, D.Y.M., Rosen, R.S., and Geha, R.S. (1974): Disorders of immunoglobulin-antibody system. In: *Primary and Secondary Immunodeficiency Disorders*, edited by R.K. Chandra, pp. 44–61. Churchill Livingstone, Edinburgh.
41. Marcu, K.B., and Cooper, M.D. (1982): New views of the immunoglobulin heavy-chain switch. *Nature*, 298:327–328.
42. Morell, A., Skvaril, F., Hitzig, W.H., and Barandum, S. (1972): IgG subclasses: development of the serum concentrations in "normal" infants and children. *Pediatrics*, 80:960–964.
43. Oxelius, V.-A. (1974): Chronic infections in a family with heredity deficiency of IgG2 and IgG4. *Clin. Exp. Immunol.*, 17:19–27.
44. Oxelius, V. (1979): IgG subclass levels in infancy and childhood. *Acta Paediatr. Scand.*, 68:23–27.
45. Oxelius, V., et al. (1981): IgG subclasses in selective IgA deficiency. Importance of IgG2-IgA deficiency. *N. Engl. J. Med.*, 304:1476–1477.
46. Pabst, H.F., and Kreth, H.W. (1980): Ontogeny of the immune response as a basis of childhood disease. *J. Pediatr.*, 97:519–534.
47. Pandey, J.P., Virella, G., Londholt, C.B., Fudenberg, H.H. Kyoung, C.V., and Gulbraith, R.M. (1979): Association between immunoglobulin allotypes and immune responses to *Haemophilus influenzae* and meningococcus polysaccharides. *Lancet*, 5:190–192.
48. Perlmutter, R., Hansburg, D., Briles, D., Nicolotti, R., and Davie, J.M. (1978): Subclass restriction of murine anti-carbohydrated antibodies. *J. Immunol.*, 121:2.
49. Perlmutter, R., Nahm, M., Schroer, K., Baker, P., and Davie, J. (1980): Susceptibility of (CBA/N × DBA/2) FI Male mice to infection with type III *Streptococcus pneumoniae*. In: *Perspectives of Immunology, 1980*, edited by E.S. Komena, p. 173. Academic Press, New York.
50. Persson, M.A.A., Hammarström, L., and Smith, C.I.E. (1985): Enzyme-linked immunosorbent assay for subclass distribution of human IgG and IgA antigen-specific antibodies. *J. Immunol. Methods*, 78:109–121.
51. Prellner, K., Kalm, O., and Pedersen, F.K. (1984): Pneumococcal antibodies and complement during and after periods of recurrent otitis. *J. Pediatr. Otorhinolaryngol.*, 7:39–49.
52. Rosen, F.S., Wedgewood, R.J., Auiti, F., Cooper, M.D., Good, R.A., Hansson, L.A., Hitzig, W.H., Matsumoto, S., Sligman, M., Soothill, J.F., and Waldman, T.A. (1983): Meeting report: Primary immunodeficiency diseases. *Clin. Immunol. Immunopathol.*, 28:450–475.
53. Rosen, F.S., Cooper, M.D., and Wedgewood, R.J.P. (1984): The primary immunodeficiencies (first of two parts). *N. Engl. J. Med.*, 311:235–242.
54. Rynnel-Dagöö, B., Freijd, A., Hammarström, L., Oxelius, V., Persson, M.A.A., and Smith, C.I.E. (1986): Pneumococcal antibodies of different immunoglobulin subclasses in normal and IgG subclass deficient individuals of various ages. *Acta Otolaryngol. (Stockh).*, 101:146–151.
55. Rynnel-Dagöö, B., Freijd, A., and Prellner, K. (1985): Antibody activity of IgG subclasses against pneumococcal polysaccharides after vaccination. *Am. J. Otolaryngol.*, 6:275–279.

56. Schur, P.H., Bowel, H., Gelfand, E.W., Chester, A.A., and Rosen, F.S. (1970): Selective gamma-G globulin deficiencies in patients with pyogenic infections. *N. Engl. J. Med.*, 288:631–634.
57. Schur, P.H., Rosen, F., and Norman, M.E. (1979): Immunoglobulin subclasses in normal children. *Pediatr. Res.*, 13:181–183.
58. Shurin, P.A., et al. (1980): Bactericidal antibody and susceptibility to otitis media caused by nontypable strains of *Haemophilus influenzae*. *J. Pediatr.*, 97:364–369.
59. Siber, G.R., Schur, P.H., Aisenberg, A.C., Weitzman, S.A., and Schiffman, G. (1980): Correlation between serum IgG-2 concentration and the antibody response to bacterial polysaccharide antigens. *N. Engl. J. Med.*, 303:178–182.
60. Siegel, R.L., Issekutz, T., Schwaber, J., Rosen, F., and Geha, R.S. (1981): Deficiency of T helper cells in transient hypogammaglobulinemia of infancy. *N. Engl. J. Med.*, 305:1307–1313.
61. Sloyer, J., Howie, V., Ploussard, J., Ammann, A., Autrian, R., and Johnston, R. (1974): Immune response to acute otitis media in children. 1. Serotypes isolated and serum and middle ear fluid antibody in pneumococcal otitis media. *Infect. Immun.*, 9:1028–1032.
62. Sloyer, J., Cate, C., Howie, V., Ploussard, J., and Johnston, R. (1975): The immune response to acute otitis media in children. II. Serum and middle ear fluid antibody in otitis media due to *Haemophilus influenzae*. *J. Infect. Dis.*, 132:685–688.
63. Sloyer, J., Howie, V., Ploussard, J., Schiffman, G., and Johnston, R. (1976): Immune response to otitis media: association between middle ear fluid antibody and the clearing of clinical infection. *J. Clin. Microbiol.*, 4:306–308.
64. Snell, G.D., Dausset, J., and Nathenson, J. (1976): Immune response genes. In: *Histocompatibility*, pp. 133–144. New York.
65. Soothill, J.F. (1983): The role of primary immunodeficiency in common disease. In: *Primary and Secondary Immunodeficiency Disorders*. edited by R.K. Chandra, pp. 37–43. Churchill Livingstone, New York.
66. Spiegelberg, H. (1974): Biological activity of immunoglobulins of different classes and subclasses. *Adv. Immunol.*, 19:259–294.
67. Terry, W., and Fahey, J. (1964): Subclasses of human globulin based on differences in the heavy polypeptide chains. *Science*, 146:400–401.
68. Tonegawa, S. (1983): Somatic generation of antibody diversity. *Nature*, 302:575–581.
69. Vogler, L.B., Pearl, E.R., Gathings, W.E., Lawton, A.R., and Cooper, M.D. (1976): Lymphocyte precursor in bone marrow in immunoglobulin deficiency disease. *Lancet*, 2:376.
70. Yount, W., et al. (1968): Studies on human antibodies. VI. Selective variations in subgroup composition and genetic markers. *J. Exp. Med.*, 127:633–646.

Immunology of the Ear, edited by J. Bernstein
and P. Ogra. Raven Press, New York © 1987.

Allergy and Middle Ear Effusions: Fact or Fiction?

Robert C. Welliver

Division of Infectious Diseases and Microbiology Laboratories, Children's Hospital of Buffalo, Buffalo, New York 14222

The nature of the association of allergy with otitis media has been made the subject of debate for decades. The question is certainly of more than academic interest. Proof that a clear-cut causal relationship exists would suggest strongly that aggressive antiallergic therapy should at least partially alleviate the number of attacks of acute otitis media experienced during childhood or, alternatively, shorten the duration of persistence of middle ear effusion. The child would therefore be spared either the morbidity of frequent ear infections or the risk of hearing loss or delay in verbal learning, which is currently believed to result from persistence of fluid in the middle ear cavity (30).

Several mechanisms (see Table 1) by which an allergic constitution might predispose to middle ear disease have been proposed (6). The simplest mechanism would be that swelling of the nasal mucosa, in response to exposure to an allergen, might spread to the eustachian tube, producing obstruction of the tube with entrapment of fluid in the middle ear. Secondly, positive pressure, developing in nasopharynx when an individual with nasal obstruction swallows, might cause reflux of nasopharyngeal secretions into the middle ear cavity via the eustachian tube. There is little evidence to support, and some to contradict, these theories. The most viable current theory is that the middle ear is capable of acting as a target organ for an IgE-mediated allergic response upon entrance of an allergen to the middle ear cavity.

The chapter will review past efforts to delineate the relationship of allergy to otitis media. These efforts have included exhaustive studies of the epidemiology, immunology, and response to antiallergic therapy of otitis media with effusion. Unless specified below, the term otitis media with effusion (OME) will refer to all forms of otitis media, including acute otitis, chronic otitis, serous otitis, and all similar terminology.

EPIDEMIOLOGIC STUDIES

Numerous publications allude to an increased incidence of otitis media among atopic individuals. In studies of individuals with persistent middle ear effusions,

TABLE 1. *Proposed mechanisms of allergy-induced middle ear effusion and results of pertinent investigations.*[a]

Mechanism	Supportive evidence	Opposing evidence
Extension of anaphylaxis in nasopharynx to eustachian tube and middle ear	Numerous anecdotal reports; correlation of middle ear effusion with nasal allergy, but not allergy at other sites	Induction of allergic response in experimental animals did not result in middle ear effusion
		Lack of benefit of antiallergic therapy
Swallowing with obstructed nasal cavity forces fluid into middle ear via eustachian tube	Essentially none	Resolution of nasal obstruction does not result in clearing of middle ear effusion
Local immediate hypersensitivity reaction in middle ear cavity	Confirmed in experimental situations when antigen enters middle ear	Still insufficient documentation of the frequency with which this occurs in humans under natural conditions
	Antigen-specific IgE production in middle ear is reasonably well-documented	

[a]See text for references.

estimates of the frequency with which an underlying allergic predisposition exists as the primary cause range from 23% to as high as 80% of cases (2,10,11, 16,20,24,34,36,44). In addition, Draper (9) studied 340 allergic patients and found the incidence of chronic middle ear effusion to be twice as great in this group as in a group of 200 nonallergic individuals. Nasal allergies seem to be particularly predictive of an increased risk for OME (9,20,24). Lecks (20) found that 84% of patients with suspected allergic OME predominantly had nasal allergy. Among those individuals with "chest allergy" (asthma) as their predominant manifestation, OME was virtually nonexistent.

Although some early studies suggested that allergy to foods played an important causal role in OME (20,44), later studies have clearly shown that sensitivity to aeroallergens (tree pollens, dust, molds) is more commonly documented in patients with OME than is sensitivity to foods (9,40). Studies such as these frequently fail to define allergy in general and, specifically, fail to determine what constitutes food allergy.

Other studies dispute a role for allergic disease as a predisposing factor for OME. Cantekin et al. (8) evaluated over 500 children with serous OME, and found that only 5% gave a history of allergic disease. Virolainen et al. (43) studied over 1,200 Finnish schoolchildren, finding that 44% had experienced at least one episode of OME previously, 6% had experienced more than five earlier episodes, and 4% currently had effusions. The frequency of reported allergy was 17% for the whole study group and was approximately the same in all subgroups with OME. When followed prospectively, 35 children subsequently developed mucoid effusions. The presence of such effusions was directly related to the frequency of occurrence of respiratory infections, but was unrelated to a history of allergy in either the patients or their families.

It is difficult to draw firm conclusions from these studies, since most seem to be biased by methods of patient selection, or else were hampered by small patient numbers or lack of adequate definitions of allergy or OME. It seems safe to say that the majority of cases of OME are unrelated to the presence of an underlying allergic diathesis. At most, a subgroup of patients may exist in whom sensitivity to environmental aeroallergens may result in persistent OME.

IMMUNOLOGY

Nature of Middle Ear Effusions

Since the presence of eosinophils in middle ear effusions might suggest that such effusions were present on an allergic basis, many investigators have attempted to quantitate the degree of eosinophils in these fluids. Most investigators have found that eosinophils are virtually never present in middle ear effusions (23,36,42), whereas Koch found eosinophils in approximately 25% of effusions (19). Other investigators found that thin, serous effusions are unlikely to have eosinophils present, but thicker mucopurulent effusions had eosinophils present in over 15% of cases (17,47).

Many studies have emphasized the different types of effusions (serous, mucinous, purulent, etc.) that can be recovered from the middle ear. This differentiation is often easily made by visual inspection of the effusions, but the significance of the classification has not been substantiated. Bacterial pathogens are recovered with a similar frequency from all types of effusions (18). In serous effusions, macrophages predominate whereas T lymphocytes are few in number and B lymphocytes are absent. In mucoid effusions, B lymphocytes predominate (3). These findings suggest that the immune response may play a role in the persistence of effusion in the middle ear, potentially by local production by B cells of IgE antibody. These speculations, however, require further proof (see below).

Total IgE Levels and OME

Stempel et al. (41) attempted to relate serum IgE levels to the occurrence of OME in a group of 24 children followed over a period of 55 child-years. The frequency with which acute otitis, serous otitis, and total otitis episodes occurred was similar in groups with IgE levels greater or less than 94 IU/ml. In contrast, wheezing was noted more frequently in the group with higher total IgE concentrations.

Tympanometry was carried out following all episodes of upper respiratory infection in the study group, but no differences were observed when high- and low-IgE groups were studied.

The middle ear mucosa is apparently immunologically totally competent (3,4,28,29). Many investigators have therefore sought to determine whether an IgE-forming apparatus is present in the middle ear (1,14,15,22,29,32). Ishikawa et al. (15) were able to detect IgE in middle ear fluids by radial diffusion assays in only 2 (6.5%) of 31 effusions. Other immunoglobulin isotypes (IgA, IgG, IgM) were almost uniformly present. Ogra et al. (29) found no IgE-forming plasma cells in middle ear mucosal biopsy specimens, although they found trace amounts of IgE in 25% of effusions. These authors concluded that IgE was present via transudation from the mucosa. Phillips et al. (32) found IgE-positive plasma cells using direct immunofluorescence on mucosal biopsy specimens. Controls for specificity were not optimal in that study.

Other investigators compared total IgE levels in samples of serum and middle ear fluid obtained simultaneously from patients with chronic ear effusions. Two earlier studies concluded that total IgE levels were higher in middle ear fluids, suggesting local production of IgE (22,32). However, these studies utilized the RIST technique to measure total IgE, a technique that has been subsequently found to yield falsely high results for IgE when studying secretions (21). Subsequent studies using the PRIST technique have demonstrated that, for most subjects, total IgE levels are lower in middle ear fluids than in serum (26,33) regardless of the nature of the effusion (serous, mucinous, etc.) or the duration of its persistence. Only a few patients had higher concentrations of IgE in middle ear fluids than in serum.

Specific IgE Levels in OME

In addition to studies of total IgE, specific IgE concentrations have been measured in middle ear effusions. Mogi et al. (27) detected house-dust mite-specific IgE in 5 (8.9%) of 56 middle ear fluids. Since this is approximately the frequency with which mite-specific IgE could be measured in the serum of a large population of individuals with and without allergies, the authors doubted that such specific IgE played a role in OME. In contrast, Bernstein et al. (2,5) found that 22% of middle ear fluids from children with serous otitis media and documented allergy gave positive RAST results to a battery of environmental allergens. Less than 1% of effusions from nonallergic children gave similar positive RAST results. Sloyer et al. (38) demonstrated antipneumococcal IgE antibody in middle ear effusions obtained from children with and without previous documented pneumococcal otitis media. Adequate blocking experiments were not carried out to ensure the specificity of the IgE, but specificity was strongly implied by the demonstration of reactivity of the fluids in classic Prausnitz-Kustner reactions. Other studies of bacteria recovered from middle ear effusions demonstrated IgE antibody bound to bacteria in 15 of 23 (65%) effusions studied (4). It should be emphasized that functional antibacterial IgE has not yet been demonstrated in any of the numerous investigations that have been performed.

Antigenic exposure at distant mucosal sites unequivocally results in an immune response in the middle ear (37). Infections with respiratory syncytial virus and the parainfluenza viruses commonly precipitate episodes of OME (12,34) and incite a virus-specific IgE response in the nasopharynx (45,46). It is quite possible, therefore, that virus-specific IgE responses occur in the middle ear. In addition, viral antigen has been demonstrated in middle ear effusions (18). Degranulating and intact mast cells (2-5 per square micron) have been observed in middle ear mucosal tissue (22,32). Although proof is lacking, nevertheless infections with the above viruses might result in middle ear disease through the interaction of viral antigen and virus-specific IgE in the middle ear cavity, with resulting mediator release from mast cells.

Experimental OME

Many outstanding investigations on laboratory animals support a pathogenic role for hypersensitivity in OME. Hopp et al. (13) induced changes in the tympanic membrane resembling those of serous otitis media by injecting bovine serum albumin into the middle ear cavity of guinea pigs previously sensitized to the antigen. Koch (19) injected horse serum into the middle ear cavity of sensitized guinea pigs, resulting in the development of an eosinophil-laden effusion as well as infiltration of the mucosa with eosinophils. Smirnov (39) injected horse serum into one ear of a sensitized guinea pig and injected bouillon into the other ear. After an intracardiac injection of streptococci, infection developed only in the ear injected with horse serum. The author concluded that infection was a result of leaking through blood vessels that became dilated as a result of a local anaphylactic reaction.

Miglets (25) transfused monkeys with serum from ragweed-sensitive humans, then injected the middle ear cavity with ragweed pollen using a long cannula passed up the eustachian tube. Effusions developed within 5 days in the injected ear only. The middle ear mucosa became edematous and was infiltrated with acute and chronic inflammatory cells but no eosinophils. No attempt was made to measure ragweed-specific IgE titers in the effusions, so it remains unclear whether the hypersensitivity was IgE-mediated.

Yamashita et al. (48) sensitized guinea pigs to ovalbumin, then inoculated either liquid ovalbumin into the middle ear cavity or powdered ovalbumin into the nasal cavity. The results of this experiment are shown in Table 2. Injection of ovalbumin into the middle ear cavity resulted in formation of an effusion containing inflammatory cells and eosinophils. The middle ear mucosa was infiltrated with similar cells, as was the proximal eustachian tube. Minimal changes were observed in the pharyngeal end of the eustachian tube, and no changes were noted in the nasopharynx. In contrast, nasopharyngeal challenge resulted in profuse rhinorrhea as well as infiltration of the nasal cavity and pharynx with inflammatory cells and eosinophils. Interestingly, no changes were observed in the eustachian

TABLE 2. *Effects of inoculation of ovalbumin into middle ear or nasopharynx of sensitized guinea pigs*[a]

Site of inoculation	Observed site	Finding
Middle ear	Middle ear	Gelatinous fluid with eosinophils; mucosa infiltrated with eosinophils
	Eustachian tube	Same as middle ear
	Nasopharynx	No abnormal findings
Nasopharynx	Middle ear	No abnormal findings
	Eustachian tube	No abnormal findings
	Nasopharynx	Profuse rhinorrhea with eosinophils; mucosa infiltrated with eosinophils

[a]See ref. 48.

tube or middle ear. Challenge of nonsensitized animals intranasally or in the middle ear caused no effusion or inflammatory infiltrate. This elegant study emphasizes that the middle ear and eustachian tube can act as "shock organs" in acute hypersensitivity reactions. However, these studies tend to exclude nasal allergy as an important predisposing mechanism for OME or eustachian tube dysfunction.

RESPONSE TO ANTIALLERGIC THERAPY

If patients with OME were to respond to antiallergic therapy, some insight would be gained into the mechanism by which effusions were formed. Results of such therapeutic trials have been disappointing, with only a few exceptions. Viscomi (44) studied 50 children with mucoid middle ear effusions that had proven resistant to surgical management. Most of these patients had evidence of seasonal or perennial rhinitis. Lingual desensitization apparently reduced the incidence of serous otitis media from 100% to 40% and reduced the need for tympanostomy tubes from 66% to 12%. Solow and Updegraff (40) also reported some benefit from allergen-avoidance modes of therapy. Neither of these studies included a simultaneous control group, and neither used an adequate documentation of allergy nor listed criteria for tube replacement. Reisman and Bernstein (33) reported six children with well-documented nasal allergies and severe recurrent secretory OME. Following immunotherapy and allergen avoidance, marked improvement in nasal symptoms but no change in ear disease were noted.

Studies of the effect of oral decongestants on middle ear effusions have not yielded beneficial results regardless of whether individuals with a history of allergy or all patients with serous effusions were evaluated (8). Decongestant-antihistamine combinations have been demonstrated to have beneficial effects on eustachian tube function in children with chronic OME. However, these benefits have not yet been translated into any appreciable improvement in the course of the effusion itself (7). Administration of corticosteroids systemically has resulted in rapid resolution of middle ear effusions (31,35), even in individuals whose effusions are refractory to surgical management (11). Steroid-treated patients with allergies do not seem to respond better than similarly treated patients without allergies (35).

CONCLUSIONS

Despite the numerous anecdotal reports testifying to the frequent occurrence of chronic OME in the allergic individuals noted above, the few controlled epidemiologic investigations of the relationship of allergy and OME have yielded equivocal results (see Table 1). The only prospective evaluation (43) does not support the existence of such an association. Immunologic studies are also somewhat equivocal, but have not been able to develop convincing evidence that IgE-mediated hypersensitivity plays a role in the development of OME. Further studies of bacterial-specific and viral-specific IgE response in the middle ear may well resolve the current confusion. Studies in animals strongly support the concept that middle ear effusions may develop as a result of immediate hypersensitivity reactions within the middle ear cavity. These same studies tend to exclude the occurrence of similar reactions in the nasopharynx alone as a cause of OME. The fact that antiallergic therapy may result in resolution of nasal symptoms of allergy without altering the nature of middle ear effusions is also evidence against the possibility that nasal allergy promotes the development of OME. It must also be concluded, therefore, that swallowing with obstructed nasal passages does not contribute to persistent OME, since resolution of the obstruction does not result in clearing of effusions.

The principal cause of most, if not all, middle ear inflammatory disease is eustachian tube dysfunction, which may or may not be related to allergy. The role of allergy and eustachian tube dysfunction is completely covered in a chapter by Bluestone (*this volume*), and there appears to be increasing evidence that nasal provocation with specific allergens may cause eustachian tube blockage and may eventually lead to middle ear disease. However, this question has not been completely resolved at the present time. In the few patients who produce allergen-specific IgE in the middle ear, appearance of the allergen in the middle ear (not simply in the nasopharynx) may result in local anaphylaxis and the development of effusions. How frequently this happens in nature, if at all, remains to be determined, but it has been suggested that perhaps in 5% to 10% of allergic children with OME the target organ may be the middle ear mucosa.

REFERENCES

1. Bernstein, J.M., Hayes, E.R., Ishikawa, T. (1972): Secretory otitis media: a histopathologic and immunochemical report. *Trans. Am. Acad. Opththalmol. Otolaryngol.*, 76:1305–1318.
2. Bernstein, J.M., and Reisman, R. (1974): The role of acute hypersensitivity in secretory otitis media. *Trans. Am. Acad. Opththalmol. Otolaryngol.*, 788:120–127.

3. Bernstein, J.M., Szymanski, C. Albini, B., Sun, M., and Ogra, P.L. (1978): Lymphocyte subpopulations in otitis media with effusion. *Pediatr. Res.*, 12:786–788.
4. Bernstein, J.M., Myers, D., Kosinski, D., Nisengard, R., and Wicher, K. (1980): Antibody coated bacteria in otitis media with effusions. *Ann. Otol. Rhinol. Laryngol.*, 89(Suppl.):104–109.
5. Bernstein, J.M., Ellis, E., and Li, P. (1981): The role of IgE-mediated hypersensitivity in otitis media with effusion. *Otolaryngol. Head Neck Surg.*, 89:874–878.
6. Bluestone, C.D. (1978): Eustachian tube function and allergy in otitis media. *Pediatrics*, 61:753–760.
7. Cantekin, E.I., Bluestone, D.C., Rockette, H.E., and Beery, Q.C. (1980): *Ann. Otol. Rhinol. Laryngol.* 89(Suppl.):290–296.
8. Cantekin, E.I., Mandel, E.M., Bluestone, C.D., Rockette, H.E., Paradise, J.L., Stool, S.E., Fria, T.J., and Rogers, K.D. (1983): Lack of efficacy of a decongestant-antihistamine combination for otitis media with effusion ("secretory" otitis media) in children. *N. Engl. J. Med.*, 308:297–301.
9. Draper, W.L. (1967): Secretory otitis media. *Laryngoscope*, 78:636–641.
10. Fernandez, A.A., and McGovern, J.P. (1965): Secretory otitis media in allergic infants and children. *South. Med. J.*, 58:581–585.
11. Heisse, J.W. (1963). Secretory otitis media: treatment with depomethyl prednisolone. *Laryngoscope*, 73:54–59.
12. Henderson, F.W., Collier, A.M, Sanyal, M.A., Watkins, J.M., Fairclough, D.L., Clyde, W.A., Jr., and Denny, F.W. (1982): A longitudinal study of respiratory viruses and bacteria in the etiology of acute otitis media with effusion. *N. Engl. J. Med.*, 306:1377–1383.
13. Hopp, E.S., Elevitch, F.R., and Pumphrey, R.E. (1954): Serous otitis media: an immune theory. *Laryngoscope*, 74:1149–1159.
14. Hussl, B., and Lim, D. (1974): Experimental middle ear effusions: an immunofluorescent study. *Ann. Otol. Rhinol. Laryngol.*, 83:332–343.
15. Ishikawa, T.M.D., Bernstein, J.M., Reisman, R.E., and Arbesman, C.E. (1972): Secretory otitis media: immunologic study of middle ear secretions. *J. Allergy Clin. Immunol.*, 50:319–325.
16. Jordan, R., (1949): Chronic serous otitis media. *Laryngoscope*, 59:1002–1015.
17. King, J.T. (1953): The condition of fluid in the middle ear: factors influencing the prognosis in 56 children. *Ann. Otol.*, 62:498–506.
18. Klein, J.O. (1980): Microbiology of otitis media. *Ann. Otol. Rhinol. Laryngol.*,89(Suppl.):98–101.
19. Koch, H. (1947): Allergical investigation of chronic otitis. *Acta Otolaryngol. (Stockh.)* 62:(Suppl.)1–201.
20. Lecks, H.J. (1961): Allergic aspects of serous otitis media in childhood. *N.Y. State J. Med.*, 61:2737–2743.
21. Lewis, D.M., Schram, J.L., Lim, D.J., Birck, H.G., and Gleich, G. (1978): Immunoglobulin E in chronic middle ear effusions. *Ann. Otol. Rhinol. Laryngol.*, 87:197–201.
22. Lim, D.J., Liu, Y.S., Schram, J., and Birck, H.G. (1976): Immunoglobulin E in chronic middle ear effusions. *Ann. Otol. Rhinol. Laryngol.*, 85 (Suppl.):117–123.
23. Lim, D.J., Lewis, D.M., Schram, J.L., and Birck, H.G. (1979) Otitis media with effusion. cytological and microbiological correlates. *Arch. Otolaryngol.*, 105:404–412.
24. McGovern, J.P., Haywood, T.J., and Fernandes, A. (1967): Allergy and secretory otitis media. *J. Am. Med. Assoc.*, 200:124–128.
25. Miglets, A. (1973): The experimental production of allergic middle ear effusion. *Laryngoscope*, 83:1355–1384.
26. Mogi, G., Maeda, S., Yoshida, T., and Watanabe, N. (1976): Immunochemistry of otitis media with effusion. *J. Infect. Dis.*, 133:126–136.
27. Mogi, G., Maeda, S., Yoshida, T., and Watanabe, N. (1976): Radioimmunoassay study of IgE antibodies in middle ear effusions. *Acta Otolaryngol. (Stockh).*, 82:26–32.
28. Mogi, G., Maeda, S., and Watanabe, N. (1980): Immunofluorescent study on middle ear mucosa. *Ann. Otol. Rhinol. Laryngol.*, 89(Suppl.): 333–338.
29. Ogra, P.L., Bernstein, J.M., Yurchak, A.M., Coppola, P.R. and Tomasi, T.B., Jr. (1974): Characteristics of secretory immune system in human middle ear: implications in otitis media. J. Immunol., 112:488–495.
30. Paradise, J.L. (1980): Otitis media in infants and children. *Pediatrics*, 65:917–943.

31. Perisco, M., Podoshin, L., and Fradis, M. (1978): Otitis media with effusion: a steroid and antibiotic therapeutic trial before surgery. *Ann. Otol. Rhinol. Laryngol.,* 87:191–196.
32. Phillips, M.J., Knight, N.J., Manning, H., Abbott, A.L., and Tripp, W.G. (1974): IgE and secretory otitis media. *Lancet,* II:1176–1178.
33. Reisman, R.E., and Bernstein, J. (1975): Allergy and secretory otitis media: clinical and immunologic studies. *Pediatr. Clin. North Am.* 22:251–256.
34. Sarkkinen, H., Ruuskanen, O., Meurman, O., Puhakka, H., Virolainen, E., and Eskola, J. (1985): Identification of respiratory virus antigens in middle ear fluids of children with acute otitis media. *J. Infect. Dis.,* 151:444–448.
35. Schwartz, R.H., Puglese, J., and Schwartz, D.M., (1980): Use of a short course of prednisone for treating middle ear effusion: a double-blind crossover study. *Ann. Otol. Rhinol. Laryngol.,* 89(Suppl.):296–300.
36. Senturia, B.H. (1960): Allergic manifestations in otologic disease. *Laryngoscope,* 70:287–297.
37. Sloyer, J.L., Jr., Howie, V.M., Ploussard, J.H., Bradac, J., Habercorn, M., and Ogra, P.L.: Immune response to acute otitis media in children. III. Implications of viral antibody in middle ear fluid. *J. Immunol.,* 118:248–250.
38. Sloyer, J.L., Jr., Ploussard, J.H., and Karr, L.J. (1980): Otitis media in the young infant: an IgE-mediated disease? *Ann. Otol. Rhinol. Laryngol.,* 89(Suppl.):133–137.
39. Smirnov, P.P. (1938): Experiences visant à obtenir l'anaphylaxie des animaux au moyen des microbes et histolysats de l'orielle humaine. *Acta Otolaryngol. (Stockh.)* 26:1–17.
40. Solow, I.A. and Updegraff, W.C. (1958): Is serous otitis media due to allergy or infection? *Ann. Allergy,* 16:297–299.
41. Stempel, D.A., Clyde, W.A., Jr., Henderson, F.W., and Collier, A.M. (1980): Serum IgE levels and the clinical expression of respiratory illnesses. *J. Pediatr.,* 97:185–190.
42. Suehs, O.W. (1952): Secretory otitis media. *Laryngoscope,* 62:998–1027.
43. Virolainen, E., Puhakka, H., Aantaa, E., Tuohimaa, P., Ruuskanen, O., and Meurman, O.H. (1980): Prevalence of secretory otitis media in seven to eight year old school children. *Ann. Otol. Rhinol. Laryngol.* 89(Suppl.):7–10.
44. Viscomi, G.J. (1974): Allergic secretory otitis media: an approach to management. *Laryngoscope,* 85:751–758.
45. Welliver, R.C., Wong, D.T., Sun, M., Middleton, E., Jr., Vaughan, R.S., and Ogra, P.L. (1981): The development of respiratory syncytial virus-specific IgE and the release of histamine in nasopharyngeal secretions after infection. *N. Eng. J. Med.,* 305:841–846.
46. Welliver, R.C., Wong, D.T., Middleton, E., Jr., Sun, M., McCarthy, N., and Ogra, P.L. (1982): Role of parainfluenza virus-specific IgE in pathogenesis of croup and wheezing subsequent to infection. *J. Pediatr.,* 101:889–896.
47. Williams, R.L. (1966): Modern concepts in clinical management of allergy in otolaryngology. *Laryngoscope,* 76:1489–1515.
48. Yamashita, T., Okazaki, N., and Kumazawa, T. (1980): Relation between nasal and middle ear allergy: experimental study. *Ann. Otol. Rhinol. Laryngol.,* 89(Suppl.):147–152.

Immunology of the Ear, edited by J. Bernstein
and P. Ogra. Raven Press, New York © 1987.

Immunobiology of Acquired Aural Cholesteatoma

Bruce J. Gantz and Michael J. Hart

Department of Otolaryngology—Head and Neck Surgery, University of Iowa, Iowa City, Iowa 52242

Acquired aural cholesteatoma is a poorly understood sequella of chronic otitis media. This disease is characterized by the invasion of keratinizing stratified squamous epithelium into the normally aerated epitympanum and mesotympanum. When this occurs, a sequence of destructive events ensues which requires surgical intervention to prevent further functional impairment and potential life-threatening complications. Bone resorption is a prominent feature of cholesteatoma and contributes to the expanding nature of the disease. Evidence suggests that the cellular and biochemical events associated with the chronic inflammatory component of the cholesteatoma induce these destructive changes. However, the specific factors that regulate the inflammatory response in this disease are unknown. It has always been assumed that the keratinizing stratified squamous epithelium played a role, but evidence in support of this concept has been lacking in the past.

Certain chronic inflammatory reactions are regulated by cell-mediated immunologic mechanisms. Recently it has been shown that stratified squamous epithelium contains immunocompetent cells (epidermal Langerhans' cells) that activate cell-mediated immunologic mechanisms. Langerhans' cells have been identified in tissue specimens of aural cholesteatoma and may be important in the evolution and regulation of this disease. Studying the cutaneous immune system and contact hypersensitivity states may lead to further comprehension of the pathophysiology of acquired aural cholesteatoma. In addition, this information may provide more appropriate measures to control the disease. This chapter will review the morphology and pathophysiology of acquired aural cholesteatoma and will explore immunologic mechanisms that may contribute to the disease process.

MICROSCOPIC FEATURES OF ACQUIRED AURAL CHOLESTEATOMA

The light microscopic features of an acquired aural cholesteatoma (Fig. 1) consist of a layer of keratinizing stratified squamous epithelium overlaying a subepithelial connective tissue zone containing an abundant chronic inflammatory infil-

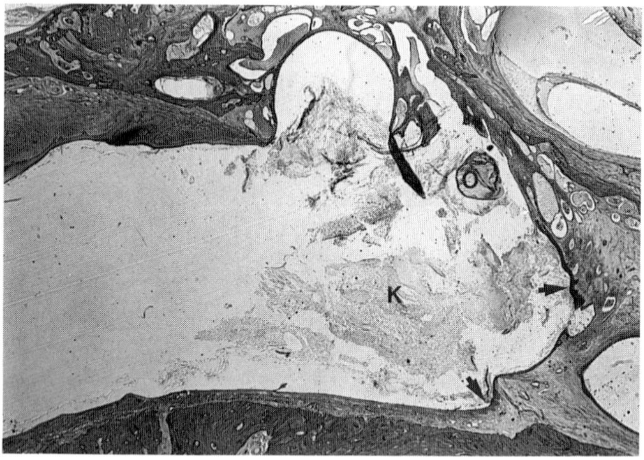

FIG. 1. Human acquired cholesteatoma. Keratinizing stratified squamous epithelium (*arrows*) lines cholesteatoma sac that extends into mesotympanum. Ossicle partially resorbed by disease (O). Keratin debris (K). (Hematoxylin and eosin, X1.)

trate. Desquamated epithelial debris accumulates in a sac-like structure created by the epithelial lining. These sac-like pockets arise predominantly in the pars flaccida region and/or the posterior superior quadrant of the tympanic membrane. It is unclear why some tympanic membrane retractions progress to develop into cholesteatomas, but there is general agreement that persistent eustachian tube dysfunction contributes to the formation (1,7). As the retraction pocket continues to expand into the recesses of the attic and antrum, the ability to remove desquamated keratin is reduced by its relatively narrow neck. A secondary infection consisting of mixed aerobic and anaerobic bacterial flora usually ensues, producing foul purulent otorrhea (6).

The subepithelial connective tissue zone always separates the epithelial layer of the cholesteatoma matrix from the underlying bone. This layer exhibits features of chronic granulation tissue with a rich vascular network and a mononuclear cell infiltrate consisting of macrophages, lymphocytes, and plasma cells (Fig. 2). In areas undergoing bone resorption, mononuclear inflammatory cells are most prominent at the resorption margin (Fig. 3). Multinucleated osteoclasts classically associated with bone breakdown are an infrequent finding in human cholesteatomas (4,10,25).

BIOCHEMISTRY AND IMMUNOBIOLOGY OF ACQUIRED AURAL CHOLESTEATOMA

Bone resorption in cholesteatoma is an active process requiring the biochemical activity of living cells. The biochemical mechanisms involved in the breakdown of bone are extremely complex and include demineralization, removal of glycopro-

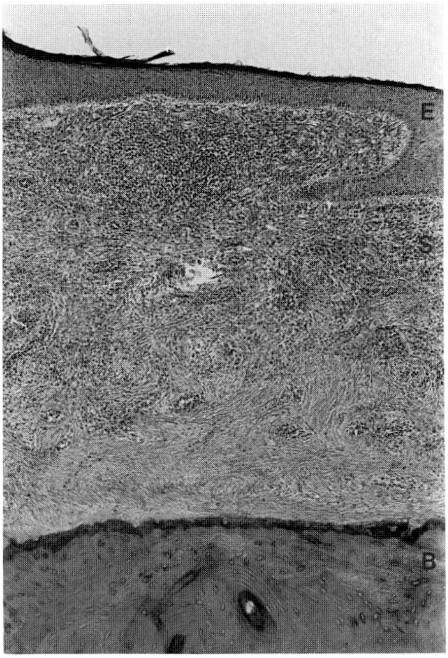

FIG. 2. Subepithelial connective tissue layer (S), consisting of chronic inflammatory cells and rich vascular network, separates the epithelium (E) of the cholesteatoma and the bone (B). (Hematoxylin and eosin, X40.)

tein ground substance, and collagenolysis. An ordered sequence of these events is required since the mineral protects the collagen from proteolytic enzyme attack (26). It is unclear what generates demineralization, but a localized lowering of the pH by acid hydrolases is suspected. Collagen hydrolysis is intitiated by the neutral protease, collagenase, but other enzymes such as elastase and cathepsin G may also participate. Following the cleavage of the collagen molecule, acid hydrolases continue the degradation process both intra- and extracellularly.

Our laboratory has been studying the granulation tissue-bone interphase to determine the precise cellular and biochemical events that promote bone destruction in acquired cholesteatoma. As mentioned previously, the cells commonly responsible for bone resorption, osteoclasts, are seldom seen at the resorption margin. In an attempt to identify the cells that were producing the biochemical environment for bone resorption, cytochemical and immunohistochemical staining techniques were employed (4,5). The predominant cell at the resorption margin, the macrophage, demonstrated both abundant intracellular acid phosphatase and extracellular collagenase. These cells also lacked the classic ''ruffled border'' associated with osteoclasts. The acid hyrolase, acid phosphatase, was also observed in osteocytes adjacent to areas of bone resorption, whereas osteocytes remote from bone degradation sites did not exhibit the enzyme. An obvious change to a secretory cytoplasmic organelle structure was also seen in osteocytes involved in the resorption process. These studies confirmed the destructive hydrolytic character of the cellular contents of acquired aural cholesteatoma, but did not explain its aggressive destructive nature when compared to chronic otitis media without cholesteatoma—especially

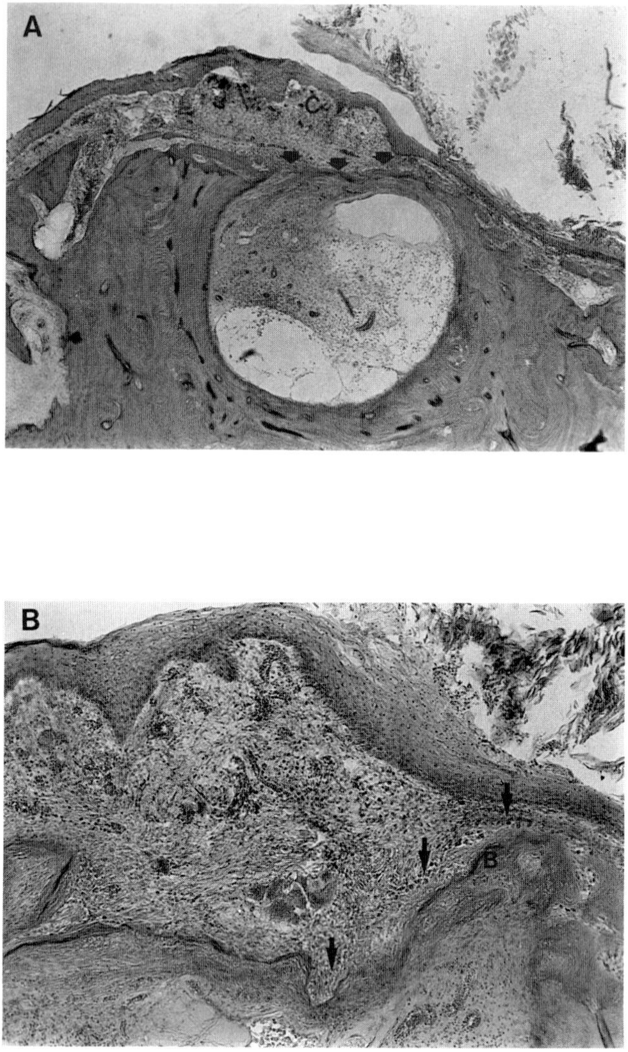

FIG. 3. Human cholesteatoma. **A**: Low-power X10 view of lateral semicircular canal fistula (*arrows*) with cholesteatoma matrix (C). **B**: High-power hematoxylin and eosin, X40 view of bone undergoing resorption with mononuclear inflammatory cells (*arrows*) along resorption margin (B). Note absence of osteoclast-like cells.

since histologically there is no apparent difference in the cellular makeup of the bone-granulation tissue zone between chronic otitis media with or without cholesteatoma (9). However, there is a vast clinical difference in the destructive activity of these two disease processes. Therefore, it is likely that the regulation of the cellular and biochemical environment of the chronic inflammatory subepithelial zone of the cholesteatoma is the key to understanding why there is much more destructive activity when keratinizing stratified squamous epithelium is involved in the disease process.

It has been recognized that chronic inflammatory states involving similar cellular features observed in acquired cholesteatoma are finely controlled by the cell-mediated immune system (13,14,27). Mononuclear phagocytes (macrophages and monocytes) and T (thymus-derived) lymphocytes are the cellular elements of cell-mediated immune mechanisms. Macrophages are known to be phagocytic but they also play an important role in the afferent and efferent limbs of the immune system. A physical interaction between macrophages and immunocompetent lymphocytes is necessary to activate the immune response. Antigen-presenting cells (macrophages, Langerhans' cells, and other mononuclear phagocytes) recognize given antigens and present them to T lymphocytes through direct physical contact. Antigen recognition occurs in association with surface class-II major histocompatability complex (MHC) glycoproteins, formerly referred to as surface I-region-associated (Ia) antigens. Surface class-II MHC glycoproteins are products of the I-region portion of DNA that migrate to the cell surface, where they are able to "associate" (mechanism unknown) with foreign antigen (Fig. 4). Helper T lymphocytes then can attach to the antigen-class-II MHC glycoprotein complex and recognize the antigen as foreign. Helper T lymphocytes cannot recognize antigens unless they are "associated" with antigen-presenting cells. This synergistic interchange activates a series of events which includes clonal propagation of lymphocytes, immunoregulatory and cytotoxic T cells, antibody formation, and secretion of inflammatory mediators (lymphokines). Lymphokines, in turn, evoke effector systems to neutralize the offending antigen by attracting new phagocytic *macrophages* to the site of antigen presentation and stimulating them to secrete hydrolytic substances. Some lymphokines also regulate the growth and differentiation of other *lymphocytes*. A number of hydrolytic enzymes have been identified and include lysosomal acid hydrolases (acid phosphatase), lysozyme, collagenase, and prostaglandins (2). In essence, a chronic inflammatory reaction is an expression of cell-mediated immune mechanisms regulated by the synergistic activity of mononuclear phagocytes and T lymphocytes that are geared to eliminate invading antigens (i.e., bacteria, foreign protein).

Similar antigen recognition and immunoregulatory functions have been recently observed in the epithelium. Epidermal Langerhans' cells, a minor cell type located in the suprabasal layer of the epidermis, have been the subject of intense investigation since it was recognized that lymphocytes cluster around these cells in contact hypersensitivity reactions (17). It is now accepted that Langerhans' cells play a prominent role in the cutaneous immune surveillance system functioning as anti-

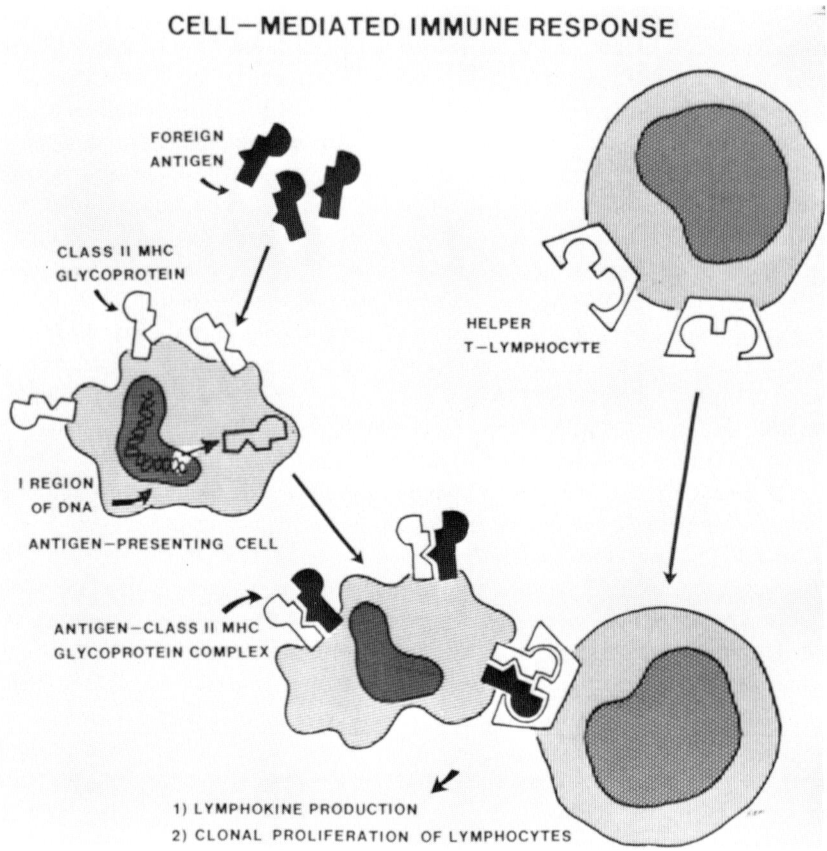

FIG. 4. Induction phase of cell-mediated immune response. Foreign antigen is recognized by mononuclear phagocyte (antigen-presenting cell). Antigen becomes associated with class-II MHC glycoprotein on the cell membrane. Class-II MHC glycoprotein is manufactured by I region of DNA. Antigen-class-II MHC glycoprotein is recognized by helper T lymphocyte. The synergistic interaction of mononuclear phagocyte and lymphocyte initiates effector phase system of cell-mediated immune response.

gen presenting cells similar to macrophages. These dendritic cells comprise 3% to 5% of the epidermal cell population, display mobility, and have unique ultrastructural cytoplasmic organelles (Birbeck granules) of unknown function (Fig. 5). Langerhans' cells are mesenchymal cells derived from, and are continuously repopulated from, a mobile pool of precursor cells originating in the bone marrow. Langerhans' cells are found in most keratinizing stratified squamous epithelium, including the external ear canal and tympanic membrane (3,10). They have not been identified in middle ear mucosa (8).

Epidermal Langerhans' cells bear surface receptors, Fc-IgG and C_3b, similar to macrophages, implicating an immunocompetence function (21). Also, some, but not all, Langerhans' cells express surface Ia antigens, or class-II MHC glycopro-

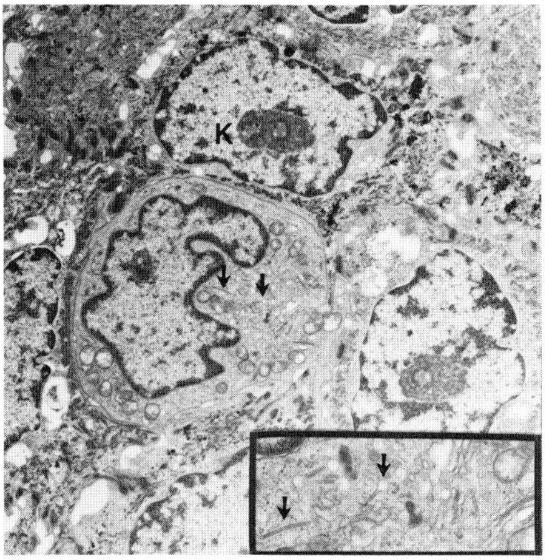

FIG. 5. Normal human ear-canal skin. Langerhans' cell (arrows point to Birbeck's granules). Cell is round with moderate lobulated nucleus. Cell membrane lacks intercellular bridges, characteristic of surrounding keratinocytes (K). (Uranyl acetate and lead citrate, X7,315.) Arrows in boxed area point to rod- and tennis-racket-shaped Birbeck's granules. (Uranyl acetate and lead citrate, X31,428.)

teins (23). In cutaneous hypersensitivity states, antigen processing and presentation is essential for induction of an immune response. It is thought that Langerhans' cells present immunologically relevant determinants to immunoreceptive helper T lymphocytes through cell-cell contact similar to other mononuclear phagocytes. Apposition of Langerhans' cells to lymphocytes has been observed in contact hypersensitivity reactions; however, following contact irritant application to the skin, this cellular apposition does not occur (17). Langerhans' cell-lymphocyte interaction can take place in the epidermis, dermis, or regional lymph node (18,20). *In vitro* and *in vivo* experimental evidence has now documented that Langerhans' cells can present antigens to T lymphocytes (22,24) and can generate a cytotoxic T-cell response (11).

Langerhans' cells may also participate in the effector limb of the immune response, but they engage in phagocytosis much less avidly than mononuclear phagocytes. Langerhans' cells with surface foreign antigen may be targets for cytotoxic T cells. Morphologic changes characteristic of increased secretory activity have been observed in Langerhans' cells at sites of contact hypersensitivity reactions. The ultrastructural cytoplasmic changes include increased prominent rough endoplasmic reticulum, Golgi apparatus, and lysosomes (19). Langerhans' cells may be the source of prostaglandin E and F at sites of contact hypersensitivity, but the evidence is indirect. Lymphokine production by Langerhans' cells has been suspected, and recently production of Interleukin-1 has been confirmed (16). The inflammatory response may also be intensified, in part, as a result of damage mediated by immune complexes and complement since these cells contain C_3b and Fc receptors. In summary, Langerhans' cells recognize antigen and present it to lymphocytes as part of the afferent limb of the cutaneous immune response. And, based on complement-dependent damage and observed morphologic changes, Langerhans' cells may also participate in a nonspecific effector response to antigen by inducing localized inflammation by releasing prostaglandins, lysosomal enzymes, and lymphokines similar to mononuclear phagocytes.

In view of what is known about the immunoregulatory function of the epithelium, are these mechanisms regulating the persistent inflammatory reaction in acquired aural cholesteatoma? One of the striking differences between normal ear canal and tympanic membrane epithelium and cholesteatoma epithelium is the increased number of epidermal Langerhans' cells in cholesteatoma (10). Veldman (28) and Gantz et al. (25) have confirmed this observation using monoclonal antibody staining techniques. We have also observed ultrastructural changes in cholesteatoma Langerhans' cells that appear similar to those that occur during contact hypersensitivity states (3). Langerhans' cells in human cholesteatomas (Fig. 6) exhibited increased Golgi apparatus, lysosomes, and prominent endoplasmic reticulum when compared to normal ear canal and tympanic membrane Langerhans' cells. These changes suggest increased secretory activity. Another important feature of the immune response was observed in acquired cholesteatomas. Langerhans' cells were found apposed to lymphocyte-like cells, suggesting cell-cell transfer of immunologic information as occurs in the afferent limb of the immune response reaction (Fig. 6). Specifically, we hypothesize that Langerhans' cells act as antigen-presenting cells in cholesteatoma, thus having similar function as in cutaneous contact hypersensitivity states.

The subepithelial granulation tissue zone of cholesteatomas has also been studied using monoclonal antibodies to determine the type of lymphocytes that participate in the inflammatory response (28,29). T lymphocytes were present in large numbers, whereas B lymphocytes were rarely seen. Analysis of the T-cell popula-

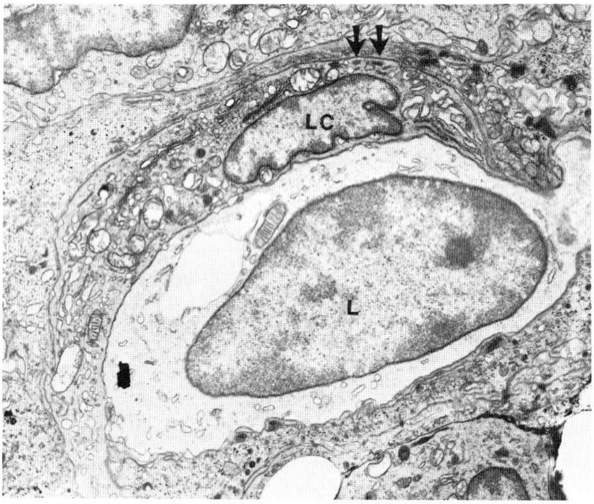

FIG. 6. Human cholesteatoma keratinizing stratified squamous epithelium. Langerhans' cell (LC) is adjacent to lymphocyte (L). The shape of the Langerhans' cell is different than a Langerhans' cell in normal epithelium, and cytoplasm contains more Golgi apparatus, mitochondria, and vacuoles, suggesting increased cellular activity. (Arrows point to Birbeck's granules.) Physical interaction of Langerhans' cell and lymphocyte suggests induction phase of cell-mediated immune response (Uranyl acetate and lead citrate, X11,070.)

tion revealed that most of these cells were cytotoxic/T-suppressor cells, but T-Helper/inducer cells were also present. These observations support the concept that cell-mediated immune mechanisms are active in acquired aural cholesteatoma. But their importance has yet to be elucidated. It seems likely that the immune response is generated against bacterial antigen or other foreign debris in the cholesteatoma sac. Langerhans' cells present this information to T lymphocytes, which activate a cytotoxic T-cell response. The combination of cytotoxic T cells, along with other mediators activated by the effector limb of the immune response, create a localized environment to destroy the offending antigen. The appearance of suppressor T cells in the subepithelial inflammatory zone is interesting and may explain the low-grade localized nature of the immune response.

It is generally assumed that eustachian tube dysfunction and chronic middle ear effusion plays an important role in cholesteatoma formation. Other questions need addressing in light of the immunoregulatory function discussed. For instance, what effect do inflammatory mediators found in chronic effusion have on the Langerhans' cells in the tympanic membrane? It has been shown experimentally that chronic inflammation, in the form of sterile granulomas, can induce proliferation of the basal epithelial cell layer of the tympanic membrane thus producing ingrowth (15). It has been speculated that Langerhans' cells may have a regulatory function controlling basal keratinocyte cell growth. If this does occur, activation of immune mechanisms may promote retraction pocket formation by stimulating keratinocyte growth in addition to activating the destructive elements of aural cholesteatomas.

Once a retraction pocket forms in the pars flaccida or posterior superior quadrant of the tympanic membrane, accumulation of keratin debris occurs because of the anatomic characteristics of the pocket (Fig. 7). The static condition induces a secondary infection. Bacteria or keratin debris can invade the stratum corneum while being recognized as antigens by the cutaneous immunoregulatory network. A cell-mediated inflammatory response is generated to eliminate the foreign antigen. The initial response fails to accomplish antigen elimination because of the persistent stasis and infection. Continued presence of the antigen most likely activates a contact hypersensitivity state. The effector limb of the immune response (Fig. 8), through lymphokine production, recruits increased numbers of macrophages to the site intensifying the inflammatory response. Hydrolytic enzyme production also increases, causing surrounding tissue breakdown, which continues expansion of the disease process.

Many of the mechanisms discussed above are unresolved, but identification of a cutaneous immune regulatory system helps to explain the aggressive and persistent nature of chronic otitis media when keratinizing stratified squamous epithelium is present. An animal model of acquired cholesteatoma is now being used to further document the role of the cutaneous immune system in this disease (12). Preliminary findings are supportive of the theory that acquired aural cholesteatoma should be considered a contact hypersensitivity epithelial disease. Future research directed toward influencing the cutaneous immune system of the ear may be helpful in eliminating this disease.

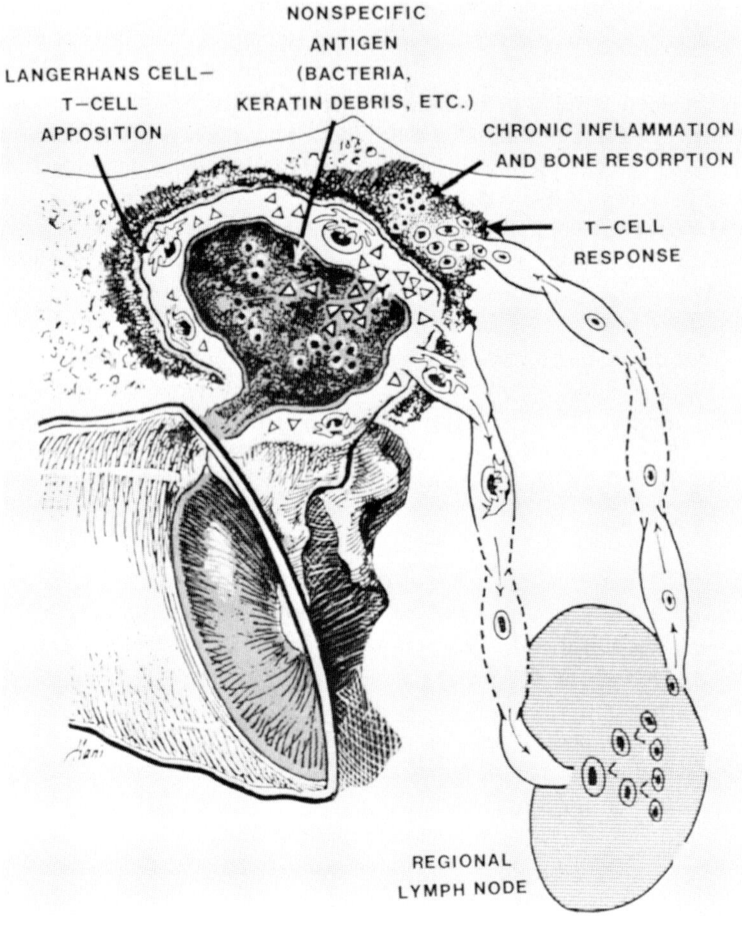

FIG. 7. Theoretical immunologic mechanisms in acquired cholesteatoma. Following mechanical formation of a tympanic-membrane retraction pocket, keratin debris accumulates in the sac. This static condition promotes bacterial infection. The bacteria or keratin debris invades the stratum corneum of the cholesteatoma epithelium and is recognized as a foreign antigen by the cutaneous immunoregulatory network (Langerhans' cells and T cells). The induction phase of the immune response generates a proliferation of cytotoxic T cells in regional lymph nodes which attempt to eliminate the offending antigen through the effector limb of the cell-mediated immune response. The combination of cytotoxic T lymphocytes and macrophages make up the chronic inflammatory infiltrate in the subepithelial layer of cholesteatoma which attempts to eliminate the antigen through hydrolytic enzyme production.

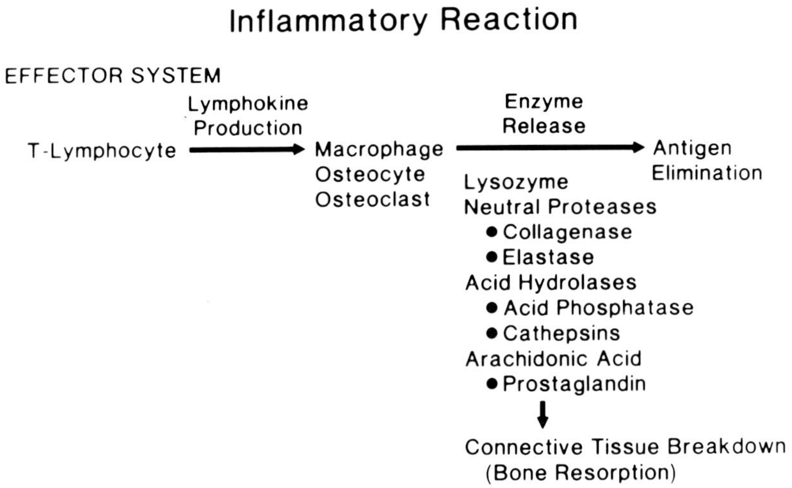

FIG. 8. Effector phase of the cell-mediated immune response.

ACKNOWLEDGMENT

The research for this chapter was funded, in part, by NIH Teacher Investigator Development Award 5 K07 NS00570 and the Deafness Research Foundation.

REFERENCES

1. Bluestone, C., Casselbrant, M., and Cantekin, E. (1982): Functional obstruction of the eustachian tube in the pathogenesis of aural cholesteatoma in children. In: *Cholesteatoma and Mastoid Surgery,* edited by J. Sade, pp. 211–214. Kugler Publications, Amsterdam.
2. Davies, P., and Bonney, R. (1979): Secretory products of mononuclear phagocytes: a brief review. *J. Reticuloendothelial Soc.,* 26:37–47.
3. Gantz, B. (1984): Epidermal Langerhans cells in cholesteatoma. *Ann. Otol Rhinol. Laryngol.,* 93:150–156.
4. Gantz, B., and Maynard, J. (1982): Ultrastructural evaluation of the biochemical events of bone resorption in human chronic otitis media. *Am. J. Otology,* 3:279–283.
5. Gantz, B., Maynard, J., Bumsted, R., Huang, C., and Abramson, M. (1979): Bone resorption in chronic otitis media. *Ann. Otol. Rhinol. Laryngol.,* 88:693–700.
6. Harker, L., and Koontz, F. (1977): Bacteriology of cholesteatoma. In: *Cholesteatoma 1st International Conference,* edited by B. McCabe, J. Sade, and M. Abramson, pp. 264–267. Aesculapius Publishing Co., Birmingham, Ala.
7. Harker, L., and Severeid, L. (1982): Cholesteatoma in the cleft palate patient. In: *Cholesteatoma and Mastoid Surgery,* edited by J. Sade, pp.37–40. Kugler Publications, Amsterdam.
8. Kawabata, I., and Paparell, M. (1969): Ultrastructure of normal human middle ear mucosa. *Ann. Otol. Rhinol. Laryngol.* 78:125–130.
9. Krane, S., Dayer, J., and Goldring, S. (1977): Aspects of bone resorption. In: *Cholesteatoma 1st International Conference,* edited by B. McCabe, J. Sade, and M. Abramson, pp.102–104. Aesculapius Publishing, Birmingham, Ala.
10. Lim, D., and Saunders, W. (1972): Acquired cholesteatoma. *Ann. Otol. Rhinol. Laryngol.,* 81:1–12.

11. Pehamberger, M.D., Stingl, L.H., Pogantsch, S., Steiner, G., Wolff, K., and Stingl, G. (1983): Epidermal cell induced generation of cytotoxic T-lymphocyte responses against alloantigens or TNP-modified syngenic cells: requirement for Ia positive Langerhans cells. *J. Invest. Dermatol.,* 81:108–124.
12. Ragheb, S., and Gantz, B. (1985): Factors influencing cholesteatoma formation in an animal model. Presented at the American Academy of Otolaryngology—Head and Neck Surgery, Annual Meeting, Atlanta, Georgia, October 20–24.
13. Rosenthal, A. (1980): Regulation of the immune response—role of the macrophage. *N. Engl. J. Med.,* 303:1153–1156.
14. Rosenwasser, L.J., Werdelin, O., Braendstrup, O., and Rosenthal, A.S. (1980): Physical and functional macrophage-lymphocyte interactions in antigen recognition by T-lymphocytes. In: *Mononuclear Phagocytes. Functional Aspects.,* edited by R. Van Furth pp.1887–1904., Marinus Nijhoff Publishers, The Hague/Boston/London.
15. Ruedi, L., and Spoendlin, H. (1959): Cholesteatoma formation in the middle ear in animal experiments. *Acta Otolaryngol. (Stockh),* 50:233.
16. Sauder, D.N., Dinarello, C.A., Morhenn, V.B. (1984): Langerhans cell production of Interleukin-1. *J. Invest. Dermatol.,* 82:605–607.
17. Silberberg, I. (1973): Apposition of mononuclear cells to Langerhans cells in contact allergic reaction. *Acta Derm. Venereol. (Stockh),* 53:1.
18. Silberberg, I. (1976): The role of Langerhans cells in allergic contact hypersensitivity. *J. Invest. Derm.,* 66:210.
19. Silberberg, I., Baer, R.L., and Rosenthal, S.H., (1974): The role of Langerhans cells in contact allergy. *Acta Derm. Venereol. (Stockh).* 54:321–333.
20. Silberberg-Sinakin, I, (1976): Antigen bearing Langerhans cells in skin, dermal lymphatics and lymph nodes. *Cell Immunol.* 25:137.
21. Stingl, G. (1977): Epidermal Langerhans cells bear Fc and C3 receptors. *Nature,* 268:245.
22. Stingl, G., Katz, S.I., Shevach, E.M., Rosenthal, A.S., and Green, I. (1978): Analogous functions of macrophages and Langerhans cells in the initiation of the immune response. *J. Invest. Dermatol.,* 71:59.
23. Streilien, J., and Bergstresser, P. (1984): Langerhans cells: antigen presenting cells of the epidermis. *Immunobiology,* 168:285–300.
24. Sullivan, S.J., Streinlein, J.W., Bergstresser, P.R., and Tigelaar, R.E. (1984): Hapten derivatized, purified epidermal Langerhans cells induce contact hypersensitivity without down regulation. *J. Invest. Derm.,* 82:440.
25. Thomsen, J., Balslev Jorgensen, M., Bretlau, P., and Kristensen, H. (1974): Bone resorption in chronic otitis media. A histological and ultrastructural study. *J. Laryngol. Otol.,* 88:983–992.
26. Thomsen, J., Tos, M., Nielsen, M., and Balslev Jorgensen, M. (1982): Bone destruction in inflammatory diseases of the ear. In: *Cholesteatoma and Mastoid Surgery.,* edited by J. Sade, pp.397–411. Kugler Publishing, Amsterdam.
27. Unanui, E. (1980): Cooperation between mononuclear phagocytes and lymphocytes in immunity *N. Engl. J. Med.* 303:977–985.
28. Veldman, J. (1985): The Langerhans T-cell microenvironment in aural cholesteatoma. In: *Immunobiology, Autoimmunity, Transplantation in Otorhinolaryngology.,* edited by J. Veldman, B. Huizing, and E. Mygind, pp.69–79. Kugler Publications, Amsterdam.
29. Veldman, J., Visser, C., Schuurman, H., de Groot, J., and Huizing, E. (1986): Immunobiology of Langerhans cells migrating into aural cholesteatoma.

Immunology of the Ear, edited by J. Bernstein and P. Ogra. Raven Press, New York © 1987.

Animal Models of Otitis Media with Effusion

G. Scott Giebink

Department of Pediatrics, University of Minnesota Medical School, Minneapolis, Minnesota 55455

Otitis media is characterized by a broad range of pathophysiologic events. Different types of middle ear inflammation are classified by duration of disease, effusion type, and characteristics of middle ear tissue histopathology. These various forms of otitis media occur along a continuum, are dynamically interrelated, and may at any one time represent an identifiable entity based on clinical findings and fluid characteristics (17).

A scheme for classifying otitis media based on the physical characteristics of middle ear fluid and on the presence of middle ear tissue pathology was suggested by Paparella (53); the classification was further defined by an Ad Hoc Committee on Definition and Classification of Otitis Media at the Second International Symposium on Recent Advances in Otitis Media with Effusion (64,65). The classification is based on duration of disease (acute, 0–3 weeks; subacute, 4–12 weeks; chronic, more than 3 months) and on effusion characteristics. Physical characteristics of effusions that are readily apparent on gross inspection include clarity (clear or cloudy) and viscosity (thin or thick). Serous effusion has been defined as a thin, clear liquid; mucoid effusion as a thick, usually cloudy liquid; and purulent effusion as a thin, cloudy liquid. The effusion of acute otitis media is most often purulent, whereas that of chronic otitis media with effusion (OME) in infants and preschool children is usually mucoid (22). In older children, mucoid and serous effusion occur with equal frequency.

RATIONALE FOR STUDYING OTITIS MEDIA IN ANIMAL MODELS

Recognizing the difficulty of studying the mechanisms of otitis media pathogenesis, as well as its natural history and treatment in humans, investigators turned to models of otitis media in animals over 60 years ago. Whereas there is a continued emphasis on relating mechanisms of disease pathogenesis learned in animal models to the human condition, it has become evident that animal models provide specific opportunities not available in human studies.

Among the advantages of otitis media animal models are the ability to control variables, to study potentially pathogenic stimuli in isolation, to make repeated observations under comparable conditions, to control the time course of the disease process, and to obtain sequential histological and biochemical information on cellular and fluid-phase events in the middle ear and adjacent tissues. Animal models provide an opportunity to study the embryogenesis and development of middle ear and eustachain tube tissues, the immune response, and the contribution of these elements to the pathogenesis of otitis media.

A number of animal models have been used to investigate possible etiologic factors and pathogenic mechanisms in otitis media, as well as to study the effect of therapeutic manipulation on pathogenesis (see Table 1). Otitis media has been induced in animals by (a) mechanical obstruction of the eustachian tube using liga-

TABLE 1. *Animal Models of Otitis Media with Effusion*

Experimental condition	Animal species	Results[a]
Mechanical eustachian tube obstruction	Squirrel monkey	SOM
	Chinchilla	SOM
	Cat	SOM → MOM
	Germfree rat	SOM
Functional eustachian tube obstruction	Dog, Rhesus monkey	SOM
Middle ear inoculation of viable bacteria		
S. pneumoniae	Chinchilla	POM → COM
H. influenzae, nontypable	Chinchilla	POM
Anaerobes	Gerbil, guinea pig	Middle ear histopathology
Middle ear inoculation of nonviable bacteria		
S. pneumoniae	Chinchilla	Mild middle ear inflammation, minimal effusion, mild COM
H. influenzae, nontypable	Chinchilla	SOM
H. influenzae, type b	Chinchilla	SOM
Nasal inoculation of viable *S. pneumoniae* with middle ear deflation	Chinchilla	POM → COM
Nasal inoculation of viable *S. pneumoniae* and influenza A virus	Chinchilla	POM → COM
Passive sensitization with human sera and middle ear challenge	Squirrel monkey, guinea pig	SOM

[a]SOM, serous otitis media; MOM, mucoid otitis media; POM, purulent otitis media; COM, chronic otitis media.

tion and cauterization of the tubal lumen or blockage with foreign objects, (b) functional obstruction of the eustachian tube after manipulating the paratubal muscles or nasopharyngeal architecture, (c) inoculating microbes or their products into the bulla or middle ear cavity, (d) inoculating foreign bodies or viscous fluids into the bulla or middle ear cavity, (e) inoculating microbes or their products into the nasopharynx, and (f) applying negative pressure to the middle ear cavity or bulla.

The role of the eustachian tube and middle ear physiology in the pathogenesis of otitis media can be studied in detail using animal models. The role of pathogenic, as well as presumably nonpathogenic, bacteria in the upper respiratory tract in the development of otitis media after eustachian tube obstruction has been demonstrated in animal models and is specifically addressed in the chapter by Kuijpers and van der Beek (*this volume*).

The variability of middle ear and systemic responses to bacterial strains of the same species but of different serotypes, including strains of *Streptococcus pneumoniae* and nontypable *Hemophilus influenzae*, has been demonstrated. Adhesion of bacteria to respiratory epithelial cells has been studied in animal models, permitting further study of the contribution of bacterial adhesion to nasopharyngeal, eustachian tube, and middle ear epithelial cells in the pathogenesis of otitis media.

Local versus systemic immune defense mechanisms can be studied in animal models. The immunoglobulin class-specific content of middle ear effusion in experimental otitis media has been measured and compared with the immunoglobulin content of human middle ear effusion (MEE). Methods to obtain macrophages from MEE during experimentally induced otitis media have been developed, suggesting that there will be a way to investigate cellular defense systems in the middle ear space. Models to study immune-complex-mediated otitis media have been developed. The availability of animal species with defined and well-characterized immunological deficiencies and the ability to restore critical elements of host defense, such as specific antibody and sensitized lymphocytes, and to deplete elements of host defense, such as complement and certain leukocyte subclasses, permit the study of the contribution of individual elements of host defense in otitis media.

Local middle ear, upper respiratory tract, and systemic immune responses to the presence of antigens in the middle ear space have been studied in animal models. Persistent otitis media and middle ear mucoperiosteal pathology have been examined after eradication of viable bacteria from the middle ear space by antibiotic treatment. That middle ear mucoperiosteal pathology can be caused solely by nonviable *S. pneumoniae* and *H. influenzae* in the middle ear space has been demonstrated, and a search is in progress to identify the subcellular products that cause middle ear pathology.

Models have been used to characterize the effect of inflammatory mediators in the middle ear. Differences and sequential changes in the enzymatic, protein, cytologic, and inflammatory mediator composition of serous, mucoid, and purulent MEE in isolation and in combination have been demonstrated.

Identification of otitis media in animal models can be accomplished by noninvasive and invasive methods. The possibility of employing invasive methods is an inherent advantage of the animal model since such procedures cannot be used in humans. Invasive methods are more comprehensive in assessing the total ear condition. The most definitive method to establish this condition is histopathological examination of temporal bones. The importance of histopathologic assessment was recently illustrated by Meyerhoff et al. (46), who reported extensive residual middle ear disease in chinchillas with normal tympanic membranes and among chinchillas with disease-free middle ears according to otoscopic and tympanometric assessment. However, progression of the disease in individual animals is best documented by inspection of the middle ear cavity through a bullar opening or tympanocentesis and aspiration of the contents of middle ear. These procedures are useful for determining the presence or absence of effusion and to perform laboratory tests on the fluid contents of the middle ear.

Animal species most frequently used for otitis media research include the Rhesus and squirrel monkey, cat, dog, guinea pig, rabbit, mouse, Mongolian gerbil, and chinchilla. The chinchilla is ideally suited as an animal model for studying purulent and serous otitis media (POM and SOM, respectively) because the chinchilla (a) is small, (b) has auditory capabilities quite similar to those of humans, (c) has a cochlea with a membranous architecture similar to the human cochlea, (d) does not manifest presbycusis in long-term studies, (e) lacks susceptibility to naturally occurring middle ear infections that are common to the guinea pig and rabbit (f) are reasonably inexpensive to obtain and maintain, (g) has a large middle ear cavity with a volume of 1.0 to 1.5 ml, and (h) has a reasonably well-characterized humoral and cellular immune system. Chinchillas have been used to develop models of (a) POM caused by *S. pneumoniae* and nontypable *H. influenzae* and (b) SOM following mechanical and functional eustachian tube obstruction. Moreover, chinchillas are susceptible to influenza A virus infection, thereby permitting study of dual respiratory virus-bacteria infections in this model.

A variety of biochemical and immunochemical studies on middle ear fluids from chinchillas with SOM and POM have been conducted and compared with human middle ear fluids. A great deal has been learned about the immunochemical response during acute otitis media using the chinchilla animal model. Moreover, the efficacy of active immunization using pnuemococcal polysaccharide vaccines in preventing vaccine-type experimental pneumococcal otitis media has been studied in the chinchilla. Recently, chinchilla immunoglobulins have been fractionated from chinchilla serum (69,70), and the specific immunoglobulin contents of middle ear fluids and serum have been studied. A sensitive enzyme-linked immunoabsorbent assay employing antisera to these immunoglobulin fractions has been developed to measure immunoglobulins and specific antibodies in middle ear fluids (6).

Animal models for studying other aspects of otitis media pathogenesis, principally, eustachian tube function, have been developed in other animal species—notably dogs, cats, and squirrel monkeys. Chinchillas have also been used for these investigations, but chronic otitis media and otitis media sequelae seem more comparable to the human disease in cat and Rhesus monkey models.

MODELS EMPLOYING MECHANICAL EUSTACHIAN TUBE OBSTRUCTION

Middle ear effusion was first produced experimentally by Beck (3) in dogs by mechanically obstructing the eustachian tube. Subsequently, a number of investigators reported different methods for creating mechanical tubal obstruction in dogs, cats, and squirrel monkeys (30,38,52,55,57,59–63,64). Using a piece of fine-grade silicone sponge, the eustachian tubes of squirrel monkeys, cats, chinchillas, and rabbits were obstructed. These middle ears manifested early negative pressure followed by widening of the subepithelial space as a result of vascular dilatation and transudation of serous fluid from the small vessels (32,33). After 1 week of eustachian tube obstruction, there was a mild inflammatory reaction in the subepithelial space with infiltration of polymorphonuclear (PMN) leukocytes, lymphocytes, and some plasma cells (32). Early metaplasia and hyperplasia of the epithelium was also identified at this time. Within 2 weeks, epithelial metaplasia advanced with marked goblet cell formation. Fibroblastic activity was identified as was osteoneogenesis in the subepithelial space. Later, MEE became viscous and contained increased levels of lactate dehydrogenase, lysozyme, hexosamine, immunoglobulins, and total protein. With prolonged eustachian tube obstruction the middle ear mucosa became almost totally metaplastic, MEE became mucoid, and fibroblastic activity and osteoneogenesis dominated the subepithelial space. Culture of the MEE was almost always sterile.

In the cat, inflammatory changes after tubal obstruction involve the entire middle ear cleft, including mucoperiosteum, middle ear muscles, and round window membrane (27,56). Early tympanostomy tube insertion after tubal ligation prevented development of MEE (7), but subtotal removal of the tympanic membrane 1 week after obstruction did not prevent the inflammatory changes seen in non-tubed ears (28). Thus, once the inflammatory process is intitiated in the middle ear, it apparently cannot be easily reversed by surgical middle ear ventilation.

The cat model has also been utilized to investigate the relationship between MEE and hearing loss (71,72). The pattern of hearing loss fluctuated between 10 dB and 40 dB over the 1 year follow-up period. Hearing loss was directly related to effusion volume and to effusion viscosity or density.

The isolated effect of tubal obstruction without the confounding variable of middle ear infection has been studied in germfree rats by Kuijpers et al. (35) and is thoroughly discussed in the chapter by Kuijpers and van der Beek (*this volume*). The high incidence of infectious middle ear disease after tubal obstruction in conventionally raised animals suggested that tubal obstruction enhanced the development of otitis media caused by both known pathogens and created circumstances for pathological behavior of nonpathogen symbionts of normal middle ear and upper respiratory flora. Tos (68) reproduced these observations in germfree rats, documenting the transformation of epithelial cells to secretory cells without infection in the middle ear mucosa.

MODELS EMPLOYING FUNCTIONAL EUSTACHIAN TUBE DYSFUNCTION

In 1930 Claus (8) induced MEE in dogs by interfering with the tensor veli palatini muscle function after severing its tendon, injecting paraffin into the muscle, and severing its attachment to the hamulus; experimental palate clefting also led to the accumulation of MEE. Subsequently, Odoi et al. (51) studied the effect of pterygoid hamulotomy and tensor veli palatini muscle excision in cats on eustachian tube function and on the middle ear condition; Misurya (49) investigated the effects of transposition of the tensor veli palatini muscle in dogs.

Excision or transection of the tensor veli palatini muscle in Rhesus monkeys also caused eustachian tube dysfunction and OME (4,5). Muscle excision led to chronic sterile MEEs. Muscle transection caused abnormal middle ear pressures, or effusion, or both, which returned to normal in some ears, but effusion was recurrent or chronic in other ears. Muscle transposition caused immediate postoperative middle ear and eustachian tube dysfunction, similar to animals with muscle excision, but function improved within a short time after surgery.

Eustachian tube dysfunction is known to occur in children with cleft palate (54), and this condition has been replicated in animal models. Palate clefting in Rhesus monkeys caused functional obstruction of eustachian tube with high negative middle ear pressures soon after surgery, and high positive middle ear pressures later (11). Nearly all animals developed recurrent OME, and the effusions were sterile for bacteria. Tubal function was more severly affected in these infant Rhesus monkeys compared with the juvenile animals (13).

Mechanical clefting of the chinchilla's soft palate also led to an abrupt fall in middle ear pressure and the appearance of MEE. Within 3 to 4 weeks, granulation tissue and osteogenesis is developed (43). These changes were avoided by intubating the tympanic membrane prior to palate clefting, suggesting that the middle ear events following palate clefting were a result of the associated eustachian tube dysfunction and subsequent absorption of middle ear gases and negative middle ear pressure (9,43,44).

MODELS EMPLOYING MIDDLE EAR INOCULATION OF VIABLE BACTERIA

Hayman (29) first demonstrated that inoculation of bacteria into the middle ear cavity of guinea pigs resulted in MEE. Friedmann (14) expanded these experiments by inoculating eight different bacterial species into the middle ears of guinea pigs. The model has been most widely used, however, to study pneumococcal otitis media.

Experimental pneumococcal otitis media has been studied in chinchillas following direct middle ear inoculation of *S. pneumoniae* types 3, 6A, 7F, 18C, and 23B (16,18,21,37,40,66). Otitis media was uniformly produced by inoculating as few as 20 colony-forming units (cfu) of viable pneumococci into the middle ear space.

Extensive study of the natural history of otitis media caused by *S. pneumoniae* showed that during the first 3 days after inoculation, bacteria remained localized in the middle ear fossa (16). Dissemination of pneumococci to peripheral blood and occasionally, then, to cerebrospinal fluid was demonstrated during the latter half of the first week after inoculation in as many as 50% of the animals infected with certain pneumococcal serotypes. Spontaneous resolution of MEE began during the second week and was associated with diminished acute mucoperiosteal inflammatory cells and increasing numbers of subepithelial fibroblasts. Clearing of pneumococci from the middle ear was nearly complete after 6 weeks although subepithelial thickening persisted.

Histologic study of temporal bones obtained from chinchillas infected by intrabullar inoculation with *S. pneumoniae* revealed almost every type of tissue pathology previously described for otitis media in humans. Positive middle ear culture and histologic changes compatible with acute inflammation (subepithelial edema, MEE, diffuse infiltration and exudation of polymorphonuclear leukocytes, subepithelial hemorrhage, and hyperemia) were identified as clearly as 2 to 3 days following direct inoculation. These acute changes persisted for approximately 2½ weeks, at which time more chronic findings, such as sterile MEE, lymphocyte infiltration, osteoneogenesis, granulation tissue, and epithelial metaplasia, appeared. Similarly, inner ear changes, when present, become intractable with time, resulting in destruction of the membranous labyrinth and labyrinthitis ossificans (42).

The response of chinchillas to direct middle ear inoculation of type b *H. influenzae* (Hib) and nontypable *H. influenzae* (NTHi) has been studied in three laboratories (12,22,34). Middle ear infection was more aggressive with universal bacteremia and meningitis after inoculation of the encapsulated Hib strain (22). After inoculation of nontypable strains, otitis media without bacteremia was observed. Sterile serous MEE persisted in one study for an average of 11 days after bacteria were cleared from the middle ear, suggesting that this may be a model for studying persistent postinfectious MEE (34).

The NTHi model has been used to examine the response of previously infected chinchillas to rechallenge with homologous and heterologous NTHi strains (12,34). Animals challenged by repeat intrabullar inoculation with the same organism after resolution of the intitial infection showed a reduced incidence of otitis media in both the previously infected ear as well as in the previously uninfected contralateral ear. A serologic response to outer-membrane protein antigens of both NTHi strains was observed, and strain-specific protective immunity was demonstrated upon rechallenge (34). Animals rechallenged with a heterologous NTHi strain had a course similar to animals experiencing the initial infection.

The NTHi model was used to determine the efficacy of sulbactam, a penicillanic acid sulfone combined with ampicillin, in treating experimental otitis media caused by a β-lactamase-producing NTHi (58). Fourteen days after inoculation, all ears in the combined treatment group were culture-negative, whereas NTHi was cultured from 70% of the effusions in the ampicillin group. Thus, the chinchilla animal model of otitis media appears to be a useful *in vivo* method for evaluating the efficacy of new antimicrobial agents.

Fulghum et al. (15) and Thore et al. (67) examined the pathogenic potential of anaerobic bacteria in the middle ear of Mongolian gerbils and guinea pigs, respectively. Direct middle ear inoculation of gerbils with *Corynebacterium* species (isolated from the ear fluid of a child with otitis media) produced striking middle ear mucoperiosteal inflammation, whereas inoculation of *Streptococcus intermedius* or *Propionibacterium acnes* produced transient, mild inflammation (15). In contrast, *P. acnes* inoculated into the middle ear of guinea pigs produced inflammation with effusion; the response to *Peptostreptococcus micros* was weak and irregular; and no effects of *Bacteroides asaccharolyticus* were observed (67). Thus, certain anaerobic bacteria may be pathogens in the human middle ear, and the contribution of anaerobes in polymicrobic infection of the middle ear remains to be determined.

MODELS EMPLOYING MIDDLE EAR INOCULATION OF NONVIABLE BACTERIA

The pattern of middle ear injury in chinchillas following inoculation of heat-killed type 23B *S. pneumoniae* was studied by Lowell et al. (39). Edema of the subepithelial space accompanied by mild inflammatory response and epithelial metaplasia was observed in the middle ear mucosa of these animals. Osteoneogenesis was seen within 3 weeks in the subepithelial space of these animals. Similarly, sterile MEE and an extensive middle ear inflammatory response was observed in chinchillas after middle ear inoculation of formalin-killed Hib and NTHi (10). The mechanism of injury from these nonviable organisms may be related to inflammatory activities of cell envelope components. In the case of pneumococcus, substances such as the peptidoglycan-teichoic acid cell wall or cell membrane or type-specific capsular polysaccharide substances may have caused inflammation. With *H. influenzae*, the likely cell-wall mediator of inflammation is endotoxin. The fact that nonviable bacteria are capable of producing middle ear inflammation in animal models suggests that bacterial cell-wall substances may persist in human middle ear tissues after antimicrobial treatment of acute otitis media and contribute to the persistence of OME.

MODELS EMPLOYING INTRANASAL INOCULATION WITH VIABLE BACTERIA

Although chinchillas can be readily colonized intranasally using *S. pneumoniae* inocula having between 10^4 and 10^7 cfu, otitis media rarely ensued unless middle ear ventilation was altered (21). In an attempt to reproduce conditions observed in humans with otitis media, negative pressure (deflation) was applied to the middle ear cavity following intranasal inoculation of pneumococcus by inserting a 23-gauge needle attached to a mercury manometer into the epitympanic bulla (19). Nearly two-thirds of the animals developed pneumococcal otitis media with purulent effusion during the following 7 days. Tympanograms showed a direct relationship between the duration of negative pressure after mechanical deflation and the development of otitis media; animals in which the pressure in the middle ear returned to normal within 4 days after deflation did not develop otitis media (23). Purulent effusion was occasionally preceded by a sterile serous effusion. Purulent effusions gradually become sterile, and by 4 weeks after inoculation, dense granulation tissue was found in the epitympanic and midtympanic space of previously infected ears. Culture of the granulation tissue, however, yielded pneumococci in only one ear. Middle ear histopathology after pneumococcal inoculation of the nares, followed by negative middle ear pressure, paralleled that observed in animals whose ears were directly inoculated with pneumococci (45).

Local and systemic immune responses were measured after nasal inoculation of pneumococci. Animals that did not develop pneumococcal otitis media had significantly higher levels of serum antibody before nasal inoculation than did animals that developed otitis. Middle ear effusions collected 3 or more weeks after inoculation from ears that had been infected previously but were sterile at the time of collection all contained high concentrations of antibody (21). Likewise, most sterile effusions obtained during the first 3 weeks after inoculation contained antibody concentrations that were equal to or greater than serum concentrations. The concentrations of antibody in effusions that harbored viable pneumococci were less than serum. These results suggested that local concentration of anti-pneumococcal antibody might be important for preventing middle ear infection and for resolving infection. To test this hypothesis, experiments have been performed to examine the ability of prior infection and of active immunization to prevent homologous pneumococcal otitis media in chinchillas.

Lewis et al. (37) and Marshak et al. (40) found that repeated pneumococcal inoculations of the middle ear rendered the ear resistant to a subsequent homologous infection. Comparing intramuscular, intranasal, and intratympanic immunization with formalinized type-3 pneumococcus, Lewis et al. (37) reported that the frequency and severity of subsequent type-3 pneumococcal otitis media was reduced only in animals previously immunized by the intratympanic route. In two other studies, unilateral middle ear inoculation with pneumococcus reduced the susceptibility of animals to subsequent ipsilateral, but not contralateral, rechallenge with the same pneumococcal strain (40,66). Middle ear effusion antibody levels were higher in previously infected than in uninfected ears, but the concentration of pneumococcal antibody in serum did not correlate with protection from subsequent pneumococcal otitis media (40).

The role of systemic vaccination with purified pneumococcal capsular polysaccharides in preventing vaccine-type pneumococcal otitis media has been studied in chinchillas and in humans (18,19,24). Subcutaneous vaccination with purified pneumococcal polysaccharide elicited a significant rise in serum antibody in approximately two-thirds of vaccinated chinchillas (24). Animals that developed increased serum antibody after vaccination and were subsequently challenged by intranasal pneumococcal inoculation with middle ear deflation showed an 87% reduction in vaccine-type pneumococcal otitis media (19).

These studies suggest that (a) pneumococcal otitis media confers local protection against subsequent otitis media caused by the homologous pneumococcal type, (b) protection following infection is a result of enhanced local, rather than systemic, defenses, yet (c) systemic parenteral immunization with the capsular polysaccharide of one type (type 7F), but not another (type 3), confers local protection against the vaccine type.

MODELS EMPLOYING INTRANASAL INOCULATION OF BACTERIA AND RESPIRATORY VIRUS

Since middle ear deflation experiments showed a direct relationship between persistent negative middle ear pressure and development of otitis media, and because observations in humans indicated that negative middle ear pressure often accompanied respiratory virus infection (61), an animal model was developed to examine the hypothesis that upper respiratory tract viral infection predisposes animals colonized intranasally with *S. pneumoniae* to pneumococcal otitis media (20). Four different influenza A virus strains were tested in the chinchilla for infectivity. A multiply passaged H1N1 laboratory strain (influenza A/NWS/33), two wild-type clinical isolates (an H3N2, A/Alaska/6/77 strain; and a H1N1, A/Hong Kong/123/77 strain), and a cold-adapted H3N2 recombinant vaccine strain (CR29) were all found to infect chinchillas (25).

Infection of chinchillas with the laboratory-passaged H1N1 strain and the wild-type H3N2 strain led to the development of high negative middle ear pressure and increasing tympanic membrane inflammation during the first week after inoculation. However, MEE was not discernible by otoscopy or tympanometry in these animals. In contrast, infection with the wild-type H1N1 strain and the CR29 vaccine strain caused little evidence of middle ear inflammation.

Infection with the laboratory-passaged H1N1 strain and the wild-type H3N2 strain caused a marked depression in PMN leukocyte chemiluminescent, chemotactic, and bactericidal activity during the latter half of the first week after virus inoculation (1,2,25). It was found that PMN phagocytic activity remained normal during infection. Thus, influenza virus appeared to alter intracellular oxidative metabolism and bactericidal activity by a mechanism independent of phagocytosis. Others have found evidence that influenza A virus impairs lysosomal granule fusion, with the phagocytic vacuole as a possible explanation for reduced PMN bactericidal activity (31).

In the presence of pneumococcal colonization of the nasopharynx, infection with the laboratory-passaged H1N1 influenza strain and wild-type H3N2 influenza strain significantly increased the incidence of pneumococcal otitis media, whereas infection with the wild-type H1N1 strain and the vaccine CR29 strain did not significantly increase the incidence of otitis (25). The greatest incidence of pneumococcal otitis media (90%) and bacteremia (40%) occurred in animals inoculated with pneumococcus 6 days after influenza virus inoculation (2).

The laboratory-passaged H1N1 influenza strain and the wild-type H3N2 strain significantly impaired the clearance of pneumococci from the nasopharynx during the first week after virus inoculation (25). Impaired bacterial clearance paralleled desquamation of ciliated epithelium in the nasopharyngeal portion of the eustachian tube (26).

Histologic study of chinchilla temporal bones following nasopharyngeal inoculation with *S. pneumoniae* and influenza A virus manifested changes of acute POM within 1 week of inoculation (46). The spectrum of acute to chronic changes was observed as time progressed, including hemorrhage, hyperemia, edema, leukocyte infiltration, granulation tissue, and osteoneogenesis (Figs. 1 and 2).

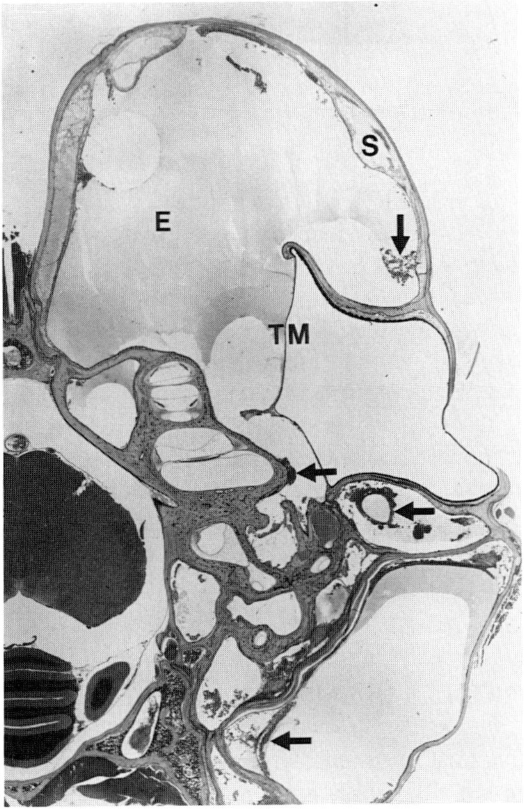

FIG. 1. Middle ear bulla of chinchilla with POM showing effusion (E), edema of the subepithelial space (S), and isolated collections of PMN leukocytes (*arrows*). The tympanic membrane (TM) in this case shows no histopathology. X7.

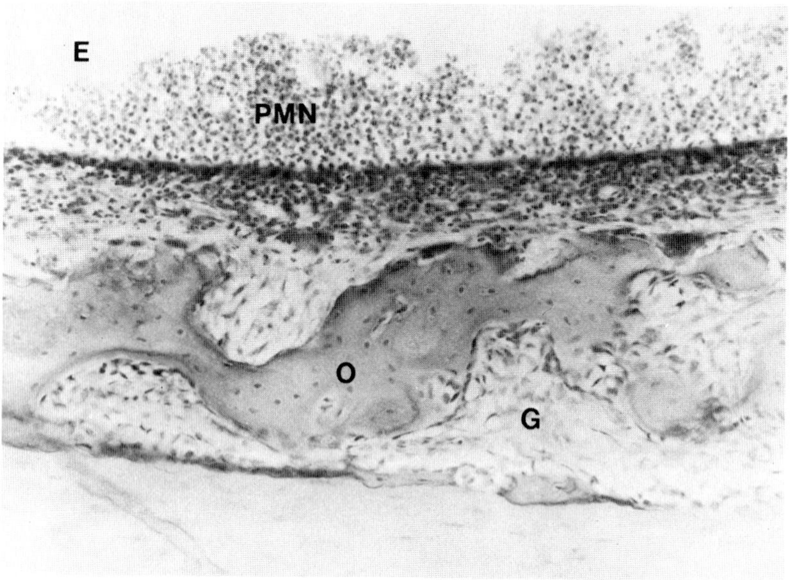

FIG. 2. Higher magnification of middle ear bulla pathology showing abundant PMN leukocytes in effusion (E), as well as osteoneogenesis (O) and granulation tissue (G) in the subepithelial space. X100.

To determine the relative contribution of the various host defense abnormalities produced by influenza A virus to otitis media pathogenesis, unilateral tympanostomy tubes were placed in the tympanic membrane of chinchillas prior to influenza virus and pneumococcus inoculation. Tympanic membrane inflammation occurred significantly more often in nontubed than tubed ears, suggesting that influenza-induced negative middle ear pressure was required for some of the inflammatory changes leading to OME. However, the incidence of culture-positive purulent effusion was similar in tubed and nontubed ears, and the temporal bone histopathology indicated that middle ear mucoperiosteal inflammatory changes were similar in tubed and nontubed ears (46). Therefore, abnormalities of middle ear ventilation were not solely responsible for the development of otitis media in this animal model.

MODELS OF IMMUNE-MEDIATED OME

A model of otitis media presumably caused by an immediate hypersensitivity response has been reported; MEE was produced in squirrel monkeys following passive sensitization with allergic human sera and challenge with various allergens (47,48). Yamashita et al. (73) reported an allergic challenge to the nasal mucosa of guinea pigs but related this model to otitis media when the bulla was directly challenged. Challenge of the nasal mucosa itself did not result in OME.

In considering the contribution of bacteria in the pathogenesis of OME, the role of immune complexes and of complement-mediated tissue damage must be considered. Immune complexes have been demonstrated in human MEE, as was C3 proactivator (41). Others have shown lowered levels of complement components in effusion, suggesting that complement activation occurred (32,36). Mravec et al. (50) injected immune complexes, prepared by mixing rabbit serum with goat anti-rabbit serum, into the middle ear bullae of chinchillas and observed intense mucoperiosteal inflammation within 24 hr; control ears inoculated with either serum or antiserum alone showed no inflammation. However the role of immune complexes is thoroughly discussed in Pellner's chapter (*this volume*), and the general opinion is that immune complexes probably do not contribute to the pathogenesis of otitis media, but more likely are found as a result of normal elimination of bacteria.

SUMMARY

The ability to control variables in animal models has led to an increased understanding of otitis media pathogenesis. Bacterial infection of the middle ear tissues and eustachian tube dysfunction are principal etiologic mechanisms. The host responses to these conditions, including local and, perhaps, systemic immune responses, appear to determine the outcome of the initial inflammation. Viral infection with respiratory viruses, such as influenza A virus, may be the basis for eustachian tube dysfunction and subsequent POM in young children, as had been demonstrated in an animal model. Based on these observations, effective strategies for treating otitis media would include antibacterial and anti-inflammatory therapies. Active or passive immunization against certain respiratory viruses or bacterial pathogens, such as *S. pneumoniae* and NTHi, might be effective in preventing otitis media.

ACKNOWLEDGMENTS

The research for this chapter was supported, in part, by grant no. AI 17160 from the National Institute of Allergy and Infectious Diseases and by grant no. NS 14538 from the National Institute of Neurological and Communicative Disorders and Stroke.

REFERENCES

1. Abramson, J.S., Giebink, G.S., Mills, E.L., and Quie, P.G. (1981): Polymorphonuclear leukocyte dysfunction during influenza virus infection in chinchillas. *J. Infect. Dis.*, 143:836–845.
2. Abramson, J.S., Giebink, G.S., and Quie, P.G. (1982): Influenza A virus-induced polymorpho-

nuclear leukocyte dysfunction in the pathogenesis of experimental pneumococcal otitis media. *Infect. Immun.*, 36:289–296.

3. Beck, K. (1919): Uber mittelohrveranderungen bei experimenteller lasion der tube. *S. Ohrenheilk.* 78:83–108.
4. Cantekin, E.I., Bluestone, D.C., Saez, C.A., Doyle, W.J. and Phillips, D.C. (1977): Normal and abnormal middle ear ventilation. *Ann. Otol. Rhinol. Laryngol.* 86(Suppl. 41): 1–15.
5. Cantekin, E.I., Phillips, D.C., Doyle, W.J., Bluestone, C.D., and Kimes, K.K. (1980): Effect of surgical alterations of the tensor veli palatini muscle on eustachian tube function. *Ann. Otol. Rhinol. Laryngol.* 89(Suppl. 68): 47–53.
6. Carlson, B.A., Giebink, G.S., Spika, J.S., and Gray, E.D. (1982): Measurement of IgG and IgM antibodies to type 3 pneumococcal capsular polysaccharide by ELISA. *J. Clin. Microbiol.*, 16:63–69.
7. Castelli, J.B., Murray, J.P., and DeFries, H.O. (1976): A semipermeable membrane for tympanic ventilation tubes: design evaluation and results in experimental middle ear effusion by eustachian tube ligation in the cat. *Trans. Am. Acad. Ophthalmol. Otolaryngol.*, 82:245–254.
8. Claus, G. (1930): Experimentelle studien uber den verschluss der tuba eustachii beim hunde. *A Hals Nasen Ohrenheilk.*, 26:143–174.
9. Cohen, J.I., and Meyerhoff, W.L. (1982): Tympanostomy tube therapy for otitis media. *Ear Hear.*, 3:96–100.
10. DeMaria, T.F., Briggs, B.R., Lim, D.J., and Okazaki, N. (1984): Experimental otitis media with effusion following middle ear inoculation of nonviable *H. influenzae*. *Ann. Otol. Rhinol. Laryngol.*, 93:52–56.
11. Doyle, W.J., Cantekin, E.I., Bluestone, C.D., Phillips, D.C., Kimes, K.K., and Siegel, M.I. (1980): Nonhuman model of cleft palate and its implications for middle ear pathology. *Ann. Otol. Rhinol. Laryngol.*, 89(Suppl. 68):41–46.
12. Doyle, W.J., Supance, J.S., Marshak, G. Cantekin, E.I., and Bluestone, C.D. (1982): An animal model of acute otitis media consequent to β-lactamase producing nontypable *Haemophilus influenzae*. *Otolaryngol. Head Neck Surg.*, 90:831–836.
13. Doyle, W.J., Ingraham, A., Mohamed, M.S., and Cantekin, E.K. (1984): A primate model of cleft palate and middle ear disease: results of a one-year postcleft follow-ip. In: *Recent Advances in Otitis Media with Effusion,* edited by D.J. Lim, C.D. Bluestone, J.O. Klein, and J.D. Nelson pp. 215–218. B.C. Decker, Philadelphia.
14. Friedman, I. (1955): The comparative pathology of otitis media: experimental and human. *J. Laryngol. Otol.*, 69:588–601.
15. Fulghum, R.S., Brinn, J.E., Smith, A.M., Daniel, H.J. III, and Loesche, P.F. (1982): Experimental otitis media in gerbils and chinchillas with *Streptococcus pneumoniae, Haemophilus influenzae,* and other aerobic and anaerobic bacteria. *Infect. Immun.*, 36:802–810.
16. Giebink, G.S., Payne, E.E., Mills, E.L., Juhn, S.K., and Quie, P.G. (1976): Experimental otitis media due to *Streptococcus pneumoniae*: immunopathogenic response in the chinchilla. *J. Infect. Dis.*, 134:595–604.
17. Giebink, G.S., and Quie, P.G. (1978): Otitis media: the spectrum of middle ear inflammation. *Ann. Rev. Med.*, 29:285–306.
18. Giebink, G.S., Schiffman, G., Petty, K., and Quie, P.G. (1978): Modification of otitis media following vaccination with the capsular polysaccharide of *Streptococcus pneumoniae* in chinchillas. *J. Infect. Dis.*, 138:480–487.
19. Giebink, G.S., Berzins, I.K., Schiffman, G., and Quie, P.G. (1979): Experimental otitis media in chinchillas following nasal colonization with type 7F *Streptococcus pneumoniae*: prevention after vaccination with pneumococcal capsular polysaccharide. *J. Infect. Dis.*, 140:716–723.
20. Giebink, G.S., Berzins, I.K., Marker, S.C., and Schiffman, G. (1980): Experimental otitis media after nasal inoculation of *Streptococcus pneumoniae* and influenza A virus in chinchillas. *Infect. Immun.*, 30:445–450.
21. Giebink, G.S., (1981): The pathogenesis of pneumococcal otitis media in chinchillas and the efficacy of vaccination in prophlyaxis. *Rev. Infect. Dis.*, 3:342–352.
22. Giebink, G.S. (1982): Experimental otitis media due to *Haemophilus influenzae* in the chinchilla. In: *Haemophilus influenzae,* edited by S.H. Sell and P.F. Wright, pp.73–80. Elsevier Science Publishing Co., New York.
23. Giebink, G.S., Heller, K.A., and Le, C.T. (1983): Prediction of serous vs. purulent otitis media by otoscopy and tympanometry in an animal model. *Laryngoscope,* 93:208–211.

24. Giebink, G.S., and Schiffman, G. (1983): Humoral immune response in chinchillas to the capsular polysaccharides of *Streptococcus pneumoniae*. Infect. *Immun.*, 39:638–644.
25. Giebink, G.S., and Wright, P.F. (1983): Different virulence of influenza A virus strains and susceptibility to pneumococcal otitis media in chinchillas. *Infect. Immun.* 41:913–920.
26. Giebink, G.S. (1984): The pathogenesis of experimental pneumococcal otitis media during respiratory virus infection in chinchillas. In: *Recent Advances in Otitis Media with Effusion,* edited by D.J. Lim, pp.107–111. B.C. Decker, Philadelphia.
27. Goycoolea, M.V., Paparella, M.M., Juhn, S.K., and Carpenter, A.M. (1980): Cells involved in the middle ear defense system. *Ann. Otol. Rhinol. Laryngol.,* 89(Suppl. 68): 121–128.
28. Goycoolea, M.V., Paparella, M.M., Juhn, S.K., and Carpenter, A.M. (1980): Otitis media with perforation of the tympanic membrane: a longitudinal experimental study. *Laryngoscope,* 90:2037–2045.
29. Haymann, L. (1912–1913): *Arch. Ohrenheilk.,* 90:267. Quoted in: Friedmann, I. (1955): The comparative pathology of otitis media: experimental and human. I. Experimental otitis of the guinea pig. *J. Laryngol. Otol.,* 69:27–50.
30. Holmgren, L. (1940): Experimental tubal occlusion. *Acta Otolaryngol. (Stockh).,* 28:587–592.
31. Jakab, G.J., Warr, G.A., and Sannes, P.L. (1980): Alveolar macrophage ingestion and phagosome-lysozyme fusion defect associated with virus pneumonia. *Infect. Immun.,* 27:960–968.
32. Juhn, S.K., Paparella, M.M., Kim, C.S., Goycoolea, M.F., and Giebink, G.S. (1977): Pathogenesis of otitis media. *Ann. Otol. Rhinol. Laryngol.,* 86:481–492.
33. Kaneko, Y., and Paparella, M.M. (1971): Middle ear epithelium in the presence of experimental effusion. *Acta. Otolaryngol.,* 72:206–214.
34. Karasic, R.B., Trumpp, C.E., Gnehm, H.E., Rice, P.A., and Pelton, S.I. (1985): Modification of otitis media in chinchillas rechallenged with nontypable *Haemophilus influenzae* and serological response to outer membrane antigens. *J. Infect. Dis.,* 151:273–279.
35. Kuijpers, W., van der Beek, J.M.H., and Willart, E.C.T. (1979): The effect of experimental tubal obstruction on the middle ear. *Acta Otolaryngol. (Stockh.),* 87:345–352.
36. Lang, R.W., Liu, Y.S., Lim, D.J., and Birck, H.G. (1976): Antimicrobial factors and bacterial correlation in chronic otitis media with effusion. *Ann. Otol. Rhinol. Laryngol.,* 85(Suppl. 25): 145–151.
37. Lewis, D.M., Schram, J.L., Meadema, S.J., and Lim, D.J. (1980): Experimental otitis media in chinchillas. *Ann. Otol. Rhinol. Laryngol.* 89(Suppl. 68): 344–350.
38. Lim, D.J., and Hussl, B. (1970): Tympanic mucosa after tubal obstruction. *Arch. Otolaryngol.,* 91:585–593.
39. Lowell, S.H., Juhn, S.K., and Giebink, G.S. (1980): Experimental otitis media following middle ear inoculation of nonviable *Streptococcus pneumoniae. Ann. Otol. Rhinol. Laryngol.,* 89:479–482.
40. Marshak, G., Cantekin, E.I., Doyle, W.J., Schiffman, G., Rohn, D.D., and Boyles, R. (1981): Recurrent pneumococcal otitis media in the chinchilla. *Arch. Otolaryngol.,* 107:532–539.
41. Maxim, P.E., Veltri, R.W., Sprinkle, P.M., and Pusateri, R.J. (1977): Chronic serous otitis media: an immune complex disease. *Trans. Am. Acad. Ophthalmol. Otolaryngol.,* 84:ORL-234–ORL-238.
42. Meyerhoff, W.L., Shea, D.A., and Giebink, G.S. (1980): Experimental pneumococcal otitis media: a histopathological study. *Otolaryngol. Head Neck Surg.,* 88:606–612.
43. Meyerhoff, W.L., Shea, D.A., and Foster, C.A. (1981): Otitis media, cleft palate, and middle ear ventilation. *Otolaryngol. Head Neck Surg.,* 89:288–293.
44. Meyerhoff, W.L. (1981): use of tympanostomy tubes in otitis media. *Ann. Otol. Rhinol. Laryngol.,* 90:537–542.
45. Meyerhoff, W.L., Giebink, G.S., and Shea, D. (1981): Pneumococcal otitis media following middle ear deflation. *Ann. Otol. Rhinol. Laryngol.,* 90:72–76.
46. Meyerhoff, W.L., Giebink, G.S., Shea, D.A., and Le, C.T. (1982): Effect of tympanostomy tubes on the pathogenesis of acute otitis media. *Am. J. Otolaryngol.,* 3:189–195.
47. Miglets, A.W. (1973): Experimental production of allergic middle ear effusions. *Laryngoscope,* 83:1355–1384.
48. Miglets, A.W., Spiegel, J., and Bronstein, H.A. (1976): Middle ear effusion in experimental hypersensitivity. *Ann. Otol. Rhinol. Laryngol.,* 85(Suppl. 25): 81–86.
49. Misurya, V.K. (1974): Surgical treatment of the abnormally patulous eustachian tube. *J. Laryngol. Otol.,* 88:877–883.

50. Mravec, J., Lewis, D.M., and Lim, D.J. (1978): Experimental otitis media with effusion: an immune complex-mediated response. *Trans. Am. Acad. Ophthalmol. Otolaryngol.*, 85:ORL-258–ORL-268.
51. Odoi, H., Proud, G.O., and Toledo, P.S. (1971): Effects of pterygoid hamulotomy upon eustachian tube function. *Laryngoscope,* 81:1242–1244.
52. Paparella, M.M., Hiraide, F., Juhn, S.K., and Kaneko, Y. (1970): Cellular events involved in middle ear fluid production. *Ann. Otol. Rhinol. Laryngol.*, 79:766–779.
53. Paparella, M.M. (1976): Middle ear effusions: definitions and terminology. *Ann. Otol. Rhinol. Laryngol.*, 85(Suppl. 25):8–11.
54. Paradise, J.L., Bluestone, C.D., and Felder, H. (1969): The universality of otitis media in 50 infants with cleft palate. *Pediatrics.* 44:35–42.
55. Proud, G.O., and Odoi, H. (1970): Effects of eustachian tube ligation. *Ann. Otol. Rhinol. Laryngol.*, 79:30–32.
56. Proud, G.O., Odoi, H., and Toledo, P.S. (1971): Bullar pressure changes in eustachian tube dysfunction. *Ann. Otol. Rhinol. Laryngol.*, 80:835–837.
57. Rankin, J.D., and Karmody, G.S. (1970): Serous otitis media: an experimental model. *Arch. Otolaryngol.*, 92:14–23.
58. Reilly, J.S., Doyle, W.J., Cantekin, E.I., Supance, J.S., Kim, H.K.C., Rohn, D.D., and Bluestone, C.D. (1983): Treatment of ampicillin resistant acute otitis media in the chinchilla. *Arch. Otolaryngol.*, 109:533–535.
59. Reiner, C.E., and Pulec, J.L. (1969): Experimental production of serous otitis media. *Ann. Otol. Rhino. Laryngol.*, 78:880–887.
60. Sade, J., Carr, C.D., and Senturia, B.H. (1959): Middle ear effusions produced experimentally in dogs. *Ann. Otol. Rhinol. Laryngol.*, 68:1017–1027.
61. Sanyal, M.A., Henderson, F.W., Stempel, E.C., Collier, A.M., and Denny, F.W. (1980): Effect of upper respiratory tract infection on eustachian tube ventilatory function in the preschool child. *J. Pediatr.*, 97:11–15.
62. Senturia, B.H., Gessent, C.F., Carr, C.D., and Baumann, E.S. (1960): Middle ear effusions: causes and treatment. *Trans. Am. Acad. Ophthalmol. Otolaryngol.*, 64:60–72.
63. Senturia, B.H., Carr, C.D., and Rosenblat, B. (1962): Middle ear effusions produced experimentally in dogs. III. Further studies concerning the pathogenesis of the effusions. *Acta Otolaryngol. (Stockh).*, 54:383–392.
64. Senturia, B.H. (1962): Pathologic changes in the muco-periosteum of the experimental animal. *Ann. Otol. Rhinol. Laryngol.*, 71:632–636.
65. Senturia, B.H., Bluestone, C.D., Klein, J.O., Lim, D.J., and Paradise, J.L. (1980): Report of the Ad Hoc Committee on Definition and Classification of Otitis Media and Otitis Media with Effusion. *Ann. Otol. Rhinol. Laryngol.*, 85(Suppl. 68): 3–4.
66. Supance, J.S., Marshak, G., Doyle, W.J., and Cantekin, E.I. (1982): A longitudinal study of the efficacy of ampicillin in the treatment of pneumococcal otitis media in a chinchilla model. *Ann. Otol. Rhinol. Laryngol.*, 91:256–260.
67. Thore, M., Burman, L.G., and Holm, S.E. (1982): *Streptococcus pneumoniae* and three species of anaerobic bacteria in experimental otitis media in guinea pigs. *J. Infect. Dis.*, 145:822–828.
68. Tos, M. (1981): Experimental tubal obstruction. Changes in middle ear mucosa elucidated by quantitative hematology. *Acta Otolaryngol. (Stockh.),* 92:51–61.
69. Watanabe, N., Briggs, B.R., and Lim, D.J. (1982): Experimental otitis media in chinchillas. I. Baseline immunologic investigation. *Ann. Otol. Rhinol. Laryngol.*, 91(Suppl. 93):3–8.
70. Watanabe, N., DeMaria, T.F., Lewis, D.M., Mogi, G., and Lim, D.J. (1982): Experimental otitis media in chinchillas. II. Comparison of the middle ear immune responses to *Streptococcus pneumoniae* types 3 and 23. *Ann. Otol. Rhinol. Laryngol.*, 91(Suppl. 93):9–16.
71. Wiederhold, M.L., Marinex, S.A., Scott, R.E.C., and DeFries, H.O. (1978): Effects of eustachian tube ligation of auditory nerve responses to clicks. *Ann. Otol. Rhinol. Laryngol.*, 87(Suppl. 45):12–20.
72. Wiederhold, M.L., Zajtchuk, J.T., Vap, J.G., and Paggi, R.E. (1980): Hearing loss in relation to physical properties of middle ear effusions. *Ann. Otol. Rhinol. Laryngol.*, 89(Suppl.68):185–189.
73. Yamashita, T., Okazaki, N., and Kumazawa, T. (1980): Relation between nasal and middle ear allergy: experimental study. *Ann. Otol. Rhinol. Laryngol.*, 89(Suppl. 68):147–151.

Immunology of the Ear, edited by J. Bernstein
and P. Ogra. Raven Press, New York © 1987.

The Immunobiology of Autoimmune Disease of the Inner Ear

Joel M. Bernstein

Departments of Otolaryngology and Pediatrics, State University of New York at Buffalo, Buffalo, New York 14214, and Division of Infectious Diseases, Buffalo, New York 14222

Recent advances in our understanding of cellular immunology, molecular biology, and genetics have influenced current thinking about autoimmunity (11). Since the turn of the century, the central dogma of immunology has always been that the body does not normally mount an immune response against itself. This phenomenon described originally by Ehrlich and Morgenroth (5) in the early twentieth century is accepted today as immunological tolerance to self-components and is obviously necessary for health. Classically, autoimmunity defines a state in which the natural unresponsiveness, or tolerance to self, terminates. As a result, antibodies or cytotoxic cells react with self constituents, thereby causing disease.

This definition implies that responses against self do not occur normally, and if they do occur, the outcome, depending on their magnitude and duration, is harmful to the host. However, it has recently become apparent that autoimmune responses are not so rare as one thought, and most importantly, that not all autoimmune responses are forbidden or harmful. Actually, certain forms of autoimmune response, such as recognition of self surface antigens coded for by the major histocompatability complex (14) and idiotype-anti-idiotype responses (6), unlike the horror autotoxicus of Ehrlich (5), appear to be essential for the diversification and the normal functioning of the intact immune system. This chapter reviews the hypothetical models of autoimmunity of the cochlear labyrinth which may occur. The next chapter (McCabe, *this volume*) will address the phenomenon of progressive sensorineural hearing loss. The three subsequent chapters will specifically deal with immunopathology of the inner ear in experimental animals, Meniere's disease, and recent advances in animal models of autoimmune disease. Finally, the otologic manifestations of systemic immunological disease, and in particular Wegener's granulomatosis, will be reviewed in the final two chapters.

To this day, the prevailing explanation for the evolution and existence of the immune system is defense against invading microorganisms (7). The word "immunity" suggests resistance to second attacks of certain infection. Broadening the concept of host defense to include resistance to malignant cells still places primary emphasis on the protective aspect of the immune system. If the immune system can be called into action to protect the host from potential threats in its environment, then clearly it must also be endowed with mechanisms to prevent an immunological attack on the host's own tissue. This need for self/non-self discrimination was appreciated very early in the history of immunology. In his clonal selection theory, Burnet (3) spoke of forbidden clones that consisted of potentially self-reactive lymphocytes, and these were eliminated as the organism developed. The concept still has some validity today, particularly since most immunologists feel that T-cell deletion that could be reactive with self is eliminated during fetal life. This concept has many experimental examples; for instance, if foreign allogenic cells are injected into an experimental animal during early development, that animal will see that foreign antigen as self and will not react against it in adult life (8). Similarly, those self-antigens that can be seen by the developing hemopoietic system during fetal development will be treated as self in the adult animal unless some mechanism exists for the breadown of this tolerance in adult life. However, self-recognition, far from being a forbidden event, now appears to be a major principle upon which the immune system is founded. In a sense then, immunology has come full circle because now not only is autoimmunity something that may not be harmful, but it is actually necessary for the sophisticated and fine adjustment of the regulation of the immune system.

IMMUNOBIOLOGY OF AUTOIMMUNITY

The combination of antigen and macrophage signals a regulator T cell (thymus-derived lymphocyte) that controls the activity of T helper and T suppressor cells. There are feedback circuits between these three T-cell subpopulations. The equilibrium established between the helper and suppressor T cells determines whether or not the B cell (bone-marrow- or bursa-derived lymphocyte) is activated to produce a mature immunoglobulin-secreting plasma cell. Depending on the regulatory equilibrium established, either antibody synthesis or immunological unresponsiveness may result. However, in order for the T cell to recognize the antigen, it must also recognize a marker for self along with the antigenic determinant, and this self-recognition unit is specified by genes contained within the so-called major histocompatability complex (MHC), which, in the human, is found on the short arm of chromosome 6 (21). The macrophage, therefore, presents to the lymphocyte the MHC antigen (type-II antigen) along with the processed foreign antigen. It is only within this context of MHC restriction that the T helper or T cytotoxic cell will recognize the antigen. Furthermore, Jerne (9) has advanced the theory that immunological control is mediated by a complementary network of membrane receptors that express idiotypic determinants on immunoglobulins. These idiotypic receptors that specifically represent the antigen-combining parts of the antibody are in themselves novel for the host and will bring forth the response of another antibody, which is called the anti-idiotype. This anti-idiotype response is believed to act as a fine adjustment of the immunological network and, in general, will down-regulate or suppress the overproduction of antibody. In this way, the immunological network is kept in equilibrium.

These are two examples of the importance of self-recognition; this is what can be called physiological autoimmunity, which may be responsible for modulation and regulation of a normal immune response.

Another example of physiological autoimmunity is that of senescence (4). The aging process, for example, gives rise to changes in the biochemical properties in the surface of the cell, e.g., the surface of cartilage or bone protein. These old and effete proteins or nucleoproteins may be constantly released into circulation. One can conceive of autoantibodies directed against aging self to be, at least in some cases, a physiological form of autoimmunity. In this way, antigen-antibody complexes consisting of senescent or altered self are eliminated by phagocytosis, particularly in the reticuloendothelial system of the body.

In the normal aging animal, therefore, an ongoing process of autoimmunity and the development of autoantibodies exists. This kind of reversible autoimmunity is frequently found in otherwise healthy people. Another type of reversible autoimmunity that can be found in healthy people would be the effect of the polyclonal activation of B cells by, for example, Epstein-Barr virus or lipopolysaccharide. These polyclonal activators may produce autoantibody, particularly if the T-regulatory system is deficient. If the duration of this T-cell dysregulation continues for a long period of time, a true autoimmune disease may occur, particularly in the human form of lupus erythematosis (12).

In general, lymphocytes, particularly T cells that could react with self-antigen, are usually eliminated during fetal life, as proposed by Burnet (2). Such autoantigens in adult life would constantly be under the control of T suppressor cells. These T suppressor cells may be antigen-specific, or idiotype-specific or they may be nonspecific. In general, these three types of lymphocytes would constantly suppress the ability of self-reacting clones of B cells to proliferate. It should be kept in mind that self-antigens such as thyroglobulin, the insulin receptor, and the acetylcholine receptor on muscles are all potential autoantigens (19). Furthermore, it is probable that there are some T cells and B cells that are also autoreactive normally. However, in the normal adult the suppressor mechanisms that have been stated above are active in down-regulating all of these potential pathways and the organism does not develop an autoimmune response (13). However, anything that can theoretically bypass this suppressor mechanism, such as cross-reacting antigen, altered antigen on the surface of a cell that may be caused by viral infection, or nonspecific polyclonal stimulation of B cells, may all bypass this suppressor mechanism and produce autoantibodies. If this system is not brought back into homeostasis and if the duration of these autoantibodies occurs for long periods of time, true autoimmune disease may occur with literal self-destruction.

One other point that needs to be emphasized before specifically addressing sensorineural deafness is the so-called genetic basis of autoimmune disease. The important discovery that the presence of a particular MHC antigen may influence the chance of developing particular diseases has resulted in a wealth of information that is of great value for analysis of the genetic basis of autoimmune disease (10). For example, it is now well known that ankylosing spondylitis is at least 87 times more common in patients with the B27 antigen (16). Dermatitis herpetiformis is 56 times more common in patients who have the DRW3 antigen (17). Chronic active hepatitis is 14 times more common in patients with DRW3, and Addison's disease is 6 times more common in those with DRW3 (17). Myesthemia gravis is 6 times more common in patients who have the B8 antigen, and lupus erythematosus appears to be related to B8, DRW2, and DRW3 (17). These genes apparently code for, or are in dysequilibrium linkage with, genes that influence the immune response and therefore they influence the probability that certain clones of lymphocytes with specificity for self-antigens arising by somatic mutation will occur. Autoimmunity, then, must be cnsidered on the basis of two general ideas: (a) There may be a defective immunoregulation that allows bypassing of normal suppressor mechanisms which, in turn, would allow autoantigen to stimulate autoreactive lymphocyte clones. An inducing agent in this regard could be viruses, and this could be common in the inner ear. (b) Autoimmunity is probably very closely related to multiple gene systems, many of which are expressed on the major histocompatability locus on the short arm of chromosome 6. The duration and strength of the immune response are all controlled in this small area of the MHC, and it has been well documented that certain autoimmune diseases are closely related to these various MHC phenotypes.

With this general background of immunobiology of autoimmunity, specific areas of the inner ear can now be addressed. One of the great shortcomings in studying inner ear autoimmunity is that there is a general inaccessibility of inner ear fluids and inner ear tissues that are required in order to make the early diagnosis of immunopathology that might be present. This is not true for almost all other autoimmune diseases that occur, for example, in the thyroid and the kidney. Nevertheless, at least four possible mechanisms for the production of autoimmune inner ear disease may be present.

The inner ear possesses a structure that has a significant alteration of blood flow and perhaps increased capillary permeability. This structure, the stria vascularis, is similar to the glomerulus of the kidney, the ciliary process of the eye, and the choroid plexus of the brain. It is certainly possible that immune complexes associated with diseases such as lupus erythematosis, rheumatoid arthritis, and other autoimmune diseases could nonspecifically deposit in the blood vessels of the stria because of the particular hemodynamic properties associated with this structure (18). It is theoretically possible for immune complexes to deposit here with resultant immunopathology and produce diseases such as strial atrophy and other metabolic diseases of the inner ear.

A second possibility is that specific antibody may be directed against altered epithelial cells in the stria, in the endolymphatic sac, in the blood vessels under the basilar membrane, or in the blood vessels in the spiral ganglia. It is known, for example, that viral infection may produce the release of gamma interferon from T helper cells and in this way stimulate epithelial cells to produce type-II antigen on their surfaces (15). This could recruit a cytotoxic or a humoral immune response and result in an autoimmune disorder.

A third mechanism producing autoimmune inner ear disease would involve T cells that are cytotoxic. Such effector cells could recognize altered epithelial cells, as mentioned above, and produce destruction. For example, it has been established now that in experimental autoimmune encephalomyelitis, T cytotoxic cells are responsible for the destruction of basic myelin with the production of neural destruction (1), and the human counterpart of this disease would be either multiple sclerosis or other demyelinating diseases.

Finally, in recent years the possibility that alterations in collagen components of the inner ear may give rise to antibody has been suggested by Yoo (20) and will be more specifically addressed in Yoo et al.'s chapter *(this volume)*. It is conceivable that viral infection of the inner ear may cause alteration of collagen, and, in this way, type-II collagen antibody may result with the development of immune complex disease, which could involve any part of the inner ear in which type-II collagen is present.

In this regard, Table 1 reviews information on the presence of autoantibody and immune complexes in various types of sensorineural hearing loss disorders in 70 patients. The data are interesting because they suggest that in 70% of cases, immune complexes are present in patients with Meniere's disease, otosclerosis, and progressive sensorineural deafness; and interestingly, in sudden deafness 70% of the patients had immune complexes that were greater than two standard deviation above the upper limit of normal in our laboratory. It is also interesting to note that in a small group of patients with Meniere's disease, there is the presence of a significant elevation of thyroglobulin antibodies as well as microsomal antibodies. Thus, Meniere's disease may be associated with Hashimoto's disease or autoimmune thyroiditis in a few patients. The presence of antinuclear antibodies was present in 23 of 77 patients, and smooth muscle antibodies were present in 33 of 77 patients. Finally, type-II collagen antibodies were present in fairly high levels in 16 (approximately 21%), of the patients.

It is important to keep in mind that autoantibodies do increase with age; and because the ages of many of these patients are very widespread, it is hard to know the significance of the findings. However, if one looks at the incidence of immune complexes, particularly in otosclerosis and Meniere's disease, one is struck by the high incidence of immune complexes in these patients, whose average age is less than 50. It also is interesting to note the high incidence of immune complexes in sudden deafness as well as progressive sensorineural hearing loss. In the aging human there is an increased incidence of circulating immune complexes. Therefore, the relationship between the pathogenesis of inner ear disease associated with immune complexes remains uncertain.

These studies and the studies of many that have been reported in the literature have not been carefully controlled, particularly in age-related studies. Secondly, it is possible that the presence of immune complexes or autoantibodies that are present in the serum of these patients may have absolutely nothing to do with the path-

TABLE 1. *Immune complexes and autoantibodies in sensorineural hearing disorders*[a]

Disease	No. of cases	Immune complexes		RF		Thyr.		Micros.		ANA		AMA	SMA		Type-II collagen	
		No.	%	No.	%	No.	%	No.	%	No.	%	No.	No.	%	No.	%
Meniere's disease	16	11	69	1	6	3	19	4	25	6	38	0	8	50	1	6
Otosclerosis	7	5	71	0		1	14	2	29	2	29	0	4	57	2	14
Progressive sensorineural hearing loss	23	16	70	0		0		0		6	26	0	11	48	5	22
Sudden deafness	13	9	70	0		0		0		4	31	0	3	23	4	31
Miscellaneous	18	10	56	0		0		0		5	28	0	7	39	4	22
Totals	77	41	53	1	1	4	5	6	8	23	30	0	33	43	16	21

[a]RF, rheumatoid factor; Thyr., thyroglobulin antibodies; Micros., microsomal antibodies; ANA, antinuclear antibodies; SMA, smooth muscle antibodies.

ogenesis of the disease. Finally, it is very important, when talking about autoimmunity and autoantibodies, that we realize that autoantibodies may not necessarily be harmful or pathological, but actually may be important in the elimination of senescent cells, and that the recognition of self is an integral and absolutely necessary part of the normal immune network as it exists today.

CONCLUSION

At least four possible mechanisms exist for autoimmune disease in the inner ear. Humoral immune mechanisms by specific or cross-reacting autoantibody may react with specific autoantigens in the inner ear. Structures such as the epithelial cells of the stria vascularis, vascular endothelium underlying the basillar membrane, spiral ganglion cells, epithelial cells of the endolymphatic sac, and perhaps even the hair cells may be involved. Another humoral immune mechanism may involve the deposition of circulating immune complexes from bacterial antibodies or viral antibody complexes. These complexes may nonspecifically deposit in the stria vascularis, just as they would in the choroid plexus of the brain or more commonly in the glomerulus of the kidney. Thirdly, cell-mediated immune responses involving cytotoxic T cells with specific targets on the various structures mentioned above may also be effector cells for autoimmune disease of the inner ear. Finally, autoantibody directed against type-II collagen may be very important, and this has already been demonstrated by a number of investigators; in over 20% of cases in our study, this autoantibody was significantly elevated.

Circulating immune complexes are elevated in patients with various types of sensorineural hearing loss and otosclerosis. Antibody to type-II collagen was associated with some patients with Meniere's disease, otosclerosis, sudden deafness, and progressive sensorineural hearing loss. Finally, other types of sensorineural hearing loss, including those related to viral infections and strial atrophy, may be caused by autoimmune disease.

REFERENCES

1. Ben-Nun, A., and Cohen, I.R. (1982): Experimental autoimmune encephalomyelitis (EAE) mediated by T cell lines: process of selection of lines and characterization of these cells. *J. Immunol.*, 129:303–308.
2. Burnet, F.M. (editor) (1969): *The Clonal Selection Theory of Acquired Immunity*. Cambridge University Press, Cambridge, Mass.
3. Burnet, F.M. (1957): A modification of Jerne's theory of antibody production using the concept of clonal selection. *Aust. J. Sci.*, 20:67.
4. Calkins, E. (1985): Antibodies and aging. A geriatrician looks at the clinical literature. In: *Antibodies: Protective, Destructive and Regulatory Role,* edited by F. Milgrom, C.J. Abeyounis, and B. Albini, pp. 389–397. Karger Press, Basel.
5. Ehrlich, P., and Morgenroth, J. (1900): Über Hämolysine. *Berl. Klin. Wochenschr.*, 37:453–458.
6. Eichmann, K. (1978): Expression and function of idiotypes on lymphocytes. *Adv. Immunol.*, 26:195.

7. Hahn, H., and Kaufmanns, S.H. (1981): The role of cell mediated immunity in bacterial infections. *Rev. Infect. Dis.,* 3:121.
8. Howard, J.G., and Mitchison, N.A. (1975): Immunological tolerance. In: *Progress in Allergy,* edited by B.H. Waksman, pp. 18–43 Karger Press, Basel.
9. Jerne, N.K. (1974): Towards a network theory of the immune system. *Ann. Immunol.,* 125:373–378.
10. Krco, C.J., and David, C.S. (1981): Genetics of the immune response: a survey. *CRC Crit. Rev. Immunol.,* 1:211.
11. McConnell, I., Munro, A., and Waldman, H. (1981): *The Immune System: A Course on the Molecular and Cellular Basis of Immunity,* 2nd ed. Blackwell Scientific Publishers, Oxford.
12. Miller, K.B., and Schwartz, R.S. (1979): Familial abnormalities of suppressor cell function in systemic lupus erythematosis. *N. Engl. J. Med.,* 301:803–809.
13. Paul, W.E., and Bena, C. (1982): Regulatory idiotypes and immune networks: a hypothesis. *Immunology Today,* 3:230–234.
14. Plough, H.L., Orr, H.T., and Strominger, J.R. (1981): Major histocompatibility antigens: the human (HLA-A,B.C) and murine H-2K, H-2D, class I molecules. *Cell,* 24:287.
15. Pober, J.S., Gimbrone, M.A., Ramzi, S.C., Reiss, C.S., Burakoff, W.P., and Aults, K.A. (1983): Ia expression by vascular endothelium is inducible by activated T cells and by human γ interferon. *J. Exp. Med.,* 157:1339–1353.
16. Roitt, I., Brostoff, J., and Mole, D. (editors) (1985): *Immunology,* Chapter 4. C.V. Mosby Co., St. Louis.
17. Roitt, I., Brostoff, J., and Mole, D. (editors) (1985): *Immunology,* Chapter 23. C.V. Mosby Co., St. Louis.
18. Roitt, I., Brostoff, J., and Mole, D. (editors) (1985): *Immunology,* Chapter 21. C.V. Mosby Co., St. Louis.
19. Theofilopoulos, A.N., and Dixon, F.J. (1982): Autoimmune diseases: immunopathology and etiopathogenesis. *Am. J. Pathol.,* 108:321–365.
20. Yoo, T.J. (1984): Etiopathogenesis of Meniere's disease: a hypothesis. *Ann. Otol. Rhinol. Laryngol.* (Suppl.), 113(93):6–12.
21. Zinkernagel, R.M., and Doherty, P.C. (1979): MHC-restricted cytotoxic T cells: studies on the biological role of polymorphic major transplantation antigens determining T cell restriction, specificity, function, and responsiveness. *Adv. Immunol.,* 27:51.

Immunology of the Ear, edited by J. Bernstein
and P. Ogra. Raven Press, New York © 1987.

Autoimmune Inner Ear Disease

Brian F. McCabe

Department of Otolaryngology—Head and Neck Surgery, University of Iowa, Iowa City, Iowa 52242

In 1979 we described a type of deafness that had not often been described and would seem distinct from other hearing losses that were sensorineural in origin (3). The disease appeared to occur in young adults, was slowly progressive over a period of months rather than hours, and was accompanied by no other systemic disease and no hereditary defects. Over a period of the last 10 years this progressive sensorineural hearing loss has been recognized more frequently. These patients were treated with immunosuppressant medications with sometimes dramatic recoveries. Because these patients improved with immunosuppressive medication, it was suggested that a distinct new entity had been recognized and was one of the few types of sensorineural hearing loss that might be treatable. Since that time it has been reported worldwide and now appears to be accepted as autoimmune inner ear disease (1,2,4; J.L. Sheehy, 1984, *personal communication*).

Fifty-six patients have now been recognized and treated as having this disorder in the series that we have presented. The diagnosis is based on the clinical course of the hearing loss, immunological tests, and the response to immunosuppression. Treatment has consisted uniformly of high doses of steroids and moderate doses of intravenous cyclophosphamide. Response to treatment has been favorable in over 95% of the cases; 52 of 56 patients have had acceptable results and 4 patients have been considered as treatment failures.

CLINICAL COURSE OF AUTOIMMUNE SENSORINEURAL DEAFNESS

The clincal course of this hearing loss has been quite uniform and is characteristic of this disorder as opposed to other types of hearing loss. The deafness in all cases has been purely sensorineural, bilateral, asymmetric, and progressive over weeks or months rather than hours or years. The time course of the hearing loss distinguishes it from other forms of sensorineural deafness such as sudden deafness, familial recessive sensorineural deafness, cochlear Meniere's disease, presenile presbycusis, noise-induced hearing loss, luetic labyrinthitis, and perilymph fistulae. In these diseases the hearing loss occurs over hours or years or has sudden shifts or fluctuations. Vestibular episodes or crises have not been a feature of this type of disease, but ataxia in the dark has been a feature of all patients who had moderate to severe disease. There was no preponderance with regard to the sex of patients, who ranged in age from 16 to 52 years. Visible tissue changes were present in only two patients. One had neovasculogenesis of the tympanic membrane and one had granulation tissue displaying a definite vasculitis in which infiltration of all layers of blood vessels with lymphocytes occurred together with fibrinoid degeneration. In all other patients, objective physical examination was normal.

LABORATORY TESTS

All patients suspected of having this disorder should have an immunological screen consisting of a sedimentation rate, antinuclear antibody testing, rheumatoid factor, and quantitive immunoglobulin determinations. If any two of these tests are abnormal, treatment described in detail below should be commenced.

A more specific laboratory test is the lymphocyte migration inhibition assay, which was positive in 12 of 20 patients with the disease. The test is fully described below. In this test, the patient's leukocytes are challenged with prepared inner-ear antigen harvested from the membranous labyrinths of patients undergoing translabyrinthine operations for other diseases. Three different controls are run in parallel; one of them uses the leukocytes of the spouse or other close relatives. Hughes et al. (1) have reported that the lymphocyte transformation test is more specific and sensitive than the lymphocyte migration inhibition assay.

TREATMENT

The therapeutic regimen is immunosuppression. Patients are hospitalized and given a daily infusion of cyclophosphamide, the dose being 2 to 3 mg/kg for 14 days. Monitoring of the white blood cell count must be performed to maintain it above 5,000 cells/μl. Dexamethasone is given orally and is commenced at a dose of 4 mg every 6 hr. The patient is then discharged for 2 weeks on dexamethasone alone and is returned to the hospital for another 2 weeks of intravenous cyclophosphamide. Dexamethasone is then continued for a period of 3 months and tapered over a period of 4 weeks. If the hearing drops during the taper then the 16-mg/day level is restored for another 3 months before a second taper is started. Most patients have required only 3 to 6 months of treatment, but some patients have required treatment for as long as 2 years.

RESULTS OF TREATMENT

All patients except four responded to treatment with moderate hearing gains. In those cases in which the hearing loss was mild to moderate, treatment would result in a return to normal or low normal hearing; however, if the hearing loss was profound in the 80- to 100-dB range, treatment would result in an improvement in thresholds to at least satisfactory rehabilitation with a hearing aid. All patients successfully treated have not had recurrence of the disease.

Vestibular symptoms and caloric tests were performed on all of these patients and, in general, paralleled the hearing loss. Thus the disease apparently is not cochlear alone, but involves the entire membranous labyrinth. The otolith organs are involved as well, particularly in patients with severe to profound losses. It is of interest that 12 patients subsequently developed other diseases considered to be autoimmune in nature: Cogan's syndrome (4), chronic ulcerative otitis (3), rheumatoid arthritis (2), carotidodynia (2), and polyarteritis nodosa (1).

DISCUSSION

Other otologists have recognized this disease, and it appears that experience with this disorder is now becoming fairly widespread. Hughes et al. (1), for example, have reported the disorder in an 8-year-old child, whereas Sheehy (J.L. Sheehy, 1984, *personal communication*), had a patient with a rather indolent form of the disease, progressing over several years, in which the hearing disorder was severe on one side and moderate on the other side. There was apparently a rapid and dramatic response to steroids. Shea's (4) report of 10% of a series of patients with rapidly progressive Meniere's disease responding with hearing gain and/or dramatic reduction in dizziness on dexamethasone treatment suggests that either this disorder can take the pattern of Meniere's disease or that some patients with Meniere's disease have an autoimmune labyrinthine disorder.

It is important to recognize these patients on presentation with their hearing loss because it is one of the few forms of sensorineural deafness for which there may be some treatment. If they are not diagnosed and treated, all hearing will probably be lost in each ear. Obviously, more specific laboratory test procedures are needed and the ones that are presently available are relatively nonspecific. It is recommended that any patients suspected of having the disease be given at least a trial of treatment with steroids.

Otolaryngologists who see a patient with a clinical picture compatible with the disease that has been described in this chapter should institute a trial treatment irrespective of the laboratory tests since these are clearly nonspecific at this point. If there is no other contraindication to the use of cytotoxic drugs or other immunosuppressive drugs, there is nothing to lose and possibly everything to gain in treating these patients with these medications. It is thus important to learn the clinical profile of the disease from the literature.

The following paragraphs specifically review the protocol for the leukocyte inhibition assay as it is performed in the laboratory of the University of Iowa, Department of Otolaryngology.

Procedure for Leukocyte Migration Inhibition Test

1. Draw 25 ml whole blood from patient into tube with preservative-free heparin (10 units per milliliter of blood). Mix well.
2. Transfer 8.0 ml heparinized blood to replicate 15-cc sterile polystyrene conical centrifuge tubes and add 2.0 ml sterile 5% dextran 250. Mix by inversion.
3. Sediment erythrocytes at 37°C. When sedimentation of erythrocytes has slowed considerably (about 30 min), remove plasma containing white blood cells into 15-cc tube and bring to 15 cc with calcium-magnesium-free Hanks buffered saline solution (BSS), pH 7.0. Centrifuge at 220*g* for 10 min.
4. Aspirate supernatant fluid to 1 ml above cell button and resuspend with a sterile siliconized Pasteur pipette. If too many red blood cells are present, add 9.0 ml of Tris-buffered NH_4Cl, pH 7.2, and incubate at 37°C for 20 min, mixing every 5 min to lyse red blood cells. Centrifuge at 220*g* for 5 to 7 min. If still heavily contamined with erythrocytes, repeat lysis.
5. Wash cell button three times with calcium-magnesium-free Hanks BSS, pH 7.0, and centrifuge at 220*g* for 5 min.
6. Resuspend cells to concentration of 1×10^8 per milliliter with RPMI 1640 medium containing 10% fetal calf serum.
7. Fill siliconized, preshortened, sterilized 50-μl micropipettes to manufacturer's mark. Plug nearest end with Critoseal (vinyl plastic putty), being careful not to have any air bubbles caught between media and plug.
8. Centrifuge micropipettes in a stationary, upright position at 700*g* for 10 min (packed cell length approximately 4 to 5 mm).
9. Prepare Sterilin leukocyte migration plate with tissue culture surface by applying silicone grease to the top rim of each well to be used and a dot of silicone grease toward the lower center of the well to hold the cut micropipette in place.
10. After centrifugation, cut Critoseal end within 2 to 4 mm from cell-media interface (length cut dependent on packed cell length). Cut approximately 1.0 mm into packed cells and place into well on top of silicone grease. Immediately add antigen suspension and media to a total volume of 430 γ per well.
11. Cover with a 22 × 22-mm coverslip that has been presoaked in 70% ethanol and flamed. Do not allow air bubbles to be left underneath coverslip.
12. Repeat steps 10 and 11 for each preparation to be tested. Completed test includes assays with: (a) no. of antigens, (b) phytohemagglutinin (PHA) (2 μg/ml, final concentration), (c) inner ear membrane antigen (approximately 5 μg/ml, final concentration), and (d) control antigen (approximately 5 μg/ml, final concentration). Each test is run in triplicate or quadruplicate.
13. Incubate 24 hr at 37°C in a 5% CO_2 air incubator. Be sure plates are on a level surface.
14. Vertically project the plate onto bond paper with "GK" slide Delineascope (Model 3689) projector. Trace the area of migration onto the bond paper.
15. Carefully cut out and weigh paper with a ±0.01-mg analytical balance (Mettler Instrument Corp., Hightstown, N.J.).

16. Calculate percentage of migration inhibition of each cell in comparison to negative control as

Percent Inhibition =

$$100\left(1-\frac{\text{Mean weight of fan in antigen-exposed cultures}}{\text{Mean weight of fan in control cultures}}\right)$$

17. Statistical analyses (*t* tests) are performed to determine the significance of the results based on weight.

Preparation of Inner Ear Membrane Antigen and Control Antigen

Inner ear membrane

1. Suspend surgically removed inner ear membrane in 1 ml PBS, pH 7.2.
2. Sonicate (Sonifier cell disrupter) inner ear membrane with five 3-min bursts at the no. 2 setting. Keep tube in ice-water bath during procedure to prevent overheating and protein denaturation (foaming at the surface).
3. Repeat sonication until opalescent suspension is obtained.
4. Store at −20°C or below.
5. When thawed at room temperature, mix well to resuspend.

Control antigen

1. Obtain 20 ml heparinized whole blood (10 units per milliliter of preservative-free heparin) from donor of the inner ear membrane for a control.
2. Separate mononuclear cells by Ficoll-Hypaque (LSM medium) density gradient.
3. Suspend and sonicate separated mononuclear cells following the above procedure.
4. Determine protein content of both antigens using the Lowrey method.

Reagents

1. Sterilin leukocyte migration plate with tissue culture surface: Superior Plastic Products Corp., Providence, Rhode Island; Sterilin Ltd., Teddington, Middlesex, England.
2. Dextran 250 (200,000–300,000 MW): Polyscience, Inc., Warrington, Pa.
3. LSM medium (Ficoll-Hypaque): Bionetic Laboratory Products, Kensington, Md.
4. Phytohemagglutinin, 2 mg/box: Burroughs Wellcome Company, Greenville, N.C.
5. 1640 RPMI complete media, 87.5 ml; 10 ml inactivated fetal calf serum (Gibco, Grand Island, N.Y.); 2.0 ml HEPES buffer (Gibco, Grand Island, N.Y.); 0.5 ml penicillin-streptomycin (Gibco, Grand Island, N.Y.).
6. Tris-NH_4Cl: 0.83% (7.47 g) ammonium chloride; 2.0594 g Trizma; 900 ml double distilled H_2O; pH adjusted to 7.2 with HCl; add HCl to double-distilled H_2O to 1,000 ml.

7. Hanks balanced salt solution without calcium or magnesium: M.A. Bioproducts, Walkersville, Md.
8. Phosphate buffered saline, pH 7.2.
9. Sonifier cell disrupter, Model W185 with Microtip: Branson Sonic Power Co., Danbury, Ct.
10. Heparin sodium injection, 1,000 USP units per milliliter, 5 ml per vial, no preservative: O'Neil, Jones and Feldman, St. Louis, Mo.
11. 15-cc Falcon 2095 tube: Scientific Co., Pittsburgh, Pa.
12. "GK" Slide Delineascope, Model 3689 with 12-in. lens attachment.
13. Prosil-28 siliconizing agent: PCR Research Chemicals Inc., Gainesville, Fl.
14. Stopcock silicone grease: Dow Corning, Midland, Mi.
15. 50-liter Accupette Pipettes: Dade Diagnostic, Inc., Aquada, Puerto Rico.
16. Critoseal: Lancer, St. Louis, Mo.

CLINICAL EXAMPLES OF AUTOIMMUNE INNER EAR DISEASE

Figures 1 through 4 represent audiograms of patients with this progressive sensorineural hearing loss. Figure 1 demonstrates the audiogram of a 24-year-old pa-

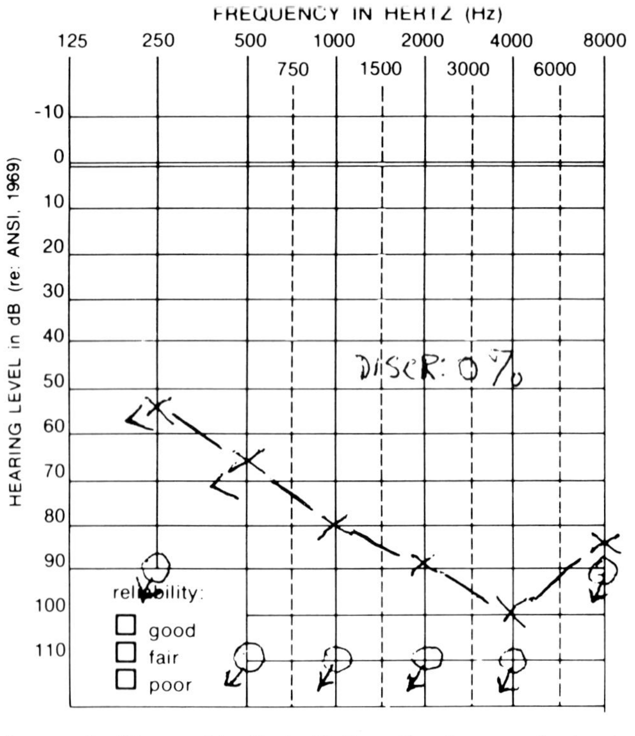

FIG. 1. Audiogram of a 24-year-old patient with 7 months of progressive hearing loss. There is no hearing at any frequency on the right. There is a profound loss in the left ear.

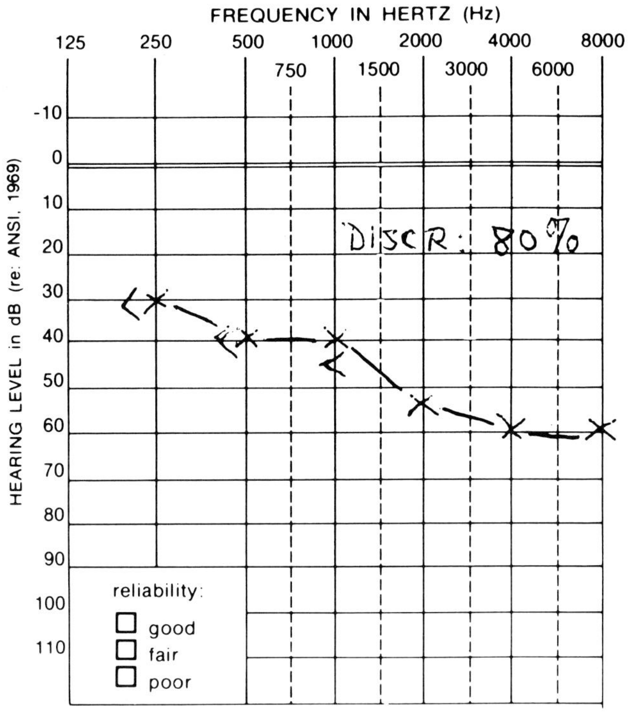

FIG. 2. Six months after commencing treatment. Note that there has been a very satisfactory response in the left ear. There has been no response on the right, demonstrating that when all hearing is gone, no recovery can be expected.

tient who had a 7-month history of progressive sensorineural hearing loss. Figure 2 demonstrates that after commencing immunosuppressive therapy there has been a very satisfactory improvement in the hearing loss in the left ear. Similarly, Figs. 3 and 4 show the results of the improvement in hearing in a 40-year-old patient with a 5-month history of hearing loss. Three months after treatment there is a significant improvement in both the pure tone hearing as well as the discrimination.

CONCLUSION

There appears to be increasing evidence that autoimmune inner ear disease may be a new entity. Progressive sensorineural hearing loss is the hallmark of this disease. Medical management consists of the use of steroids and immunosuppressive drugs. Plasmaphoresis may be reserved for selected cases. It is very important to recognize these patients because they have one of the few forms of sensorineural hearing disorders for which a medical treatment is available.

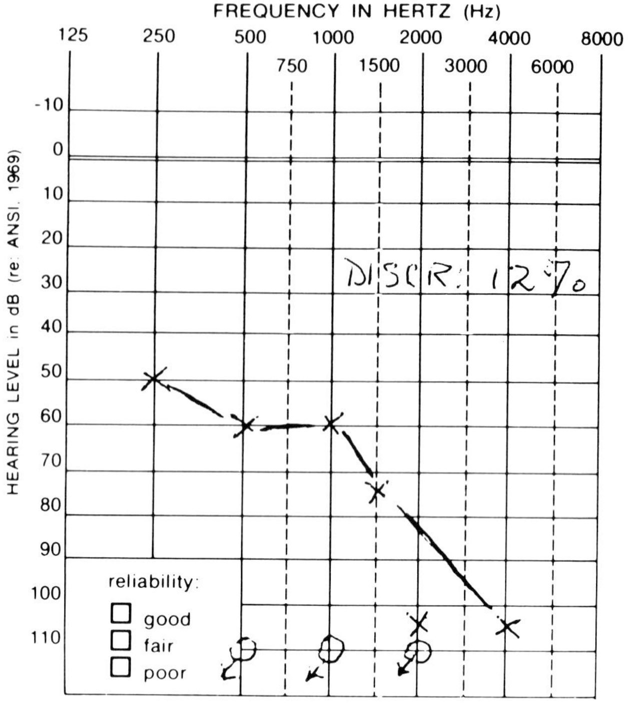

FIG. 3. Audiogram of a 40-year-old patient with a 5-month history of hearing loss. The discrimination is so poor that the patient is unable to tolerate a hearing aid.

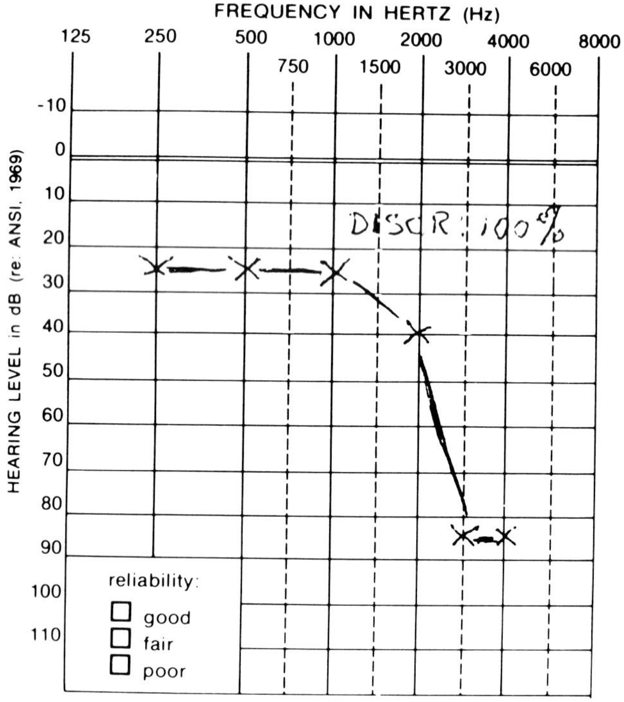

FIG. 4. Three months after treatment. There is a significant improvement in both the hearing loss and discrimination on the left side.

REFERENCES

1. Hughes, G.B., Kinney, S.E., Barna, B.P., and Calabrese, L.H. (1984): Practical versus theoretical management of autoimmune inner ear disease. *Laryngoscope,* 94:758–767.
2. Maini, R.N., Roffe, L.M., Magrath, I.T., and Dumonde, D.C. (1973): Standardization of the leukocyte migration test. *Int. Arch. Allergy,* 45:308–321.
3. McCabe, B. (1979): Autoimmune sensorineural hearing loss. *Ann. Otol. Rhinol. Laryngol.,* 88:585–589.
4. Shea, J.J. (1982): Autoimmune sensorineural hearing loss as an aggravating factor in Meniere's disease. Presented at the Barany Society Meeting, Basel, Switzerland, June 1982.

Immunology of the Ear, edited by J. Bernstein and P. Ogra. Raven Press, New York © 1987.

Immunopathology of the Inner Ear

Jeffrey P. Harris

Department of Surgery, Division of Otolaryngology, University of California, San Diego, School of Medicine, La Jolla, California, 92093, and Veterans Administration Medical Center, San Diego, California 92161

It is well recognized today that the secretory immune system functions to protect the middle ear from the penetration of bacteria and aids in the clearing of infections from this site (19,27,31,34,35). Furthermore, immune injury has been postulated as a contributory mechanism in a variety of middle ear disease states (4,5,13,33). Until recently, it was not known whether the inner ear is similarly protected and/or susceptible to immune injury, or whether it exists encased within its bony capsule as one of the body's immunoprivileged sites. This chapter will examine the basic immune responses elicited from the inner ear when challenged with an antigen or pathogen and the consequence of these responses on cochlear morphology and function.

ANATOMICAL CONSIDERATIONS

At first glance the inner ear does not appear to possess the necessary cellular constituents for the development of immune reactions. There are no collections of lymphoid tissue, no lamina propria plasma cells, and no clearly discernible lymphatics that drain the membranous labyrinth. However, although the candidates for these functions are not readily apparent, more and more evidence is accumulating which indicates that the inner ear may indeed possess the necessary components for a functioning immune system. Rask-Andersen and Stahle (24) demonstrated that the endolymphatic sac contains interacting lymphocytes and macrophages, which therefore suggests a possible role for this site in the host defense of the inner ear. The presence of epithelial cells, an occasional lymphocyte, and macrophages can be seen in the lumen of the "nonstimulated" normal endolymphatic sac (Fig. 1). Furthermore, the identification of perisacular lymphatics provides evidence that makes this site extremely attractive as the regional site for antigen processing and perhaps the elaboration of local inner ear immune reactions. Arnold et al. (1,2) have demonstrated that the endolymphatic sac in humans can be stained with antisera to secretory component and secretory immunoglobulin A (sIgA). This finding may indicate that the host defense of the inner ear may involve the

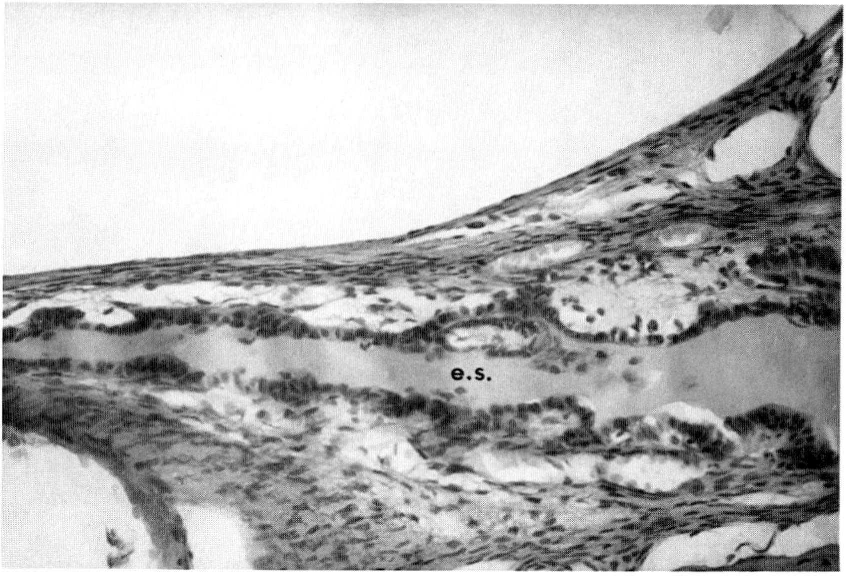

FIG. 1. Normal guinea pig endolymphatic sac (e.s.) in which occasional lymphocytes and macrophages can be identified within the lumen and the perisaccular connective tissue.

secretory immune system, known to play a predominant role in middle ear immunity as well.

An understanding of the fate of antigen challenge within the inner ear may provide some insight as to the mechanism by which host sensitization occurs. Saijo and Kimura (26) studied the distribution of horseradish peroxidase (HRP) following its injection into the middle ear space and the perilymphatic compartment. HRP was eventually seen within the endolymphatic sac lumen and subepithelial layer of the endolymphatic duct and sac. From obliteration studies of the endolymphatic duct, they hypothesized that the HRP traversed Reissner's and saccular membranes to enter the vestibular aqueduct en route to the endolymphatic sac. In other tracer studies, labeled substances that are introduced into the perilymphatic space appear to rapidly enter the spiral ligament, which may act as a "lymphatic" to host circulation. Consideration should also be given to the cochlear aqueduct since it is in continuity with the cerebrospinal fluid (CSF) and might be an additional route of antigen either entering or leaving the inner ear. If antigen were to leave the inner ear via the cochlear aqueduct and enter the CSF, it would then come under the influence of central nervous system (CNS) immunity. Thus, the distribution of antigen that gains entrance to the inner ear may do so via the endolymphatic sac and its draining lymphatics, the spiral ligament on into the systemic circulation, and/or the cochlear aqueduct into the CSF. Whether regional lymph nodes such as the retropharyngeal, deep cervical, or postauricular nodes are integrally involved in inner ear immune responses is yet to be determined.

IMMUNOBIOLOGY OF THE NONSTIMULATED INNER EAR

An initial step toward the understanding of the inner ear immune system would be to study the components of the immune response under normal "nonstimulated" conditions. A number of human and animal studies have examined the composition of perilymph and have found that it contains immunoglobulins as well as other blood proteins (2,6,7,23). IgG has been found to be the most prevalent immunoglobulin class in the inner ear under nonstimulated conditions; however, IgM and IgA have also been identified (21,23). These immunoglobulins appear to enter the inner ear by a process of filtration across the blood-labyrinthine barrier and are found in approximately one one-thousandth the concentration found in serum (9,16,22). However, if the inner ear is truly a secretory site, then the concentration of sIgA would be expected to be much higher in comparison to the other immunoglobulins found in the perilymph. This question has not been directly addressed; however, it appears that the levels of IgA found in the previously mentioned studies were too low to be consistent with it being the predominant immunoglobulin that is normally found in other secretory sites. It should be stated that in these studies perilymph, not endolymph, was measured, so perhaps this could explain the discrepancy.

Immunohistochemical examination of the normal temporal bone for possible sites of immune processing have shown no evidence of immunocompetent cells outside of the endolymphatic sac (1; J.P. Harris, *unpublished observation*). The presence of tissue-bound IgG can also be demonstrated, but there are no associated plasma cells suggesting that its presence is the result of serum transudation.

These basic observations concerning the immune status of the nonstimulated inner ear leads one to conclude that aside from the potential role of the endolymphatic sac, the major influence of immunity on the inner ear would be derived from either systemic or CNS immunity. In 1982, Mogi et al. (21) immunized animals systemically with egg albumin and showed that serum antibody was transferred to the perilymph at a level two to five times greater than it was to the CSF. Additionally, the mean perilymph IgG and albumin levels were two to four times higher than they were in CSF. These results suggested that the inner ear may have an independently functioning immune system or that it has the capacity to concentrate proteins more effectively than the CSF. In subsequent studies, Harris inoculated keyhole limpet hemocyanin (KLH) into the perilymphatic compartment of either nonsensitized (primary response) or KLH-sensitized (secondary response) guinea pigs and measured the resulting inner ear and serum anti-KLH antibody levels (9). A significant rise in serum antibody was seen over a 4-week period in the nonsensitized animals receiving a single inoculation into the inner ear. Inner ear anti-KLH antibody levels were found 7 weeks later to be greater than what one would expect from just the passive transfer of serum immunoglobulin across the blood labyrinthine barrier. In the secondarily immunized group of animals, the perilymph antibody rise was much greater than in the primary response group and significantly greater than the corresponding CSF antibody titers. These experiments demonstrated that the inner ear was not an immunoprivileged site since it responded to antigen stimulation and served as an effective site for the afferent limb of the immune response. However, this experiment was not able to determine whether the rise in inner ear antibody was a result of increased vascular permeability, contributions from the adjacent CSF, or local production within the inner ear.

In order to determine if the inner ear were the source of antibody, a second series of experiments were performed in which a serum reference was established by systemically immunizing animals to bovine serum albumin (BSA) (20). In these studies, animals that had circulating levels of anti-BSA were then immunized with only KLH into the inner ear and the resulting anti-BSA and anti-KLH antibody levels in the serum and perilymph were measured. Thus, if there were an increase in vascular permeability causing a nonspecific rise in antibody, one would then expect to see a corresponding rise in anti-BSA as well as anti-KLH antibody. The results of this study revealed a significant rise in the perilymph anti-KLH antibody levels without a corresponding increase in anti-BSA (20) (see Fig. 2) Furthermore, the inner ear immune response to KLH was significantly greater than the CSF anti-KLH levels. Thus these results demonstrated that the observed increase in perilymph antibody was not the result of CNS immunity but rather local production within the inner ear itself. This further suggested that this response either emanated from the stimulation of immunocompetent cells residing within the inner ear or that these cells migrated out of the systemic circulation into the inner ear upon antigen challenge.

Assessment of the ability of the inner ear to process antigen and confer systemic immunity on the host was examined in experiments in which a single antigen inoculation was performed into the inner ear, the middle ear, or the peritoneal cavity (12). The development of systemic humoral and cellular immunity was then compared for each of these sites. The inner ear and peritoneal routes of antigen presentation resulted in a parallel rise in serum antibody over a 3-week period. In contrast, the middle ear route resulted in a weak, transient antibody response within 2 weeks. The acquisition of cell-mediated immunity occurred earliest (day 14) in the group receiving antigen intraperitoneally. A significant but smaller proliferative response was also seen in the group receiving antigen via the inner ear route on days 14 to 21. In contrast, the middle ear route failed to result in cell-mediated immunity. These studies indicate that the inner ear is an effective route of antigen processing which subsequently results in the acquisition of systemic humoral and cellular immunity.

In order to assess the morphological changes associated with immune stimulation of the inner ear, Woolf and Harris (36) examined the temporal bones of animals with primary and secondary inner ear immune responses. Primary immune responses were associated with a fibromyxoid infiltrate primarily within the scala tympani of the basal turn of the cochlea and preservation of sensory and neural structures throughout the membranous labyrinth (see Fig. 3). Scattered throughout this infiltrate were lymphocytes, macrophages, and plasma cells. In contrast, the cochleae of secondary response animals showed severe inflammatory reactions in

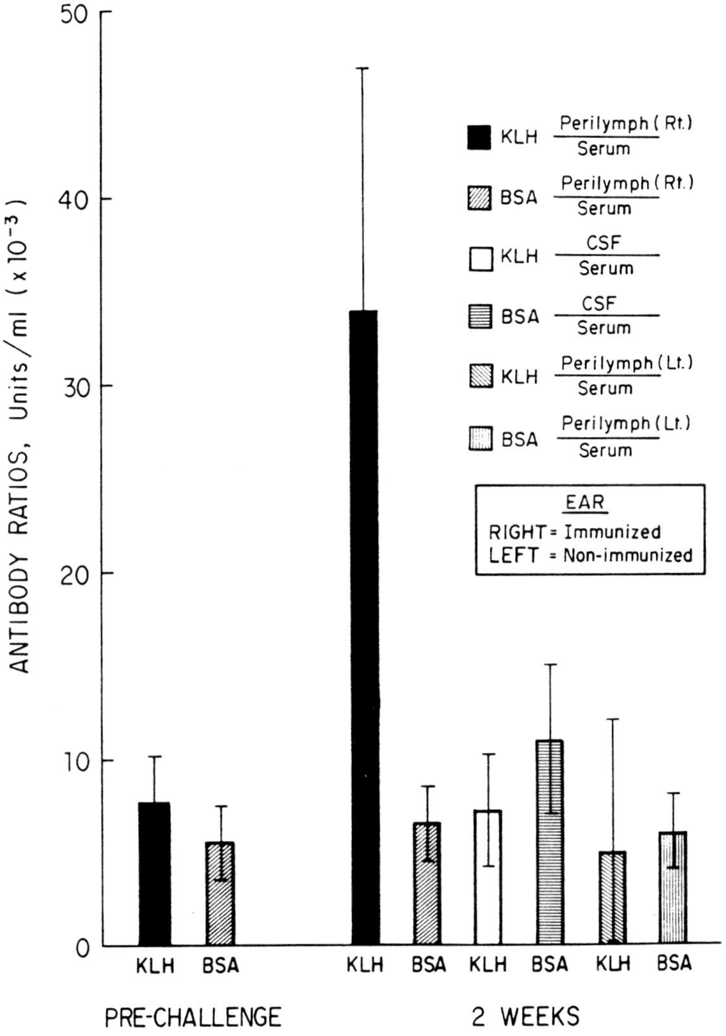

FIG. 2. Effect of KLH inner ear inoculation in animals systemically sensitized to KLH and BSA. Antibody ratios are significantly increased for perilymph anti-KLH ratio only. (From ref. 9a.)

all turns (see Fig. 4). These inflammatory changes consisted of tremendous numbers of plasma cells within the scalae tympani, hemorrhage throughout all scalae, perilabyrinthine fibrosis and osteoneogenesis, and degeneration of sensory and neural structures to varying degrees. Although hydrops was not a predominant feature, it was evident in a few temporal bones.

The temporal bone findings in a dying patient with deafness and polyarteritis nodosa was reported by Jenkins et al. (15). They observed fibro-osseous proliferation within the scala tympani and associated degeneration of the sensory and neu-

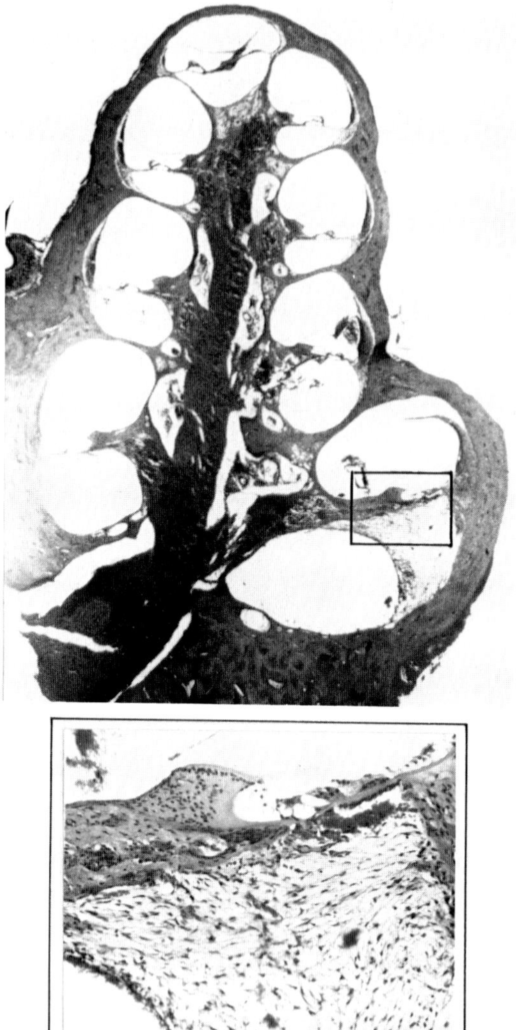

FIG. 3. Histopathology of a primary inner ear immune response to KLH. Fibromyxoid response is seen in the basal turn of the cochlea with scattered plasma cells and preservation of the sensory and neural structures.

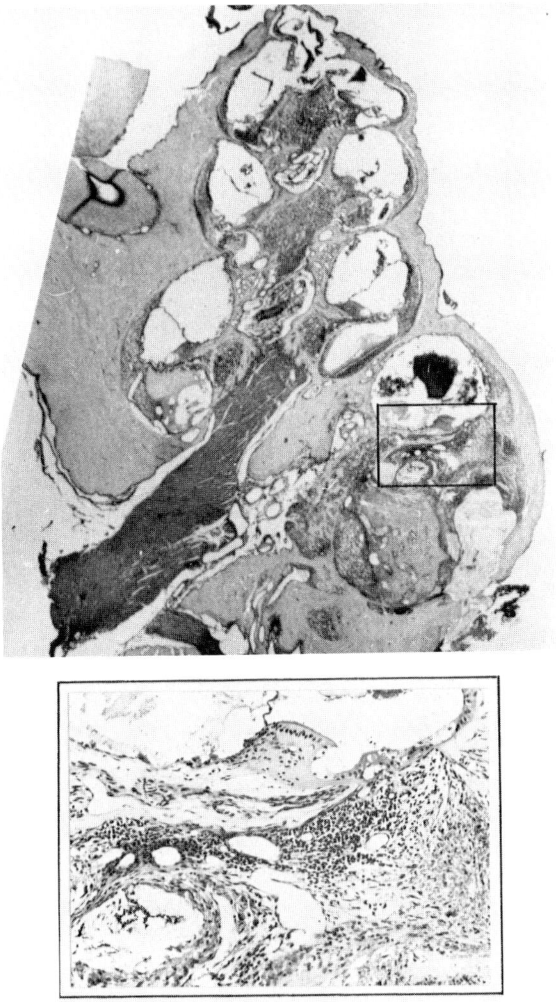

FIG. 4. Histopathology of a secondary inner ear immune response to KLH. Severe inflammatory response is seen throughout the cochlea with numerous plasma cells interspersed within fibro-osseous tissue.

ral structures (see Fig. 5). This histopathology was strikingly similar to that seen in our secondary inner ear immune response subjects and suggested the possibility that a similar mechanism of injury was at play in both the clinical and this experimental situation.

ENDOLYMPHATIC SAC AS AN IMMUNE SITE

The suggestion that the endolymphatic sac might be involved in the defense of the inner ear was first made by Lim and Silver in 1974 (18). The observation of

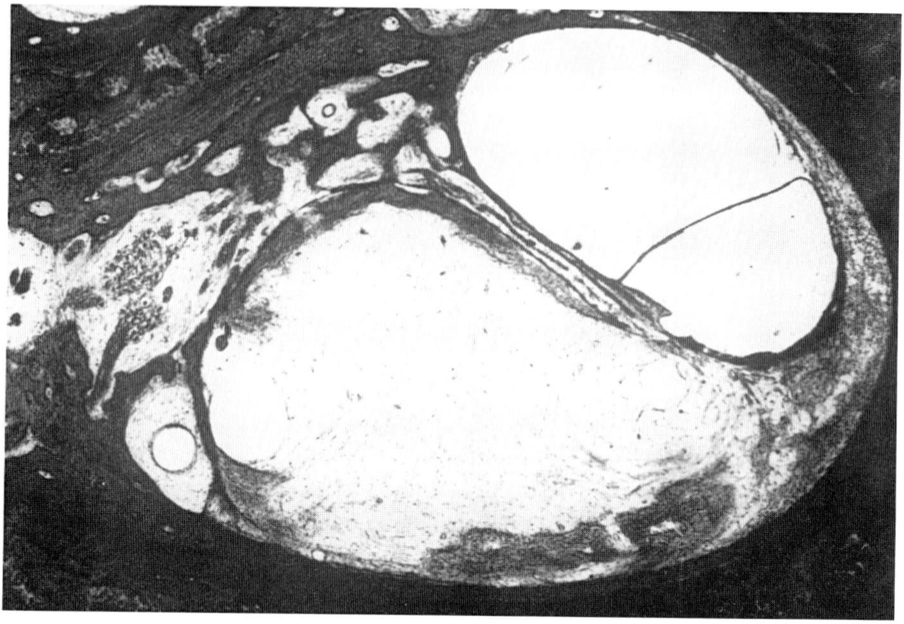

FIG. 5. Temporal bone findings in a dying patient with sudden hearing loss and polyarteritis nodosa. Proliferation of fibro-osseous tissue in the scala tympani and degeneration of sensory and neural elements was observed. (From ref. 15)

lymphocyte-macrophage interaction in the endolymphatic sac by Rask-Andersen and Stahle was an important additional piece of evidence that this site within the inner ear may in fact serve other physiological functions (24). In order to investigate the role of the endolymphatic sac in inner ear immune mechanisms, this site was examined following immune stimulation of animals undergoing secondary inner ear immune responses (Tomiyama and Harris, *unpublished observations*). In these animals, an obvious increase in the number of plasma cells both within the sac and in the perisacular connective tissue was seen (see Fig. 6). The endolymphatic duct showed a similar, but less dramatic, increase in the number of inflammatory cells. One such tissue section revealed a collection of lymphocytes surrounding a capillary in the perisaccular space. This perivascular cuffing is suggestive that lymphocytes are leaving the circulation and collecting in the region of the endolymphatic duct and sac.

Since the endolymphatic sac is considered to be a possible candidate for the site of antigen processing and inner ear immune responses, Tomiyama and Harris (30) performed an experiment in which one group of animals had their endolymphatic sacs obliterated and the other underwent sham operations. Endolymphatic sac obliteration was accomplished through an intradural approach, by first employing silver nitrate as a chemical cautery injected into the sac and then surgically removing the sac and drilling away the operculum and the underlying sac and duct. After

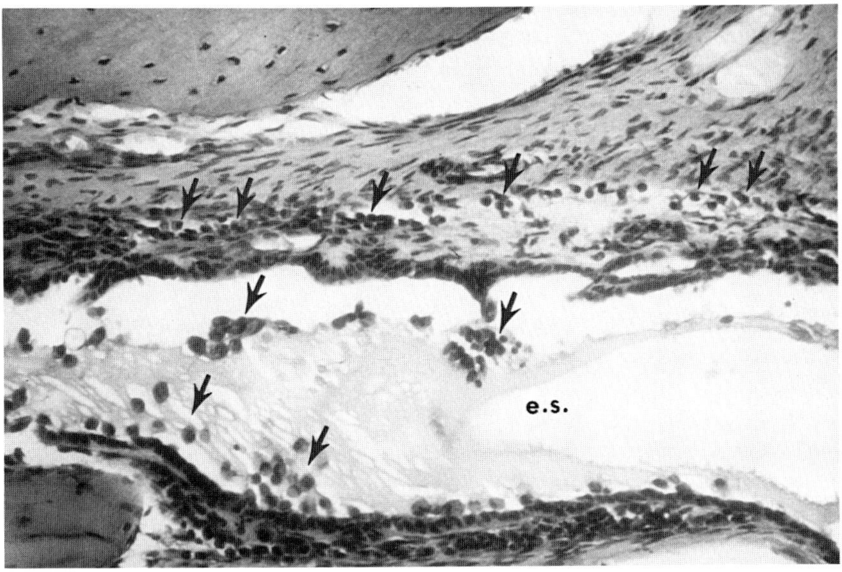

FIG. 6. Endolymphatic sac (e.s.) from a guinea pig with a secondary inner ear immune response to KLH. Note the abundance of plasma cells in the perisaccular connective tissue and within the sac lumen *(arrows).*

a recovery period, both groups of animals were further divided into primary and secondary immune response subgroups. The primary response groups were then inoculated with KLH into the perilymphatic space. Two weeks following antigen challenge, serum anti-KLH levels of sham-operated animals were significantly greater than those of endolymphatic-sac-obliterated animals. This difference could be demonstrated at day 21; however, by day 28 there was no longer a significant difference between the two groups. At this time, the perilymph was also sampled in both groups and no significant differences could be demonstrated. After systemic presensitizations with KLH and BSA, the secondary response animals received KLH challenge into their inner ears when high seurm titers had been achieved. Two weeks later, the sham-operated animals had significantly greater perilymph antibody levels than the endolymphatic-sac-obliterated animals, but no differences could be demonstrated for their serum levels. These results suggest that the endolymphatic sac must participate in the generation of both systemic and local antibody responses following inner ear antigen challenge. If the mechanism of the sac's function in these responses is antigen processing by macrophage-lymphocyte interaction, then its obliteration would modify the resulting antibody responses by altering the afferent limb of the immune system within the inner ear. The results obtained in these experiments are consistent with this operational construct for the sac.

Recently, Morgenstern *(personal communication)* performed similar experiments in systemically immunized endolymphatic-sac-obliterated animals and measured antibody development in both the perilymph and endolymph. He was able to demonstrate a decrease in the endolymph antibody levels of sac-obliterated versus normal animals. Both studies taken together indicate that the sac must play a role in the immunodefense of the inner ear. With the proliferation of plasma cells seen following antigen entry into the inner ear and the diminution of developing inner ear and systemic antibody levels following its obliteration, there seems little doubt that it serves as more than a resorptive site within the ear—possibly in a fashion analogous to the intestinal tract, which serves a resorptive as well as an immunologic role for the body.

EFFECT OF INNER EAR RESPONSES ON HEARING

Since there is mounting clinical evidence that immune responses may adversely affect hearing (14,17,20,32) we undertook a study to determine what the effect of primary and secondary inner ear immune responses would be on cochlear function (36). Utilizing a similar paradigm as previously outlined for immunizing the perilymphatic compartment of sensitized and nonsensitized animals, their hearing was monitored electrophysiologically both before and at various times following inner ear inoculation with antigen (KLH). Following primary inner ear immune responses, mild physiological changes were seen in association with this gradually mounting immune response (see Fig. 7). Eight to 14 days following the inoculation, mean 8th nerve action potential (AP) recordings showed no significant change from the control subjects, whereas cochlear microphonic (CM) recordings demonstrated a small but significant deterioration beyond what was attributable to injection artifact. At day 30, these animals showed no difference in either AP or CM compared with controls. In contrast, the secondary immune response group showed significant increases in both AP and CM thresholds over a 30-day period compared to the primary response animals and the control group.

Clearly, the conclusion from these experiments is that the inner ear is capable of handling a slowly mounting primary inner ear immune response, whereas it suffers what appears to be irreversible damage from a vigorous secondary immune response. Clinically, this might be important in a situation in which an organism (bacterium or virus) or other antigenic material (i.e., prosthetic materials or substances used during stapedectomy) gains entrance to the inner ear, thus setting up conditions for a primary immune response. Although characteristic immune reactions may occur within the inner ear, they do not result in significant or permanent hearing deficits. However, when a substance is reintroduced to the inner ear once there has been sensitization to this antigen or organism, the secondary immune response that develops causes significant and probably permanent hearing loss. An attractive hypothesis for the development of sudden hearing losses caused by viruses or hearing losses resulting from "reparative" granulomas following stapedectomy is that we are really witnessing secondary inner ear immune responses that are unleashed because of re-exposure to the offending antigen during subsequent infection (or reactivation of a latent virus) or surgery.

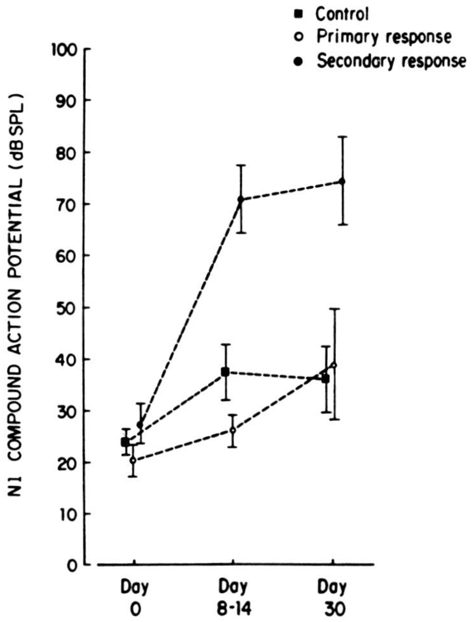

FIG. 7. Comparison of 8th nerve action potential thresholds (mean ±1 SD) for control, primary, and secondary inner ear immune response animals on days 0, 8–14, and 30. Only the secondary immune response animals showed significant changes in action potential thresholds at days 8–14 and 30 postinoculation ($p < 0.001$ *t*-test). (From ref. 36.)

PROTECTIVE ROLE OF INNER EAR IMMUNITY

Although much has been written on the potential harm that immunity can cause to the inner ear, one should not lose sight of the fact that the immune system evolved to protect the host from a hostile environment. Thus, if the inner ear truly has an immune system, then one must be able to demonstrate its functional capacity to protect the inner ear from virulent organisms. To investigate this further, Harris and co-workers (11,37) established a model of cytomegaloviral labyrinthitis in the guinea pig. In animals with no prior exposure to this virus, inoculation of the perilymphatic compartment with a live viral suspension resulted in deafness within 8 days. The histopathological changes associated with this decline in cochlear function included tremendous inflammatory infiltrates, hemorrhage and fibrosis in the scalae, degeneration of sensory and neural elements throughout the cochlea, and the presence of characteristic cells with inclusions lining the scala tympani and within the spiral ganglion cells. In contrast, those animals with immunity to cytomegalovirus (CMV) following systemic presensitization with live virus were protected from a subsequent inoculation with the live viral suspension. In addition to preservation of cochlear function, these animals showed normal morphology 8 days following inner ear challenge. This protection was correlated with a rise in specific anti-CMV antibody levels within the perilymph. Thus, these experiments demonstrated for the first time that inner ear immunity may play a protective role by neutralizing a virulent organism. Furthermore, these experiments confirm that inner ear immunity does in fact exist functionally and is not merely an observation artificially created by the experimental technique.

EFFECT OF MIDDLE EAR IMMUNE RESPONSES ON INNER EAR ANTIBODY LEVELS

Studies of middle ear immunity have demonstrated that antibody, complement, and inflammatory mediators are involved in the generation and perpetuation of the effusion associated with otitis media with effusion (OME) (4,10,22,27). Furthermore, studies have shown the semipermeable nature of the round window membrane to substances instilled into the middle ear (8,25). Since the association of sensorineural hearing loss with chronic otitis media has been suggested, it is conceivable that substances elaborated during middle ear inflammation can cross the round window membrane and exert an effect upon the inner ear. Suzuki (28) demonstrated that in the presence of acute middle ear inflammation there was an increase in the protein concentration within the inner ear. With this in mind, Harris and Ryan (10) performed a study to determine if antibody and/or antigen from an immunologically induced middle ear effusion could pass into the perilymphatic space. Animals were systemically sensitized to both KLH and BSA until high antibody titers were achieved. The middle ear cleft was then challenged on two successive weeks, resulting in a vigorous immune response with effusion and mucosal inflammation. Antibody levels against KLH and BSA were then compared in serum, middle ear effusions, and perilymph. Anti-KLH levels in the inner ear were found to increase substantially on the inflamed side, whereas the anti-BSA levels did not, indicating its local, rather than serum, origin. This study suggested that antibody and/or antigen within the middle ear penetrated the inner ear. In subsequent experiments, injection of KLH into the middle ear did not result in the detection of KLH within the perilymph; however, inoculation of anti-KLH immunoglobulin into the middle ears of nonimmunized animals resulted in an increase of antibody in the perilymph. Thus, it appears that in these circumstances, antibody but not antigen was able to pass into the inner ear from the middle ear space. This may be a size-dependent phenomenon, so that if an antigen with a smaller molecular weight had been selected, then perhaps both antibody and antigen would have been detected. What this also suggests is that the presence of inflammation was not the sole requirement for the passage of substances into the inner ear, but may in fact enhance it.

The passage of antibody from a middle ear effusion into the inner ear was not associated with any morphological changes within the inner ear and thus appeared to be a well-tolerated process. The passage of specific antibody into the inner ear might serve an important protective function in an ear that harbors potential pathogens; perchance those organisms violate the normal barriers isolating the inner ear. However, what subtle or long-term effects the presence of antibody or its corresponding antigen might have on inner ear function is unknown. It is conceivable that antigen-antibody interaction might have adverse effects which, over time, could cause inner ear dysfunction. This phenomenon may contribute to the occurrence of sensorineural hearing loss associated with chronic otitis media.

EXPERIMENTAL ALLERGIC LABYRINTHITIS

The concept that the inner ear may also be the target of autoimmune conditions follows from extensive experimental studies conducted on other organ systems. Such animal models have been established for experimental allergic encephalomyelitis (EAE), allergic neuritis, myasthenia gravis and allergic thyroiditis, to name a few. In 1961, Beickert (3) performed the first study to examine this possibility in relation to the inner ear. Utilizing guinea pigs immunized to inner ear antigen, he was able to demonstrate lesions within the cochlea. In 1963, Terayama and Sasaki (29) immunized guinea pigs with isologous cochlear tissue in Freund's adjuvant and were also able to produce isolated lesions within the cochleae and alterations in the Preyer's reflex. Neither study was able to document the development of anticochlea antibodies nor the presence of perivascular infiltrates. These observations were essentially ignored at the time because of (a) limited technological resources that did not allow the researchers to extend their findings and (b) a general disregard for autoimmune conditions. Since that time, Yoo et al. (38,39) have reported the development of an animal model with inner ear injury secondary to type-II collagen anti-immunity. A full discussion of this condition is covered in Yoo et al.'s chapter *(this volume)*. Recently, Harris et al. (9b) investigated the possible creation of an animal model of autoimmune inner ear dysfunction resulting from exposure to heterologous cochlear tissue. Immunizing guinea pigs with fresh bovine cochlear antigen in Freund's adjuvant, these animals developed significant hearing loss compared to a control group of animals (defined as an increase in 8th nerve action potential threshold that was greater than two standard deviations above the mean for the control ears tested). In the experimental group of animals, the presence of anticochlear antibodies were uniformly detected and 32% of those ears tested (12 of 38) had significant hearing losses. Histological evidence of immunological injury was seen, as characterized by spiral ganglion cell degeneration, perivascular infiltration by plasma cells, edema, and hemorrhage. Interestingly, some animals showed unilateral hearing losses, whereas others had bilateral losses of varying degrees. This finding is reminiscent of the clinical picture of autoimmune sensorineural hearing loss as described by McCabe (20). The etiology of autoimmunity is unknown, but one theory suggests that the tissues that are involved in this process are either of ectodermal or endodermal origin and are viewed as foreign by the immune system, which is mesodermal. Since the entire membranous labyrinth is of ectodermal origin, this would be consistent with the concept that the inner ear is a potential site of an autoimmune process.

CONCLUSION

The inner ear is a sensory organ that certainly comes under the influence of host immunity. Experiments have shown that the immune reactions that develop within the inner ear may be protective of cochlear function, yet under certain circumstances these responses can result in immune-mediated injury. To assume that the inner ear has a unique immune system that is different or that operates in isolation from systemic immunity is unfounded. More reasonable is the view that there are immune responses that can occur locally within the inner ear; however, the population of immunocompetent cells that are responsible for these responses probably arise outside of the ear and migrate to the site of antigen challenge. The hypothesis that the potential of the endolymphatic sac is the site where antigens are processed and presented for immune processing is attractive and deserves further investigation. Evidence showing that the endolymphatic sac is ultimately involved in the development of inner ear responses suggests that this site may then become a bystander to immune-related injury and ultimately result in its own dysfunction. Such a hypothesis is appealing in light of the known histopathological findings seen in the endolymphatic sacs of Meniere's disease patients, which include perisaccular fibrosis and loss of vascularity. Whether this condition or others ultimately prove to be related to immunity is as yet undetermined; however, the continued investigation of immune responses and the damage it causes to the inner ear will serve as a tool to better understand the physiology of hearing and balance.

ACKNOWLEDGMENTS

The author wishes to acknowledge the contributions of Drs. Nigel Woolf, Elizabeth Keithley, Allen Ryan, and Shunichi Tomiyama for portions of this work and the excellent technical efforts made by Patricia Sharp, Roberta Dupre, Eric Silva, and William Cornell.

This research has been supported by the Research Service of the Veterans Administration, a Teacher Investigator Development Award #NS00606 from the NIH, NIH grants NS18643 and NS21485, and a grant from the Deafness Research Foundation.

REFERENCES

1. Arnold, W., Altermatt, H.-J., and Gebbers, J.O. (1984): Demonstration of immunoglobulins (SIgA, IgG) in the human endolymphatic sac. *Laryngol. Rhinol. Otol. (Stuttg.)* 63:464–467.
2. Arnold, W., Pfaltz, R., and Altermatt, H.-J. (1985): Evidence of serum antibodies against inner ear tissues in the blood of patients with certain sensorineural hearing disorders. *Acta Otolaryngol. (Stockh.)*, 99:347–444.
3. Beickert, P. (1961): Zur frage der empfindungsschwerhorigkeit und autoallergie. *Z. Laryngol.*, 54:837–842.
4. Bernstein, J.M., Tomasi, T.B., and Ogra, P.L. (1974): The immunochemistry of middle ear effusions. *Arch. Otolaryngol.*, 99:320–326.

5. Bernstein, J.M., Szymanski, C., Albini, B., Sun, M., and Ogra, P.L. (1978): Lymphocyte subpopulations in otitis media with effusion. *Pediatr. Res.*, 12:786–788.
6. Chevance, L.G., Galli, A., and Jeanmarie, J. (1960): Immunoelectrophoretic study of human perilymph. *Acta Otolaryngol.*, 52:41–46.
7. Fritsch, J.H., and Jolliff, C.R. (1966): Protein components of human perilymph. *Ann. Otol. Rhinol. Laryngol.*, 75:1070–1076.
8. Goycoolea, M.V., Paparella, M.M., Goldberg, B., and Carpenter, A.M. (1982): Permeability of the round window membrane in otitis media. *Arch. Otolaryngol.*, 106:430–436.
9. Harris, J.P. (1983): Immunology of the inner ear: response of the inner ear to antigen challenge. *Otolaryngol. Head Neck Surg.*, 91:17–23.
9a.Harris, J.P. (1984): Immunology of the inner ear: evidence of local antibody production. *Ann. Otol. Rhinol. Laryngol.*, 93:157–162.
9b.Harris, J.P. (1987): Experimental autoimmune sensorineural hearing loss. Laryngoscope, 97(1):63–76.
10. Harris, J.P., and Ryan, A.F. (1985): Effect of a middle ear immune response on inner ear antibody levels. *Ann. Otol. Rhinol. Laryngol.*, 94:202–206.
11. Harris, J.P., Woolf, N.K., Ryan, A.F., et al. (1984): Immunologic and electrophysiologic response to cytomegalovirus inner ear infection. *J. Infect. Dis.* 150:523–530.
12. Harris, J.P., Woolf, N.K., and Ryan, A.F. (1985): Elaboration of systemic immunity following inner ear immunization. *Am. J. Otolaryngol.*, 6:148–152.
13. Hopp, E.S., Elevitch, E.R., Pumphrey, R.E., Irving, T.E., and Hoffman, P.W. (1965): Serous otitis media—"immune" theory. *Laryngoscope*, 74:1149–1159.
14. Hughes, G.B., Kinney, S.E., Barna, B.P., et al. (1983): Autoimmune reactivity in Cogan's syndrome: a preliminary report. *Otolaryngol. Head Neck Surg.*, 91:24.
15. Jenkins, H.A., Pollak, A.M., and Fisch, U. (1981): Polyarteritis nodosa as a cause of sudden deafness. A human temporal bone study. *Am. J. Otolaryngol.*, 2:99–107.
16. Juhn, S.K., and Rybak, L. (1981): Nature of the blood-labyrinth barrier. In: *Meniere's Disease: Pathogenesis, Diagnosis and Treatment*, edited by K.-H. Vosteen, H. Schuknecht, et al., pp. 59–67. Thieme-Stratton, Stuttgart.
17. Kanzaki, J., and Ouchi, T. (1983): Steroid-responsive bilateral sensorineural hearing loss and immune complexes. *Arch. Otol. Rhinol. Laryngol.*, 230:5–9.
18. Lim, D., and Silver, P. (1974): The endolymphatic duct system. A light and electron microscopic investigation. In: *Proceedings of Barany Society Meeting, Los Angeles, California*, edited by J. Pulec, p. 390.
19. Liu, Y.S., Lim, D.J., Lang, R.W., and Birck, H.G. (1975): Chronic middle ear effusions: immunochemical and bacteriological investigation. *Arch. Otolaryngol.*, 101:278–286.
20. McCabe, B.F. (1979): Autoimmune sensorineural hearing loss. *Ann. Otol. Rhinol. Laryngol.*, 88:585–589.
21. Mogi, G., Lim, D., and Watanabe, N. (1982): Immunologic study on the inner ear. *Arch. Otolaryngol.*, 108:270–275.
22. Mogi, G., Maeda, S., Yoshida, T., and Watanabe, N. (1976): Immunochemistry of otitis media with effusion. *J. Infect. Dis*, 133:125–136.
23. Palva, T., and Raunio, V. (1981): Disc electrophoretic studies of human perilymph. *Ann. Otol. Rhinol. Laryngol.*, 76:23–26.
24. Rask-Andersen, H., and Stahle, J. (1980): Immunodefense of the inner ear? *Acta Otolaryngol.*, 89:283–294.
25. Rhodes, R. (1980): Round window membrane permeability to horseradish peroxidase: an electromicroscopy study. Thesis, University of Minnesota, Minneapolis.
26. Saijo, S., and Kimura, R.S. (1984): Distribution of HRP in the inner ear after injection into the middle ear cavity. *Acta Otolaryngol.(Stockh.)*, 97:593–610.
27. Sloyer, J.L., Howie, V.M., Ploussard, J.H., Amman, A.J., Austrian, R., and Johnston, R. (1974): Immune response to acute otitis media in children. I. Serotypes isolated and serum and middle ear fluid antibody in pneumococcal otitis media. *Infect. Immun.*, 9:1028–1032.
28. Suzuki, Y. (1977): Immunological studies on inner ear fluids under the influence of acute middle ear inflammation. *J. Otolaryngol. (Japan)*, 6:618–626.
29. Terayama, Y., and Sasaki, Y. (1963): Studies on experimental allergic (isoimmune)labyrinthitis in guinea pigs. *Acta Otolaryngol.(Stockh.)*, 58:49–64.
30. Tomiyama, S., and Harris, J.P. (1985): Specific antibody production in the endolymphatic sac

obliterated guinea pig following inner ear antigen challenge. AAO-ARO Research Forum, Atlanta, Georgia, October.
31. Tubara, E.S., and Freter, R. (1972): Source and protective function of coproantibodies in intestinal disease. *Am. J. Clin. Nutr.*, 25:1357–1363.
32. Veldman, J.E., Roord, J.J., O'Connor, J.J., et al. (1984): Autoimmunity and inner ear disorders: an immune complex mediated sensorineural hearing loss. *Laryngoscope*, 94:501–507.
33. Veltri, R.W., and Sprinkle, P.M. (1976): Secretory otitis media. An immune complex disease. *Ann. Otol. Rhinol. Laryngol.*, Suppl. 25:135–139.
34. Walker, W.A., Isselbacher, K.J., and Bloch, K.J. (1974): Immunologic control of soluble protein absorption from the small intestine: a gut-surface phenomenon. *Am. J. Clin. Nutr.*, 27:1434–1440.
35. Williams, R.C., and Gibbons, R.J. (1972): Inhibition of bacterial adherence by secretory immunoglobulin A: a mechanism of antigen disposal. *Science*, 177:697–699.
36. Woolf, N.K., and Harris, J.P. (1986): Cochlear pathophysiology associated with inner ear immune responses. *Acta Otolaryngol.*, 102:353–364.
37. Woolf, N.K., Harris, J.P., Ryan, A.F., et al. (1985): Hearing loss in experimental cytomegalovirus infection of the inner ear of the guinea pig: prevention by systemic immunity. *Ann. Otol. Rhinol. Laryngol.*, 94:350–356.
38. Yoo, T.J., Stuart, J.M., Kang, A.H., Townes, A., Tomoda, K., and Dixit, S.: Type II collagen autoimmunity in otosclerosis and Meniere's disease. *Science*, 217:1153–1155.
39. Yoo, T.J., Tomoda, K., Stuart, J.M., Kang, A.H., Townes, A.S., and Cremer, N.A. (1983): Type II collagen-induced autoimmune sensorineural hearing loss and vestibular dysfunction in rats. *Ann. Otol. Rhinol. Laryngol.*, 92:267–271.

Immunology of the Ear, edited by J. Bernstein
and P. Ogra. Raven Press, New York © 1987.

Immunological Factors in Meniere's Disease

Allen F. Ryan

Department of Surgery, Division of Otolaryngology, University of California, San Diego, School of Medicine, La Jolla, California 92093, and Research Service, Veterans Administration Medical Center, San Diego, California 92161

Meniere's disease was first described by Prosper Meniere in 1861 (37). Several years earlier, he had encountered a spectacular case of sudden hearing loss and vertigo. Postmortem examination of this patient revealed a blood-tinged "plastic lymph" in the labyrinth as the only pathological finding. Based upon this and a similar case, as well as upon the earlier studies of Flourens (14) on the labyrinth of the pigeon, Meniere correctly identified the co-occurrence of (a) tinnitus, (b) fluctuant hearing loss, and (c) repeated attacks of vertigo as symptoms of a disease of the labyrinth (37). In the intervening years, this identification has been repeatedly confirmed. Modern diagnosis also often includes a fourth symptom, a feeling of fullness in the ear (58). This cluster of symptoms is usually regarded as a single disease entity. There is some controversy on this point, however, and some authors prefer to refer to the condition as Meniere's syndrome (41).

Attempts to apply more specific descriptive and diagnostic criteria have been frustrated by the capriciousness and variability of Meniere's disease. However, it is generally accepted that the condition is most frequently unilateral and that hearing losses are primarily low frequency at the onset of symptoms, spreading to include high frequencies as the duration of the disease increases (41).

Little progress has been made in identifying the etiology of Meniere's disease. In the most significant advance, Hallpike and Cairns (23) and Yamakawa (64) established a relationship between Meniere's disease and endolymphatic hydrops. Although the exact relationship between the symptoms of the disease and distension of the membranous labyrinth has yet to be established, a central role for hydrops is now accepted. In a small percentage of cases, the symptoms of Meniere's disease can be brought about by a specific and identifiable condition, such as syphilis, viral infection, or vascular disease (41,58). However, in the vast majority of cases no cause can be established. The term Meniere's disease has now come to mean the idiopathic occurrence of the symptoms originally described by Meniere.

Many explanations of the etiology of Meniere's disease have been postulated, often paralleling advances in medical science and technology in other fields. They have frequently been linked to specific therapies reported to be successful in ameliorating the symptoms, and often the course, of the disease. However, the evidence offered in support of such treatments has typically consisted of patient testimonials and the impressions of treating physicians. This has made critical evaluation of the proposed etiologies difficult. With each new explanation there has been the hope that a definitive etiology for the disease would be established. However, over an extended period of time, none of the etiologies and associated treatments have been widely accepted.

Given this history, it is not surprising that immunological causes for Meniere's disease have been proposed and that they have recently been renewed, given the tremendous advances in immunology which have occurred in recent decades. However, as with other proposed etiologies, it is necessary to exercise caution in drawing conclusions about Meniere's disease. Given the fluctuating nature and slow progression of the symptoms, establishing a cause-and-effect relationship with this disease should be expected to be quite difficult.

ALLERGY

The involvement of allergy in vestibular disorders was suggested as early as the 1890s by Quincke (47). In 1923, Duke (11) postulated a relationship between allergy and Meniere's disease. Since that time there have been a number of studies and case reports linking allergy and Meniere's disease.

Evaluation of the role played by allergy has been made difficult by the differing defintions of the term allergy. Allergy is generally defined as immediate hypersensitivity, mediated by the interaction of antigens with immunoglobin E (IgE), as in the most prevalent example of inhalant allergy. Several studies have investigated the possible role of IgE in Meniere's disease. Elevated levels of IgE have not been found to be associated with this disease (54), nor have abnormal levels of histamine or serotonin (40). Sensitivity to inhalant allergens is also frequently associated with Meniere's disease (5,6,13,53,60,61).

The term allergy has also been used to denote hypersensitivity to ingested foods. A large number of case reports have presented anecdotal evidence that management of food hypersensitivity can lead to improvements in the symptoms of Meniere's disease (5,6,10,13,42,43,52,53,60,61). However, there have been no large-scale controlled studies of food hypersensitivity management of Meniere's disease. This reaction does not appear to be mediated by IgE. The mediating factors have yet to be identified, although it has been suggested that reactions to food antigens may be produced by a type-III immune reaction, i.e., complement fixation induced by antigen/IgG interactions (58). Thus it is not yet clear that hypersensitivity to foods is an immunological phenomenon.

Most authors agree that allergy, in whatever form proposed, does not account for more than a small fraction of Meniere's disease patients, estimated at 14% from one large patient sample (44).

AUTOIMMUNITY

It has recently been proposed that Meniere's disease may, in certain cases, be an autoimmune disease. McCabe (36) first suggested in 1979 that certain forms of sensorineural hearing loss have an autoimmune origin, based primarily upon the response these patients showed to steroid therapy. One category that he identified as being of autoimmune origin was bilateral Meniere disease. Laboratory tests for autoimmune disease were largely negative, leading to the suggestion that the condition was localized to the inner ear. Subsequent studies by Hughes et al. (30,31) suggested that a fraction of Meniere's disease patients can be confirmed as autoimmune, based upon a positive lymphocyte blastogenesis response to human inner ear tissue. Again, the majority of these patients showed symptoms bilaterally.

A potential problem with the data of Hughes et al. is that the positive values obtained in his blastogenesis assay were relatively low, all falling below 3.0. Such low values are not generally accepted as indicating positive T-cell (thymus-derived cell) sensitization. Harris and Ryan (26) recently attempted to confirm the observation of Hughes et al., but did not observe any instances of positive lymphocyte transformation in a sample of 14 Meniere's disease patients (Table 1).

Arnold (2) tested the sera of patients with progressive cochleovestibular disturbance and reported that a large proportion showed IgG antibodies directed against human inner ear tissues. Elies and Plester (12) have reported similar findings for Meniere's disease patients. Although additional control data are required to confirm the specificity of these observations, they are suggestive of humorally mediated autoimmunity.

The hypothesis of autoimmune inner ear disease has been examined experimentally by Harada et al. (24), who immunized normal guinea pigs and guinea pigs genetically deficient in the complement component C4 with homogenates of rabbit stria vascularis. In some of the normal guinea pigs, cochlear hydrops were observed, whereas all C4-deficient animals showed normal inner ear histology. These data suggest that autoimmune damage to the inner ear might be mediated by the interaction of antigen and antibody, with complement fixation and resultant local tissue damage.

TABLE 1. *Lymphocyte blastogenesis responses to inner ear and skin antigens in Meniere's disease patients and normal controls*

		Stimulation index				
			Inner ear antigen		skin antigen	
Patients	*n*	PHA[a]	4 μg	500 μg	4 μg	500 μg
Meniere's disease	14	52.8	0.95	0.98	1.17	1.05
Control	11	43.9	0.90	0.95	1.19	1.12

[a]PHA, phytohemagglutin.

Yoo and co-workers (49,65,66) have hypothesized that autoimmunity to type-II collagen causes a cluster of otological disorders, including otosclerosis, eustachian salpingitis, sensorineural hearing loss, and Meniere's disease. They have observed hydrops in experimental animals immunized with type-II collagen (49,65). In addition, elevated serum titers against type-II collagen were observed in patients with Meniere's disease (66). Harris et al. (27) induced type-II collagen autoimmunity in animals, producing a severe arthritis, but failed to note any inner or middle ear abnormalities. A strain difference between the rats used in the two studies may have contributed to the discrepancy in experimental outcomes.

Clinical forms of collagen autoimmunity have not been associated with Meniere's disease. Disseminated collagen autoimmunity occurs in relapsing polychondritis, and more localized collagen disease is present in Cogan's syndrome. Although auditory and vestibular symptoms have been shown to be present in a small proportion of patients with polychondritis, and in most patients with Cogan's syndrome, the symptoms are more consistent with sudden hearing loss than with Meniere's disease (7–9,28). The proportion of rheumatoid arthritis patients exhibiting Meniere's disease is not greater than in the normal population (18,29,55).

Although the evidence for autoimmune involvement in Meniere's disease is mixed, there is reason to suspect an autoimmune etiology for a small proportion of patients, especially those with bilateral symptoms.

IMMUNE COMPLEX DISEASE

In recent reports, Brookes (4) and Veldman et al. (56) reported that a number of patients with sensorineural hearing loss, including some cases consistent with Meniere's disease, showed elevated levels of circulating immune complexes. Immune complex reactions, which may be related to autoimmunity or a response to exogenous antigens such as microorganisms or drugs, can result in a variety of vascular reactions that could impact on the inner ear.

Based on these observations, Brookes suggested that deposition of immune complexes in the vessels of the stria vascularis results in cochlear damage and sensorineural hearing loss. This mechanism could be a final common pathway for cochlear damage in a variety of disorders, e.g., autoimmune disease and viral infections, which result in the formation of circulating immune complexes.

Whereas Brookes limited his suggestion to the stria vascularis, it is also possible that complex deposition in vessels associated with the endolymphatic sac could lead to damage to this organ, with resultant hydrops and Meniere's symptoms.

If immune complex deposition is an etiology in Meniere's disease, one might expect a high incidence of related symptoms in patients with disseminated immune complex disease, such as systemic lupus erythematosis and serum sickness. The evidence for this is not convincing (15,17,45,55).

OTHER IMMUNE FACTORS

Another possible immune etiology is that response to antigens that gain access to the inner ear, such as microorganisms or drugs, might cause damage to cochlear tissues by inducing local inflammation. This could be by activation of complement or arachidonic acid metabolism, delayed hypersensitivity, or other forms of immune-recruited inflammation. Both immunoglobulins (24,25,39) and lymphocytes (48,55a) have been demonstrated at various locations in the inner ear, providing a substrate for such reactions.

This hypothesis has been examined in animal experiments. Kumagami et al. (33) introduced antigens into the stylomastoid foramen of guinea pigs. Within 1 to 2 hr they measured hearing loss and observed hydrops in the cochlea. Woolf and Harris (62) injected antigen directly into the cochlea of guinea pigs and measured its effects on hearing for up to 6 hr post-injection. They observed no acute change in auditory thresholds. However, after several days, in concert with a mounting inner ear immune response, the animals' hearing declined and occasional basal turn hydrops was noted. Tomiyama and Harris (55a) observed the accumulation of plasma cells in the perisaccular connective tissue in animals undergoing inner ear immune responses. Furthermore, if the endolymphatic sac was obliterated, a significant reduction in perilymph antibody titers was found. These studies suggest the important role of the sac in the development of inner ear immune responses and also the potential for it to be injured by such responses locally in the sac.

A small number of papers have reported that nonspecific tests of immune responsiveness, such as serum immunoglobulin levels, are abnormal in Meniere's disease patients (55,59). Such studies indicate at least an involvement of immune responses in Meniere's disease.

Several authors have suggested that damage to the inner ear may be linked to viruses, and that idiopathic conditions such as Meniere's disease may represent subacute or circumscribed viral infection (16,57). Reactivation of latent viruses could account for recurrent disease. In this case, one might expect increases in circulating antibodies against viruses to be associated with Meniere's disease. Williams and Lowery (59) have recently reported that Meniere's disease patients show significantly elevated lymphocyte blastogenesis responses and serum titers to several common viruses, when compared to control patients.

CONCLUSIONS

There have been many published reports that link immunity and Meniere's disease, with a variety of proposed immune-related etiologies. Given the lack of large, long-term studies of immunity and immunotherapy in this condition, a conclusion that immunity plays an important role in Meniere's disease is premature.

Given the fluctuant nature of symptoms and the capricious course of the disease, both large numbers of patients and long-term follow-up would be necessary to produce reliable and convincing results. However, the evidence is provocative and is sufficient to suggest possible mechanisms of immune mediation. The most promising of these mechanisms may be the one that involves damage to the region of the endolymphatic sac.

It has long been suspected that endolymph flows from the inner ear to the endolymphatic sac and that the endolymphatic sac functions both to resorb endolymph and to concentrate and dispose of waste products in endolymph (19,63). Endolymph within the sac has been shown to contain much higher levels of protein than the remainder of the endolymphatic compartment (38). Destruction of the endolymphatic sac in animals leads to hydrops (32), although it does not appear to lead to the symptoms of Meniere's disease. Damage to the sac has been observed in Meniere's disease patients (20,50,51).

More recently, Lim and Silver (35) have suggested that the endolymphatic sac is a site of immunologic defense of the inner ear. Raske-Andersen et al. (48) supported this hypothesis when they reported lymphocyte/macrophage interactions and plasma cells within the sac and described a system of lymphatic channels containing lymphocytes and macrophages in the connective tissue surrounding the sac. Tomiyama and Harris (1986, *unpublished observation*) provided experimental evidence that obliteration of the sac reduces immune responses produced by the introduction of antigen into the inner ear. An immunologic role for the sac is consistent with the concept of endolymphatic flow from the inner ear to the sac (19,63), with concentration and disposal of waste products and foreign material. The presence of immunoglobulins and lymphocytes at relatively high levels could predispose the sac to immune injury, compared to the remainder of the inner ear.

Vascular specializations might also make immune injury to the sac more likely. Gussen (22) has suggested that vascular damage in the region of the sac could play an important etiological role in Meniere's disease. Inner ear symptoms similar to Meniere's disease have been reported in systemic vascular disease (21,55). It is possible that the vessels of this region may be particularly sensitive to damage by immune reactions, as are vessels in other organs, such as the kidney (46), that are involved in resorptive function. Capillary endothelial cells in the sac region could have receptors for (a) immune complexes, related to the transport of antigen/antibody reaction products from the sac or (b) lymphocytes, related to local lymphocyte traffic. These could predispose the sac region to damage by lymphocytes and antibodies. Damage to the epithelium of the sac itself, to cells of the subepithelial connective tissue which also appear to be specialized for transport (1,34), or to any lymphatic channels present (1) could also occur by a similar mechanism.

It is important to keep in mind that it is also quite possible that the majority, if not all, of Meniere's disease occurs independently of immune-mediated damage. As recently pointed out by Bernstein et al. (3), the presence of specific immunoglobulins or lymphocytes may represent only a normal immune response to related or even unrelated disease, rather than a pathogenetic mechanism. Immunity may well be involved in the prevention or control of Meniere's disease. If localized viral infection is an important etiological mechanism, for example, immune responses may play a central role in amelioration. In this case, immune responses could be useful in diagnosis and possible treatment of Meniere's disease.

ACKNOWLEDGMENTS

This research was supported by the Research Service of the Veterans Administration, by grants NS14389 and NS18643 from the NIH/NINCDS, and by the Duaei Hearing Research Fund.

REFERENCES

1. Arnold, W., Morgenstern, C., and Miyamoto, H. (1981): Morphology and function of the endolymphatic sac. In: *Meniere's Disease: Pathogenesis, Diagnosis and Treatment,* edited by K.-H. Vosteen, H. Schuknecht, C.R. Pfaltz, J. Wersall, R.S. Kimura, C. Morgenstern, and S.K. Juhn, pp. 110–114. Thieme-Stratton, New York.
2. Arnold, W.J. (1985): Experimental and clinical approach to autoimmune diseases of the inner ear. In: *Immunobiology, Autoimmunity, Transplantation, in Otorhinolaryngology,* edited by J.E. Veldman, B.F. McCabe, E.H. Huizing, and N. Mygind, pp. 131–137. Kugler Publications, Amsterdam/Berkeley.
3. Bernstein, J.M., Schatz, M. and Zeiger, R. (1984): Immunologic ear disease in adults. *Clin. Rev. Allergy,* 2:349–375.
4. Brookes, G.B. (1985): Immune complex-associated deafness: preliminary communication. *J. R. Soc. Med.,* 78:47–55.
5. Bryan, W.T.K., and Bryan M.P. (1972): Clinical examples of resolution of some idiopathic and other chronic disease by careful allergic management. *Laryngoscope,* 82:1231–1238.
6. Clemis, M.D. (1975): Allergy as a cause of fluctuant hearing loss. *Otolaryngol. Clin. North Am.,* 8:375–383.
7. Cody, D.T.R., and Sones, D.A. (1971): Relapsing polychondritis: audiovestibular manifestations. *Laryngoscope,* 81:1208–1222.
8. Cody, D.T.R., and Williams, H.L. (1960): Cogan's syndrome. *Laryngoscope,* 70:447–478.
9. Cogan, D.G., and Dickersin, G.R. (1964): Nonsyphilitic interstitial keratitis with vestibuloauditory symptoms: a case with fatal aortitis. *Arch. Ophthalmol.,* 71:172–175.
10. Derlacki, E.L. (1982): Otologic allergy. *Am. J. Otolaryngol.,* 3:379–383.
11. Duke, W.W. (1923): Meniere's syndrome caused by allergy. *JAMA* 81:2179–2181.
12. Elies, W., and Plester, D. (1985): Sensorineural hearing loss and immunity. In: *Immunobiology, Autoimmunity, Transplantation, in Otorhinolaryngology,* edited by J.E. Veldman, B.F. McCabe, E.H. Huizing, and N. Mygind, pp. 111–117. Kugler Publications, Amsterdam/Berkeley.
13. Endicott, J.N., and Stucker, F.J. (1977): Allergy in Meniere's disease related fluctuating hearing loss preliminary findings in a double-blind crossover clinical study. *Laryngoscope,* 87:1650–1657.
14. Flourens, P. (1824): *Recherches Experimentales sur les Propriétés et les Fonctions du Systeme nerveux dans les Animaux Vertebres.* Crevot, Paris.
15. Ford, F.R. (1952): *Disease of the Nervous System in Infancy, Childhood and Adolescence.* Charles C Thomas, Springfield, Ill.
16. Forquer, B.D., and Brackmann, B.E. (1980): Eustachian tube dysfunction and Meniere's disease: a report of 341 cases. *Amer. J. Otolaryngol.,* 1:160–162.
17. Girsch, L.S. (1981): Current neurological trends with allergic implications. *Immunol. Allergy Pract.,* 3:185–194.
18. Goodwill, C.J., Lord, I.J., and Knill-Jones, R.P. (1972): Hearing in rheumatoid arthritis. *Ann. Rheum. Dis.,* 31:170–173.
19. Guild, S.R. (1927): The circulation of the endolymph. *Amer. J. Anat.* 39:57–81.

20. Gussen, R. (1972): Abnormalities of the endolymphatic sac system. *Ann. Otol. Rhinol. Laryngol.*, 81:235–240.
21. Gussen, R. (1977): Polyarteritis nodosa and deafness. A human temporal bone study. *Arch. Otorhinolaryngol.*, 217:263–271.
22. Gussen, R. (1982): Vascular mechanisms in Meniere's disease. Theoretical considerations. *Arch. Otolaryngol.*, 108:544–549.
23. Hallpike, C.S., and Cairns, H. (1938): Observations on the pathology of Meniere's syndrome. *Proc. R. Soc. Med.*, 31:1317–1336.
24. Harada, T., Matsunaga, T, Hong, K., and Inoue, K. (1984): Endolymphatic hydrops and III type allergic reaction. *Acta Otolaryngol.*, 97:450–459.
25. Harris, J.P. (1984): Immunology of the inner ear: evidence of local antibody production. *Ann. Otol. Rhinol. Laryngol.*, 93:157–162.
26. Harris, J.P., and Ryan, A.F. (1986): Autoimmunity in the pathogenesis of Meniere's disease. *(submitted for publication).*
27. Harris, J.P., Woolf, N.K. and Ryan, A.F. (1986): A reexamination of experimental type II collagen autoimmunity: middle and inner ear morphology and function. *Ann. Otol. Rhinol. Laryngol.*, 95:176–180.
28. Haynes, B.F., Kaiser-Kupfer, M.I., Mason, P., and Fauci, A.S. (1980): Cogan syndrome: studies in thirteen patients, long-term follow up, and a review of the literature. *Medicine*, 59:426–441.
29. Heyworth, T., Liyanage, S.P. (1972): A pilot survey of hearing loss in patients with rheumatoid arthritis. *Scand. J. Rheumatol.*, 1:81–83.
30. Hughes, G.B., Kinney, S.E., Barna, B.P., and Calabrese, L.H. (1985): Autoimmune Meniere's syndrome. In: *Immunobiology, Autoimmunity, Transplantation, in Otorhinolaryngology*, edited by J.E. Veldman, B.F. McCabe, E.H. Huizing, and N. Mygind, pp. 119–129. Kugler Publications, Amsterdam/Berkeley.
31. Hughes, G.B., Kinney, S.E., Barna, B.P., and Calabrese, L.H. (1983): Autoimmune reactivity in Meniere's disease: a preliminary report. *Laryngoscope*, 93:410–417.
32. Kimura, R., and Schuknecht, H.F. (1965): Membranous hydrops in the inner ear of the guinea pig after obliteration of the endolymphatic sac. *Pract. Otorhinolaryngol.*, 27:343–345.
33. Kumagami, H., Nishida, H., and Dohl, K. (1976): Experimental labyrinthine lesions through styloid foramen. *ORL J. Otorhinolaryngol. Relat. Spec.*, 38:334–343.
34. Lim, D.J., and Glasscock, M.E. (1981): Fine morphology of the endolymphatic sac in Meniere's disease. In: *Meniere's Disease: Pathogenesis, Diagnosis and Treatment*, edited by K.-H. Vosteen, H. Schuknecht, C.R. Pfaltz, J. Wersall, R.S. Kimura, C. Morgenstern, and S.K. Juhn, pp. 115–127. Thieme-Stratton, New York.
35. Lim, D., and Silver, P. (1974): The endolymphatic duct system. A light and electron microscopic investigation. *Presented at the Barany Society Meeting*, Los Angeles, California.
36. McCabe, B. (1979): Autoimmune sensorineural hearing loss. *Ann. Otol. Rhinol. Laryngol.*, 88:585–589.
37. Meniere, P. (1861): Pathologie auriculaire: memories sur des lesiones de l'orielle interne donnant lieu à des symptomes de congestion cerebrale apoplectiforme. *Gazette Med. Paris*, 16:597–601.
38. Miyamoto, H., and Morgenstern, C. (1981): Role of electrolytes in different parts of the endolymphatic space. In: *Meniere's Disease: Pathogenesis, Diagnosis and Treatment*, edited by K.-H. Vosteen, H. Schuknecht, C.R. Pfaltz, J. Wersall, R.S. Kimura, C. Morgenstern, and S.K. Juhn, pp. 110–114. Thieme-Stratton, New York.
39. Mogi, G., Watanabe, N., and Lim, D.J. (1985): Inner ear immunology: immunoglobulin composition of inner ear fluids. In: *Immunobiology Autoimmunity, Transplantation, in Otorhinolaryngology*, edited by J.E. Veldman, B.F. McCabe, E.H. Huizing, and N. Mygind, pp. 139–146. Kugler Publications, Amsterdam/Berkeley.
40. Nikolaev, M.P., and Tsyrulnikova, L.G. (1976): Concerning the allergic genesis of Meniere's disease. *Vestn. Otorinolaringol.*, 3:33–37.
41. Pfaltz, C.R., and Matefi, L. (1981): Meniere's disease—or syndrome? A critical review of diagnose criteria. In: *Meniere's Disease: Pathogenesis, Diagnosis and Treatment*, edited by K.-H. Vosteen, H. Schuknecht, C.R. Pfaltz, J. Wersall, R.S. Kimura, C. Morgenstern, and S.K. Juhn, pp. 1–15. Thieme-Stratton, New York.
42. Powers, W.H. (1971): Allergic phenomena in the inner ear. *Otolaryngol. Clin. North Am.*,

4:557–564.
43. Powers, W.H. (1975): The role of allergy in fluctuating hearing loss. *Otolaryngol. Clin. North Am.,* 8:493–500.
44. Pulec, J.L., and House, W.F. (1973): Meniere's disease study: three-year progress report. *Equilibrium Res.,* 3:156–160.
45. Pruszewewicz, A., Obrebowski, A., Swiudzinski, P., and Rydzewski, B. (1979): Localization of the site of hearing organ damage in serological incompatibility. *Otolaryngol. Pol.,* 33:421–429.
46. Quick, C.A. (1975): Antigenic causes of hearing loss. *Otolaryngol. Clin. North Am.,* 8:385–394.
47. Quincke, H.I. (1893): Ueber Meningitis serosa. *Samml. Klin. Vortr.: Innere Med.,* 23:655–694.
48. Rask-Andersen, H., Bredberg, G., and Stahle, J. (1981): Structure and function of the endolymphatic duct. In: *Meniere's Disease: Pathogenesis, Diagnosis and Treatment,* edited by K.-H. Vosteen, H. Schuknecht, C.R., Pfaltz, J. Wersall, R.S. Kimura, C. Morgenstern, and S.K. Juhn, pp. 99–109. Thieme-Stratton, New York.
49. Schiff, M., and Yoo, T.J. (1985): Immunologic aspects of otologic disease: an overview. *Laryngoscope,* 95:259–269.
50. Schuknecht, H.F. (1975): Pathophysiology of Meniere's disease. *Otolaryngol. Clin. North Am.,* 8:507–514.
51. Schuknecht, H.F. (1978): A critical evaluation of treatments for Meniere's disease. *J. Cont. Ed. ORL Allergy,* 40:15–30.
52. Shambaugh, G.E., Jr., and Wiet, R.J. (1980): The diagnosis and evaluation of allergic disorders with food intolerance in Meniere's disease. *Otolaryngol. Clin. North Am.,* 13:671–679.
53. Shaver, E.F. (1975): Allergic management of Meniere's disease. *Arch. Otolaryngol.,* 101:96–99.
54. Stahle, J. (1976): Allergy, immunology, psychosomatic, hypo- and hypertonus. *Arch. Otorhinolaryngol.,* 212:287–292
55. Stephens, S.D.G., Luxon, L., and Hinchcliffe, R. (1982): Immunological disorders and auditory lesions. *Audiology,* 21:128–148.
55a. Tomiyama, S., and Harris, J.P. (1986): The endolymphatic sac: its importance in inner ear immune responses. *Laryngoscope,* 96:685–691.
56. Veldman, J.E., Roord, J.J., O'Connor, A.F., and Shea, J.J. (1984): Autoimmunity and inner ear disorders: an immune complex mediated sensorineural hearing loss. *Laryngoscope,* 94:501–507.
57. Veltri, R.W., Wilson, W.R., Sprinkle, P.M., Rodman, S.M., and Kavash, D.A. (1981): The implications of virus in idiopathic sudden hearing loss; primary infection or reactivation of latent viruses? *Otolaryngol. Head and Neck Surg.,* 89:137–141.
58. Williams, H.L. (1965): A review of the literature as to the physiologic dysfunction of Meniere's disease: a new hypothesis as to its fundamental cause. *Laryngoscope,* 75:1661–1689.
59. Williams, L.L., and Lowery, H.W. (1987): Evidence of persistent viral infection in Meniere's disease. *Arch. Otolaryngol. (in press).*
60. Wilson, W.H. (1972): Antigenic excitation in Meniere's disease. *Laryngoscope,* 82:1726–1735.
61. Wilson, W.H. (1974): Fungal derivatives as antigenic excitants of episodic vertigo. *Laryngoscope,* 84:1585–1598.
62. Woolf, N.K., and Harris, J.P. (1986): Cochlear pathophysiology associated with inner ear immune responses. *Acta Otolaryngol.,* 102:353–364.
63. Yamakawa, K. (1928): Die Wirkung der arsenigen Saure: auf das Ohr. *Arch. Ohrenheilk,* 123:238–248.
64. Yamakawa, K. (1938): Uber die pathologische Veranderung bei einem Meniere's-kranken. *J. Otol. Rhinol. Laryngol. Soc. Japan,* 4:2310–2312.
65. Yoo, T.J. (1984): Etiopathogenesis of Meniere's disease: a hypothesis. *Ann. Otol. Rhinol. Laryngol.* (Suppl.), 113:6–12.
66. Yoo, T.J., Stuart, J.M., Kang, A.H., Townes, A.S., Tomoda, K., and Dixit, S. (1982): Type II collagen autoimmunity in otosclerosis and Meniere's disease. *Science,* 217:1153–1155.

Immunology of the Ear, edited by J. Bernstein and P. Ogra. Raven Press, New York © 1987.

Animal Model of Autoimmune Ear Disease

*[†]T.J. Yoo, R.A. Floyd, and H. Kitano

*Departments of Medicine, *Microbiology and Immunology, and [†]Neurosciences Program, University of Tennessee, Memphis, Tennessee 38163*

The pathogenesis of autoimmunity involves various genetic, immunological, and viral factors interacting through complicated mechanisms that are still poorly understood. Recent evidence suggests that immunological disturbances may be associated with some causes of auditory dysfunction (2,3,17). There are several diseases associated with hearing loss; these include Meniere's disease, otosclerosis, autoimmune sensory hearing loss, and other forms of sudden hearing loss (Table 1).

Cogan's syndrome, which consists of interstitial keratitis and vestibuloauditory disorder progressing to profound hearing loss, was well described in 1945 by Cogan (6). In 1960, Cody and Williams implied this was a collagen disease. Their treatment included high doses of corticosteroid, under the assumption that the improvement of hearing produced by this drug was lost when the doses were reduced (5).

In 1958, Lehnhardt (15) reported cases of bilateral sudden hearing loss and proposed an etiological hypothesis that the degenerated organ of Corti could induce anticochlear antibody that would react with another intact organ of Corti. In 1959, Kikuchi (14) reported several cases of hearing loss as sympathetic otitis in which hearing in the opposite ear had been markedly influenced by the operation of the other ear. In 1961, Beickert (4) was the first to publish the experimental data concerning autoimmune reaction in the cochlea. He injected an anti-guinea-pig cochlea antibody, produced in the duck, into a guinea pig. In 1964, Sasaki and Terayama (20) produced experimental allergic labyrinthitis in guinea pigs by the immunization of guinea pig cochlea tissue emulsified with Freund's adjuvant. They found degenerative changes in the spiral ganglia and stria vascularis, hemorrhages in the scala tympani, and disintegration of the organ of Corti. They noted acoustic threshold shifts, although they could not demonstrate any anticochlear antibody.

In the past 6 years, a unique animal model of ear disease has been developed and partially characterized. Animals immunized with native type-II collagen developed sensory hearing loss, vestibular dysfunction, degeneration in the spiral ganglion, crista ampullaris, vacuolar degeneration in the utricles, endolymphatic hydrops, and otospongiosis-like lesions (Table 2) (7,22–25,28,29). Preliminary

TABLE 1. *Ear diseases with immunologic features*

External ear	Auricular chondritis Relapsing polychondritis
Tympanic membrane	Tympanosclerosis
Eustachian tube	Autoimmune salpingitis
Middle ear	Otosclerosis Secretory otitis media Necrotizing otitis media Cholesteatoma
Inner ear	Autoimmune sensorineural hearing loss Meniere's disease Otosclerosis Cochlear vasculitis Sudden hearing loss
Retrocochlea	Autoimmune CNS disease

TABLE 2. *Collagen-induced ear disease*

Sensorineural hearing loss
Vestibular dysfunction
Spiral ganglion degeneration
Atrophy of organ of Corti
Cochlear vasculitis
Salpingitis and chondritis
Otospongiosis-like lesion
Endolymphatic hydrops

data suggest that this is associated with both cellular and humoral immune response to native type-II collagen. In addition, the immunopathological changes in this model are similar to human conditions. Furthermore, we are able to transfer this pathology by serum or lymphoid cells, thus fulfilling the requirement of autoimmune phenomena.

TYPE-II COLLAGEN AUTOIMMUNE RESPONSE AS A BASIC PATHOGENESIS OF EAR LESIONS

Well-established criteria for immunologists who wish to determine the relationship of immunological phenomena to disease etiology include the following: (a) the autoimmune response must be regularly associated with the disease; (b) a replica of the disease must be inducible in laboratory animals; (c) immunopathological changes in the natural and experimental disease should parallel each other; and (d) transfer of the autoimmune illness should be possible by the transfer of serum or lymphoid cells from the diseased individual to a normal recipient. Though studies in this regard are preliminary, these criteria have been fulfilled for certain ear diseases.

Although there are several ear diseases in which an immunological reaction might play a role, it is not clear at this time to what extent autoimmune responses are responsible for human ear lesions.

However, type-II collagen autoimmunity has been proven to exist in relapsing polychondritis in which auricular chondritis and cochlear and vestibular lesions also occur in approximately 50% of patients (19). About 20% of patients with autoimmune sensorineural hearing loss (AISNHL) have shown either type-II or type-IV collagen immunity (30); they also had positive responses in a migration inhibition assay when labyrinthine membranes were used as antigens (30,31). Though the exact biochemical properties of these labyrinthine antigens have not been characterized, preliminary studies show that they contain type-II collagens (36). This speculation is based on three studies performed in our laboratory: (a) the presence of hydroxyproline and proline in amino acid analysis of this tissue (Table 3), (b) immunoperoxidase or immunofluorescent staining using monoclonal antibodies against type-II collagens, and (c) transblot technique.

TABLE 3. *Amino acid composition of human labyrinthine membrane*

Amino acid	Residues calculated per thousand[a]
Hydroxyproline	42.6
Asparagine	79.3
Threonine	28.4
Serine	39.6
Glutamine	95.8
Proline	95.1
Glycine	216.0
Alanine	102.9
Cysteine-2	6.2
Valine	45.9
Methionine	10.2
Isoleucine	25.6
Leucine	51.1
Tyrosine	12.9
Phenylalanine	31.4
Hydroxylysine	7.8
Lysine	43.4
Histidine	13.2
Arginine	47.9

[a]These results indicate that, in nature, 45% of the proteins are collagen because of the presence of hydroxyproline residues. If they were all collagens, then we would have about 20 residues of hydroxylysine. Therefore, these data are not incompatible with the presence of type-II collagen (which contains enough hydroxylysine) in the samples. Immunofluorescence or immunoperoxidase data show the presence of type-II collagen using monoclonal antibody against type-II collagen.

The underlying causes for AISNHL are probably multiple because at least some of these patients have type-II collagen autoimmunity. Preliminary evidence suggests that some experimental animals develop AISNHL without type-II collagen autoimmunity and show autoantibodies diverted against other tissue components of the inner ear.

Some otosclerosis patients have type-II collagen autoimmunity (24) and the presence of immune complexes in their lesions (13), which are also found in some patients with an idiopathic form of Meniere's disease (13). The levels of antibodies to type-II collagen are higher in Meniere's disease, suggesting a possible role for type-II collagen autoimmunity in the etiology of Meniere's disease (24). Histopathological study of the membranous labyrinth of the guinea pig hydrops model has shown fluorescent deposits on the epithelium lining, suggesting the presence of immune deposits in these areas (22,28).

The stimultaneous occurrence of Meniere's disease and otosclerosis may support type-II collagen autoimmunity (11). Autoimmune responses to type-II collagen in inner ear tissue could result in the deposition of immunoglobulin, complement, and other immune injuries in the endolymphatic duct that could impair the resorption mechanism of the endolymph, resulting in endolymphatic hydrops.

Although the importance of the antibodies to type-II collagen in Meniere's disease patients is not known, it appears that antibodies to type-II collagen can cause hearing loss and endolymphatic hydrops in guinea pigs. The stimulus for the natural development of autoimmunity in this type of pathology remains unknown.

ANIMAL MODELS

Collagen-Induced Ear Disease Model for the AISNHL, Spiral Ganglion Degeneration, and Cochlear Vasculitis

Autoimmune sensorineural hearing loss had been induced in rats by immunizing them with native bovine type-II collagen. Type-I, type-III, and denatured type-II collagen, administered by an identical immunization procedure, does not induce disease. Evidence of sensorineural hearing loss has been obtained by measuring the brain-stem-evoked potential and observing the histopathological changes consisting of cochlear nerve degeneration and perineural vasculitis in affected animals. Immunized animals have high levels of antibodies to native type-II collagen. Some have mild atrophy of the organ of Corti (25). This also occurs in chinchillas (8), guinea pigs (28), and monkeys (33). Female inbred Lewis and outbred Wistar rats, Hartley and strain-13 guinea pigs (Fig. 1a and b), and DBA-1 mice have also been used (32).

After measuring the auditory brainstem response (ABR) and obtaining sera for antibody determinations, the temporal bones are examined. Perivascular abnormalities are observed in the cochlear arteries. A large number of mononuclear cells infiltrated around the artery; the vessel is thickened and the endothelial cells are

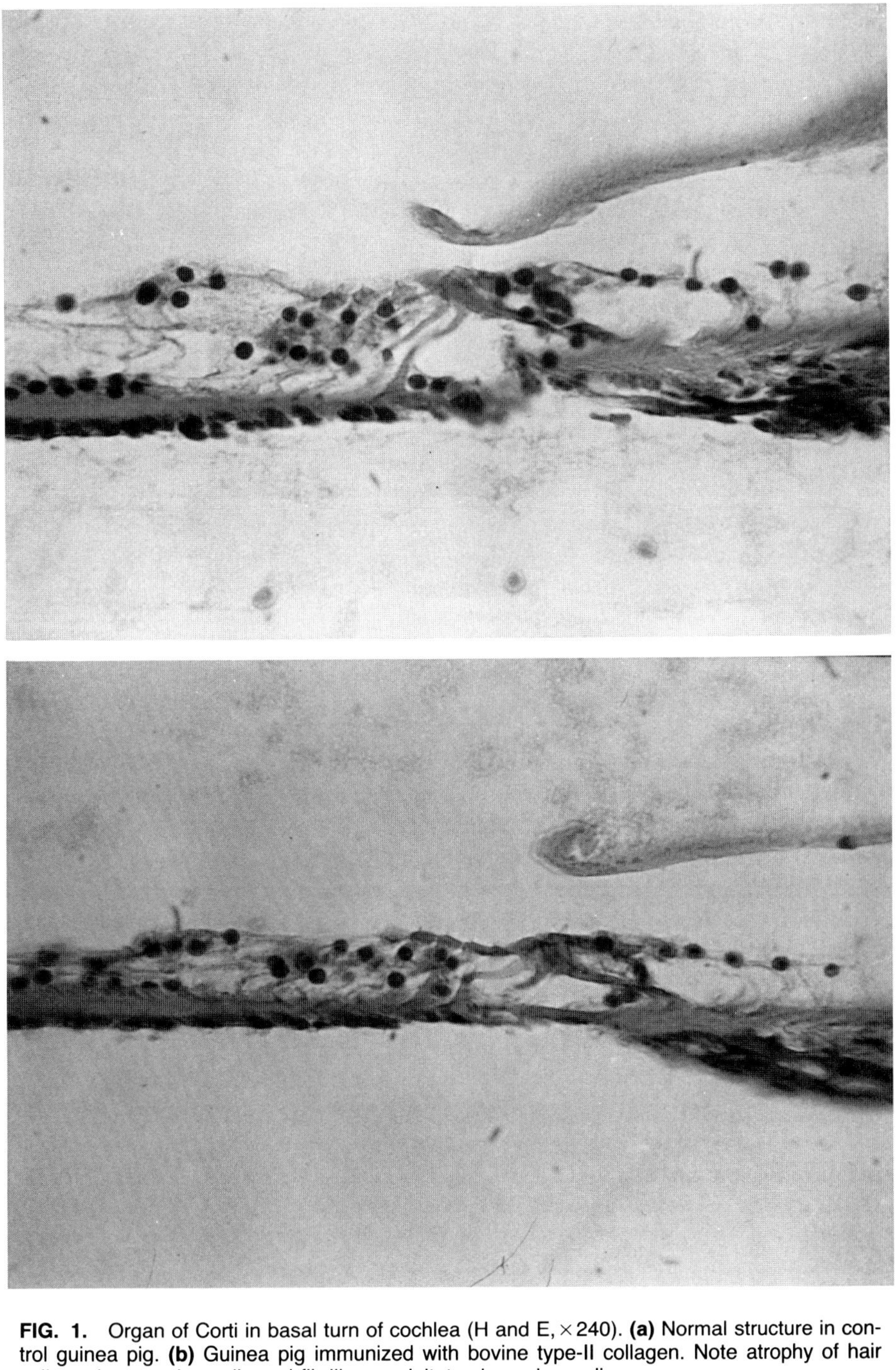

FIG. 1. Organ of Corti in basal turn of cochlea (H and E, ×240). **(a)** Normal structure in control guinea pig. **(b)** Guinea pig immunized with bovine type-II collagen. Note atrophy of hair cells and supporting cells and fibrillar precipitates in scala media.

increased. Mild fibrosis is found in the perivascular area (Fig. 2a and b). Immunofluorescence reveals the deposition of fluorescent substances in the vessel wall, perivascular fibrous tissue, and surrounding bone tissue of the cochlear artery in all rats. Spiral ganglion cell degeneration is also observed. There is vacuolar degeneration of the cochlear neurons throughout most of the cochlea of the type-II collagen-immunized rats. The ganglion cell bodies are swollen, the cytoplasm is clear, and the nuclei are pyknotic and displaced toward the axonal poles of the cells (Fig. 3a and b). Nerve fibers show slight atrophic changes. Pathological changes are relatively conspicuous in the apical turn relative to the basal turn. Immunofluorescence studies did not show pathology in the area of the spiral ganglion. The organ of Corti, stria vascularis, and the cochlear nerve also have normal histologies revealed on both regular hematoxylin-and-eosin (H and E)-stained sections and immunofluorescence sections. These results are from the animals immunized for less than 1 month's duration. However, when these animals are examined 2 or 3 months after the initial immunization, mild atrophic changes are observed in the cochlear nerve, organ of Corti, and stria vascularis. Hair cells are still present but slightly atrophied. No apparent pathological changes are observed in the vestibular sensory organ and nerve other than those previously mentioned.

The ABR of the control rats and immunized rats shows that amplitude and latency differed significantly. This also occurs in chinchillas, guinea pigs, and monkeys.

GUINEA PIG MODEL OF AUTOIMMUNE HYDROPS AND SACCULAR DEGENERATION

Endolymphatic hydrops have been induced in guinea pigs by immunization with native bovine type-II collagen. Histopathological changes consist of moderate distension of Reissner's membrane, spiral ganglion degeneration, atrophy of the organ of Corti, and a mild atrophy of the surface epithelium in the endolymphatic duct (27). These findings suggest that an immune response may be directed against type-II collagen, which is found in the membranous labyrinth, subepithelial layer of the endolymphatic duct, spiral ligament, and the enchondral layer of the otic capsule. (Fig. 4) (27).

The animal model for hydrops has some limitations. The histology of the saccule and utricle are normal, except for some vacuolar degeneration in a few of the animals, which may represent an early lesion. Most animals show atrophy of the neurosensory element of the inner ear, which is not usually present in patients with Meniere's disease.

The guinea pig is the only species that exhibits endolymphatic hydrops. A limited number of other experimental animal species have been investigated without finding hydrops. These include the mouse, rat, chinchilla, rabbit, monkey, gerbil, and cat.

Although this model has these intrinsic limitations, it still may be useful in defining the pathogenesis of Meniere's disease in humans. This model provides a new theory for the mechanism of the Meniere's disease attack (23).

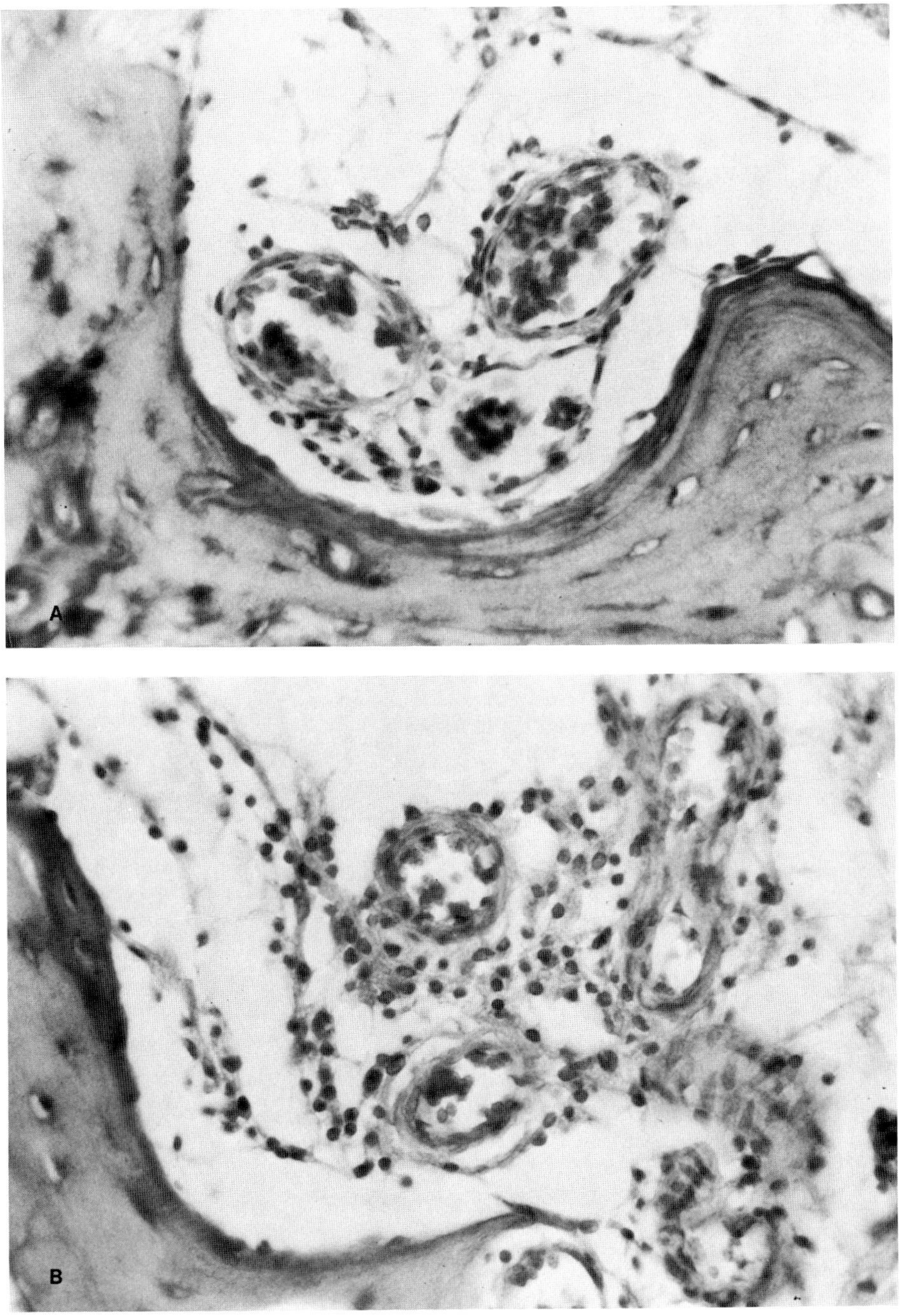

FIG. 2. **(a)** Cochlear arteries and veins from normal rat. **(b)** Inflamed cochlear artery in autoimmune sensorineural hearing loss in rat. (H and E, ×240; micrograph ×3,840.)

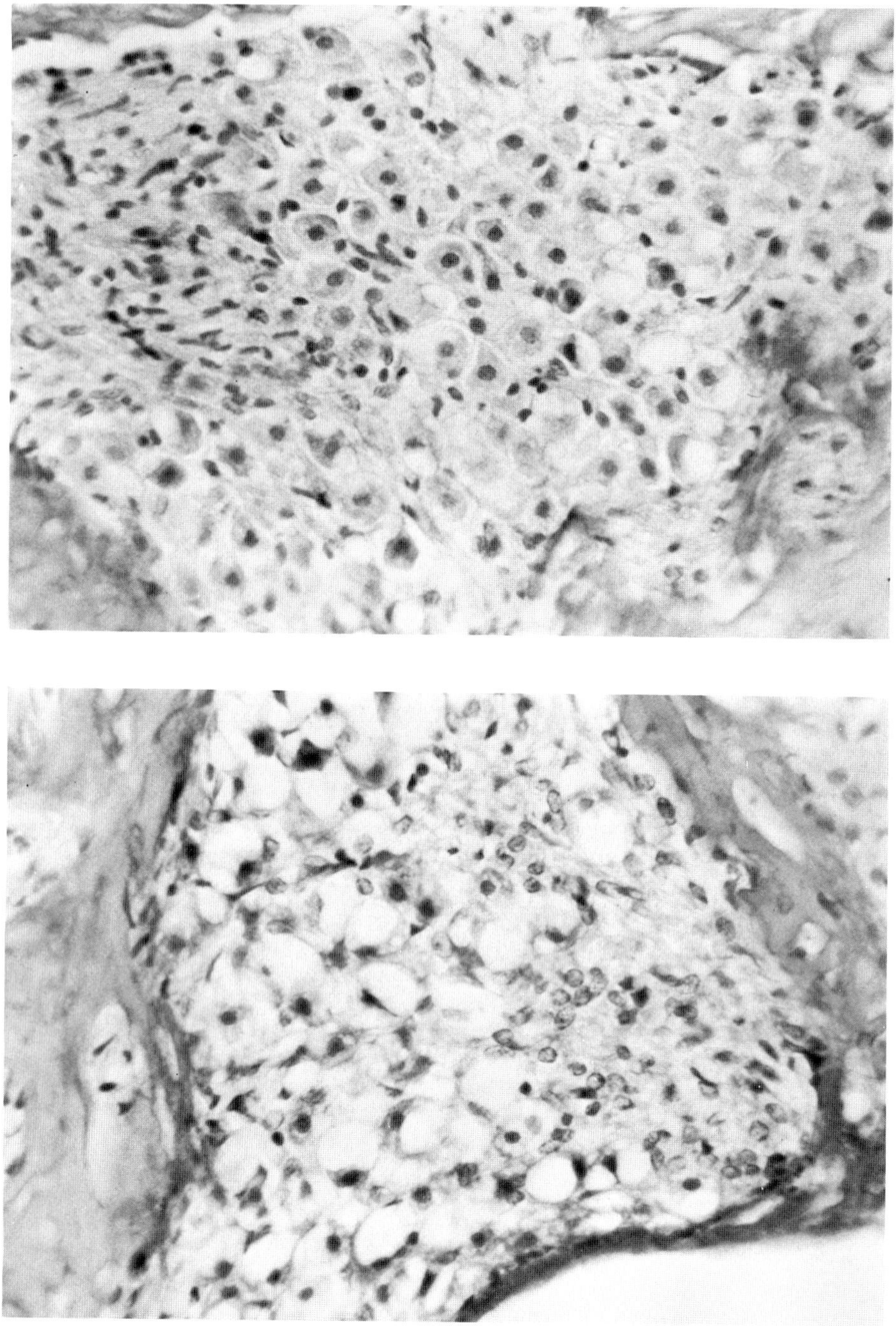

FIG. 3. **(a)** Spiral ganglion from normal ear. **(b)** Degenerated spiral ganglion in ear with autoimmune sensorineural hearing loss.

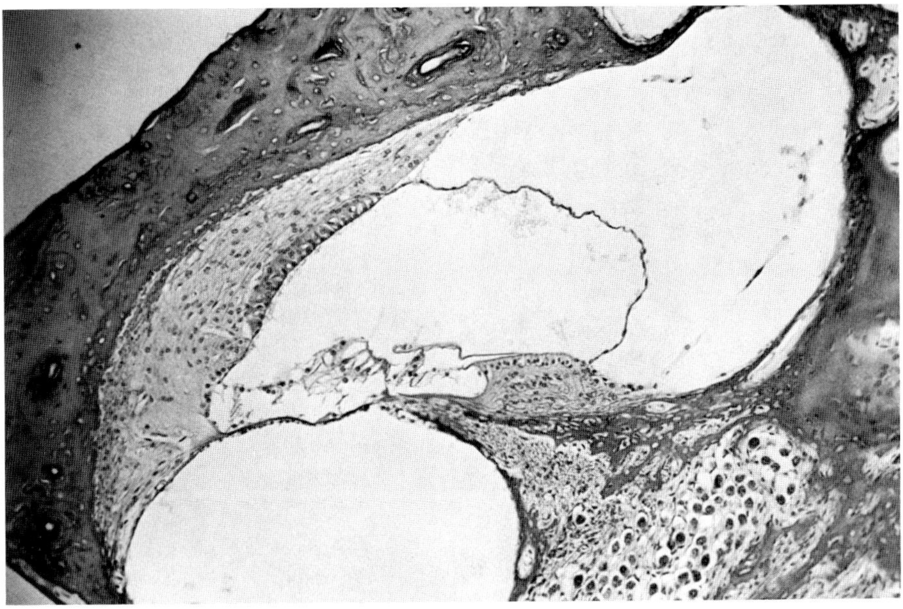

FIG. 4. Moderate extension of Reissner's membrane in a guinea pig immunized with native bovine type-II collagen. (H and E, ×240.)

The experimental results, using animal models, indicate that the inner ear fluid from immunized animals has antibody activity against type-II collagen antigen (29). Type-II collagen antibody might be responsible for some of the immune injuries associated with inner ear disease. The correlation of antibody levels and pathological changes in the inner ear are seen in Table 4. Results of the skin test for the measurement of cell-mediated immunity correlates well with the pathological changes (Table 5) (9).

ANIMAL MODEL FOR DEGENERATION OF THE CRISTA AMPULLARIS AND VESTIBULAR DYSFUNCTION

In this model, the animal develops vacuolar degeneration of the crista ampullaris with vestibular dysfunction. Type-II collagen exists in the crista ampullaris (25).

OTOSPONGIOSIS-LIKE LESIONS

Otosclerosis is a poorly understood pathological condition that causes hearing loss by affecting the otic capsules of the labyrinth and the stapes. Characteristic

TABLE 4. *Correlation of antibody levels and pathological changes in the inner ear of guinea pigs immunized with type-II collagen*

Guinea pig strain	No. of animals	Weeks after Immunization with type-II collagen	ELISA[a] (absorbance) (Mean = SD)	Endolymphatic hydrops[b]	Degeneration of spiral ganglion cells[b]		Atrophy of organ of Corti[b]	Atrophy of stria vascularis[b]
					Apical turn	Basal turn		
Hartley	7	2	0.324 ± 0.078	–	–	–	–	–
	8	4	0.829 ± 0.087	+	+ +	+	+ +	+
Strain 13	9	2	0.676 ± 0.192	–	+	+	+	+
	9	4	1.037 ± 0.170	+	+ +	+ +	+	+

[a]ELISA background less than 0.009.
[b]– no lesion; + mild lesion; + + severe lesion.

TABLE 5. *Guinea pig skin test reaction*

Type	Immunizing antigen	Skin testing antigen	Size of skin reaction (mm)
Strain 13			
1	nCII[a]	nCII	15 × 17
2	nCII	nCII	12 × 14
3	nCII	nCII	17 × 25
4	nBII[b]	nBII	6 × 9
5	nBII	nBII	6 × 6
6	nBII	nBII	10 × 10
Hartley			
7	nCII	nCII	16 × 20
8	nCII	nCII	16 × 16
9	nCII	nCII	17 × 18
10	nBII	nBII	12 × 12
11	nBII	nBII	9 × 8

[a]nCII, native chick type-II collagen.
[b]nBII, native bovine type-II collagen.

histopathological changes of otosclerosis have been described in fetuses and in very young children as well as in adults of all ages. Although genetic and basic histological patterns have been identified in otosclerosis, there is no agreement as to its etiology or precise pathogenesis (16).

An experimental model of otospongiosis-like lesion in rats following immunization with native type-II collagen has been described. Immunized rats develop spongiotic changes in the external meatal bone near the tympanic annulus and in the middle layer of the cochlear capsule. It is proposed that these changes are the result of collagen autoimmunity in this animal model and may shed some new light on the possible pathogenesis of human otosclerosis (23,37).

Spongiotic changes are observed in the anterior border of the external meatus bone near the tympanic annulus of the type-II collagen-immunized rat. Lesions are not found in the rats immunized with type-I collagen. In normal rats this area consists of woven and lamellar bone. In type-II collagen-immunized rats there are spongiotic vascular lesions characterized by numerous osteocytes and osteoblasts (dark staining is probably a result of chemical alteration of ground substance) and wider vascular spaces with fibrosis (Fig. 5). These distinctive pathological features resemble the spongification of bone that is seen in human otosclerosis (26).

The early lesion of spongiotic change is observed in the middle layer of the cochlear capsule. Macrophages and osteoclastic cells invade the widely vascular space and erode perivascular bone. The surrounding interstitial bone is acellular and nonviable and contains degenerated lacunae. However, spongiotic changes are not clearly recognized in the oval window and other areas (26).

Immunofluorescent studies demonstrate deposition of fluorescent substance on the bone matrix and vessel wall within the area of spongiosis, which is separated from normal bone by a defined boundary. There are no fluorescent substances in

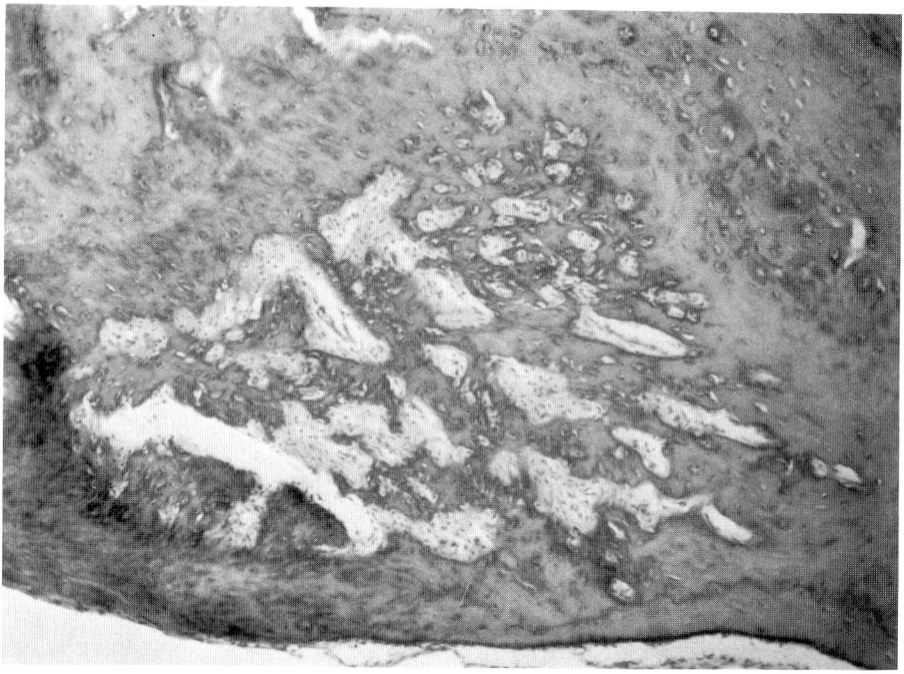

FIG. 5. Spongiotic change in rat by immunizing with native type-II collagen. (×71.)

the adjacent bone or in the temporal bone of control animals. The temporal bones of rats with collagen-immunized spongiosis are further characterized by a strong deposition of green fluorescent substances on the endochondral layer of the otic capsule. In normal rats, there is no fluorescent substance in this area. In the sections stained with H and E, there are no differences between the control and collagen-immunized rats except the thin blue staining on the surface of the lacunae and canaliculae. In addition, the walls of the vascular channels are slightly more prominent in immunized as compared to normal rats. These results have been confirmed by other investigators (1).

Ossicular joints of immunized and control rats have normal histology in both H and E and immunofluorescence sections, whereas the bone tissue of ossicles from the type-II collagen-immunized rats have a deposition of green fluorescent substances around lacunae, canaliculae, and vascular channels (26).

TRANSFER OF DISEASE

Cell Transfer of Collagen-Induced Autoimmune Ear Disease (CIAED)

The transfer of ear diseases by passive transfer of immunocytes from donor animals that have been sensitized with type-II collagen has been attempted. Guinea pigs are used in these studies, and 1×10^8 spleen cells from sensitized strain-2 or sensitized strain-13 guinea pigs have been given to the corresponding strain of guinea pigs; 4×10^7 cells have been given to healthy Hartley guinea pigs from sensitized guinea pigs. The animals are killed between 30 and 50 days after cell transfer. The temporal bone pathology has been examined and antibody activity against type-II collagen is also measured. The most prominent finding from the guinea pig experiment is the degeneration of spiral ganglion cells. One animal had developed mild to moderate endolymphatic hydrops in all turns. The saccule and crista ampullaris showed degeneration of sensory hair cells with vacuolization. The vessel walls of the modiolus seemed to be thicker than those of the controls. The lesions were more prominent in the guinea pigs that received cells from donors with high antibody titers against native bovine type-II collagen. Immunofluorescence studies of the guinea pig showed anti-Ig or anti-C3 fluorescent deposits on the otic capsule, footplate of stapes (one animal), perivascular area, and the subepithelial area of the endolymphatic duct. One animal had endolymphatic hydrops. The antibody level in the recipient guinea pig showed a mild elevation (9). Control animals that received normal lymphocytes did not have these lesions.

Thus, these studies show that ear lesions can be transferred by sensitized cells and that lesions are a result of injury mediated by immunological mechanisms. Further studies are necessary to define the precise role of the components of the immune system (cellular versus humoral) in the production of ear immune injury. The following are the pathological lesions observed in recipient guinea pigs.

Cochlea. The organ of Corti shows degeneration in the upper turns of the cochlea where the outer hair cells were missing. In the lower turns, although the supporting cells sometimes show a vacuolated degeneration, the hair cells are relatively well preserved.

Spiral ganglion. Spiral ganglion cells demonstrate severe vacuolated degeneration in which the cell bodies are swollen. The cytoplasm is clear, and the nuclei are pyknotic and displaced toward the axonal poles of the cells. Nerve fibers show atrophic changes. The degeneration of spiral ganglion is more extensive in the upper turns than in the lower turns. In the upper turns, more than 50% of the ganglion cells are degenerated. These ganglion cells are surrounded by ear structures that contain type-II collagen.

Cochlear vessels. Cochlear vessels show a thickening of their walls in which endothelial cells seem to predominate. Moderate fibrosis is found in the perivascular area.

Saccule. The saccular macula shows slight vacuolated degeneration in which the cell bodies are swollen and the cytoplasm is clear.

Serum Transfer of CIAED in Rats

To fulfill the immunological criteria of autoimmune disease, transfer of CIAED in animals was performed using serum from immunized animals. Wistar rats were immunized with native bovine type-II collagen. Antisera were fractionated with ammonium sulfate, dialyzed, lyophilized and reconstituted into a quarter of the volume of the original antisera. About 2.5 of 3 ml of this gamma-globulin fraction was given.

Fifty days later, the recipient animals were killed for histological examination. The recipients had a mildly elevated antibody titer [0.125 + 0.095 by the enzymed-linked immunosorbent assay (ELISA)]. Some spiral ganglion cells showed a mild vacuolated degeneration in which the cytoplasm was clear and the nuclei were pyknotic and necrotic. The cochlear vessels showed a thickening of their walls. Several mononuclear cells were observed around the vessels, and a mild fibrosis was found in the perivascular area. The organ of Corti had mild changes in which some supporting cells seemed to be swollen, but the hair cells were preserved. In the saccule, there was a loss of approximately half of the hair cells and supporting cells. The crista ampullaris seemed almost normal. Thus CIAED, which was transferable by immune sera, fulfilled one of the immunological criteria of ear disease. We have not done this experiment on guinea pigs.

INDUCTION OF TOLERANCE

We were able to induce a tolerance by pretreating rats with type-II collagen in varying doses prior to immunization with the antigen in an attempt to induce lesions. Four months after type-II collagen immunization, these rats had not developed ear disease. These phenomena, so far, are antigen-specific, thus indicating another support of an immunological mechanism for the induction of inner ear disease in these animal models (10).

ANATOMIC BASIS OF TYPE-II COLLAGEN AUTOIMMUNE INJURY IN THE EAR

The occurrence of diverse ear lesions in the animal models can be understood if one assumes that the immunization produced sensitized lymphocytes and antibodies capable of attacking the region where type-II collagen is an important structural component. With this in mind, extensive studies of the distribution of type-II collagen in the ears of humans, monkeys, cats, rats, chinchillas, mice, gerbils, guinea pigs, frogs, and guinea pig fetuses have been undertaken.

Collagen Distribution in the Middle and Inner Ear

Type-II collagen-specific hybridoma monoclonal antibody was applied to localize type-II collagen in the inner and middle ear. In the cochlea, positive staining to type-II collagen is observed in the endochondral layer and globular interossei in the cochlear capsule; the cribriform base and Rosenthal's canal in the modiolus, and the spiral ligament and limbus. In the vestibule, staining occurred in the endochondral layer and globular interossei in osseous labyrinth; the macula utriculi and sacculi, the semicircular canal membrane, the crista ampullaris, and the subepithelial connective tissues in the endolymphatic duct. In the external and middle ear, positive staining to type-II collagen was observed in the meatus and tympanic annulus, the interossicular joints; the stapes footplate; the endochondral layer and globular interossei in the otic capsules; and the eustachian tube cartilage. The facial nerve, outer layers of tympanic membrane, middle ear muscles, mucosa, and glands did not stain. None of the control sections showed specific staining in this study. These findings, as seen in the rats, were similar to findings observed in the guinea pig. Human stapes bones also show similar results. Only the human temporal bone shows the presence of the fissula antefenestrum as a type-II collagen structure. It was never found in the other animals tested (34).

Collagen Distribution in the Guinea Pig Fetus

The guinea pig fetus was stained with a monoclonal antibody against type-II collagen. In the 20-day old fetus, positive staining to type-II collagen was observed in the primitive temporal bone, primitive ossicles, primitive otic capsule, primitive cochlear duct, primitive spiral ganglion area, semicircular canal membrane, crista ampullaris, utricle, and saccular macula. In the 30-day old fetus, in addition to the findings in the 20-day fetus, staining occurred in the cartilage plate in the auricle and external ear meatus, tympanic membrane, endolymphatic duct, limbus, spiral ligament, and the basilar membrane. In addition to the findings in the 30-day-old fetus, the 50-day fetus showed staining of the tympanic annulus, eustachian tube cartilage, Rosenthal's canal, cribriform base, interossicular joint, the endochondral layer, and the globular interossei in the otic capsule. Because cartilage develops into bone in the otic capsule, the ossicles, and the primitive temporal bone, the positive and negative staining are mixed in these areas. Thus, these studies indicate the presence of type-II collagens in various locations of ear tissue (34).

Monoclonal antibody against streptococcal M protein was used as a negative sera.

ANTIGENIC STRUCTURAL BASIS OF THE INDUCTION OF CIAED

The preliminary finding of cyanogen bromide-cleaved peptide (CB-11) from type-II collagen produced by cyanogen bromide cleavages seems to play an important role in the collagen-induced arthritis in mice (21). The role of the peptide CB-11 or other peptides (CB-6 to CB-10 and CB-13) in the production of CIAED is being investigated. These studies might shed some light on the epitope-related phenomena in the production of CIAED. If, indeed, one or several different epitopes are responsible for the production of arthritis and CIAED, CIAED alone, or arthritis alone, it would add a great deal of understanding to these immunological phenomena.

Cyanogen bromide peptides were made according to the method of Miller (18). Cyanogen bromide was added to type-II collagen and isolated by column chromatography. This denatured protein was renatured by stepwise cooling according to the methods of Igarashi et al. (12).

These peptides were used for ELISA techniques. The CB-11 peptides correlated with the production of arthritis in mice (21). Preliminary studies with mice sera showed that CIAED is associated with antibodies reacting against CB-11 peptides. Differential binding with these peptides in various animals is associated with different anatomic lesions (e.g., joint and ear diseases).

Four or five DBA-lJ mice, which received 10 μg of CB-11 peptide in complete Freund's adjuvant, showed evidence of hearing loss 3 months after immunization. These animals received only primary immunization and had no arthritis by gross and microscopic examination, thus indicating some differences in the induction between joint and ear lesions; with the peptide, the threshold of the immune response for the ear disease was lower than that for arthritis. Mice (5 of 10) showed joint disease only after booster immunization. These studies are preliminary, and further studies are needed before any definite conclusions can be reached.

OTHER INFLUENCING FACTORS

Collagen-induced autoimmune ear disease occurs in several different animal species. Rats and guinea pigs were the most extensively studied animals, but CIAED can also be induced in monkeys and mice. The lesions of CIAED were mild in chinchillas, rabbits, and cats. Type-II collagen immune responses have been studied extensively in mice in terms of the induction of arthritis. The immune response gene to type-II collagen is linked to $H2^q$ loci. In the rat, it is also linked to AgB loci. Wistar outbred rats and Lewis rats produce these ear lesions. Wistar rats have an immune response to type-II collagen and show only a mild degree of changes in the organ of Corti. In the guinea pig, Hartley and strain-13 types are better responders for the production of CIAED. Strain 2 produces less severe lesions. The type of lesion also depends on the degree of immune responses and animal species; e.g., only guinea pigs showed any endolymphatic hydrops. Otospongiosis-like lesions were observed only in rats and, to a lesser degree, in monkeys.

In general, animals immunized with antigens in complete Freund's adjuvant showed relatively more severe lesions than animals immunized with antigens in incomplete Freund's adjuvant. The duration of the immunization seems to be a more important factor in producting severe lesions. The strain, and even the source of the animals, are very important factors in autoimmune ear disease, as is the condition of the host animals.

Recently, Cremer et al. (7) reported that subclinical or clinical mycoplasma infection in the rat markedly reduced the incidence and severity of lesions in type-II collagen-induced arthritis. Sialoductal adenovirus, widely distributed among laboratory rats, has also been implicated as a non-lesion-producing factor in rats by many researchers. As a result of complications in disease induction associated with certain viral infections, several investigators now use laminar flow rooms to ensure induction of pathological lesions at the maximum level.

We have also recently observed that none of the type-II collagen-immunized Lewis rats had developed arthritis or hearing loss in one experiment. These rats are being followed closely at the present time.

The nature of antigens is also important. Chicken type-II collagen seems better than bovine for the induction of ear lesions. The native confirmation is needed in the rat model, but it does not seem to be an important factor in the guinea pig and mouse models. Other factors that might affect the induction of ear lesions include infection or trauma. Although many factors influence the induction and severity of CIAED, these animal models provide us with an excellent new avenue of inner ear research.

ACKNOWLEDGMENTS

The research for this chapter was supported by grants from the Deafness Research Foundation, American Otologic Society, National Hearing Association, and Medical Research Funds granted by the Veterans Administration.

REFERENCES

1. Abramson, M., Huang, C.C., and Saporta, D. (1985): Type II collagen induced bone resorption in the temporal bone of rats: histological and immunohistochemical studies. *Arch. Otorhinolaryngol.*, 242:183–188.
2. Arnold, W., and Pfaltz, C.R., and Altermatt, H.J. (1985): Evidence of serum antibodies against inner ear tissues in the blood of patients with certain sensorineural hearing disorders. *Acta Otolaryngol.*, 99:437–444.
3. Barna, B.P., Calabrese, L.M., Hughes, G.B., and Kinney, S.E. (1983): Autoimmune reactivity in Meniere's disease: preliminary report. *Laryngoscope,* 93:410.
4. Beickert, V.P. (1961): Zur frage der empfindungs schwerhorigkeit under autoallergie. *Laryngol. Rhinol. Otolaryngol.* 40:837–842.
5. Cody, D.T. and Willians, H.L. (1960): Cogan's syndrome. *Laryngoscope,* 70:447–478.
6. Cogan, D.G. (1945): Syndrome of nonsyphilitic interstitial keratitis and vestibuloauditory symptoms. *Arch. Ophthal.*, 33:144.
7. Cremer, M.A., Leary, S.L., and Taurog, J.D. (1984): Infection with mycoplasma pulmonis modulates adjuvant- and collagen-induced arthritis in Lewis rats. *Arthritis Rheum.*, 27:943–946.
8. Floyd, R.A., Ishibe, T., Kuo, C.Y., Sudo, N., Yazawa, Y., and Yoo, T.J. (1984): Type II collagen-induced inner ear diseases in chinchillas. *Midwinter Assoc. Res. Otolaryngol.*, Abstract No. 21.
9. Floyd, R.A., Ishibe, T., Yazawa, Y., and Yoo, T.J. (1983): Cell transfer of CIAED in guinea pig. *Assoc. Res. Otolaryngol.*, Abstract No. 31.
10. Floyd, R.A., Cremer, M., Sudo, N., Takeda, T., Ishibe, T., and Yoo, T.J. (1985): Induction of tolerance to type II collagen autoimmune ear disease in rats. *Fed. Proc.*, Abstract No. 3185, 44:955.
11. Friedman, I. (1974): *Pathology of the Ear. Blackwell Scientific Publication,* p. 475. Oxford University Press, New York.

12. Igarashi, S., Kang, A.H., and Trelstad, R.L. (1973): Physical chemical properties of chick cartilage collagen. *Biochem. Biophys. Acta,* 295:514–519.
13. Ishibe, T., Shea, J.J., and Yoo, T.J. (1985): Immunohistochemical studies in Meniere's disease, otosclerosis and tympanosclerosis. *Assoc. Res. Otolaryngol.,* 92:103–108.
14. Kikuchi, M. (1959): On the "sympathetic otitis." *Practica Otologica Kyoto,* 52:600.
15. Lehnhardt, E. (1958): Plotzliche Horstorungen, auf beiden seiten gleichzeitig oder nacheinander aufgetreten. *Z. Laryngol. Rhinol. Otolaryngol.,* 37:1.
16. Lindsay, J.R. (1980): Otosclerosis. In: *Otolaryngology, Vol. 2,* edited by M.M. Paparella and D.A. Schumrick, pp. 1617–1643. W. B. Saunders, Philadelphia.
17. McCabe, B.F. (1979): Autoimmune sensorineural hearing loss. *Ann. Otol. Rhinol. Laryngol.,* 88(5):585–589.
18. Miller, E.J. (1971): Isolation and characterization of the cyanogen bromide peptides from the 1(II) chain of chick cartilage collagen. *Biochemistry,* 10:3030–3035.
19. Pearson, C.M. (1980): Relapsing polychondritis: clinical and immunologic features. In: *Clinical Immunology, Vol. 2,* edited by C. W. Parker, pp. 774–783. W. B. Saunders Co., Philadelphia.
20. Sasaki, Y., and Terayama, Y. (1964): Studies on experimental allergic (isoimmune) labyrinthitis in guinea pigs. *Acta Otol. Laryngol.,* 58:49–64.
21. Terato, K., Hasty, K.A., Cremer, M.A., Stuart, J.M., Torones, A.S., and Kang, A.H. (1985): Collagen induced arthritis in mice: localization of arthrogenic determinant to a fragment of type II collagen molecule. *J. Exp. Med.,* 162:637–646.
22. Yoo, T.J. (1984): Etiopathogenesis of Meniere's disease: a hypothesis. *Ann. Otol. Rhinol. Laryngol.* (Suppl.), 113(93):6–12.
23. Yoo, T.J. (1984): Etiopathogenesis of otosclerosis: a hypothesis. *Ann. Otol. Rhinol. Laryngol.,* 93:28–33.
24. Yoo, T.J., Kang, A.H., Stuart, J.M., Tomoda, K., Townes, A.S., and Dixit, S. (1982): Type II collagen autoimmunity in otosclerosis and Meniere's disease. *Science,* 217:1153–1155.
25. Yoo, T.J., Kang, A.H., Stuart, J.M., Tomoda, K., Towners, A.S., and Cremer, M.A. (1983): Type II collagen induced autoimmune sensorineural hearing loss and vestibular dysfunction in rats. *Ann. Otol. Rhinol. Laryngol.,* 92:267–271.
26. Yoo, T.J., Tomoda, K., Stuart, J.M., Kang, A.H., and Townes, A.S. (1983): Type II collagen-induced autoimmune otospongiosis: a preliminary report. *Ann. Otol. Rhinol. Laryngol.,* 92:103–108.
27. Yoo, T.J., Yazawa, Y., Tomoda, K., Floyd, R. (1983): Type II collagen-induced autoimmune endolymphatic hydrops in guinea pigs. *Science,* 222:65–67.
28. Yoo, T.J., Tomoda, K., and Hernandez, A.D. (1984): Type II collagen-induced autoimmune inner ear lesions in guinea pigs. *Ann. Otol. Rhinol. Laryngol.* (Suppl.), 113(93):3–5.
29. Yoo, T.J., Yazawa, Y., Tomoda, K., Floyd, R. (1984): Antibody in perilymph from rats with type II collagen-induced autoimmune inner ear disease. *Ann. Otol. Rhinol. Laryngol.* (Suppl.), 113(93):1–2.
30. Yoo, T.J., Shea, J.J., Shulman, A., PerLee, J., Gardner, G., and McCabe, B. (1985): Autoimmune sensorineural hearing loss: treatment update. *J. Otol. Laryngol.,* 6:96–100.
31. Yoo, T.J., Floyd, R., Ishibe, T., Shea, J.J. and Bowman, C. (1985): Immunologic testing of certain ear diseses. *Am. J. Otolaryngol.,* 6(1):96–100.
32. Yoo, T.J., Floyd, R.A., Ha, S.C., Ishibe, T., Stuart, J., Sudo, N., Takeda, T., Tomoda, K., Yazawa, Y., and Choe, I.S. (1985): Influencing factors of collagen induced autoimmune ear disease. *Am. J. Otolaryngol.,* 6:209–216.
33. Yoo, T.J., Stuart, J.M., Takeda, T., Sudo, N., Floyd, R., Ishibe, T., Olson, G., Orchik, D., Shea, J., and Kang, A.H. (1985): Induction of type II collagen autoimmune arthritis and ear disease in monkeys. *N.Y. Acad. Sci.,* 475:341–342.
34. Yoo, T.J., Tomeda, K. (1986): Type II collagen distribution in rodents. *(Submitted for publication.)*
35. Yoo, T.J., Takeda, T., Sudo, N., and Stuart, J. (1987): An epitope of type II collagen which induced inner ear lesion. *(Submitted for publication.)*
36. Yoo, T.J., Chiang, T., Dixit, S., Sudo, N., Takeda, T., Ishibe, T., Seyer, J., Shea, J.J., Causse, J.B., Causse, J. (1987): Collagen components of bovine fetal and guinea pig cochlea bone and human stapes. *Ann. Otol. Rhino. Laryngol. (in press).*
37. Yoo, T.J., Shea, J.J., and Floyd, R. (1987): Enchondral cartilage rests collagen autoimmunity as a pathogenic mechanism of otosclerosis. *Am. J. Otolaryngol. (in press).*

Immunology of the Ear, edited by J. Bernstein and P. Ogra. Raven Press, New York © 1987.

Otologic Manifestations of Systemic Immunologic Diseases

Michael Schatz and Robert S. Zeiger

Department of Allergy-Immunology, Kaiser Permanente Medical Center, San Diego, California 92120

Systemic immunologic disorders associated with reported otologic manifestations include immunodeficiency disorders, Wegener's granulomatosis, the polyarteritis nodosa group of systemic necrotizing vasculitides, Sjogren syndrome, and sarcoidosis. Other chapters in this volume discuss immunodeficiency disorders (see chapter by Rynnel-Dagöo and Freijd) and Wegener's granulomatosis (see chapter by Faden and Piėdra). This chapter will review the otologic manifestations of the other three systemic immunologic disorders listed above.

POLYARTERITIS NODOSA GROUP OF SYSTEMIC NECROTIZING VASCULITIDES

The polyarteritis nodosa group of systemic necrotizing vasculitides has the following characteristics: (a) necrotizing vasculitis in multiple organs, (b) usual lack of spontaneous remission, and (c) tendency to rapidly cause irreversible organ system dysfunction if therapy is delayed and sometimes in spite of therapy (8). This group of disorders includes classic polyarteritis nodosa, allergic granulomatosis (Churg-Strauss syndrome), and an "overlap syndrome" (4). *Classic polyarteritis nodosa* involves small and medium-sized muscular arteries with polymorphonuclear leukocyte infiltration followed by mononuclear cell infiltration in all layers of the vessel wall. Clinically, renal disease, hypertension, gastrointestinal tract involvement, and mononeuritis multiplex are prominent, whereas the lungs are usually spared (9). *Allergic granulomatosis* is characterized clinically by prominent lung involvement associated with severe asthma, a strong allergic history, and peripheral eosinophilia, and is characterized pathologically by intravascular and extravascular granulomata, eosinophilic tissue infiltration, and involvement of blood vessels of various types and sizes (small and medium-sized muscular arteries, veins, arterioles, and venules) (3,9). The *"overlap syndrome"* describes patients who exhibit clinical and pathological characteristics of both classic polyarteritis nodosa and allergic granulomatosis and therefore do not fit precisely into either of the first two categories (9). The etiology of this group of vasculitides is unknown in most cases, but a systemic immune complex reaction to an undefined antigen is the suspected pathogenesis (9).

Otologic involvement has been occasionally reported in patients fitting into the polyarteritis nodosa group of systemic necrotizing vasculitides (1,3,16,22–25). In their classic review of polyarteritis nodosa, Rose and Spencer (22) described 32 patients with "polyarteritis nodosa with lung involvement," a syndrome similar to or identical to what was previously described as allergic granulomatosis by Churg and Strauss (3), and 66 patients with polyarteritis nodosa without lung involvement, apparently corresponding to what is currently classified as classic polyarteritis nodosa. These authors reported granulomata of the middle ear in 2 of 32 patients with lung involvement, and granulomata of the nose in an additional 3 patients, but the clinical correlates of these granulomata were not reported. In their study, nasal and otologic involvement was not described in the 66 patients with polyarteritis nodosa without lung involvement.

Sale and Patterson (24) have recently described a patient with well-documented allergic granulomatosis and otologic manifestations. After a 4.5 year remission, their patient with proven allergic granulomatosis presented with unilateral conductive hearing loss, nasal obstruction without mucosal ulceration or saddle nose deformity, and maxillary sinus clouding associated with fever, asthma, palpable purpura, pulmonary infiltrates, and peripheral eosinophilia. The auditory findings, as well as the other presenting features, resolved rapidly with corticosteriod therapy. Whether the conductive hearing loss associated with the recurrent allergic granulomatosis in this patient resulted from eustachian tube dysfunction caused by nasopharyngeal involvement or from direct middle ear infiltrative disease could not be determined. However, this patient and the patients described by Rose and Spencer (22) demonstrate that patients with allergic granulomatosis may have pathologic nasal or middle ear involvement that occasionally may manifest itself clinically as auditory dysfunction.

In 1974, Sargeant and Christian (25) described seven patients with biopsy-proven systemic necrotizing vasculitis without features of allergic granulomatosis that began 2 weeks to 10 months after refractory, but usually improving, otitis media with effusion. The characteristics of these patients are shown in Table 1. All patients required myringotomy for otologic involvement that was bilateral initially or eventually in six of seven patients, and five of seven patients required tympanostomy tubes. Most patients exhibited anergy, neurologic disease, renal disease, and a positive test for rheumatoid factor. High blood pressure was notably absent in this series. The outcome of the otologic involvement in the five surviving patients was variable: one patient had recurrent otitis media with effusion with increased activity of the vasculitis, one patient had chronic hearing impairment, and the other three had normal hearing.

Three earlier reported cases also documented the development of systemic necrotizing vasculitis shortly after otitis media with effusion (7,11,21). In a more recent report (16), a patient with systemic necrotizing vasculitis also manifested inner ear deafness, and electromyolagromography revealed the absence of caloric irritability of both labyrinths. Postmortem examination of the left os petrosum re-

TABLE 1. *Features of seven patients with systemic necrotizing vasculitis following otitis media with effusion*[a]

Feature	Number of patients
Bilateral involvement (initially or eventually)	6
Required myringotomy	7
Tympanostomy tubes	5
Anergy	7
Neurologic disease	6
Renal disease	6
Rheumatoid factor	6
Scleritis	4
Skin lesions	3
High blood pressure	2
Surviving patients	5

[a]Data from ref. 25.

vealed inflammation and fibrosis of the perineurium of the acoustic nerve and the surrounding tissue as well as evidence of necrotic blood vessels.

There are at least two possible explanations for the association of otitis media with effusion with the systemic necrotizing vasculitis in these patients. Firstly the initial otitis media may be caused by an infectious agent, most likely a virus, which is capable of subsequently initiating an immune response leading to systemic necrotizing vasculitis. Consistent with this hypothesis are (a) the finding of antibody against respiratory syncytial virus in two patients in Sargeant and Christian's series (25) and (b) the finding of antibody against rubella in the patient described by Jonkers et al. (16). The second possible explanation is that the vasculitis initially involves the nasopharynx, eustachian tube, middle ear, or inner ear, leading to auditory abnormalities as the presenting complaint. Supporting this hypothesis is the documentation of direct otologic involvement in other systemic vasculitides (Wegener's granulomatosis and allergic granulomatosis), the correlation of the severity of the ear disease with systemic disease activity in at least one patient (25), and the pathologic findings in the os petrosum of another patient described above. Whatever the responsible mechanisms, refractory (particularly bilateral) otitis media with effusion must be considered as a possible premonitory manifestation of systemic vasculitis.

The diagnosis of systemic necrotizing vasculitis should be suspected on clinical grounds and then confirmed by biopsy of involved tissue (9). Alternatively, the diagnosis of classic polyarteritis nodosa can be made on the basis of the presence of characteristic aneurysmal dilations on visceral angiography in a patient with a suggestive clinical picture but without readily accessible tissue for biopsy (9). Corticosteroids alone or combined with immunosuppressive agents often induces remissions in patients with systemic necrotizing vasculitis (9). From the data available, it appears that when otologic manifestations are present, they often improve, either spontaneously or following effective treatment of the underlying vasculitis.

SJOGREN'S SYNDROME AND SICCA SYNDROME

Sjogren's syndrome is the triad of keratoconjunctivitis sicca (dry eyes), xerostomia (dry mouth), and a connective tissue disorder, most commonly rheumatoid arthritis. The term "sicca syndrome" refers to the first two features only. The pathogenesis of Sjogren's syndrome appears to be related to the lymphoid infiltrates that may be found in the salivary glands, lacrimal glands, and mucus-secreting glands of the conjunctiva, nasal cavity, pharynx, larynx, and trachea. Glandular atrophy may apparently result from these infiltrates (12). Although the etiology of Sjogren's syndrome is unknown, an immunologic pathogenesis is suggested by the lymphoid infiltrates, the association with connective tissue disorders, and the abundance of serum autoantibodies found in such patients (20).

Otologic symptoms and signs are not uncommon in patients with Sjogren's syndrome. Doig et al. (6) have reviewed the otolaryngologic aspects of Sjogren's syndrome in 22 patients with the sicca syndrome and in 31 patients with the complete Sjogren's syndrome associated with rheumatoid arthritis (Table 2). Significant deafness was observed in 18% to 19% of patients, and tympanic membrane perforation occurred in 6% to 9%. All of the patients with the sicca syndrome had a conductive component to their deafness, whereas approximately one-half of the patients with the complete Sjogren's syndrome had a conductive component. In contrast, Doig et al. described 21 patients with rheumatoid arthritis alone in whom 9 had significant deafness; only 1 of these patients demonstrated a conductive component. These authors concluded that the prevalence of conductive hearing loss in the sicca syndrome suggests that dryness and resulting dysfunction of eustachian tube and middle ear mucosa may be responsible for the hearing loss in these patients. On the other hand, the tendency toward sensorineural deafness in the patients with rheumatoid arthritis is most likely a result of the ototoxic medication used in the treatment of their illness. In patients with the sicca complex plus rheumatoid arthritis (the complete Sjogren's syndrome), both factors are likely to contribute to the occurrence of deafness.

Although the otolaryngologic abnormalities in Sjogren's syndrome are generally

TABLE 2. *Incidence of otologic manifestations in Sjogren's syndrome*[a]

Parameter	Sicca syndrome		Sjogren's syndrome	
	Number of patients	Percentage	Number of patients	Percentage
Total number of patients	22		31	
Grade-3 deafness	4	18	6	19
Conductive	3	14	2	6
Mixed	1	4	1	3
Sensorineural	0	0	3	10
Perforated tympanic membrane	2	9	2	6

[a]Data from ref. 6.

attributed to insufficient exocrine and mucosal glandular function, three patients with Sjogren's syndrome have been reported in whom the conductive deafness was caused by definable eustachian tube obstruction. Doig et al. (6) described two patients with established Sjogren's syndrome in whom the onset of acute deafness was associated with findings of exudative otitis media. Nasopharyngeal examination revealed large crusts covering the eustachian tubes and, following the removal of these crusts, rapid recovery of hearing ensued. Michael et al. (19) described a patient with long-standing Sjogren's syndrome who presented with unilateral otitis media with effusion. Nasopharyngeal examination revealed a mass in the region of the eustachian tube, and lymphoid hyperplasia was demonstrated on biopsy of this mass. Thus, although patients with the sicca complex may demonstrate decreased hearing as a result of presumed mucosal dryness and dysfunction, correctable eustachian tube obstruction must be excluded in subjects with the sicca complex who present with otitis media with effusion.

The diagnosis of the sicca syndrome or Sjogren's syndrome is usually suspected on clinical grounds. Keratoconjunctivitis sicca is confirmed by the presence of abnormalities in at least two of the following three tests: Schirmer test, break-up time, or quantitative rose-bengal dye test (20). Xerostomia is defined by the presence of abnormalities in at least two of the following three tests: lower lip biopsy, sialometry, and salivary gland scintigraphy or sialography (20).

Once an obstructing lesion has been excluded, there is no specific treatment available for the conductive deafness associated with the sicca syndrome. However, saline irrigation may be useful in patients with nasopharyngeal disease. In addition, for a patient with severe otologic manifestations associated with the sicca syndrome, consideration may be given to the use of bromhexine, which has been reported to be useful particularly for the ophthalmologic manifestations of the sicca syndrome (20). Because the incidence of malignant lymphoproliferative disorders is increased in patients with Sjogren's syndrome, one of the other objectives of management of patients with Sjogren's syndrome is to detect complicating lymphoid neoplasms as early as possible (20).

SARCOIDOSIS

Sarcoidosis is a multisystemic disorder, characterized by noncaseating granulomata, which can occur in any organ of the body and which most commonly involves the lymph nodes, lungs, skin, and eyes (18,26). The etiology of sarcoidosis is unknown, but the presence of multiple immunologic aberrations is well established (15,26).

Otologic manifestations are seen occasionally in patients with sarcoidosis. The most common otologic manifestation of sarcoidosis is neurosensory deafness, which is often associated with vestibular dysfunction (13,17). It has been reported that the eighth cranial nerve is the fourth most commonly affected cranial nerve in sarcoidosis (5). The deafness may be unilateral or bilateral, may fluctuate (14), and may vary from a minimal to a profound loss (17). A conductive component to the hearing loss has been reported in some cases (17). There appears to be no characteristic pattern of low or high frequency involvement (17), and there also appears to be no consistent site of involvement along the nerve axis as determined clinically using modern audiological techniques. Otologic manifestations in sarcoidosis commonly occur in association with uveitis and facial nerve palsy (13,14).

The involvement of the vestibuloacoustic system in patients with sarcoidosis has been attributed most commonly to a posterior fossa granulomatous meningitis that directly infiltrates the eighth cranial nerve or causes compression from involvement of adjacent intracranial structures (7,13). However, pathologic material from a patient recently reported by Babin et al. (2) has suggested a different potential mechanism. These authors found a lymphocytic infiltrate in all areas of the internal auditory canal, particularly distributed intraneuronally and perivascularly, associated with noncaseating granulomata. They also found loss of nerve fibers in cochlear and vestibular nerves associated with degeneration of the neuroepithelium of the inner ear and stria vascularis of the cochlea, but without marked lymphoid infiltration or granuloma formation within these structures. The authors interpret these findings to suggest that the perivascular intraneuronal lymphocytic infiltration leads either to reversible neuropraxia or to neural degeneration caused by vascular occlusion with subsequent ischemia of distal functional elements.

Fishman and Canalis (10) have presented a patient whose initial manifestation of sarcoidosis was bilateral hearing loss resulting from a unique mechanism. Otologic examination revealed bilateral retracted tympanic membranes and the presence of middle ear fluid. Examination of the nasopharynx revealed a smooth mucosa-covered mass in the center of the vault. Biopsy of the mass revealed noncaseating granulomata, and subsequent evaluation revealed other laboratory stigmata of sarcoidosis. Treatment with steroids led to a decrease in size of the nasopharyngeal mass and clearing of the otitis media with effusion.

The diagnosis of sarcoidosis is usually made on the basis of consistent clinical and radiologic findings supported by histologic evidence of noncaseating epithelioid granulomata and negative bacterial and fungal studies of biopsied tissue, sputum, and other appropriate body fluids (18,26). Although the Kveim-Siltzback skin test has been considered a specific and reliable diagnostic test, this antigen is not currently widely available (26).

Systemic corticosteroids are considered to be the most effective available therapeutic agents for sarcoidosis (18). Nasopharyngeal lesions apparently respond to systemic steroid therapy. Corticosteroid therapy also appears to reduce hearing loss and vestibular symptoms in most affected patients, but some degree of hearing loss and asymptomatic vestibular abnormalities usually persist even after steroid therapy (13,17).

REFERENCES

1. Allison, D.J., and Breltie, R.P. (1979): Polyarteritis nodosa: a clinical and angiographic analysis of 17 cases. *Semin. Arthritis Rheum.*, 3:184–189.

2. Babin, R.W., Liu, C., and Aschenbrener, C. (1984): Histopathology of neurosensory deafness in sarcoidosis. *Ann. Otol. Rhinol. Laryngol.*, 93:389–393.
3. Churg, J., and Strauss, L. (1951): Allergic granulomatosis, allergic angiitis, and periarteritis nodosa. *Am. J. Pathol.*, 27:277–301.
4. Conn, D.L., McDuffie, F.C., Hillary, K.E., and Schroeter, A. (1976): Immunologic mechanisms in systemic vasculitis. *Mayo Clin. Proc.*, 51:511–518.
5. Delaney, P. (1977): Neurologic manifestations in sarcoidosis. *Ann. Int. Med.*, 87:336–345.
6. Doig, J.A., Whaley, K., Dick, W.C., Nuki, G., Williamson, J., and Buchanan, W.W. (1971): Otolaryngological aspects of Sjogren's syndrome. *Br. Med. J.*, 4:460–463.
7. Dudley, G.P., and Goodman, M. (1969): Periarteritis nodosa and bilateral facial paralysis. *Arch. Otolaryngol.*, 90:139–146.
8. Fauci, A.S. (1979): Vasculitis: new insights amid old enigmas. *Am. J. Med.*, 67:916–918.
9. Fauci, A.S. (1983): Vasculitis. *J. Allergy Clin. Immunol.*, 72:211–223.
10. Fishman, S.M., and Canalis, R.F. (1979): Nasopharyngeal sarcoidosis. *Ear Nose Throat J.*, 58:4–9.
11. Herberts, G., Hillerdal, O., and Ranstrom, S. (1957): Rhinitis, sinusitis and otitis as initial symptoms in periarteritis nodosa. *Acta Otolaryngol (Stockh.)*, 48:204–218.
12. Hughs, G.R.V., and Whaley, K. (1972): Sjogren's syndrome. *Br. Med. J.*, 4:533–536.
13. Hybels, R.L., and Rice, D.H. (1976): Neuro-otologic manifestations of sarcoidosis. *Laryngoscope*, 86:1873–1878.
14. Jahrsdoerfer, R.A., Thompson, E.G., Johns, M.E.E., and Cantrell, R.W. (1981): Sarcoidosis and fluctuating hearing loss. *Ann. Otol.*, 90:161.
15. James, D.G., and Williams, W.J. (1982): Immunology of sarcoidosis. *Am. J. Med.*, 72:5–8.
16. Jonkers, G.H., Kwadijk, E.M., and Tio, L. (1975): Necrotizing polyarteritis and serous otitis media. *Neth. J. Med.*, 18:142–144.
17. Kane, K. (1976): Deafness in sarcoidosis. *J. Laryngol. Otol.*, 90:531–537.
18. Kerdel, K.A., and Moschella, S.L. (1984): Sarcoidosis. *J. Am. Acad. Derm.*, 11:1–19.
19. Michael, R.G., Hughes, L.A., and Hudson, W.R. (1976): Sjogren's syndrome and serous otitis media. *Laryngoscope*, 7:996–1003.
20. Montorpe, R., Frost-Larsen, K., Isager, H., and Prause, J.V. (1981): Sjogren's syndrome. *Allergy*, 36:139–153.
21. Peiterson, E., and Carlsen, B.H. (1966): Hearing impairment as the initial signs of polyarteritis nodosa. *Acta. Otolaryngol. (Stockh.)*, 61:189–195.
22. Rose, G.A., and Spencer, H. (1957): Polyarteritis nodosa. *Q. J. Med.* 26:43–80.
23. Sack, M., Cassidy, J.J., and Bole, G.G. (1975): Prognostic factors in polyarteritis. *J. Rheumatol.*, 2:411–420.
24. Sale, S., and Patterson, R. (1981): Recurrent Churg-Strauss vasculitis with exophthalmos, hearing loss, nasal obstruction, amyloid deposits, hyperimmunoglobulinemia E and circulating immune complexes. *Arch. Intern. Med.*, 141:1363–1365.
25. Sergeant, J.S., and Christian, C.L. (1974): Necrotizing vasculitis after acute serous otitis media. *Ann. Intern. Med.*, 81:195–199.
26. Sharma, O.P. (1984): *Sarcoidosis: Clinical Management*. Butterworths, London.

Immunology of the Ear, edited by J. Bernstein
and P. Ogra. Raven Press, New York © 1987.

Wegener's Granulomatosis and Other Granulomatous Diseases of the Ear

Howard S. Faden and Pedro Piedra

Department of Pediatrics, State University of New York at Buffalo, School of Medicine, Buffalo, New York 14214, and Children's Hospital of Buffalo, Buffalo, New York 14222

The purpose of this chapter is to review the subject of granulomatous diseases that may involve the structures of the ear. However, the list of distinctive disorders in which granuloma formation occurs is extensive and all too inclusive to be discussed in its entirety in this chapter. Therefore, we have selected several disorders for in-depth review. Wegener's granulomatosis and related disorders will be discussed first, followed by histiocytosis X, tuberculosis, and syphilis.

GRANULOMA FORMATION

Granulomata are organized collections of mononuclear phagocytes. The monocytes that participate in the formation of granulomata first migrate and then mature into tissue macrophages before evolving into highly specialized epithelioid cells. Other cell types, including T (thymus-derived) and B (bone marrow-derived) lymphocytes, may be present in the periphery of some types of granuloma. Granulomata form in response to a failure of the acute inflammatory process to rid the body of an unwanted substance. The nature of the inciting agent dictates the types of granuloma that form. For example, inert materials trigger the formation of granuloma around the particle; the particle is distributed in almost all of the mononuclear phagocytes. This type of granuloma exhibits a low turnover rate of cells. The granuloma enlarges primarily by cell proliferation. In contrast, the granulomata that form in response to facultative or obligate intracellular parasites (Table 1), such as mycobacterial organisms, have a high rate of turnover. These granulomata change in character because of an influx of many cell types and often reflect immunologic amplification. The presence of this type of granuloma is associated with augmented levels of cellular and humoral immunity to the inciting antigen. The cells inside granulomata are in an activated state and as such release a variety of substances designed to attract other cellular elements and to destroy the inciting antigen. In the early phase of granuloma formation, one finds T-helper cells present; whereas in the resolving phase, T-suppressor cells are more often encoun-

TABLE 1. *Infectious agents associated with granuloma formation*

Bacteria	Fungi	Parasites
Actinomyces	Blastomyces	Leishmania
Brucella	Histoplasma	Schistosoma
Francisella	Sporotricha	Toxoplasma
Klebsiella		
Nocardia		
Mycobacteria		
Treponema		

tered. The ultimate destruction of the foreign material leads to the resolution of the granuloma.

WEGENER'S GRANULOMATOSIS

Wegener's granulomatosis (WG) is a necrotizing vasculitis that is recognized for its distinctive clinicopathologic manifestations. The characteristic features of WG, which differentiate it from other vasculitides, include nectrotizing granulomatous vasculitis of the upper and lower respiratory tract, disseminated small vessel vasculitis, and focal necrotizing glomerulonephritis (8). In addition, a limited form of WG has been described; it is similar to WG but without renal involvement (2).

The etiology of WG is not known, although a hypersensitivity reaction to an unidentified antigen is suspected. Recent studies have suggested an association between viral and bacterial infections and relapse of disease in patients who had been in remission with WG (6,25). Circulating immune complexes (IC) have been documented in patients with active disease and in infection-provoked relapse; their role in WG remains speculative.

In WG, as in most necrotizing vasculitides, immunopathogenic mechanisms are associated with the disease process. A prevailing theory proposes the formation of IC after exposure to antigen and during a period of antigen excess. The antigen-antibody complex thus formed is ineffectively cleared by the reticuloendothelial system, creating a potential source of IC to be entrapped in blood vessel walls. The IC in the vessel wall indirectly causes vascular damage by activating the complement cascade, which, in turn, initiates and amplifies the inflammatory response.

Other mechanisms may be responsible for vascular damage. A poorly understood immunopathogenic event, cell-mediated immune reactivity, may elicit the formation of granulomata. It is proposed that sensitized lymphocytes are triggered by circulating antigens to release macrophage inhibitory factor and other lymphokines. Migration inhibitory factor causes a ''homing in'' and accumulation of monocytes with macrophage transformation in and around vessels (31). The activated macrophage releases lysosomal contents that are capable of causing vascular damage. Macrophage phagocytosis of IC may also induce granuloma formation (10).

In WG there is a slightly greater predilection for males. It may affect any age group, although it is rarely seen in the first decade of life. The incidence peaks during the fourth and fifth decades. Prior to effective treatment, WG was fatal; mean survival approached 5 months (17).

The characteristic triad in WG of necrotizing granulomatous vasculitis in the respiratory tract, small vessel vasculitis, and necrotizing glomerulonephritis may present in a highly variable manner. Sometimes there is a long history of nasal congestion with a persistent serosanguinous discharge. In other situations, there is a sudden onset of disease in both the upper and lower respiratory tract as well as progressive glomerulonephritis. However, in a majority of patients there is nasal and paranasal symptomatology such as rhinorrhea, mucosal ulceration, diffuse nasal crusting, sinus pain and, on occasion, nasal deformity. Lower airway involvement manifests as cough, hemoptysis, and pleuritic pain. Other symptoms may include arthralgia, myalgia, hearing deficit, vision impairment, skin ulceration, fever, weight loss, and poor appetite. It is unusual to find advanced renal disease on initial presentation. In the pediatric population, WG is a rare entity. It is often difficult to recognize WG early in its course in children because of its atypical presentation and slow progression (12).

Nose and paransal sinuses are involved in greater than 90% of patients. The usual presentation is a mucopurulent rhinitis associated with mucosal crusting. On occasion, necrosis of the septal cartilage occurs. Sinusitis is seen in patients with chronic rhinitis. Bacterial superinfection is a frequent complication in patients with severe sinusitis. The prevailing bacterial etiologic agent is *Staphylococcus aureus* (17).

The lungs are also involved in greater than 90% of the cases. Multiple bilateral nodular infiltrates that tend to cavitate are commonly seen on chest radiographs. Pleural effusion may be found in 20% of the cases. Pulmonary calcification is extremely rare, as is hilar adenopathy.

Biopsy-proven renal involvement may be found in 85% of patients. The spectrum of disease ranges from mild focal segmental glomerulonephritis with minimal renal dysfunction to fulminant diffuse necrotizing glomerulonephritis with a clinical picture of renal failure. Whereas extra renal disease generally precedes renal involvement, renal disease often progresses rapidly into severe glomerulonephritis within days to weeks of presentation (9).

Otologic involvement occurs in 20% to 40% of cases (13,18,21). Otitis media (OM) is common and occurs in 25% of patients. The pathophysiology of OM relates to eustachian tube dysfunction and blockage resulting from inflammation caused by chronic rhinitis. Serous OM is the most common form of ear disease in WG. Conservative medical management is ineffective in eradication of the effusion; however, effective therapy of WG results in the resolution of the middle ear disease. Purulent OM often complicates serous OM in patients with WG. The predominant organisms involved are *Staphylococcus aureus* and *Pseudomonas aeruginosa*. In patients with protracted disease, perforation of the tympanic membrane, mastoiditis, and cranial nerve, palsy may occur (13).

In addition to complications from eustachian tube dysfunction, the ear may be a primary site for granuloma formation. The anatomic pathology includes spontaneous defects of the earlobe, otitis externa, and hearing loss. Multiple factors appear to play a role in hearing loss. Cochlear vessel involvement, granulomata compression of the acoustic nerve, and immune complex deposition in the cochlea have all been implicated in this process (1).

Laboratory tests are not helpful in making a diagnosis of WG, although they may be useful in excluding other diseases. The hemoglobin profile may show a normochromic-normocytic anemia. The white blood cell count may be normal or elevated, but leukopenia is rare. The erythrocyte sedimentation rate is typically elevated and may be used to monitor the response to therapy. Parameters of renal function may need to be followed. Hypergammaglobulinemia is often documented. Cell-mediated immunity remains intact. Rheumatoid factor and antinuclear antibody are not detectable. In addition, special staining and extensive culturing of biopsy material are negative for bacteria, mycobacteria, and fungi. The histopathologic findings in the diseased tissues consists of necrotizing granulomata with giant cell formation and vasculitis involving both small arteries and veins; eosinophils are rarely present. Repeated tissue samples from the upper respiratory tract are often required in order to establish the correct diagnosis since as many as 50% of the biopsies exhibit nonspecific acute and chronic inflammation with necrosis (9). Renal biopsy is not helpful in establishing a diagnosis of WG because vasculitis and graulomata are rarely seen. However, the finding of focal glomerulonephritis in a patient with upper and/or lower respiratory disease suggests the diagnosis of WG.

Wegener's granulomatosis is one of the few vasculitides with a characteristic clinicopathologic picture. Still, other diseases have the potential to masquerade as WG. Since the therapy for each of the diseases varies widely, it is crucial to distinguish WG from other vasculitides and granulomatous processes prior to initiating treatment. Infectious etiologies are excluded by performing appropriate histiologic stains and cultures on the biopsy material. Destructive midline facial lesions (Tables 2 and 3), once known as *lethal midline granuloma*, are distinguished by the focally destructive nature and histopathologic findings. Such entities include T-cell lymphoma, polymorphic reticulosis/lymphomatoid granulomatosis, and idiopathic midline destructive disease. Others, such as sarcoidosis, polyarteritis nodosa, allergic granulomatosis, and angiitis need to be considered and excluded (14,17,30).

Prior to the discovery of effective therapy, the clinical course of patients with WG was rapidly downhill, with a 90% death rate within 2 years after onset of the disease (8). The use of cytotoxic agents and steroids has produced complete remission in over 90% of the patients (9). Fauci et al. (9) demonstrated that treatment with cyclophosphamide at 2 mg/kg of body weight each day and prednisone at 1 mg/kg of body weight each day was very effective in inducing and maintaining remissions. Cyclophosphamide at 4 to 5 mg/kg of body weight per day may be used initially in a rapidly progressive case. Lymphocyte count reduction is monitored to guide therapy.

TABLE 2. *Prominent sites of involvement in "lethal midline granulomas"*[a]

Sites of involvement	Wegener's granulomatosis	Idiopathic midline destructive disease	Polymorphic reticulosis lymphomatoid granulomatosis	Lymphoma
Ear	+	+	+	−
Joint	++	−	−	−
Kidney	+++	−	+	++++
Liver/spleen	−	−	+	++++
Lung	++++	−	+++	++++
Lymphnode	−	−	+	++++
Nose/pharynx/sinus	++++	++++	+++	++++
Orbit	+	+	+	++
Skin	+	+	++	+++

[a]Frequency of involvement: − to ++++, absent to frequent.

TABLE 3. *Characteristic histopathologic changes in "lethal midline granulomas"*[a]

Histopathology	Wegener's granulomatosis	Idiopathic midline destructive disease	Polymorphic reticulosis lymphomatoid granulomatosis	Lymphoma
Acute and chronic inflammation/necrosis	+	+	+	+
Angiocentric/angiodestructive changes	−	−	+	−
Glomerulonephritis	+	−	−	−
Granuloma	+	+	+	−
Malignant lymphoid cellular infiltrate	−	−	−	+
Polymorphic cellular and immature infiltrate	−	−	+	−
Vasculitis	+	−	−	−

[a]Histopathologic changes: +, present; −, absent.

Recently, DeRemee et al (6,7) demonstrated the benefit of trimethoprim-sulfamethoxazole (TMX) in controlling and/or ameliorating the disease in a select group of patients who had an indolent course or did not appear to improve when given cyclophosphamide with or without steroids. They speculated that the usefulness of TMX was attributable to its antimicrobial activity or its immunosuppressant attributes as a folic acid antagonist.

HISTIOCYTOSIS X

Histiocytosis X represents a group of disorders of unknown etiology characterized by a proliferation of histiocytes with eosinophilic infiltration. Historically the group has been divided into three major categories: (a) eosinophilic granuloma, a localized bony lesion(s); (b) Letterer-Siwe syndrome, a progressive, multisystem, frequently fatal illness; and (c) Hand-Schüller-Christian syndrome, a chronic multisystem form of disease. The lesions of histiocytosis contain a collection of histiocytes and appears as a xanthoma with lipid-filled cells surrounded by a fibrous barrier in the latter stages of development. The predominant histiocytic cell type appears to be the Langerhans' cell. These cells are dendritic monocytes that appear to play some role in antigen processing for T lymphocytes (23). As the cells disintegrate, they leave free cholesterol crystals and giant cells. The foamy appearance of the cells has suggested a disorder of lipid metabolism. Although the etiology of the disease remains unknown, infection, hypersensitivity, immune disorder, and neoplasm have all been suggested.

In eosinophilic granuloma, the disease is characterized by pain, tenderness, and swelling over the bony lesion(s). Radiographs of the bone reveal lytic destruction. The diagnosis is established by biopsy, as in all forms of histiocytosis X. Many of the lesions resolve spontaneously, whereas others require curettage or low-dose radiation for eradication.

In contrast to the slow, somewhat limited, disorder of eosinophilic granuloma, Letterer-Siwe syndrome is dramatic and explosive. It occurs primarily in infants who exhibit fever, rash, hepatosplenomegaly, lymphadenopathy, bony lesions, and anemia. The skin lesions may resemble seborrheic dermatitis. In the past, this form of the disease was often fatal. Mortality is directly related to the extent of the disease and the age of the patient. Patients younger than 2 years of age generally do poorly. Involvement of lung, liver, spleen, and bone marrow is associated with a poor prognosis. Treatment with various cytotoxic agents may induce remissions and increase the survival rate.

The more chronic form of the disease, Hand-Schüller-Christian syndrome, has traditionally been associated with exophthalmos, as a result of bony involvement, diabetes insipidus, and osteolytic lesions of the skull. Lymphadenopathy, splenomegaly, and/or hepatomegaly may occur in up to 50% of the patients. Many of the same findings in Letterer-Siwe syndrome also may be found in this form of the disorder, but in a more subdued manner.

Anywhere from 2% to 62% of patients with histiocytosis X have aural involvement (19,27,29). For example, OM may be the presenting sign in one-third of the cases of Hand-Schüller-Christian syndrome (29). The middle ear process is chronic in nature and is the result of direct involvement of the temporal bone. The bony disease may remain silent for a long time and only becomes symptomatic when the lesion begins expanding. Patients with ear involvement complain of otorrhea, pain, and postauricular swelling. Otoscopy may reveal granulation tissue in the external canal. Most of the patients with chronic OM are children less than 3 years of age (19,27,29). The initial presentation may be misdiagnosed as otitis externa that is resistant to antimicrobial treatment. It may also be confused with the clinical picture of cholesteatoma. However, cholesteatomas tend to occur in children over the age of 3 years (5). Although both disorders may exhibit nonspecific radiographic changes in the temporal bone, such as radiolucency, blurring of osseous structures, and decreased pneumatization of the mastoids, cholesteatomas tend to cause bony erosion whereas histiocytosis X causes lytic destruction (5). Another distinguishing feature found almost exclusively in patients with histiocytosis X is an elevated erythrocyte sedimentation rate (5). The definitive diagnosis is most often made by biopsy.

TUBERCULOSIS

Tuberculosis is an infection caused by the bacterium *Mycobacterium tuberculosis*. The disease is characterized by the formation of caseating granulomata and may affect every organ system in the body, although it primarily causes lung damage.

Mycobacterium tuberculosis is an obligate parasite. Humans are the only reservoir for the organism. It is an aerobic, non-spore-forming, nonmotile bacillus that stains with a variety of special stains such as Ziehl-Neelsen or Kinyon and is characteristically acid-fast. Culture of the organism requires 4 to 6 weeks of incubation. In addition to *M. tuberculosis*, there are other pathogenic species: *M. bovis*, a strain common to cows, uncommonly produces disease in humans today, whereas atypical forms of mycobacteria, such as *M. scrofulacium*, continue to cause human infections.

The incidence, morbidity, and mortality attributable to tuberculosis have declined dramatically since the introduction of effective chemotherapy in the 1940s and 1950s. Improved living conditions, such as less crowding and better sanitation, have also contributed significantly to the lessening of importance of tuberculosis. There were 23,846 cases of tuberculosis reported to the Center for Disease Control in 1983, which is a rate of 10.2 cases per 100,000 population (4). The number of cases has declined by approximately 5% to 6% each year in the United States. The rate of disease is highest for nonwhite males over 65 years of age and lowest for children between ages 10 and 14 years (4). The immigration of Asian refugees to the United States in the 1970s accounted for a noticeable increase in the number of cases of tuberculosis in the recent past. The number of deaths attributable to tuberculosis has declined to about 2,000 each year (4).

Infection with *M. tuberculosis* induces a strong cell-mediated immune response that can be detected easily with intracutaneous deposition of old tuberculin (OT) or a purified protein derivative (PPD). Positive skin-test reactivity appears 4 to 6 weeks after the onset of infection and remains positive for as long as the immune system remains intact.

The vast majority of infections are asymptomatic, with no evidence that infection ever occurred except for the positive skin test. In other cases, it presents as a pneumonia with hilar adenopathy and which may resolve spontaneously. The diagnosis is frequently suggested by the slow rate of resolution of the pulmonary infiltrate. Most of the cases of tuberculosis in adults represent reactivation of a previous infection. The reason for the organism's ability to resist destruction over long periods may reside in its capacity to prevent fusion of the phagocytic and lysosomal vacuoles within pulmonary macrophages and to escape from the phagocytic vacuole into the cytoplasm of the cell (11,24).

Progression of pulmonary tuberculosis leads to a variety of constitutional symptoms, including anorexia, weight loss, night sweats, and fever. Cough tends to be chronic and may result in hemoptysis. Some persons will go to a physician for symptoms related to extrapulmonary disease. One group of extrapulmonary infections results from spread via the respiratory tract such as mouth sores, hoarseness, chronic OM and gastrointestinal symptoms; whereas another group of extrapulmonary infections is related to spread by the lymphatic or hematogenous routes during the early phase of the primary infection. These include meningitis, osteomyelitis, hepatitis, pericarditis, peritonitis, renal tuberculosis, and other less common forms of infection. Otitis media may occur by the hematogenous route as well as by contiguous spread from a nearby site of infection.

The diagnosis of tuberculosis of the middle ear may be difficult in the absence of some of the more dramatic systemic symptoms mentioned in earlier paragraphs. Because of the declining incidence of tuberculosis in general, one may not even include it in the differential diagnosis of chronic OM. In years past, almost half of the chronic suppurative OM seen in young infants may have been caused by *M. tuberculosis* (15). Patients characteristically present with chronic otorrhea. Most of the subjects are children less than 12 years of age. Pain is typically absent. Hearing loss occurs early and may be especially profound compared to other forms of OM. Early in the course of infection, exudate is absent and the tympanic membrane is dull and red. The diagnosis maybe suspected when the acute form of the disorder does not respond to normal modes of therapy for common forms of bacterial OM. Later, multiple small perforations are noted. These progress to form one large extensive perforation. Cervical adenopathy and pulmonary lesions may be found in more than 50% of the cases (22). The majority of patients also have positive skin tests (22). Adults may develop vestibular involvement. Almost one-third of patients exhibit facial paralysis as a complication of the middle ear infection.

Treatment of tuberculosis has improved dramatically over the years. Prior to chemotherapy, patients were encouraged to stay in fresh air and in sanitaria that were specifically designed for individuals with tuberculosis. The introduction of streptomycin as an antituberculous agent led to the sudden realization that tuberculosis was treatable. But, it was the introduction of isoniazid in 1952 that crystallized the idea the infection was curable. Today, most forms of tuberculosis may be treated with combination therapy of isoniazid and rifampin. Certain clinical diseases require a more complex therapeutic approach. Failures in therapy primarily occur because of poor compliance or isoniazid resistance. Despite effective antituberculous therapy, many of the complications of the infection, such as hearing loss, persist.

SYPHILIS

Syphilis is a disease of historical significance. Once a very common disorder, syphilis today is significantly less prevalent. Approximately 32,698 cases were identified in 1983 (3). It is caused by a spirochete, *Treponema pallidium* and is transmitted mostly by sexual contact. *T. pallidium* is one of a group of pathogenic spirochetes that cannot be cultured easily *in vitro*. The organism can be identified in the exudates of early lesions by examination with dark-field light microscopy. More often, the diagnosis is established serologically and by the clinical course of the illness.

Although syphilis is most frequently transmitted through sexual contact, it may also be transmitted by kissing, inoculation, blood transfusion, and by the transplacental route. Approximately 239 congenital infections were reported in 1983 (3).

The infection progresses through several stages of evolution. The incubation period lasts approximately 3 weeks. As little as several organisms may initiate the infection, but symptoms do not develop until a sufficient density of organisms has been reached. The primary lesion of syphilis is a single painless chancre, but multiple ulcers have been described. The lesions are most often found on the genitals. The secondary stage of the disease is characterized by bacteremia and dissemination to any organ systems in the body. It is during this phase that many of the constitutional symptoms such as fever, malaise, and anorexia appear. The rash of syphilis characteristically involves the palms and soles. The infection next progresses to a quiescent stage known as the latent period. Relapse of symptoms may occur during this period. If the disease is untreated, the spirochites migrate into the vasovasorum of blood vessels and produce an inflammatory response consisting of mononuclear cells. This ultimately leads to obliterative arteritis. The resultant vascular insufficiency causes tissue destruction that is most noticeable in the aorta and CNS in the late stage of the disease. Exaggerated immune responses are probably responsible, in part, for the dramatic gummatous lesions seen in teriary syphilis. These indolent lesions are commonly found in bones, skin, and other organs and only become manifest many years after the initial infection.

Congenital syphilis is a rather unique form of the infection. The mother is most likely to transmit the agent to the fetus early in the course of her infection. Invasion of the fetus uncommonly occurs prior to the fourth month of gestation. Babies infected *in utero* may be asymptomatic at birth. Nonspecific symptoms of intrauterine infection include jaundice, petechiae, maculopapular rash, and hepatosplenomegaly. A bloody nasal discharge, referred to as snuffles, is characteristic of syphilis. If the child survives the early period and is untreated, the infection becomes latent. As the child grows, late manifestations of the disease may appear such as saber shin, tooth abnormalities, and interstitial keratitis. Because of the decline in the occurrence of syphilis in adults, early diagnosis of congenital infection may be difficult (20).

Otologic abnormalities have been reported in congenital as well as in acquired infections. Individuals with congenital infections manifest ear problems at an earlier age, 37 ± 11 years, than those with acquired infections, 50 ± 14 years (28).

However, the time from infection to the onset of the otologic problem is shorter in the acquired form of disease. Syphilis may be suspected as a cause of the aural problem in the congenital group because other stigmata of congenital syphilis may be present in a high proportion of the subjects (28). For example, interstitial keratitis occurs in almost 80% of the subjects (28). In acquired infections, the diagnosis is commonly made during routine serologic screening. Tinnitis is the presenting sign in half of the individuals (28). Hearing loss is also common. Up to 38% of congenital syphilitics experience hearing loss (16). Although most of the individuals experience a gradual onset of hearing loss, 16% have a sudden loss (28). The degree of hearing loss may fluctuate and is most frequently unilateral. Eighteen percent of individuals manifest bilateral loss (28). Vestibular disease is also frequent. For example, 42% of individuals complain of episodic vertigo and 29% present with rotary nystagmus (28).

The pathogenesis of the otologic abnormalities is similar to luetic disease in other organ systems. The spirochete may directly invade the temporal bone. The immune response leads to granuloma formation in various tissues, including the nerves and perivascular structures. Bony destruction with sequestra formation may be evident. Involvement of the semicircular canals, cochlea, and other parts of the temporal bone occur. Spirochetes have not been isolated from middle ear effusions, although fusion of the bony ossicles may occur as part of the clinical picture.

Despite the inordinately long period of infection and extent of tissue damage, treatment of otitic syphilis may prove beneficial. Investigation of 26 subjects with early syphilis and abnormalities in either pure-tone audiometry, or brain-stem evoked potential, revealed improvement in audiometry in two of 11 and in brainstem evoked potentials in four of seven subjects 3 to 24 months after initiation of therapy (26). In the case of brain-stem evoked potentials, the return was to normality (26). Treatment of late syphilis may also lead to an improvement in a small number of individuals with otologic problems (28).

REFERENCES

1. Bradley, P.J. (1983): Wegener's granulomatosis of the ear. *J. Laryngol. Otol.*, 97:623–626.
2. Carrington, C.B., and Liebow, A.A. (1966): Limited forms of angiitis and granulmatosis of Wegener's type. *Am. J. Med.*, 41:497–527.
3. Center for Disease Control (1984): Annual summary 1983: reported morbidity and mortality in the United States. *MMWR,* 32:53–56.
4. Center for Disease Control (1984): Annual Summary 1983: reported morbidity and mortality in the United States. *MMWR,* 32:62–65.
5. Coutte, A., Pederson, B., Bartholdy, N., and Thommesen, P. (1984): Recurrent otitis media as a presenting symptom in children with special reference to cholesteatoma. *Clin. Otolaryngol.*, 9:111–114.
6. DeRemee, R.A., McDonald, T.J., and Weiland, L.H. (1985): Wegener's granulomatosis: observation on treatment with antimicrobial agents. *Mayo Clin. Proc.*, 53:634–640.
7. DeRemee, R.A., Weiland, L.H., and McDonald, T.J. (1978): Polymorphic reticulosis, lymphomatoid granulamatosis, Two diseases or one? *Mayo Clin. Proc.*, 53:634–640.
8. Fauci, A.S., Haynes, B.F., and Katz, P. (1978): The spectrum of vasculitis: clinical, pathologic, immunologic and therapeutic considerations. *Ann. Intern. Med.*, 89:660–676.

9. Fauci, A.S., Haynes, B.F., Katz, P., and Wolff, S.M. (1983): Wegener's granulomatosis: prospective clinical and therapeutic experience with 85 patients for 21 years. *Ann. Intern. Med.*, 98:76–85.
10. Fauci, A.S., and Wolff, S.M. (1977): Wegener's granulomatous and related diseases. *DM*, 23(7).
11. Goren, M.B., Hart, P., Young, M., and Armstrong, J.A. (1976): Prevention of phagosome-lysosome fusion in cultured macrophages by sulfatides of *Mycobacterium tuberculosis*. *Proc. Natl. Acad. Sci. USA*, 73:2510–2514.
12. Hall, S.L., Miller, L.C., Duggan, E., Mauer, S.M., Beatty, E.C., and Hellerstein, S. (1985): Wegener's granulomatosis in pediatric patients. *J Pediatr.*, 106:739–744.
13. Illium, P., Thorling, K., and Denmark, A. (1982): Otological manifestations of Wegener's granulomatosis. *Laryngoscope*, 92:801–804.
14. Ishii, Y., Yamanaka, N., Ogawa, K., Yoshida, Y., Takami, T., Masuir, A., Isago, H., Kataura, A., and Kikuchi, K. (1982): Nasal T-cell lymphoma as a type of so-called lethal midline granuloma. *Cancer*, 50:2336–2344.
15. Jeang, M.K., and Fletcher, E.C. (1983): Tuberculosis otitis media. *JAMA*, 249:2231–2232.
16. Karmody, C.S., and Schuknecht, H.F. (1966): Deafness in congenital syphilis. *Arch. Otolaryngol.*, 83:44–53.
17. Kornblut, A.D., Wolff, S.M., DeFries, H.O., and Fauci, A.S. (1980): Wegener's granulomatosis. *Laryngoscope*, 90:1453–1465.
18. Kornblut, A.D., Wolff, S.M., and Fauci, A.S. (1982): Ear disease in patients with Wegener's granulomatosis. *Laryngoscope*, 92:713–717.
19. Lucaya, J. (1971): Histiocytosis X. *Am. J. Dis. Child.*, 121:289–295.
20. Mascola, L., Pelosi, R., Blount, J., Alexander, C.E., and Cates, W. (1985): Congenital syphilis revisited. *Am. J. Dis. Child.* 139:575–580.
21. McCaffrey, T.V., McDonald, T.J., Facer, G.W., and DeRemee, R.A. (1980): Otologic manifestations of Wegener's granulomatosis. *Otolaryngol. Head Neck Surg.*, 88:586–593.
22. Muntoz, M.A., Schwartz, R.H., Grundfast, K.M., and Baumgartner, R.C. (1983): Tuberculosis of the middle ear and mastoid. *Pediatr. Infect. Dis.*, 2:234–236.
23. Murphy, G.F. (1985): Cell membrane glycoproteins and Langerhans cells. *Hum. Pathol.*, 16:103–112.
24. Myrivik, Q.N., Leake, E.S., and Wright, M.J. (1984): Disruption of phagosomal membranes of normal alveolar macrophages by the H37RV strain of *Mycobacterium tuberculosis*. *Am. Rev. Respir. Dis.*, 129:322–328.
25. Pinching, A.J., Rees, A.J., Pussell, B.A., Lockwood, G.M., Mitchison, R.S., and Peters, D.K. (1980): Relapses in Wegener's granulomatosis: the role of infection. *Br. Med. J.*, 281:836–838.
26. Rosenhall, U., Lowhagen, G.B., and Roupe, G. (1984): Auditory function in early syphilis. *J. Laryngol. Otol.*, 98:567–572.
27. Smith, R.J.H., and Evans, J.N.G. (1984): Head and neck manifestations of histiocytosis X. *Laryngoscope*, 94:395–399.
28. Stockelberg, J.M., and McDonald, T.J. (1984): Otologic involvement in late syphilis. *Laryngoscope*, 94:753–757.
29. Tos, M. (1966): Survey of Hand-Schuller-Christian disease in otolaryngology. *Acta Otolaryngol.*, 62:217–228.
30. Tsokos, M., Fauci, A.S., and Costa, J. (1982): Idiopathic midline destructive disease (IMMD). A subgroup of patients with the "midline granuloma syndrome." *Am. J. Clin. Pathol.*, 77:162–168.
31. Waksman, B.H. (1971): Delayed (cellular) hypersensitivity. In: *Immunologic Diseases, Vol. 1*, edited by M. Samtes, p. 220. Little, Brown and Co., Boston.

Subject Index

A23187, mast cell degranulation and, 167
Achromobacter xylosoxidans, 242
Acid hydrolase, in aural cholesteatoma, 393
Acid phosphatase, 157, 336, 341
  in aural cholesteatoma, 393, 395
Acinetobacter, 242
Acquired aural cholesteatoma, 391–401
  acid phosphatase in, 395
  bone resorption, 392
  cellular contents in, 393
  collagenase in, 395
  lysozyme in, 395
  microscopic features, 391–392
  prostaglandins in, 395
Addison's disease, 422
Adenoid hyperplasia, 88
  immunoglobulin G production in, 91
  nasopharyngeal tonsils in, 91
Adenoids, development, in immunodeficiency diseases, 371
Adenosine triphosphate, mast cell degranulation and, 167
Adenotonsillectomy, antibody activity after, 261
Adenovirus(es), 137, 250, 251
  acute otitis media and, 253
  IgA antibodies, 268–269
Agammaglobulinemia, 372
Albumin, diurnal variation, 262
Alkaline phosphatase, 341
Alkylamines, 154
Allergic granulomatosis, 481
Allergic labyrinthitis, experimental, 449
Allergic rhinitis, 124
  histamine and, 325
  Toynbee phenomenon and, 51
Allergy, 92
  defined, 454
  Eustachian tube dysfunction and, 49–52, 280
  Meniere's disease and, 454
  otitis media and, 49, 381
Alport's syndrome, 18
Anaphylatoxins, mast cell degranulation and, 167
Anaphylaxis, platelet-activating factor and, 164
Ankylosing spondylitis, 422
Antibody deficiency syndrome, 371
Antibody-dependent cellular cytotoxicity, 140
Antigens, transplantation, 186
Antihistamines, 154, 155
Arysulfatase, inflammatory cell, 157
Atelectasis, 205
Aural cholesteatoma, *see* Acquired aural cholesteatoma
Auricular chondritis, 464
Autoimmune disease, *see also* Autoimmunity
  animal model, 463–477
  cellular transfer, 474–475
  collagen type-II induced, 463–477
  ear, animal model of, 463–479
  genetic basis, 421–422
  inner ear, 419–433
  sensorineural deafness, 427–429; *see also* Sensorineural hearing loss
  serum transfer, 475–476
Autoimmune thyroiditis, 423
Autoimmunity
  aging and, 421
  defined, 419
  hypothetical models, 419
  inner ear, 11
  mechanisms, 423
  Meniere's disease and, 455
  pathogenesis, 463
  sensorineural hearing loss and, 13, 16
  sex hormones and, 144
  to type II collagen, 456

B cell
activation
polysaccharide antigen-induced, 366
protein antigen-induced, 366
in bronchus-associated lymphoid tissue, 112, 115–116
differentiation, 363
IgD and, 267
differentiation to immunoglobulin-producing immunocytes, 73–75
dysfunction, IgA deficiency in, 269
generation of, 71–72
HLA-DR determinants, 75
immunoglobulin D and, 84
macrophages and activity of, 291
respiratory tract, 120–122
subpopulation, 303
tonsillar, 70
Bacillus catarrhalis, 353
Bacteroides, enzyme activity, 270
Basophils, 124
vs mast cells, 165
morphologic features, 165
Biopsy, 306
Boyle-Davis gag, 262
Bradykinin, 325, 333–334
chymase and, 158
Breast, lymphoid tissue in, 142
Bronchus-associated lymphoid tissue, 63, 109, 110–120, 135, 282
antigen uptake, 113–114
B cell in, 112, 115–116, 284
blood supply, 112
as enriched source of IgA precursors, 115
first drawing of, 110
follicle-associated epithelium, 113
follicular dendritic cells, 112
function, 113–120
vs gut-associated lymphoid tissue, 145, 260
high endothelial venules, 109, 111
interdigitating dendritic cells, 112
lymphatic structures, 112
lymphoblasts in, 112
lymphoepithelium, 110
microfold cells, 111
middle ear as part of, 147
morphology, 111–113
ontogeny, 110–111
as part of a common mucosal immunological system, 115–119
reticulin framework, 111
similarity to Peyer's patches, 110
T cell in, 112, 119
Bruton's disease, 372
Burimamide, 154

Chondritis, auricular, 464
Cogan's syndrome, 463
Collagen, type II, ear disease induced by, 463
C-reactive protein, 311, 348
in acute purulent otitis media, 354
Calcium ion, ciliary motion and, 8
Capnocytophaga, enzyme activity, 270
Carotidodynia, 429
Cat, as model for investigating hearing loss and middle ear effusion, 407
Cathepsins, 324
Cerebral palsy, 11
Charcot Leydin crystals, 173
Chemotactic factors, 158–159
Chemotaxis
inflammation and, 287
neutrophil, 290
Children, snoring in, 11, 14
Chinchilla, as ideal model for experimental otitis media, 406
Chlamydia, otitis media and, 253
Chlamydia trachomatis, 238
Cholesteatoma, 205; *see also* Acquired aural cholesteatoma
Chondroitin sulfate, 156
Chronic maxillary sinusitis, ciliary beat and, 9
Churg–Strauss syndrome, 481
Chymase
bradykinin and, 158
collagen and, 158
heparin and, 158
Ciliary motion, 8–9
calcium ion depletion and, 8

regulation of, 9–10
Cimetidine, 154
Cleft palate, 408
Clostridium, 237
Cochlea, 13–19
organ of Corti, 13–17
stria vascularis, 17–19
Cogan's syndrome, 429
Collagen
chymase degradation, 158
type II, autoimmunity to, 456
Collagenase, 169, 324
in aural cholesteatoma, 395
Colostrum, secretory IgA in, 263–264
Complement(s)
activation, 345–348
alternative pathway, 347–348
classical pathway, 346–347
in disease, 350–351
dysfunction, 354
in acute purulent otitis media, 353–355
biological activities, 348–349
CI
aberrations, 355, 357
in acute purulent otitis media, 353
Clq, 323
binding capacity for whole bacteria, 353
Clr, 323
Cls, 323
C3b
in pneumococcal otitis media, 352
receptor, 164
in chronic otitis media with effusion, 357–359
Complement system, components, 345; *see also* Complement(s)
Compound 48/80, mast cell degranulation and, 167
Concanavalin A, mast cell degranulation and, 167
Corynebacterium, 410
Coxsackie virus, 137, 250
Coxsackie A virus, IgA antibodies, 269
Creatine phosphokinase, 321
Crista ampullaris, dark cells, 22
Cyclophosphamide, 427, 428
in Wegener's granulomatosis, 492
Cyproheptadine, 154, 155

Deafness, *see* Hearing loss; Sensorineural hearing loss; Sudden deafness
Delayed-type hypersensitivity, 222
Dermatitis herpetiformis, 422
Dexamethasone, 428
Dextran, mast cell degranulation and, 167
Dilator tubal muscle, 43
Dimaprit, 154
Diplococcus pneumoniae, 80
Dithiothreitol, 321
Donnan equilibrium, hydration of mucus and, 8
Ductus reuniens, 24

Ear, *see also* Inner ear; Middle ear
autoimmune disease, *see* Autoimmune disease, inner ear
external, auricular chondritis, 464
involvement in
histiocytosis, 494–495
tuberculosis, 496
Ear disease
collagen-induced, 464
transfer, 474
Ear Tissue Banks, 196
Echovirus, 137
Elastase, 169, 324
ELISA, *see* Enzyme-linked immunosorbent assay
Endolymph
primary source, 22
protein concentration, 24
Endolymphatic duct, 24–29
Endolymphatic hydrops, guinea pig model, 468
Endolymphatic sac, 22, 27–29, 443
as an immune organ, 11
lymphocyte in, 29, 30, 437
macrophages in, 29, 30, 437
microvilli, 27
pars intraduralis, 29
pars rugosa, 27

Endolymphatic sac *(contd.)*
size and shape, 27
subepithelial connective tissue, 29
Endotoxin, 323
Enterovirus, 145, 253
Enzyme-linked immunosorbent assay (ELISA), 249, 263, 264, 269
model for computation of standard curve, 265
Eosinophil, 172–173
basic protein, 172
Charcot Leydin crystals and, 173
enzymes, 173
granules, 172
in middle ear effusion, 383
receptor, immunoglobulin, 173
Eosinophil-releasing factor, 172
Eosinophilopoietin, 172
Epstein–Barr virus, 84
Ergot alkaloids, 155
Erythrocyte-antibody-complement rosetting, 303
Escherichia coli, 80, 137
Estradiol, anti-*Candida* antibodies and, 144
Estrogen, 143
Ethanolamines, 154
Ethylenediamines, 154
Eustachian tube, 1–11
abnormal patency, 46, 48
adrenergic innervation, 5
autonomic nervous system and, 4
cholinergic innervation, 5
drainage function, 45–46
dysfunction, 46–47
allergy and, 49–52, 280
animal models, 408
cholesteatoma formation and, 399
cleft palate and, 408
otitis media and, 47–48, 280
Wegener's granulomatosis and, 492
endodermal origin, 206
epithelium, 208
function, 208
animal models for study, 406
function testing, 52–57
indications for, 58–59
manometry, 53
modified inflation–deflation test, 56–57
nine-step inflation–deflation tympanometric test, 54–56
patulous Eustachian tube test, 54
Politzer maneuver, 53
Toynbee test, 54
for tubal patency, 53
tympanometry, 52–53
Valsalva maneuver, 53
innervation, 42–43
length, 39
levator veli palatini, 3
lower portion, 1
morphology, 39
muscles associated with function of, 43–44
obstruction, 46, 48
experimental, 210–211
otitis media with effusion and, 205
role of infection in experimental, 211–220
osseous, 39
parasympathetic ganglion block and, 4
as part of a system, 39
patency, 205
peptidergic innervation, 5
phosphatidylcholine synthesis in, 10
physiologic functions, 44–46
protective function, 45
salpingitis, 456, 464
seromucinous gland, 3
stellate ganglion block and, 4
tensor veli palatini, 3
ventilation function, 45

Fibrinogen, catabolism, inflammatory products from, 331
Fluorometric assay, 332
Follicle-associated epithelium, 113
Follicle dendritic cells, 112
antigen–antibody complexes on surface, 113
Fossa of Rosenmuller, 42

β-D-Galactosidase, inflammatory cell, 157
Glucosidase, 324

Glucuronidase, inflammatory cell, 157
Glycoproteins, 321
Granuloma
  formation, 489
  reparative, 446
Granuloproteases, 324
Gut-associated lymphoid tissue, 63, 135, 282
  antibody-dependent cellular cytotoxicity, 140
  B cell in, 284
  vs bronchus-associated lymphoid tissue, 145, 260
  middle ear as part of, 147

Hageman factor, 164, 333
Hand–Schuller–Christian syndrome, 494
Hashimoto's disease, Meniere's disease and, 423
Hearing loss, *see also* Sensorineural hearing loss
  inner ear secondary immune response and, 446
  middle ear effusion and, 407
Hemophilus influenzae, 80, 91, 234, 235–236, 352
  encapsulated from, 368
  enzyme activity, 270
    IgA resistance to, 284
  immunity, 367
  pathogenicity, mechanism of, 121
  strains, 405
  unencapsulated form, 368
  vaccination, 269
Heparin(s)
  anticomplementary activity, 157
  chymase and, 158
  from mast cell, 155
  plasminogen activator and, 157
  as storage matrix for mediators of inflammation, 156
Herpes simplex virus, 253
β-Hexosaminidase, inflammatory cell, 157
Hexamethonium, mucociliary activity and, 9
High endothelial venules, 109, 111
  hyperplasia, 112
Histaminase, 173
Histamine, 153–154, 332–333
  in allergic rhinitis, 325
  antagonists, 154
  catabolism products, 154
  chemotaxis and, 159
  formation, 153
  mast cell and, 153
  in middle ear effusion, 332
  in otitis media with effusion, 333
  receptors, 154
  release
    substance P and, 333
    vasoactive intestinal peptide and, 333
Histiocytosis X, 494–495
  ear involvement, 494
HLA-antigens, classes, 186
HLA-DR
  expression of, 67
  guidance function in immune response, 66
Hypereosinophilic syndrome, 172
Hypergammaglobulinemia, 492
Hypogammaglobulinemia, 255, 372
  prematurity and, 369
Hypotympanum, 2

Immotile cilia syndrome, 6
Immune complexes, 349–350
  assays, 357–358
  in chronic otitis media with effusion, 357–358
  complement binding sites, 346
  formation
    prerequisites for, 357
    rheumatoid factors and, 348
  identification, 323
  Meniere's disease and, 423, 424, 456
  in middle ear effusions, 357
  otitis media with effusion and, 323
  in otosclerosis, 423, 424
  precipitation, 348
  sensorineural hearing loss and, 423, 424, 456
  in sudden deafness, 423, 424
  Wegener's granulomatosis and, 490

Immune deficiency, CI aberrations in, 355
Immune response
  maturation, 368
  in otitis media, 373–377
Immunity
  cellular, defects of, 370
  inner ear, 447–448; *see also immune terms under* Inner ear
Immunization
  against pneumococcal antigen, 375
  IgGI production and, 376
  poor response, 367
  recommendation, 269
Immunocompetence, *see also* Immune response
  defined, 36
  genetic control, 364–365
Immunoelectrophoresis, 263, 371
Immunodeficiency diseases, 370–373, *see also* Immune deficiency; Immunodeficiency syndrome(s)
  agammaglobulinemia, 372
  diagnosis, 371
  hypogammaglobulinemia, transient, 372
  IgA deficiency, selective, 372–373
  IgG deficiency, selective, 373
  incidence, 370
  recurrent otitis media and, 371
  screening test for, 371
  sinusitis, 371
Immunodeficiency syndrome, 270, 365
  lymphoid tissue development in, 371
Immunoglobulin(s), *see also specific immunoglobulins*
  plasma, diffusion to secretions, 263
  secretory, 5, 260, 261
    models for transport, 261
    nasopharyngeal secretions, 265, 268
    plasma/serum, 265
    quantitation, 261–266
    ratio to total immunoglobulins, 266
    saliva, 265
  synthesis, polyclonal, 294
Immunoglobulin A (IgA)
  deficiency
    B cell dysfunction and, 269
    IgM and, 270
    selective, 372–373
  diurnal variation in, 262
  function, 120
  immune complexes, removal of, 139
  immunocytes, tonsillar, 80–81
  immunoregulation, 115
  lamina propria, 120
  lymphoblasts, 141
  middle ear production, 147
  nasopharyngeal secretions vs saliva, 266
  polymeric without secretory component, bile transport, 117
  precursor cells, 260
  proteases, 270–274
    characteristics, 271
    in vivo activity, 271–274
    resistance, 284
  radioimmunodiffusion analysis, 279
  resistance to proteolysis, 121
  saliva vs nasopharyngeal secretions, 266
  secretory, 120, 286
    antibacterial activity, 137
    antibodies, 137
    antiviral activity, 137
    bacterium-induced cleavage, 270–274
    colostrum, 264
    composition, 107
    molecule, stability, 261
    proteolysis and, 271
    quantitation, 261
    ratio to IgA, 262
    tissues that contain, 108
  synthesis, 140, 287
    middle ear mucosa, 283
  upper respiratory tract, 266
Immunoglobulin D (IgD), 84
  B cell differentiation and, 267
  immunocytes, 268
  IgM and, 267
  in middle ear effusions, 268
  mucosal transport, evidence of, 267
  synthesis, 268
Immunoglobulin E (IgE), 118–119, 259
  assays, 280
  eosinophil receptor, 173

hypersensitivity, 280, 289
as mucosal antibody, 118
otitis media with effusion, 125, 383
precursors, 118
role in, 121–122
wheezing and levels of, 383
Immunoglobulin G (IgG)
antibody, 287
diurnal variation, 262
eosinophil receptor, 173
function, 121
mucosal transport, evidence of, 267
nasopharyngeal, ratio to plasma IgG, 267
in neonates, 368
radioimmunodiffusion analysis, 279
receptor, mast cell, 164
sex hormones and production of, 144
subclasses, 365–366
tissue-bound, 439
Immunoglobulin M (IgM)
function, 122
IgA deficiency and, 270
IgD and, 267
in middle ear effusion, 280
in neonates, 368
radioimmunodiffusion analysis, 279
in respiratory secretions, 122
secretory, 135, 261
purification, 265
quantification, 261
ratio to IgM, 266
sex hormones and production of, 144
Immunonephelometry, 264
Immunoprecipitation, 263
Immunotherapy, 386
Impromidine, 154
Infant, antibody production in, 368, 369
Inflammation
chemotaxis and, 287
lactic acid dehydrogenase as indicator of, 336
lysozyme as indicator of, 325
mediators, 153–173, 325–326, 332–341
bradykinin, 164
cellular, 164–173, 301–317; *see also* Inflammatory cells
chemotactic factor, 158–159
histamine, 153–154
kinins, 164
leukotrienes, 161–163
lysosomal enzymes, 157–158
platelet-activating factor, 163–164
prostaglandins, 159–161
proteoglycans, 155–157
serotonin, 154–155
thromboxanes, 159–161
Inflammatory cell(s), 301–317
lysozyme, 324
middle ear effusion and, 302–303
Inflammatory factor of anaphylaxis, 159
Influenza virus, 250, 251
acute otitis media and, 253
neutropenia and, 255
Influenza A virus, IgA antibodies, 269
Inner ear, 11–30
antibody levels, effect of middle ear immune responses on, 448–449
antigen entering, 438
autoimmune disease, 419–433
autoimmunity, 11
blood supply, 422
cochlea, 13–19; *see also* Cochlea
collagen type-II distribution in, 476–477
diseases with immunologic features, 464
endolymphatic sac, 11
fluid system, 22–24
immune responses
effect on hearing, 446
involvement of regional lymph nodes in, 438
immune stimulation, morphological changes, 440
immune system, 11
immunity, protective role, 447–448
primary immune response, 446
secondary immune response, 446
vestibular labyrinth, 19–22
Interdigitating dendritic cells, 112
γ-Interferon, 368
Interleukin, 1, 169
Isoniazid, 496
Isoprenaline, *see* Isoproterenol
Isoproterenol, mucociliary activity and, 9

J chain
function, 80
incorporation into immunoglobulins, 261
production, 80–82

Kallikrein, 164, 325, 334
Kallikrein–kinin system, 325–326
activation, 333
Kininase, 173
Kininogens, 164
Kinins, 164, 325
Kveim–Siltzback skin test, 486

Labyrinthine membrane, amino acid composition, 465
Labyrinthitis
allergic, experimental, 449
strial atrophy and, 19
Lacrimal gland, 142
IgD immunocytes in, 268
Lactic acid dehydrogenase, 321
as indicator of inflammation, 336
Lamina propria, as major source of IgA plasma cells, 120
Letterer–Suive syndrome, 494
Leucine aminopeptidase, 341
Leukocyte imigration inhibition assay, protocol, 430–432
Leukotrienes, 161–163, 337–338
sources, 162
Levator veli palatini, 43
Limulus assay, 323
Lipopolysaccharide, 323
Lipoxin A, 163
Listeria monocytogenes, 122
Lupus erythematosus, 422, 456
Lymphocyte(s)
in endolymphatic sac, 29, 30, 437
growth and differentiation, 395
in respiratory tract, 123
subpopulations, 303–305
Lymphocyte migration inhibition assay, 428
Lymphocytosis, 310
Lymphoepithelium, antigen access to, 145
Lymphoid tissue
bronchus-associated, 109
conjunctival, 135
genital tract, 135
immune reactions in, 188
immunodeficiency syndromes and development of, 371
mammary gland, 135
mucous-associated, 107
Lymphokines, 122
function, 395
Lysophospholypase, 173
Lysosomal enzymes, 339
Lysozymes, 340–341
in aural cholesteatoma, 395
as indicator of inflammation, 325
in inflammatory cells, 324

Macrophage(s), 169–170
angiotensin-converting enzyme and, 170
B cell activity and, 291
in endolymphatic sac, 29, 30, 437
middle ear, 292
motility, 169
vs neutrophils, 169
otitis media with effusion and, 292, 294
phagocytic activity, 169
processing of foreign material by, 66
prostaglandins and, 161
proteolytic enzymes released by, 169
in respiratory tract, 109, 123
T cell activity and, 291
Macrophage inhibition factor, 122
Major histocompatibility complex, 66, 143, 420
Malic dehydrogenase, 341
Mammary gland
homing mechanism, 143
IgD immunocytes in, 268
Manometry, 53
Mast cells, 124
activation in otitis media with effusion, 333
activation through IgE receptors, 167
vs basophils, 165
C3b receptor, 164

degranulation
chemically induced, 167
following activation, 166
granules, 166
heparin, 155
histamine and, 153
IgG receptor, 164
intraepithelial, 166
morphologic features, 165
organelles, 166
prostaglandin biosynthesis and, 161
in secretory otitis media, 311
sites, 166
species variation, 166
Mast cell protease II, 158
Mastoiditis
otitis media and, 242
Wegener's granulomatosis and, 491
Measles
antibody activity against, middle ear, 147
labyrinthitis and, 19
Measles virus
acute otitis media and, 254–255
cell-mediated immunity and, 255
hypogammaglobulinemia and, 255
pharyngitis coryza and, 254
Meniere's disease, 453–461
autoantibodies in, 13
autoimmunity and, 455
diagnosis, 453
endolymphatic hydrops and, 453
endolymphatic sac and, 27
etiology, 453
type II collagen immunity and, 466
Hashimoto's disease, 423
immune complexes and, 423, 424, 456
otosclerosis and, 466
pathogenesis, 471
tinnitus and, 453
vertigo and, 453
Meningitis, 363
acute otitis media and, 249
Methacholine, mucociliary activity and, 9
2-Methylhistamine, 154
Metiamide, 154
Microfold cell, antigen uptake, 113
Middle ear
B cell precursors in, 283
collagen type II distribution in, 476–477
diseases with immunologic features, 464
effusion, *see* Middle effusion
embryological development, 206
immune reactivity, 146–147
IgA synthesis in, 283
implants, 194–195
infection, facial paralysis, 496
inflammation
mediators, 332–341
otitis media with effusion and, 206
macrophage, 292
natural killer cell, 295
secretory component in, 283
as target organ for IgE-mediated allergic response, 381
tuberculosis, 496
Middle ear cavity, negative pressure, 259
Middle ear effusion, 125, 319–329, 331
animal models, 408–410
aspirates, 301
B cell preponderance in, 291
C1r–C1s complexes in, 323
cathepsins in, 324
cause of, 283
composition, 319
creatine phosphokinase in, 321
endotoxin-positive, 323
enzymes in, 321, 324
eosinophils in, 383
evacuation, 311
experimental, induction of, 407
glycoproteins in, 321
glycosidase in, 324
granulocyte protease activity, 290
granuloproteases in, 324
hearing loss and, 407
IgA antibodies in, 269
IgE-mediated hypersensitivity and, 280
IgM in, 280
immune complexes in, 357
immunoglobulins, 147, 279–281
in acute otitis media, 269
inflammatory cells in, 302–303
histamine in, 332

Middle ear effusion *(contd.)*
lactic acid dehydrogenase in, 321
Limulus assay, 323
natural killer cells in, 311
oral decongestants and, 386
protein composition, 319–321
ratio of secretory immunoglobulins to total immunoglobulins in, 266
rheumatoid factor in, 323
T cell in, 305
types of, 383
virus-specific antibodies in, 286
virus-specific IgA antibodies in, 269
Middle ear fluid, *see also* Middle ear effusion
bacterial culture, 231
bacteriologic findings in, 239
Hemophilus influenzae isolated from, 235
Streptococcus pneumoniae isolated from, 234
viral antigen in, 249, 251
Modified inflation–deflation test, 56–57
Monoclonal antibody(ies), 305–306
Monocyte(s), 169–170
prostaglandins and, 161
serotonin stimulation of, 155
Mononucleosis, 95
Mucociliary transporting system
ciliary beat and, 9
mucous blanket, 6
regulation, factors affecting, 6
rheological properties of mucus and, 9
Mucosa-associated lymphoid tissue, 107
lymphocyte clusters, 111
nurse cells, 111
as source of IgE precursors, 118
Mucosal immunity, antigen stimulation, 287
Mucus
composition, 7
hydration, 8
structure, 8
Mumps, antibody activity against, middle ear, 147
Mumps virus, 253
Mycobacterium fortuitum, 242
Mycobacterium tuberculosis, 242
Mycoplasma, otitis media and, 253
Mycoplasma pneumoniae, 211
Myeloperoxidase, 169
Myringoplasty, 180–182

Nasopharyngeal secretions
IgA antibodies in, 269
IgA cleavage products in, 272
IgG in, 267
as most enriched source of secretory immunoglobulins, 268
virus-specific antibodies in, 286
virus-specific IgA antibodies in, 268–269
Nasopharynx, 259–278
bacterial colonization, 239
IgE mediated hypersensitivity in, 280
otitis media and bacteriologic findings in, 239
secretion, *see also* Nasopharyngeal secretions
collecting, 262
Natural killer cell
activity tonsillar lymphocytes, 77
middle ear, 295
in middle ear effusion, 311
Necrotizing vasculitis, systemic, 483–484
diagnosis, 483
Neisseria gonorrhoeae, enzyme activity, 270
Neisseria meningitidis, enzyme activity, 270
Neonate
activity production in, 368–369
immunoglobulin G in, 368
immunoglobulin M in, 368
Neutropenia, 255
Neutrophil, 170–172
C5a-inactivating activity, 171
chemotaxis, 290
granule content, 171, 172
half-life, 171
vs macrophages, 169
prostaglandins and, 161
Neutrophil chemotactic factor
Nine-step inflation-deflation tympanometric test, 54–56
Northern California Transplant, 196

Oral decongestants, 386
Organ of Corti, 13–17
  degeneration, anticochlear antibody in, 463
  inner hair cells, 13
    as mechanoreceptors, 15
    vs outer hair cells, 15
  outer hair cells, 13
    vs inner hair cells, 15
    as mechanoreceptors, 15
Ossicle, transportation, 184
Ossiculoplasty, 183–186
Otalgia, 50
Otic ganglion, 42
Otitis media
  acute, 50, 231–238, 345
    adenoviruses and, 253
    antibody activity in, 238
    Branhamella catarrhalis in, 236
    Hemophilus influenzae in, 235
    immune response in, 269
    in infants and children, 231–234
    in infants less than 6 weeks, 231, 234
    influenza virus and, 253
    measles virus and, 254–255
    meningitis and, 249
    pathogenesis, 326
    prephase, 272
    recurrent, 270, 272, 284, 354
    respiratory syncytial virus and, 253
    Streptococcus pneumoniae in, 234
    viral illness and, 249, 352
  acute purulent, complement profile, 353–355
  age-related incidence of, 251
  allergy and, 49, 381
  bacterial, 47, 496
  bullous, with mycoplasmal pneumonia, 253
  chlamydia and, 253
  chronic, 9, 319
    immune complexes in, 357–358
    pathogenesis, 322
  complement and, 351–359
  with effusion, 47, 125, 279–299
    animal models, 403–415; *see also* Otitis media, experimental
    antiallergic therapy in, 386
    antibodies in, 286–287
    C-reactive protein in, 311
    chronic, 241–242, 294, 301, 302, 311, 345, 357
    ciliary beat and, 9
    eustachian tube obstruction and, 205
    experimental, 385–386
    histamine in, 333
    immune complex injury and, 222–223
    immune complexes and, 323
    immune-mediated, animal model, 414–415
    immunoglobulin E and, 125, 221–222, 383, 384
    immunotherapy, 386
    local reaction, 282
    macrophage in, 292, 294
    mast cell activation, 333
    middle ear and, 287
    middle ear aspirates, 302–303
    middle ear immunity and, 448
    middle ear inflammation and, 206
    oral decongestants, 386
    prognosis, 279
    recurrent, 323
    Sjogren's syndrome and, 485
    systemic necrotizing vasculitis following, 452–453
  transudation theory, 205
  eustachian tube dysfunction and, 47–48, 280
  experimental
    animal used, 406
    chinchilla as ideal model, reasons, 406
    identification, 406
    induction of, 404
  immune response in, 373–374
  incidence, among atopic individuals, 381
  inflammatory process in, 289
  mastoiditis and, 242
  mycoplasma and, 253
  negative middle ear pressure and the development of, 412
  pathogenesis, 290
    mechanism, 403

Otitis media *(contd.)*
Toynbee phenomenon and, 52
pneumococcal, 352
purulent vs serous, 324
recurrent, 239, 241, 286, 319, 363, 371
immunodeficiency disease and, 371
reflux, 47, 51
secretory, 209–210
bacteriologic findings, 272
inflammatory cell subpopulations in, 301–317
rheological properties of mucus and, 9
serous vs purulent, 324
tubotympanum cilia and, 6
viral, 249–257
in Wegener's granulomatosis, 49
Otitis Media at the Second International Symposium, 403
Otitis-prone condition, 373; *see also* Otitis media, recurrent
immunology, 374–375
Otoconia, 19
Otological grafts, 195
Otorrhea, 392
Otosclerosis, 456
characteristic histopathological changes, 471, 473
immune complexes in, 423, 424
Meniere's disease and, 466
Overlap syndrome, 481
Oxymetazoline, mucociliary activity and, 9

Parainfluenza, 250, 251
Parainfluenza virus, 253
IgA antibodies, 269
Parotid gland, IgD immunocytes in, 268
Patulous Eustachian tube test, 54
Peptococcus, 237
Peptostreptococcus, 237
Peptostreptococcus micros, 410
Perilymph
chemical composition, 23
immunoglobulins, source of, 24
Peyer's patches, 142
follicle-associated epithelium, 113
IgA precursors in, 115, 260
Pharyngeal plexus, 42
Pharyngitis coryza, measles virus and, 254
Phenothiazines, 154, 155
Phenylepinephrine, mucociliary activity and, 9
Phosphatidylcholine, synthesis, 10
Phospholipase D, 173
Phosphorylcholine, 367
Piperazines, 154
Plasminogen, catabolism, inflammatory products from, 331
Plasminogen activator, 170
heparins and, 157
Plasminogen–plasmin system, 334–335
Platelet-activating factor, 163–164, 338–339
anaphylaxis and, 164
chemical structure, 163
hypotensive activity, 338
Pneumococcal infections, immunity, 367
Pneumonia, 363
Poliovirus, 137
antibody activity against
middle ear, 147
post-adenotonsillectomy, 261
IgA antibodies, 269
serum antibody activity, 144
vaccine, viral replication following oral administration, 268
Politzer maneuver, 53
Polyarteritis nodosa, 429, 481–483
Prausnitz–Kustner reaction, 384
Prematurity, hypogammaglobulinema and, 369
Prenalterol, mucociliary activity and, 9
Progesterone, 143
anti-Candida antibodies and, 144
Prolactin, 143
Propranolol, mucociliary activity and, 9
Proprionibacterium acnes, 237, 410
Prostaglandins, 159–160, 335–337
in aural cholesteatoma, 395
biologic effects, 161, 326
biosynthesis, 160
catabolism, 160
isolation, 160

Proteases, 270–274
  characteristics, 271
  in vivo activity, 271–274
  resistance, 284
Proteoglycans, 155–157; *see also* Heparins
  structure, 155
Proteolysis, 324
  elastase and, 324
Protympanum, 39
2-Pyridylethylamine, 154

Radioimmunodiffusion, 279
Raji cell test, 357
Reissner's membrane, 23
Respiratory burst, 171
Respiratory syncytial virus, 145, 250, 251
  acute otitis media and, 253
  IgA antibodies, 269
Respiratory tract
  cell-mediated immunity in, 122
  lymphocytes in, 109, 123
  lymphoid tissue, 107–133
  macrophages in, 123
  mast cells in, 124
  mucosal tissue, secretions, 107
  as part of a common mucosal immunologic system, 107–108
  T cells in, antigen-specific, 122
  upper, 107
Rheumatoid arthritis, 429
Rheumatoid factor, 323
  immune complex formation and, 348
Rhinitis, allergic, *see* Allergic rhinitis
Rhinovirus, 253
  IgA antibodies, 269
Rifampin, 496
Rotavirus, 145, 251
Rubella, antibody activity against, middle ear, 147
Rubella virus, 145

Saccule, location, 19
Salbutamol, mucociliary activity and, 9
Saliva, flow rate, vs nasopharyngeal secretions, 266
Salivary gland, lymphoid tissue in, 142
Salpingopharyngeus, 43
Sarcoidosis, 485–486
  diagnosis, 486
  hearing loss in, 485
  otologic manifestation, 485
  sensorineural deafness in, 485
Secretory complement, 81–82
  antigenic determinants, 263
Secretory component, combination with immunoglobulin, 260, 261
Sensorineural hearing loss, 342, 456
  audiogram in, 432–434
  autoimmunity and, 13, 16
  carotidodynia and, 429
  Cogan's syndrome and, 429
  collagen-induced ear disease model for, 466, 467
  cyclophosphamide in, 427, 428
  dexamethsone in, 428
  diagnosis, 427
  differential diagnosis, 427
  immune complexes and, 423, 424, 456
  polyarteritis nodosa and, 429
  rheumatoid arthritis and, 429
  in sarcoidosis, 485
  steroid therapy in, 427
  treatment, 427, 428
    effectiveness, 428–429
  ulcerative otitis, 429
Serotonin, 154–155
  allergic reactions and, 155
  antagonists, 155
  biosynthesis, 154
  monocyte stimulation, 155
  pharmacologic effects, 155
  platelet, 154
Serum sickness, 456
Sex hormones, autoimmunity and, 144
Shigella, 137
Sicca syndrome, 484–485
  diagnosis, 485
  otologic manifestations, 484
  tympanic membrane perforation in, 484
Sinusitis
  chronic maxillary, *see* Chronic maxillary sinusitis
  immunodeficiency disease and, 371

Sjogren's syndrome, 484–485
  diagnosis, 485
  malignant lymphoproliferative disorders, 485
  otitis media with effusion in, 485
  otologic symptoms, 484
  tympanic membrane perforation, 484
Slow-reacting substance, 161, 337
Sphenopalatine nerve, 42
Stapedectomy, reparative granuloma and, 446
Staphylococcus aureus, 80, 234
Staphylococcus epidermis, 237
Streptococcus, 137
Streptococcus intermedius, 410
Streptococcus mitior, enzyme activity, 270
Streptococcus pneumoniae, 231, 234
  enzyme activity, 270
    IgA resistance to, 284
  pathogenicity, mechanism of, 121
  strains, 405
Streptococcus pyogenes, M protein, antibody against, 283
Streptococcus sanguis, enzyme activity, 270
Streptomycin, 496
Sudden deafness, immune complexes in, 423, 424
Superoxide dismutase, inflammatory cell, 157
Syphilis, 497–498
  congenital, labyrinthitis and, 19
  otologic abnormalities, 497
Symposium on Acute Otitis Media and Secretory Otitis Media, 289

T cell, 122–123
  in bronchus-associated lymphoid tissue, 112, 119–120
  IgA immunoregulation and, 115
  macrophages and activity of, 291
  in middle ear effusion, 305
  in respiratory tract, 109
  role in B cell differentiation, 75
  subpopulation, 303, 307, 311
  tonsillar, 70, 75
Tensor tympani, 43
Tensor veli palatini, 43
Testosterone, 143
Thromboxane A_2, biosynthesis, 161
Thromboxane synthetase, 161
Thyroiditis, autoimmune, 423
Tinnitus, 453
Tonsil
  B-cell activity, disease-induced alterations in, 89–90
  B cell populations, 70
  CD4-positive, 77
  development, in immunodeficiency diseases, 371
  function
    age-associated changes in, 87–88
    disease-associated changes in, 88–92
  idiopathic hyperplasia, 88
  immunoglobulin production in, 77–78
  lingual, 65
  mononucleosis affecting, 95
  nasopharyngeal, 65, 260–261, 280
    IgD immunocytes in, 268
    immunoglobulin-producing cells, 78
    secretory immune system, 83
  palatine, 63, 260, 280
    changing functions in, 92–94
    immunoglobulin-producing cells, 78
  as precursor source for secretory IgA system, 85
  T cell population, 70
Tonsillectomy
  disease susceptibility and, 94
  serum immunoglobulin and, 95
Tonsillitis
  B cell maturity in, 90
  hyperplastic, 88
  recurrent, 84, 88, 91
Torus tubarius, 42
Toynbee phenomenon, 48
  allergic rhinitis and, 51
Toynbee test, 54
Transaminase, 341
Treponema pallidium, 497
Trimethroprim-sulfamethoxazole, 493
Tryptase, 158
Tuberculosis, 495–496
  diagnosis, 496
  treatment, 496
Tubotympanum
  heterogeneity, cellular, 6

immune system, 10–11
immunoglobulin-forming cells in, 11
morphological and functional aspects, 206–209
mucociliary transporting system, 6–8
secretions, 10
Tympanic membrane, *see also* Tympanum
atelectasis, 47
neovasculogenesis, 428
perforation
in Sicca syndrome, 484
in Sjogren's syndrome, 484
in Wegener's granulomatosis, 491
Tympanometry, 52–53, 384
nine-step, 54–56
Tympano-ossicular block graft, 189
Tympanoplasty, 179–204
allograft, 186–201
animal models, 189–192
antibody formation after, 193
immune responses in, 189–194
staged, 180
Tympanosclerosis, 205, 464
Tympanostomy, 311, 386
Tympanum, 1
ciliated cells in, 2
perforation, 254

Ulcerative otitis, 429
Utricle, 19
Utriculoendolymphatic valve of Bast, 25

Valsalva maneuver, 53
Vertigo, 453
Vestibular labyrinth, 19–22
crista ampullaris, 22
dark cells, 22
gravity receptors, 19
macula, 19–22
sensory cells, 19
Vibrio cholerae, 137
Viral infection, 280
acute otitis media and, 249, 352
intestinal origin of antibody activity in, 144–145
respiratory origin of antibody activity in, 144–145

Waldeyer's ring, 261
Wegener's granulomatosis, 490–493
characteristic features, 490
diagnosis, 492
differential diagnosis, 492
etiology, 490
Eustachian tube dysfunction and, 492
hypergammaglobulinemia, 492
immune complexes and, 490
mastoiditis and, 491
otitis media in, 491
pathogenesis, 490
treatment, 492–493
tympanic membrane perforation in, 491
Wheezing, IgE level and, 383